Pursuing Health
and Wellness

Second Edition

Pursuing Health and Wellness
Healthy Societies, Healthy People

Alexander Segall
Christopher J. Fries

OXFORD
UNIVERSITY PRESS

OXFORD
UNIVERSITY PRESS

Oxford University Press is a department of the University of Oxford.
It furthers the University's objective of excellence in research, scholarship,
and education by publishing worldwide. Oxford is a registered trade mark of
Oxford University Press in the UK and in certain other countries.

Published in Canada by
Oxford University Press
8 Sampson Mews, Suite 204,
Don Mills, Ontario M3C 0H5 Canada

www.oupcanada.com

Copyright © Oxford University Press Canada 2017

The moral rights of the authors have been asserted

Database right Oxford University Press (maker)

First Edition published in 2011

All rights reserved. No part of this publication may be reproduced, stored in
a retrieval system, or transmitted, in any form or by any means, without the
prior permission in writing of Oxford University Press, or as expressly permitted
by law, by licence, or under terms agreed with the appropriate reprographics
rights organization. Enquiries concerning reproduction outside the scope of the
above should be sent to the Permissions Department at the address above
or through the following url: www.oupcanada.com/permission/permission_request.php

Every effort has been made to determine and contact copyright holders.
In the case of any omissions, the publisher will be pleased to make
suitable acknowledgement in future editions.

Library and Archives Canada Cataloguing in Publication

Segall, Alexander, 1943-, author
Pursuing health and wellness : healthy societies, healthy people
/ Alexander Segall, Christopher J. Fries. -- Second edition.

Includes bibliographical references and index.
ISBN 978-0-19-901433-0 (paperback)

1. Health--Social aspects. 2. Medical care. 3. Social medicine.
I. Fries, Christopher J. (Christopher John), author II. Title.

RA418.S411 2016   362.1   C2016-902885-2

Cover image: Shioguchi/Getty Images

Oxford University Press is committed to our environment.
This book is printed on Forest Stewardship Council® certified paper
and comes from responsible sources.

MIX
Paper from
responsible sources
FSC
www.fsc.org   FSC® C014174

Printed and bound in the United States of America

1 2 3 4 — 20 19 18 17

Contents

Preface   xii
Acknowledgments   xv

Part One Understanding Health and Wellness Sociologically   1

1 Introducing Health Sociology   2

Introduction: The Mystery of Good Health   2
Health as a Social Construction   4
Health Consciousness: Producing Health versus Consuming Health Care   7
The Origins of Medical Sociology   13
The Scope of Medical Sociology   15
From Medical Sociology toward Health Sociology   18
Health Sociology in Canada   23
   The Social Determinants of Health   24
   Health and Illness Behaviour   25
   The Health-Care System   25
Chapter Summary   26
Study Questions   27
Recommended Readings   27
Recommended Websites   28
Recommended Audiovisual Sources   28

2 Applying the Sociological Imagination to Health and Illness   29

Applying Sociological Paradigms to Theorize Health and Illness   29
Health and Illness as "Social Roles"—The Structural Functionalist Paradigm   30
Health and Illness as "Professional Constructs"—The Conflict Paradigm   36
Health and Illness as "Interpersonal Meanings"—The Symbolic Interactionist Paradigm   41
Health and Illness as "Gendered Experiences"—The Feminist Paradigm   44
Health and Illness as "Embodied Cultural Facts"—The Sociology of the Body Paradigm   48
Health and Illness as "Unfolding across Time"—The Importance of Adopting an Intersectional Life Course Perspective   58
Chapter Summary   61
Study Questions   62
Recommended Readings   62

Recommended Website 62
Recommended Audiovisual Sources 62

3 Measuring the Dimensions of Health 63

The Meaning and Measurement of Health 63
Differentiating Personal and Population Health 65
Adopting a Salutogenic Approach for Understanding the Dimensions of Health 66
The Meaning of Ill Health (Sickness) and Good Health (Wellness) 68
    Sickness: The Presence of Disease and the Experience of Illness 68
    Wellness: More Than the Absence of Disease and Illness 70
    The Process of Health Status Designation: Separating the Dimensions of Health 72
Understanding the Difference between Health Inputs and Health Outcomes 75
Health Status Indicators 76
    Single-Item Measures: Global Self-Rated Health 77
    Composite Measures: The Health Utilities Index 80
Indicators of Ill Health: Limits to the Standard Approach 81
    Morbidity and Mortality 81
    Disability and Utilization of Health Services 83
    What Can We Learn about Health from Disease and Death Rates? 83
Indicators of Good Health: The Challenge of Measuring Wellness 84
    Sense of Coherence 85
    Canadian Index of Wellbeing 87
    Health Expectancy: Estimating Future Health Status and Quality of Life 87
The Need for a Mixed-Methods Approach to Measuring Health: Surveys, Statistics, and Stories 89
    Population Health Surveys: The Canadian Experience 90
    Health Diary Studies and Illness Narrative Accounts: The Importance of Digging Deeper 93
Chapter Summary 96
Study Questions 97
Recommended Readings 97
Recommended Websites 98

Part Two Exploring the Factors That Shape Health and Wellness 99

4 Making People Healthy: General Determinants of Health and Wellness 101

What Makes People Healthy? Two Different Answers 101
Personal and Structural Health Determinants 104

The Major Determinants of Population Health:
   An Overview of the Four Key Factors   106
      Biology   106
      Lifestyle Behaviour   107
      Environment   109
      Use of Formal Health-Care Services   119
The Relative Importance of Health Determinants   120
      Upstream and Downstream Health Determinants: Jason's Story   120
      Primary and Secondary Determinants: Moving Upstream   121
      Understanding the Cumulative Effects of Health Determinants:
         A Life Course Approach   123
      Estimating the Health Benefits of Major Determinants   124
The Determinants of Good Health and Ill Health   125
Chapter Summary   128
Study Questions   130
Recommended Readings   130
Recommended Websites   130
Recommended Audiovisual Sources   130

5   Addressing Sources of Inequality and Health Disparities: Socioeconomic Status   131

Understanding Social Inequality   131
Social Determinants of Health Disparities: Income, Occupation,
   and Education   133
      Income   134
      Occupation   136
      Education   139
The Social Gradient and Health   142
Explanations of the Social Gradient in Health   147
      Materialist and Neo-materialist Explanations   148
      Cultural Behavioural Explanations   148
      Psychosocial Explanations   151
Income Inequality and Population Health: More to the Story   153
Reducing Socioeconomic Differences in Health:
   Is It Possible to Close the Gap?   158
Toward an Intersectional Theory of Health and Socioeconomic Status across
   the Life Course   162
Chapter Summary   166
Study Questions   167
Recommended Readings   167
Recommended Websites   167
Recommended Audiovisual Sources   168

6 Addressing Sources of Inequality and Health Disparities: Gender 169

Health and Gender 169
The Importance of Sex- and Gender-Based Analysis in Health Research 171
Gender Differences in Health 173
- Women Live Longer Than Men 174
- The Genders Differ in Major Causes of Death 176
- Women Are Diagnosed as Suffering from More Ill Health Than Men 177
- Women Make More Frequent Use of Formal Health Care Than Men 178
- Gender Differences in the Social Determinants of Health 180

Explanations of Gender Differences in Health and Illness 182
- The Role Accumulation Hypothesis 183
- The Role Strain Hypothesis 183
- The Social Acceptability Hypothesis 184
- The Risk-Taking Hypothesis 186

Toward an Intersectional Theory of Health and Gender across the Life Course 189
Chapter Summary 191
Study Questions 192
Recommended Readings 192
Recommended Websites 192

7 Addressing Sources of Inequality and Health Disparities: Ethnicity 193

Health and Ethnicity 193
Ethnic Differences in Health 195
- Aboriginal Peoples Have Poorer Health Outcomes Because of Social Exclusion and Racism 196
- The Healthy Immigrant Effect Deteriorates over Time 206
- Ethnic Differences in the Perception and Understanding of Symptoms 210
- Ethnic Differences in Health-Care Behaviour 212
- Ethnic Differences in the Social Determinants of Health 213

Explanations of Ethnic Differences in Health and Illness 216
- Biological Determinist Explanations 216
- Cultural Behavioural Explanations 218
- Socioeconomic Explanations 219
- Ethnicity, Religion, and Health 220

Toward an Intersectional Theory of Health and Ethnicity across the Life Course 222
Chapter Summary 223
Study Questions 224
Recommended Readings 224

Recommended Websites   225
Recommended Audiovisual Sources   225

8   Unravelling the Mystery of Health: An Intersectional Model of Health across the Life Course   226

Intersectionality and Health Disparities   226
Lifestyle Behaviours and Health   229
    Smoking   229
    Alcohol Use   230
    Physical Activity   230
    Obesity   231
    Unsafe Sex   233
Individualized Health Promotion   234
    The Individualization of Health Lifestyles   236
    Health Lifestyles or Health Behaviours?   243
Theorizing the Intersectionality of Health   247
    Health Lifestyles and the Structure–Agency Issue   247
    Pierre Bourdieu and a Relational Theory of Health Lifestyles   250
An Intersectional Model of Health and Health Lifestyles across the Life Course   258
Chapter Summary   262
Study Questions   264
Recommended Readings   264
Recommended Website   264
Recommended Audiovisual Sources   264

Part Three Pursuing Health and Wellness   265

9   Discovering the Hidden Depths of Health Care: Lay Beliefs, Social Support, and Informal Care   267

The Iceberg of Health Care   267
Hidden Components of the Health-Care System   268
    Lay Beliefs about Health Maintenance and Illness Management   270
    Popular and Professional Health Belief Systems   281
    Self-Care Beliefs and Behaviour   285
    Social Support, Helping Networks, and Health   295
Informal Care and Illness as Embodied Experience: Making Sense of Sickness and Maintaining a Healthy Self-Identity   301
    A Narrative Account: The Meaning and Management of Pain   302
    Chronic Illness Work   308
Chapter Summary   310
Study Questions   311
Recommended Readings   311
Recommended Websites   312

10   Medicalizing Beings and Bodies: The Link between Population Health and Biomedical Care   313

The Origins of the Biomedical Model   315
     Bedside Medicine   315
     Hospital Medicine   318
     Laboratory Medicine   319
Basic Ideas of the Biomedical Model   320
     Mind–Body Dualism   322
     Physical Reductionism   322
     Specific Etiology   323
     The Machine Metaphor   324
     Therapeutic Focus on Individualized Regimen and Control   326
Medical Dominance of the Health-Care System   328
Medicalizing Beings and Bodies   331
     Explanations for Medicalization   334
Chapter Summary   352
Study Questions   353
Recommended Readings   353
Recommended Websites   354
Recommended Audiovisual Sources   354

11   Moving beyond Biomedicine: Medical Pluralism   355

The Social Construction of Healing: A Sociological Perspective on Medical Pluralism   356
     The Historical Persistence of Medical Pluralism   358
     Avoiding the "Stereotypes of Marginality" in Social Studies of Alternative Medicine   361
     Labelling Alternative Medicine   362
     Three Streams of Complementary Alternative Medicine Research   363
Explanations for the Revival of Medical Pluralism   365
     The Demographic Transition and Population Aging   365
     Dissatisfaction with Biomedicine   366
     The Postmodern Condition   366
     Individualization and Consumerism   367
Crossing Cultures in Pursuit of Health and Wellness: Choosing Healing Practices   368
     Medical Consumerism, the Marketing of Ethnicity, and the Revival of Medical Pluralism   369
Integrative Medicine: Prospects for a New Medicine   372
Chapter Summary   375
Study Questions   376

Recommended Readings   376
Recommended Website   376
Recommended Audiovisual Sources   376

12   Achieving Healthy Futures   377

Toward a Sociological Understanding of Healthy Societies and Healthy People   377
   Studying Health: Alternative Sociological Paradigms   378
   Developing an Intersectional Model of Health across the Life Course   379
   Measuring the Dimensions of Health: A Mixed-Methods Approach   380
Social Determinants of Health: Reflections on What We Have Learned   381
   Structural and Personal Determinants of Health   382
   Sources of Social Inequality and Health Disparities: Intersections of Socioeconomic Status, Gender, and Ethnicity   382
   Life Chances and Health Choices: The Structure–Agency Question   383
Shared Responsibility for Making Societies and People Healthy   384
   Personal Responsibility: Informal Care and Health   384
   Professional Responsibility: Formal Care and Health   386
   Public Responsibility: The Governance of Health   386
   Health Policy Initiatives: Lalonde and Beyond   388
The Ongoing Pursuit of Health and Wellness: Some Unanswered Questions   393
   How Does the Vision of a Healthy Society Differ from the Reality of Health-Care Reform?   393
   Is It Possible to Redress Social Inequalities in Health?   396
   Why Is It So Difficult to Implement Healthy Public Policy?   399
   Is Wellness Always Good for Your Health?   403
   What Is Required to Remake the Medicalized Society into a Salutogenic Society?   406
Study Questions   409
Recommended Readings   409
Recommended Websites   410

Glossary   411
References   418
Index   455

Preface

Our culture is preoccupied with pursuing health and wellness. Think, for example, how prominent "health" is in our everyday language: we regularly discuss topics such as healthy living, healthy eating, healthy environments, healthy arguments, healthy activity, healthy buildings, healthy relationships, healthy workplaces, healthy bodies, healthy kids, healthy communities, healthy recipes, healthy minds, healthy aging, healthy schools, healthy families, healthy weight, healthy balance, healthy habits, healthy beginnings, and healthy endings. We use the term "health" to refer to these and many more aspects of everyday life. We routinely greet people with the familiar "Hi. How are you?" inquiring about their health status. The marketplace is crowded with products and services promising better health and higher levels of wellness. Governments try to further raise health consciousness in order to get individuals to behave in ways that are intended to promote personal health and avoid potential health risks. Healthy living is synonymous with desire, virtue, vitality, beauty, and goodness. "If you have your health, you have everything," the saying goes. The pursuit of good health pervades our wellness-oriented culture!

Despite its universality, health is also intensely personal—seemingly a private matter and a personal value. We closely safeguard information regarding our personal health, carefully considering to whom we should disclose our health concerns. Medical records are subject to some of society's strictest privacy laws. Additionally, like all things of value in our culture, health is unequally distributed within society, as are the conditions necessary for achieving wellness. Not everyone is healthy or has equal access to the resources that make people well. We are left wondering whether it is possible to address social inequalities in health. Too often, the vision of achieving healthy futures gives way to never-ending debates focused on reforming the formal health-care system, repairing medicare, and consuming health-care products and services rather than producing population health. The dominance of biomedicine leads to medicalizing beings and bodies, while the goal of making people healthy gets lost amidst anxiety over the threat and treatment of illness. Some people try moving beyond biomedicine by using complementary and alternative forms of health care. It is easy to conclude that health is both public and private. It is everywhere in our culture, and yet not all members of our society share it equally. The pursuit of health and wellness truly seems a mystery that leaves us uncertain as to whether it is possible to make societies and people healthy.

By applying the sociological imagination, this book unravels the mysteries surrounding the pursuit of health and wellness. Rather than considering health as merely the absence of disease, we need to recognize that health and illness are relational concepts and that the pursuit of health is a lifelong process. Standard approaches to understanding health in terms of illness are limited in that they focus on the distribution of disease and the consumption of medical products and formal health-care services. Rather than focusing on producing health, these approaches concentrate on disease and death rates and consuming health care provided by medical practitioners (e.g., doctors) and institutions (e.g., hospitals). However, this book shows that sickness is only the tip of the iceberg when it comes to studying health! Researchers often overlook the hidden depths of health care and the contributions that lay beliefs, social support, and informal care make to the pursuit of health and wellness. As a result, we know more about what makes us sick than we do about what makes us healthy. This book adopts an alternative perspective, consistent with a shift in the social and behavioural health sciences, and concentrates on exploring salutary factors that shape health and wellness across the life course. The focus is explicitly on health rather than on illness. We will discover both the structural and the personal factors that contribute to pursuing health and wellness while learning about the importance of healthy societies for healthy people.

No single theory or associated methodology can completely unravel the mystery of health in all of its dimensions. Because of the multi-dimensional nature of health, this book considers major theoretical paradigms used by sociologists for understanding health and makes a case for adopting an eclectic approach using mixed methods to measure the dimensions of health across the life course. Extensive coverage is given to the latest research perspectives on health, combining intersectional analysis and a life course perspective. Detailed and up-to-date information is provided on the social determinants of health and the upstream factors that shape the health of both populations and individuals over time. We present the latest evidence from international and Canadian health researchers on factors that affect health. An intersectional model of health incorporating a life course perspective is outlined to guide future research. Most important, this book is written in straightforward, easy-to-read language, with student-friendly sociological analyses of current events relating to the pursuit of health and wellness. Each chapter summarizes research in a manner that allows an undergraduate student to understand the major issues. It critically evaluates the existing body of knowledge and identifies gaps as well as implications for future research. Chapters conclude with a brief summary of the main points raised in the discussion, sample study questions, suggestions for further reading, and Internet resources. Throughout the text, biographic content boxes personalize the insights of some of the most renowned scholars of health, medicine, and the body. After reading this book, you will understand that it is possible to create healthy societies and healthy people, and you will gain a better appreciation of factors that shape your pursuit of health and wellness!

The first edition of this book was a major scholarly undertaking requiring the devotion of considerable resources between 2007 and 2011. It was highly successful and was adopted as a required textbook in health sociology and health studies courses in a number of universities and colleges across Canada. We have found it very gratifying to see the way that *Pursuing Health and Wellness* contributed to the teaching of health sociology and health studies courses throughout Canada. As experienced university professors, we are well aware that textbooks represent a significant expense for our students. With this in mind, we wanted to produce a second edition that would be a meaningful revision. We believe that the second edition of *Pursuing Health and Wellness* represents just that: a novel contribution to this field of study, which builds upon and extends the first edition.

The research literature and evidence upon which this book rests has been significantly revised and updated from that of the first edition. Beyond that, the new edition further develops an intersectional life course perspective on the pursuit of health and wellness, a perspective that is integrated throughout the chapters. We have included classroom-tested, easy-to-read and student-friendly, leading-edge sociological discussions of contemporary issues such as digital health technologies, the controversy over vaccination, the inquiry into the death of Brian Sinclair, health literacy, and personalized medicine. We have also increased the number of biographic content boxes that were a popular feature in the first edition. The extensive analysis of upstream social determinants of health now includes a more wide-ranging discussion of income inequality and health. We have also expanded the discussion of the importance of sex- and gender-based analysis in health research, including consideration of lesbian, gay, bisexual, and transgender (LGBT) health issues. A new chapter devoted exclusively to ethnicity and health provides more detailed coverage of Aboriginal health, including consideration of residential schools and intergenerational trauma, racialization and racism in health care, and Indigenous knowledge of health and wellness.

Overall, this edition represents a novel contribution to our understanding of the lifelong pursuit of health and wellness and provides a clear answer to one of the critical questions instructors are often asked by their students: "Is this new edition of the book significantly different from the earlier one?" The answer is an emphatic "Yes!"

Acknowledgments

We would like to start by thanking the Oxford University Press staff who contributed in many different ways to this book. Jodi Lewchuk provided critical support and encouragement during the initial stages of preparing the second edition, while Tanuja Weerasooriya provided valuable assistance in completing the manuscript. Dorothy Turnbull's careful editing improved the readability of the book. We also sincerely appreciate the insightful and instructive comments that we received from the reviewers, who included Doug Weizhen of the University of Waterloo, Steven Prus of Carleton University, and Fiona Whittington-Walsh of Kwantlen Polytechnic University. Their feedback helped to guide our revisions of the first edition.

We would also like to thank our graduate student research assistants, Veronika Eliasova and Mansa Assam at the University of Manitoba, who assisted us by carrying out literature searches.

Finally, we want to express our appreciation to the instructors in health studies and health sociology programs throughout Canada who adopted the first edition, many of whom generously shared suggestions for the revised edition. We have considered your comments carefully and worked hard to use them to improve the text. We thank you!

> To Maxine, for the courage you displayed in dealing with the challenges you encountered in your personal pursuit of health and wellness.
> To Kevin, Sheryl, Justin, and Hayden and to Nicole, Dave, Jordan, and Greg. Sharing each others' lives is the true joy of family.
> —A.S.

> In memory of my mother, Margo Jean Fries (1947–2015), who continues to inspire me to understand that health is a journey, not a destination, just like life. I love and miss you, Mom.
> —C.J.F.

Part One
Understanding Health and Wellness Sociologically

Part One, Understanding Health and Wellness Sociologically, contains three chapters. Chapter 1, Introducing Health Sociology, begins with a discussion of the mystery of good health and the importance of recognizing that health is a social construct. The concept of health consciousness is then introduced, and an effort is made to clarify the distinction between producing health and consuming health care. This introductory discussion is followed by a brief review of the origins of medical sociology and the factors that contributed to the convergence of sociology and medicine. After outlining the scope of early medical sociology, the focus shifts to the transition from medical to health sociology and the development of health sociology in Canada. The first chapter concludes by emphasizing the need for a more theoretically oriented sociological approach to understanding the pursuit of health and wellness.

Chapter 2, Applying the Sociological Imagination to Health and Illness, provides a discussion of sociological paradigms for studying health and illness. After summarizing traditional theoretical perspectives (i.e., health and illness as viewed from structural functionalist, conflict, and interactionist paradigms), the chapter discusses feminist social theory and health and illness as gendered experiences, as well as the sociology of the body paradigm, which highlights the perspective that health and illness constitute embodied cultural facts. The chapter concludes by emphasizing the importance of adopting an intersectional life course perspective for understanding health and illness sociologically.

Chapter 3, Measuring the Dimensions of Health, addresses the need for a better understanding of the relationship between meaning and measurement, the distinction between good health (wellness) and ill health (sickness), and the process of health status designation. The multi-dimensional nature of health is emphasized, and challenges facing population health assessment are outlined, including the difficulties involved in measuring both ill health (the traditional approach) and good health (the positive aspects of health and well-being). The salutogenic model of health is introduced as a conceptual framework for studying salutary factors that protect and promote good health. The chapter clarifies the difference between health inputs, health status, and health outcomes and then reviews the advantages and disadvantages of a number of indicators typically used in measuring the health status of Canadians. Chapter 3 ends with a call for a mixed-methods approach to researching the good health dimension of wellness (and the ill health dimension of sickness), combining standard quantitative methods, such as population health surveys, with more qualitative methods, such as illness narrative accounts and health diary studies.

1 Introducing Health Sociology

Learning Objectives

In this chapter, you will be introduced to a sociological perspective on health and will gain a better understanding of

- health as a "social construction";
- the difference between a sociological understanding of health and wellness and one based on "biological determinism";
- the cultural bases of "health consciousness";
- the scope of traditional medical sociology and efforts to transform the field into health sociology; and
- the development of health sociology in Canada.

Introduction: The Mystery of Good Health

Have you ever wondered how it is possible for anyone to stay healthy? When we are young, we typically get "normal" childhood diseases such as chicken pox. As children and adults, we continually face the threat of contagious illnesses that are "going around." For example, in our daily lives we routinely encounter people who have "common" cold symptoms, such as difficulty breathing or a sore throat. Plus, there is the annual challenge of the flu season. The older we get, the more likely we are to have to deal with the increasing prevalence of chronic conditions such as arthritis or hypertension (high blood pressure). Today we routinely hear about the potential threat of pandemics such as the Zika virus, Ebola, Acquired Immunodeficiency Syndrome (AIDS), Middle East Respiratory Syndrome (MERS), and Avian Influenza A (H7N9). Finally, we are learning more about how threats to the environment are also threats to human health. Despite the many risks, most people manage to stay well and to lead healthy and productive lives!

What types of factors contribute to good health? How do people manage to protect their health and stay well? An important health sociologist named Aaron Antonovsky consistently argued (1996; 1987; 1979) that health researchers need to focus attention on finding answers to these questions if they hope to be able to unravel what he described as the mystery of good health. At present, we know a great deal about what makes us sick (as illustrated by the cartoon below), but in contrast, we have a very limited understanding of what keeps us well. The types of risk factors that contribute to ill health are quite familiar to us (e.g., cigarettes and fast food), but the "very rare condition of good health" is still somewhat a mystery!

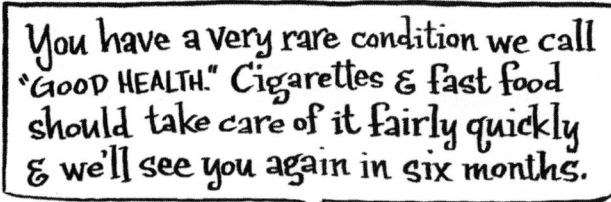

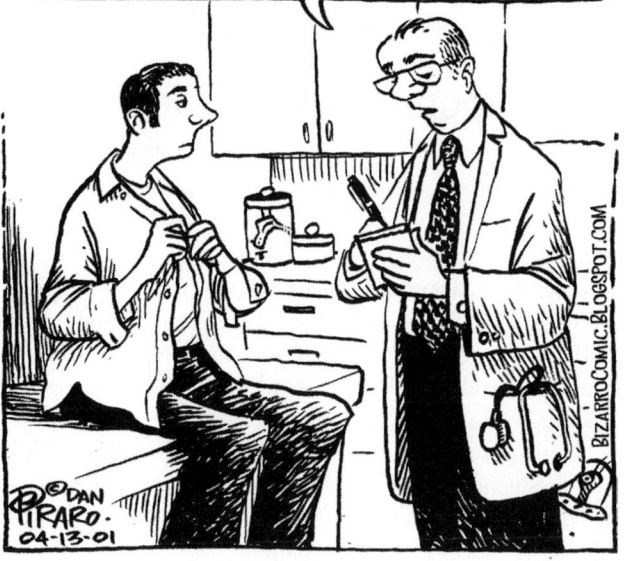

Antonovsky (1979) introduced the **salutogenic model of health** in an effort to shift our focus from ill health to the salutary factors that protect or enhance good health. His intention was to formulate an approach that would contribute to an improved understanding of the "origins" of good health and the social conditions that facilitate health-protective behaviours. By focusing on health instead of illness, Antonovsky was hopeful that the salutogenic model would provide a guide for identifying and understanding the factors that make populations healthy. We will examine the features of this model more closely later in the book when we discuss the importance of this approach for understanding the dimensions of health (Chapter 3) and the determinants of good health versus ill health (Chapter 4). For the present, it is sufficient to acknowledge the influence of the salutogenic model on the approach adopted in this book for exploring the meaning of good health and the social factors that contribute to the successful pursuit of health and wellness.

The primary purpose of this book is to provide a critical sociological framework for understanding the health and health-care behaviour of Canadians. First and foremost, the book focuses explicitly on health rather than illness. Traditionally, medical sociology focused primarily on the distribution of disease, the organization of formal medical services, and the role of medical practitioners (e.g., doctors) and institutions (e.g., hospitals) in caring for the sick. While acknowledging the traditional medical sociology approach, we shift our thinking about health and illness to a health sociology perspective, considering not only people's efforts to maintain "health" but also the more general pursuit of "wellness." Drawing on the scientific literature available, it seems that while the two terms are sometimes used interchangeably, the concept of wellness is much broader than health and actually subsumes good health. For example, Bruhn and colleagues (1977, 210) argue that while the meanings of good health and wellness differ, it is important to realize that "good health is a continual process that can evolve into wellness." In other words, good health is a necessary, but not a sufficient, condition to attain wellness. **Wellness** is an inclusive concept that incorporates not only good health but also quality of life and satisfaction with general living conditions (Corbin and Pangrazi 2001; Evans and Stoddart 1990). By providing a critical analysis informed by sociological theory and research, this book will help you to understand the factors that shape the lifelong pursuit of health and wellness by Canadians.

Health as a Social Construction

No social study that does not come back to the problems of biography, of history and of their intersections within a society has completed its intellectual journey.
—C. Wright Mills, *The Sociological Imagination*, 1959

This quotation is from the sociologist C. Wright Mills, who wrote a very important book in which he explained that the task and promise of sociology are to understand the dual process wherein society affects individual behaviour, which, in turn, in its totality affects society. The task of social science is to understand how objective structures of society (e.g., social roles, norms, institutions) influence individual, subjective behaviour (e.g., personal health-care behaviour) and, in turn, how the totality of social behaviour serves to reproduce the reality that is society. One place to begin our introduction to health sociology is by looking at how sociologists follow Mills' advice to define and understand health. In this effort, we will contrast the sociological understanding of health and wellness with an understanding based on biology, popular in our culture.

Although most people have some idea about what it means to be in good health, health is not as straightforward a concept to understand as it may appear. Usually, it is not until sickness intrudes into a person's life that health and its importance become clear to the unfortunate sufferer and her friends, family, and loved ones (Calnan and Williams 1991; Idler 1979). It may be in the ironic nature of health that it is best understood when it is gone, with health defined in opposition to illness. This notion of health is too vague, however, to satisfy the social scientist trying to gain a more precise understanding of the meaning of good health and the processes by which people pursue health and wellness.

In the classic book *Man, Medicine and Environment* (1968), Pulitzer Prize–winning biologist René Dubos makes the point that the desire for health is perhaps the most fundamental for any organism, and this is certainly no less the case for what Dubos describes in a later book as "the human animal" (1969). Yet when it comes to health, our social nature means that it occupies a unique place for human beings. Unlike animals, humans' pursuit of health is far more than an instinctual drive for survival and cannot be satisfactorily understood as such. For us, health and wellness are much more than biophysical conditions and are never experienced or understood simply at this level. The basic idea behind the sociological understanding of health is reflected in the quotation from Mills: People's locations in the social world affect their behaviour and, ultimately, their health and illness. To illustrate, aspects of our behaviour, such as living in automotive-intensive suburban cities or polluting the environment, shape our society, which, in turn, affects our health. The idea that society shapes and is shaped by human behaviour is an important sociological insight. Understanding biography, history, and their intersections is the mandate of sociology. Health sociologists systematically study the social aspects and differing interests in society that affect the human pursuit of good health and wellness. Chapter 2 presents a number of sociological paradigms for studying health.

According to the sociological approach, health represents a fundamental part of everyday life that is shaped by society and social relations. This perspective is reflected by a groundbreaking international policy document titled the *Ottawa Charter for Health Promotion*, released by the World Health Organization in 1986. The *Ottawa Charter* provides guidelines that governments throughout the world were encouraged to adopt for their population health promotion strategies. The first International Conference on Health Promotion meeting, held in Ottawa, "was primarily a response to growing expectations for a new public health movement around the world" (World Health Organization 1986, 1). In the *Ottawa Charter*, international experts chose to define **health** as

> a resource for everyday life, not the objective of living. Health is a positive concept emphasizing social and personal resources, as well as physical capacities. Therefore, health promotion is not just the responsibility of the health sector, but goes beyond healthy lifestyles to well-being (World Health Organization 1986, 1).

What was so novel about defining health in this way, rather than in relation to illness, was that these experts identified a wide range of social, political, and environmental factors that influence health and well-being beyond biology alone. More specifically, they argued that "the fundamental conditions and resources for health are: peace, shelter, education, food, income, a stable eco-system, sustainable resources, social justice, and equity" (World Health Organization 1986, 1). This broad view of health allowed the authors of the *Ottawa Charter* to write: "Professional and social groups and health personnel have a major responsibility to mediate between differing interests in society for the pursuit of health" (1986, 2).

Although health may be viewed as a crucial resource for living, obviously we do not all experience health and wellness in the same way. Sociologists point out that our pursuit of health has important social dimensions and reflects differing locations within the structures of society. In keeping with the definition of health in the *Ottawa Charter*, health sociology understands health as a social construction; that is, both the health and the illness of our bodies and the manner in which we understand these concepts are influenced by social factors.

While the term "social construction" has a long history in sociological thought, probably the most noteworthy treatment comes from Peter Berger and Thomas Luckmann's *The Social Construction of Reality: A Treatise in the Sociology of Knowledge*. This book, published in 1966, remains "one of the most widely read and influential books in contemporary sociology" (Ritzer 1992, 387). The purpose of Berger and Luckmann's book was to explore the ways in which people in the course of their everyday lives and social interactions construct subjective meanings that, in turn, serve as the basis of the social reality that is society. Reality is seen to be creatively shaped by people through social interaction. For the sociologist, aspects of our reality such as the meaning of good health are said to be socially constructed. This sociological understanding of health as a social construction can be contrasted with the way in which a doctor, for example, understands health and illness.

In medical and biological understandings of health, human beings are often described as little more than discrete bundles of biochemical and mechanical processes, and health is defined clinically by physiological processes operating within the limits of certain predefined, scientifically measurable parameters. For example, when you go to your family doctor for a physical examination, she will measure your blood pressure using technological instruments such as a sphygmomanometer and stethoscope: an inflatable arm cuff to restrict blood flow connected to a mercury manometer to read your level of blood pressure and a device to listen to sounds within the body. If, after repeated measurements, your blood pressure readings continue to fall within the high range, you will be diagnosed with hypertension, or high blood pressure, a medical condition affecting an estimated 5 million Canadians (or 19 per cent of Canadian adults aged 20 to 79 years) that can lead to stroke, heart attack, or kidney failure (Wilkins et al. 2010). Regardless of how you may report feeling, you are labelled "healthy" if your physiological markers are within the predefined parameters and "diseased" if they are not. Indeed, hypertension is known as "the silent killer" because a person with high blood pressure experiences no symptoms.

Commenting on the biomedical conception of health, McKee notes that "in contrast with the World Health Organization's definition of health as 'physical, mental, and social well-being, not merely the absence of disease or infirmity,' health tends to be defined in functional rather than experiential terms, as the absence of disease" (1988, 776). In other words, illness, scientifically labelled as disease, is understood by biomedicine in a functional rather than an experiential way. As a result, disease becomes reified. That is, disease is treated as a thing with a clearly defined reality all its own: "This approach, which posits a disease as a thing with an identity of its own, is known as the ontological definition of disease. Thus, the disease and its associated symptoms become the focus of attention, rather than the whole patient" (Berliner and Salmon 1979, 35).

Understanding human beings in terms of biological functioning has a long history in Western thought and is described as **biological determinism**, or the belief that human behaviour can best be explained in terms of the innate biological properties of individuals, such as genes and biochemical processes. "Ultimately, all human behaviour—hence all human society—is governed by a chain of determinants that runs from the gene to the individual to the sum of behaviours of all individuals. The determinists would have it, then, that human nature is fixed by our genes" (Rose, Lewontin, and Kamen 1984, 6). In the West, science has offered us this view of ourselves and a complex set of medical practices and technologies based upon it, and we have, by and large, accepted this biologically deterministic view of health (Lewontin 1991).

For the sociologist, however, **health** is not understood solely as a biophysical state experienced in the same manner by all people in all times and places but, rather, as a socially constructed life course experience that varies over time according to different social, cultural, and economic life circumstances. Conrad and Barker (2010) reviewed the different ways that sociologists have used a social constructionist approach for studying health and illness over the past 50 years and highlight a number of key findings. For example, they point out that all illnesses are socially constructed experiences. Furthermore, "some illnesses are particularly embedded with cultural meaning" (2010, S76) that is not directly related to the nature of the condition but which shapes both the ways individuals experience illness and societal responses. Finally, medical knowledge is shaped by social relations rather than solely based on biological facts. Taken together, this is what it means when sociologists refer to health and illness as socially constructed.

To fully understand health in a sociological perspective, therefore, you have to take into account individual differences and cultural dimensions involved in health, as well as the healthiness of society. People's awareness of health and their responses to illness vary not only from individual to individual because of the uniqueness of each person's biography but also from culture to culture. Health sociology, then, is the subfield of sociology that attempts to understand the social and cultural contexts within which the meaning of good health is interpreted, illness is recognized and treated, and the pursuit of health and wellness occurs.

Health Consciousness: Producing Health versus Consuming Health Care

"Hi, how are you?" This familiar phrase is typically used to start conversations with others. Why do we generally ask others about their health and wellness when we greet them? The obvious answer is that this custom is part of our cultural tradition (like a handshake) and is learned through socialization in settings such as the family and school. However, this is not a complete explanation of why we inquire about the health status of others when we meet and greet them. Asking about health is a way of acknowledging our interest in the other person and establishing a basis for social interaction. The cultural practice of starting conversations with a question about health reflects the fundamental value we attach to good health in our society.

A number of years ago, Lau, Hartman, and Ware (1986) developed a short measure of health as a value. The measure requires the person to rank the relative importance of health (i.e., physical, mental, and social well-being) compared to other aspects of life. In addition, respondents are asked to indicate the extent to which they agree with common health-related expressions such as "If you don't have your health, you don't have anything" or "There is nothing more important than good health." Results generally indicate that health is the most highly ranked value held by members of the study population. Subsequent research has shown that people in Western culture regard an individual commitment to health and wellness as a moral virtue (Conrad 1994). Reviewing the centrality of health as a moral value, Conrad (2012, 479) explains that "To be against a culture and policies that revere health is to be against one of the central values of our society." There is growing evidence that we increasingly value health and wellness highly.

We certainly spend a great deal of time talking about health. We not only regularly ask about the health of others, but we also constantly disclose information about our own health to family members, friends, and co-workers. Stop and think about how many of your daily conversations at home, at school, or at work focus on health-related topics. How much time do you spend each day talking about health? Gould (1990, 233) contends that "people who think about health also talk about it." In other words, our level of health consciousness may be reflected, in part, by the extent to which we talk about health.

Health consciousness can be defined as the degree to which an individual is aware of and attentive to health. This awareness is

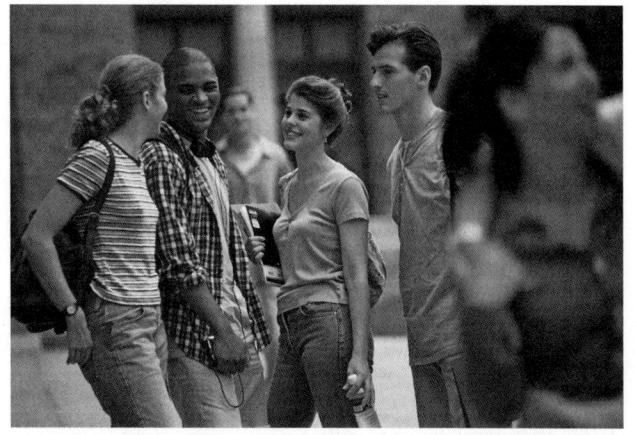

How often do you discuss health with your friends and family?

a fundamental aspect of everyday social life and involves an ongoing process of monitoring our health status, assessing and interpreting the condition of our minds and bodies, and engaging in a wide variety of health actions as a routine part of our social practice. Indeed, Ayo (2012, 100) asserts that a careful examination of the pursuit of health and wellness reveals "that health consciousness has become deeply engrained within our social fabric." As we will discuss in Chapter 8 when we consider health promotion and lifestyle behaviours more closely, health consciousness, or the degree to which we focus on our health, is likely related to everyday personal practices such as our eating habits and the extent to which we pay attention to health information (Kaskutas and Greenfield 1997). To assess your level of health consciousness, try answering the questions in Box 1.1.

Today we are bombarded by an ever-increasing amount of health information from a wide diversity of sources. Most newspapers and popular magazines have regular health columns, such as the popular health advice column by Dr Gifford-Jones syndicated in more than 60 Canadian newspapers. As well, a tremendous number of specialized publications focus entirely on health, fitness, and diet. Just browse in your favourite bookstore, and you will see this point vividly illustrated in the amount of shelf space devoted to books on health, wellness, fitness, or nutrition. Among daytime television's most popular shows are those that feature medical experts offering health advice, such as "Dr. Oz" and "The Doctors." A review by Hoffman and Tam (2013) demonstrates that in our health-conscious culture, celebrities have become a major source of health advice. In fact, an Ontario-based study found that people placed as much faith in celebrity

Box 1.1 Self-Assessed Level of Health Consciousness

Are you a health-conscious person? To assess your personal level of health consciousness, answer the following questions.

Do you

- read health-oriented magazines and books?
- listen to radio talk shows or watch television shows about health?
- search the Internet for health-related information?
- have health apps on your smartphone?
- take vitamins and/or supplements?
- shop in health food stores?
- try to avoid cholesterol?
- read the inserts that come in drug packages?
- read ingredient labels on food packages?
- check the expiry dates on products?

The more questions you checked, the higher you score on this measure of health consciousness. Positive responses suggest that you are the type of person who is self-conscious about health, attentive to inner feelings about health, and usually aware of changes in your health.

sources of health information, such as Dr Gifford-Jones and Dr Oz, as they do in their own family physicians (Clarke et al. 2007)!

Global communication technologies such as the Internet offer a variety of health-related advice and information. **E-health** refers to the application of communication and information technologies to health care (Nettleton, Burrows, and O'Malley 2005). A study carried out by Grandinetti in 2000 reported that more than 70,000 websites offer health information, and according to Nielsen Online, such websites are among the fastest-growing categories of online sites (Nielsen//NetRatings 2008). A Statistics Canada survey shows that one-third of Canadians use the Internet for health information (Underhill and McKeown 2008). Google, along with the US Centers for Disease Control and Prevention, are developing a means of detecting flu outbreaks by tracking online search queries (Ginsberg et al. 2009). Online platforms such as Web 2.0, Twitter, Facebook, blogs, and wikis have facilitated the formation of online support communities for those living with illness to share stories and coping strategies as well as social support. According to Ziebland and Wyke (2012), when we read other people's accounts of their experiences with health and illness and participate in the creation of health information through blogging and contributing to social networks, we gain a greater understanding of our own health and healthcare management. In this way, they suggest, "the Internet fundamentally shapes our experiences of the everyday, including our experiences of health and illness" (2012, 220). Rabinow (1996) coined the term "biosociality" to characterize the forms of collective identification around health that are taking shape as a result of developments in biotechnology and information technology.

Mainstream websites such as webMD.com and mayoclinic.com provide easy access to a wealth of health information. Box 1.2 shows the top five webmd search terms for 2011. However, the reliability of some health information on the Internet needs to be questioned. A US study found that in nine out of ten cases for the most costly medical conditions, the information posted on Wikipedia contradicted peer-reviewed research (Hasty et al. 2014). Pharmaceutical companies

Box 1.2   WebMD Top Mobile Search Terms in 2011

By Miranda Hitti
WebMD Feature Reviewed by Hansa D. Ghargava, MD

According to the WebMD website, "You are on the go, and so is your need for health information." Find out what WebMD users were most likely to be looking for in 2011. The list just might surprise you. The year's most popular search topics were:

1. Ringworm
2. Hemorrhoids
3. Turf Toe
4. Strep Throat
5. Pregnancy Symptoms

Source: www.webmd.com/news/year-in-health/default.htm.

are exploiting the Internet for commercial gain through a marketing strategy of partnering with patient support groups in order to influence the content of information on the groups' websites (Moynihan and Cassels 2005). There is also evidence that the so-called digital divide plays a role in health information–seeking on the Internet in that people who are socially marginalized in terms of income, age, minority status, education, or literacy have less effective access to information technology. Those who have higher incomes and education or are younger and healthier are more likely to consult online health-information sources (Cotten and Gupta 2004). Websites such as ratemds.com perpetuate a consumerist ethos toward health care by allowing patients to anonymously rate physicians on "punctuality," "helpfulness," "knowledge," and "overall quality" while viewing others' ratings of their own physicians. Some researchers have lauded the apparent democratization of information on the Internet because it presumably levels the playing field between patients and physicians (Hardey 1999; Loader et al. 2002). Others (Nettleton, Burrows, and O'Malley 2005; Seale 2003) have cautioned that the Internet is increasingly structured in a manner that reinforces the dominance of biomedical authority.

In 2011, Canadians spent $29.4 billion out-of-pocket on products and services such as dental care, eye care, and prescription medicines (CIHI 2013a). In addition, as health-conscious consumers we spend billions more in the active pursuit of good health and wellness, purchasing a wide range of health-related products and services. To illustrate, supermarkets, drugstores, and major department stores surround us with products that promise health benefits. The health-conscious consumer is encouraged to buy vitamins, minerals, and supplements to protect her health and to eat "better-for-you" foods that claim to be low in (or free of) cholesterol, caffeine, sodium, and fat or to be certified 100 per cent organic (Agriculture and Agri-food Canada 2011). It seems that new products (with names including such terms as "natural," "smart," or "sensible") show up on store shelves each day, claiming to play an important part in healthy living and, therefore, good for our health. We can apparently simplify the selection process by going directly to "health food" stores that offer natural health products such as echinacea and St John's wort. Or we can do our grocery shopping at an increasing number of specialty stores offering a range of food products that have presumably been organically grown or are free of chemical additives. Retailers are aware that good nutrition is a vital aspect of good health. This dimension of health-protective behaviour reflects the prevalent notion that "you are what you eat."

Many other types of products are available to the health-conscious individual. For example, a wide variety of home exercise equipment is on the market today. Think about the television advertisements you have seen recently. We can purchase stationary bicycles, treadmills, stair climbers, rowing machines, and weightlifting equipment to use at home and become more physically fit. For those who prefer to exercise in the company of others, there is an almost overwhelming selection of health and fitness clubs that one can join. This is a growth industry, since physical activity, like nutrition, is an important aspect of healthy behaviour.

Related to e-health is the development of **m-health** (as illustrated by Box 1.3), which refers to the use of mobile electronic technologies such as smartphones and specialized health-related apps to monitor and promote health (Lupton 2012b). Both government and commercial interests envision the potential of such technologies to promote health consciousness. Noting that while governments in the past attempted to provide health-related information through low-tech communications and advertisements, Lupton (2012b, 230) contends that "The use of mobile devices in health promotion endeavours represents a significant shift in the methods of health promotion." She argues that m-health technologies allow people to monitor and share aspects of their health status and behaviour, such as diet and exercise, with others, both their own social network and their

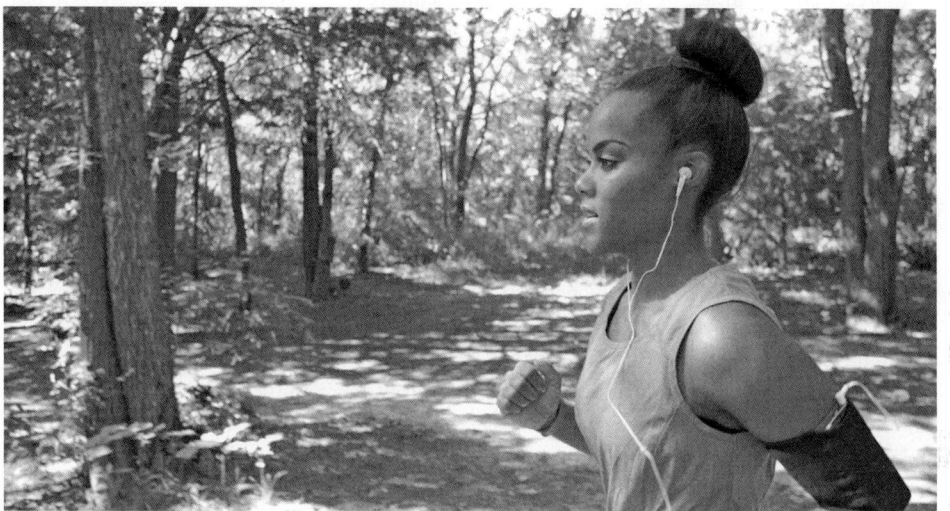

> **Box 1.3   M-health**
>
> Mobile devices now come equipped with sensor technology and apps that allow users to monitor, track, and share personal health data such as physical activity, heart rate, caloric intake, hours of sleep, body weight, and glucose level.
>
> Do you use m-health apps to share your health behaviour on Twitter or Facebook? Are there any drawbacks to such sharing of personal health information?

health-care professionals. All things considered, it is clear that the highly health-conscious individual has increasing access to a wealth of readily available health-related information and technology.

Sociologists describe Western societies as having a **consumer culture** in which the products and services we buy make statements about our identity and place in the social world. In the consumer culture of the West, a dominant characteristic of advanced capitalist society is the consumption of goods and services not necessarily for their "use value" but because of the kinds of statements they make about the individual consumer's self-identity (Bocock 1993). Consumption is a meaningful act that is linked with our sense of self, or our identity. In other words, what we buy reflects who we are. This is especially true for health-care products and services, because they are so closely connected with our bodies. As Shilling remarks, "Growing numbers of people are increasingly concerned with the health, shape and appearance of their own bodies as expressions of individual identity" (2003, 1). In this context, consumer culture and the media support a tendency to view health as a commodity and encourage health-care consumers who want to preserve their investments in the commodity of health to purchase health-care products and services. Health sociologists describe this as **medical consumerism**. Commenting on this situation, Baudrillard states that "health today is not so much a biological imperative linked to survival as a social imperative linked to status" (1998, 135). Health-conscious consumers are faced with a wide range of products and services promising to improve their health, and the choices they make distinguish them from others who won't or can't look after their health by purchasing health-care commodities. In the wellness-oriented culture of the West, how one chooses to pursue, or neglect, "the nebulous product of health" (Freund, McGuire, and Podhurst 2003, 220) acts as a cultural basis for judging the moral value both of our own self and of others. Increasingly, we judge self-worth by how people look after their bodies.

While the relationship between producing health and consuming health care has been questioned by sociology for some time (e.g., Evans and Stoddart 1990; Freidson 1970a, 1970b; McKee 1988), "wellness" as a socially constructed way of understanding health and well-being is of more recent origin (i.e., since the mid-1980s; Sointu 2005). Based on research investigating the content of British daily newspapers, Sointu (2005) tracks a movement in the language of well-being from "the body politic" to "the body personal." The current use of the term "wellness" reflects "a changed relationship between citizens and the state from that which characterized many, if not most, liberal democratic societies in the past" (Henderson and Peterson 2002, 1). Whereas under old welfare state models the government was accorded primacy in the production of health and healthy citizens, the new wellness culture tells us that as consumers, we are individually responsible for producing our health by consuming health care. In their critical synthesis of favourable and critical perspectives on well-being, Carlisle and Hanlon (2008, 267) note that "Well-being is now a highly valuable and valued commodity in Western consumer culture and is heavily and cleverly marketed—and willingly paid for by those able to do so, as part of what many uncritically take to be the good life in capitalist society." As we will learn, this individualization of health is a key component of medical consumerism.

So how can you tell if a particular advertisement is an instance of health promotion or medical consumerism? As we will learn in Chapter 8, the two concepts are empirically and theoretically interrelated, with the line between them sometimes unclear. For now, however, the key difference is that with health promotion, the government is attempting to encourage the health of the population as a productive human resource (i.e., healthy workers are more productive workers who cost less in terms of health care and days lost due to illness), while with medical consumerism, a private firm holds a financial interest in selling a particular health-care product or service. The connections between medical consumerism, the new public health, the individuation of health, and government health promotion initiatives will be explored in more detail in the concluding chapter (Chapter 12).

The health-conscious consumer today also faces the challenge of assessing the extent to which the services offered by an ever-widening range of health practitioners will assist him or her in producing health and wellness. As we will learn in Chapter 11, in addition to the services offered by health-care providers such as medical doctors, dentists, and pharmacists, we now have the option of consulting complementary or alternative healers, such as chiropractors, homeopaths, naturopaths, herbalists, and others, who claim to offer more holistic and natural health-care products and services. Thus, health-care consumers face the daunting task of sorting through the competing claims by an increasing number of alternative practitioners that their services provide effective care for the physical, psychological, social, and spiritual dimensions of health and well-being.

It should be obvious that health and wellness are important human values and that health-related concerns occupy a great deal of our time, attention, effort, and money. As embodied social beings, or individual social actors with biological bodies, health is an issue for everybody in society. It is, therefore, not surprising that social scientists, such as sociologists, psychologists, anthropologists, geographers, and economists, have shown a great deal of interest in health and health-care behaviour. The remainder of this chapter will first briefly review the types of factors that originally gave rise to the field of medical sociology and eventually transformed it into health sociology. Special attention will then be devoted to the development of health sociology in Canada.

The Origins of Medical Sociology

But it is particularly necessary, in my opinion, for one who discusses this art to discuss things familiar to ordinary folk. For the subject of inquiry and discussion is simply and solely the sufferings of these same ordinary folk when they are sick or in pain.

Ancient Medicine—The Hippocratic Corpus, ca 400 BCE

When did people first begin to think sociologically about health, illness, and medicine? Answering this question is not as straightforward as you might think. The above quotation is from the remains of an ancient library called the *Hippocratic Corpus* containing medical texts originally attributed to the Greek physician Hippocrates, but historians now know that they were in all likelihood written between the sixth and fourth centuries BCE by a group of medical thinkers (Bulgar and Barbato 2000). Examining these very old texts reveals that the people of Ancient Greece, much like people today, spent a lot of time thinking about the issues of health and illness. Indeed, the *Hippocratic Corpus* makes reference to factors health sociologists now describe as social determinants of health and illness. (Part Two of this text examines the factors that shape health and wellness.) While the term "medical sociology" was first introduced in the last decades of the nineteenth century (Bloom 2002), medical sociology is relatively new as a separate area of academic study. Prior to 1950, very few sociologists had used the health-care field as a setting in which to explore sociological research questions. Usually, scholars trace the emergence of the field of medical sociology to 1950s America when more sociologists became involved in studying organized medicine, the recruitment and training of health professionals, and pathways to care. Early research in the field concentrated on factors that influence the decision to seek medical care and the nature of doctor–patient relationships. The 1970s and 1980s witnessed a dramatic expansion in the field, as reflected by the appearance of many medical sociology textbooks (in the United States) and the publication of new international journals devoted to the sociological study of health and illness. The 1990s saw increasing interest in exploring the determinants of population health and steady growth in health services research as behavioural scientists examined the impact of ongoing efforts to reform health-care delivery systems in countries such as Canada and the United States. At the dawn of the twenty-first century, medical sociology was characterized as

> a field of study fully institutionalized in every sense. There is an organized demand for teaching and research; there are professional associations and scholarly journals specifically devoted to the field; within the university, its main locus of activity, as well as in government and private organizations, medical sociology is supported with financial and other rewards for performance (Bloom 2000, 11).

While it is accurate to say that medical sociology as a subfield of the academic discipline of sociology emerged in the latter half of the twentieth century, the origins of thinking sociologically about health, illness, and medicine really go back much further. For example, in a book entitled *The Birth of the Clinic*, the French social philosopher and historian Michel Foucault (1973) showed how efforts to understand and control morbidity resulted in a convergence of medical and social science. Morbidity refers to the distribution of disease in human groups and will be examined in more detail in Chapter 3 when we discuss some of the challenges involved in trying to measure population health. Controlling morbidity relied upon having knowledge about different social groups that facilitated mapping the distribution of disease (i.e., who got sick with what). Sociological research methods, such as the social survey, made this kind of knowledge of the population possible. As such, the effort to deal with morbidity actually contributed to the emergence of what we now call social science. Note that this is a very different account of the origins not just of medical sociology but of sociology as an academic discipline. Usually, we trace the origins of sociology to the French Enlightenment and scholars such as Montesquieu (1689–1755) and Auguste Comte (1798–1857), but for Foucault, social science arose as part of medical efforts to deal with morbidity.

What contributed to the convergence of sociology and medicine in the first place? A variety of factors have been identified (e.g., the public health movement and the emergence of social medicine), but the one factor that is consistently acknowledged to be of primary importance is the fundamental change that has occurred over the years in morbidity patterns. For the purposes of the present discussion, it is simply a matter of recognizing that the major diseases that affected the health of your grandparents' generation when they were growing up differ from those that are prevalent today. To illustrate, the past century was characterized by the so-called conquest of epidemic diseases such as smallpox. Over the years, the contribution of infectious diseases as a major cause of death has decreased significantly. Today, chronic degenerative diseases, such as heart disease, cancer, and arthritis, have replaced infectious diseases as the most prevalent conditions with which we have to contend. The twentieth century witnessed the control, for the most part, of epidemics of acute infectious diseases such as polio. At the same time, it is important to note that there has been a reappearance, to some extent, of infectious diseases such as tuberculosis among people living in certain social and physical environments (e.g., those living in poverty). In addition, with globalization we have witnessed the spread of new and devastating infectious diseases such as AIDS and SARS (Ali and Keil 2008). Overall, however, the evidence generally indicates that prevalent morbidity patterns have changed. The decline in infectious disease is the result of both advances in the scientific basis of biomedical practice (e.g., antibiotics, immunization) and significant environmental improvements in living conditions, access to safe water, and sanitation.

As a result of this major shift in morbidity patterns, the nature of medical practice and the structure of the health-care system also changed over the twentieth century. The focus of formal health-care services slowly broadened to include not just the biophysical basis of disease but also the psychosocial context of illness. (These issues will be examined in detail later in the book. Chapter 10 includes a discussion of contemporary health care and its link to population health, as well as the increasing role that medicine plays in everyday life.) In other words, while it remains important to search for the biological cause(s) of diseases such as cancer, there has been a growing recognition that it is equally important to broaden the search to include the social and psychological determinants of health. For example, according to the US President's Cancer Panel (2007), nearly two-thirds of cancer deaths could have been prevented by changes in lifestyle. Clearly, the social context must be taken into account if we hope to be able to fully understand health and illness. Part Two of this book is devoted to a thorough examination of a range of personal and structural factors that shape our health status. For example, Chapter 4 provides an overview of the general determinants that make people healthy. The point of the present discussion is that the shift that occurred in morbidity patterns was eventually accompanied by a growing awareness, perhaps most famously articulated by the Canadian-born physician (and one of the founding figures of modern biomedicine) Sir William Osler, who noted that "it is many times much more important to know what patient has the disease than what kind of disease the patient has" (1906, 758–9).

As the focus of the health-care field began to shift away from exclusively concentrating on the underlying biological basis of ill health to include psychosocial aspects, the opportunity arose for social sciences to make a meaningful contribution to our understanding of the pursuit of health and wellness. Simply stated, it was as though an intellectual door opened at this point in time. Gradually, this led to recognition on the part of health-care providers and planners that social and behavioural sciences had developed a body of knowledge and research expertise that could contribute to an improved understanding of the complex nature of contemporary health and wellness. The shift in morbidity patterns was thus followed by a shift in focus from disease pathology to concern for the whole person and, ultimately, the social context within which good health and ill health are experienced. In other words, there was a progressive convergence in the research interests of sociology and medicine and the eventual emergence of medical sociology as a legitimate field of study.

The Scope of Medical Sociology

Medical sociology, like the general discipline of sociology, encompasses many different areas of concern about human behaviour. In fact, research in the field of medical sociology cuts across almost all of the traditional areas of sociological investigation, such as family dynamics, gender roles, ethnic relations, the environment, education, and the impact of social inequality on behavioural patterns within the context of health and health care. In summary, four general areas of analysis may be identified within the field of medical sociology (as illustrated in Box 1.4).

First, medical sociology is interested in the differential distribution of disease in human groups. This field is typically described as **social epidemiology**, or the study of social factors that place individuals and populations at risk for illness and disease. According to social epidemiology, diseases are neither uniform nor random in their occurrence but rather are socially produced and influenced. In other words, while disease is a universal phenomenon that affects all people everywhere, we do not all experience exactly the same types of diseases throughout our lifetime. We know that to some extent, certain diseases are predictable based on hereditary factors (e.g., muscular dystrophy) and personal lifestyle practices such as smoking (e.g., lung cancer). At the same time, health disparities are related to different sources of social inequality.

Box 1.4 Dominant Issues in Medical Sociology

- The differential distribution of disease (i.e., social epidemiology)
- Social patterning of health and illness beliefs and behaviour
- Social institutions for treating disease
- Social organization and delivery of health services

For example, diseases are often observed to be more or less common among members of various social groups, such as social classes (Chapter 5), genders (Chapter 6), and ethnic groups (Chapter 7). Thus, we might ask, for example, why do people in different social classes experience different diseases throughout their lifetime? In searching for answers to this type of question, medical sociology is actively involved in investigating the impact of social determinants, such as income and education, on our health status.

A second major area of interest for medical sociology is the social patterning of health and illness beliefs and behaviours. Regardless of the specific condition, when disease does occur, people tend to view their health problems from the perspective of their particular social and cultural contexts. Based in part on these different perspectives, they tend to respond to disease and experience illness in socially patterned ways. To illustrate this point, think about how you would answer the following questions: Do women and men have similar beliefs about health and illness and engage in similar help-seeking behaviours? Does a backache mean the same thing to an office worker as it does to a manual labourer? Do the members of different ethnic groups feel the same way about displaying their emotions when in pain? Available research evidence clearly demonstrates that the answer to each of these questions is no! Medical sociologists have demonstrated that social and cultural factors such as social class, gender, ethnicity, and age shape our beliefs about health and our behavioural responses to illness. In summary, the evidence indicates that within any given society, there are important socio-cultural differences in lay beliefs about the nature of ill health and patterns of help-seeking behaviour. Chapter 5 presents Canadian and international evidence clearly demonstrating that income, education, and occupation continue to play important roles in shaping health status and health behaviour. Chapters 6 and 7 further explore the link between social status and health status by critically examining the evidence and alternative explanations for differences in health between the genders and ethnic groups.

Third, medical sociology has devoted a great deal of attention to exploring the social institutions that people have developed to help them deal with illness when it occurs. Because illness is a fundamental aspect of human existence, people in all societies have developed a variety of formal institutions for understanding and systematically treating disease. These institutions range from the traditional folk healer (e.g., "medicine man" or "shaman") to the current scientifically based health-care professions and the modern hospital. Medical sociology has carefully documented the development of medical knowledge and practice.

The final area of interest for medical sociology can be broadly identified as the social organization and delivery of health-care services. Today, the treatment of disease involves much more than the direct application of medical knowledge and expertise through medical institutions such as the doctor's office and the hospital. In contemporary society, the institutions that provide health care are part of a complex set of relationships involving a number of other public and private organizations. For example, the services provided by health-care professionals are influenced, to a great extent, by pharmaceutical companies, medical technology manufacturers, health insurance companies, and government health policies and programs (e.g., medicare). The basic point is that medical institutions for treating disease are related to, and in turn partly controlled by, a number of other social institutions (in Canada, government departments of health in particular). As a result, the type of health care available to the public is directly affected (e.g., ongoing controversies about the supply of family physicians). These issues are discussed in more detail in Chapter 12 when we turn our attention to health reform and the need to reorient health-care services to focus on population health behaviour rather than patient illness behaviour.

Substantial growth in the field of medical sociology over the past few decades has clearly demonstrated that the study of the impact of disease on human behaviour and the ways in which people respond to illness are important areas for the application of sociological knowledge and research methods. What are the major accomplishments of this field of inquiry? In summary, medical sociology, along with other behavioural sciences, has contributed to an improved understanding of

- the different beliefs and attitudes that various segments of the population have toward health, illness, the body, and medical care;
- the social role of the patient (i.e., the sick role) and the nature of interaction between patients and formal health-care providers;
- the socialization process through which health-care providers, such as physicians and nurses, acquire the outlook, standards, and competence necessary to carry out their professional roles;
- the social structure, culture, and functioning of hospitals;
- how biomedicine attained and struggles to maintain its position of dominance within the health-care sector;
- the efforts by health occupations such as nursing, pharmacology, and chiropractic to achieve increased professional status; and
- the ongoing struggles of complementary and alternative healers, such as homeopaths and naturopaths, to gain legitimacy as formal health-care providers.

In other words, we have learned a great deal about the social dimensions of health. Indeed, it has been suggested that the major contribution of medical sociology has been the explicitly social point of view that it provides for the study of health and illness. The emergence of medical sociology as a special field of study has reinforced the importance of broadening research perspectives in health and health care to include an analysis of not only disease pathology in the individual and the personal experience of illness but also the impact of the social environment on health status and the structural determinants of population health (e.g., income, occupation). Researchers (Rosich and Hankin 2010; Hankin and Wright 2010) recently attempted to summarize the key findings of medical sociology over the past 50 years and concluded that sociological analysis has contributed in fundamental ways to our understanding of health issues and "the broad contextual factors and conditions in society that affect, health, illness, and health care" (Rosich and Hankin 2010, S2).

At the same time, gaps still exist in the accumulated body of knowledge. One limitation of medical sociology stems from its almost exclusive focus on the impact and treatment of disease and organized responses to illness. This reflects the fact that medical sociology initially defined itself primarily in relation to the profession of medicine. The determinants of good health and the behavioural dimensions of self-health management (e.g., self-care behaviour) received little research attention in the early stages of the development of medical sociology. This realization precipitated a period of self-examination and critical reflection in the middle to latter part of the 1970s, which resulted in the start of an ongoing transformation of the field from "medical sociology" to "health sociology." Consequently, it is important to recognize that "the focus on what contributes to well-being and keeps individuals and societies healthy is a relatively new sociological endeavour" (McDaniel 2013, 2).

From Medical Sociology toward Health Sociology

Following Twaddle (1982), the transformation of medical sociology into health sociology can be understood as occurring in stages. At an early stage in the development of medical sociology, Straus (1957) suggested that the field could be divided into two patterns of research: sociology in medicine and sociology of medicine (as illustrated in Figure 1.1). Though some would like to forget the distinction between the sociology in medicine and the sociology of medicine, viewing it as a holdover from medical sociology's past that has given way to a more integrative and interdisciplinary health sociology, this distinction is still in common usage today.

While there is a significant difference between the two perspectives, it is important to realize that sociology in medicine and the sociology of medicine are not mutually exclusive. The distinction between these two perspectives simply captures the dual focus of medical sociology on both applied (practical) and basic (theoretical) health research issues. As medical sociology transitions into health sociology, many of the studies carried out in the field have combined the two patterns of research in an attempt to provide an empirical basis for restructuring the health-care delivery system while, at the same time, advancing our understanding of health and illness behaviour. As Straus (1999) more recently reminded us, if medical sociology is to overcome some of its past limitations and successfully transform itself into health sociology, the distinction between sociology in medicine and the sociology of medicine is worth holding on to, if for no other reason than that it reminds us to be mindful of the inherent tensions between biological and psychosocial explanations of health and illness.

Medical sociology first undertook research that can be described by the term **sociology in medicine** (the "insider's" viewpoint) with the application of sociological knowledge and research methods to the clarification of practical problems that had been identified by the medical profession or other health-care occupations. Timmermans (2013, 1) explains that "These social scientists have hitched their wagon to the broader health mandate: aiming to provide knowledge that directly benefits health and, more often, health care. They study social aspects of health—such as health beliefs, patient–doctor interactions, compliance, or cultural sensitivity—to improve health care delivery and utilization." In other words, the sociology in medicine perspective is devoted primarily to the search for applied solutions to medically defined problems such as finding

Sociology + Medicine → Sociology *in* Medicine "Applied"

Sociology + Medicine → Sociology *of* Medicine "Basic"

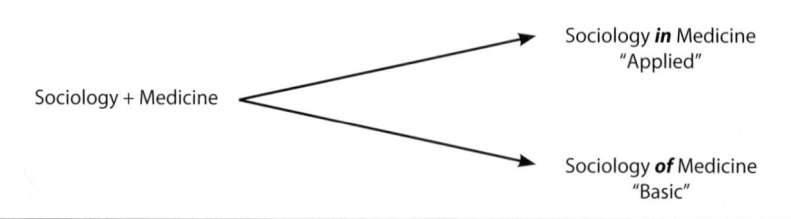

Figure 1.1 The Dual Focus of Medical Sociology

ways to improve the effectiveness of patient care. To illustrate, the medical sociologist who adopts this perspective might investigate pathways to medical care (e.g., how quickly people bring their health problems to the attention of a physician) or study the extent to which patients take their medication as prescribed by their doctor. The purpose of this research is essentially to help increase patient compliance with medical directives. This type of research has been described as having a **medico-centric bias**: an approach to understanding health, illness, and the body in a manner that privileges the medical perspective and is characterized by viewing the medical profession favourably as a social institution concerned merely with treating disease and improving health (Twaddle 1982). Just as sociologists use the term "ethnocentric" to denote using the values and norms of one's own culture as a standard by which to judge and understand other cultures, health sociologists use the term "medico-centric" to describe using the values and norms of biomedicine to judge and understand health, illness, and the body.

During the 1970s, medical sociology was subjected to increasing criticism that it was medico-centric. For example, Pflanz (1974; 1975) commented critically on the present and future state of medical sociology, as well as the nature of the close relationship between sociologists and physicians in the conduct of health research. According to Pflanz, at this stage in its growth medical sociology had failed to develop useful theories and effective predictive models for explaining the impact of social inequality on the distribution of disease and differences in the utilization of health-care services. He argued that instead of questioning medical values (e.g., the benefits of formal health care), medical sociology had essentially adopted them. In fact, Pflanz (1975) suggested that medical sociology was caught between the values of medicine (which play an important part in defining the research questions to be pursued) and the value system of the government (which influences the funding decisions of research-granting agencies). Pflanz went as far as to accuse medical sociology of having been co-opted by the profession of medicine. He contended that in carrying out research under the powerful influence of the medical profession, the medical sociologist had become a propaganda agent for medical values. In his words, "Seduced by the magic spell of medicine, involved in the medicalization of society and of sociology itself, he becomes, whether he likes it or not, the public relations man of the medical organization in which and for which he works" (Pflanz 1975, 9).

During this period, Johnson (1975) also reviewed the development of medical sociology and characterized the field as theoretically weak. Basically, he agreed with Pflanz's criticism that much of the research in medical sociology failed to be guided by either established sociological theories or new conceptual thinking. Johnson raised questions such as the following: Is medical sociology too detached from the mainstream of sociological theory? Is medical sociology over-identified with the medical model and health policy issues? In response, Johnson argued that research in medical sociology was constrained by the fact that the medical profession defined the nature of the health problems that were worthy of study through its "power to allow or refuse researchers access to medical situations and personnel" (1975, 229) and through its control of funding agencies. Johnson echoed Pflanz's (1975) call for greater autonomy in order to facilitate medical sociology's efforts to become a more credible and independent field of study.

In addition, there was a call for fundamental changes in the research emphasis of the sociological analysis of health and health care. A review by Gold (1977) of articles published in the *Journal of Health and Social Behavior* (the journal of the Medical Sociology Section of the American Sociological Association) between 1960 and 1976 suggested that during this period, the study of patient populations constituted the mainstream of research activity within medical sociology.

According to Gold's content analysis, this research emphasis was evidence of medico-centric bias. She pointed to examples of researchers who uncritically accepted medical definitions of health problems and attempted to interpret social conditions that influence health within the biomedical model. By conducting sociological analysis within the medical framework, medical sociology's primary function was to provide empirical evidence to assist organized medicine in its efforts to make compliant patients out of diverse populations. In this way, warned Gold, "The medical sociologist who incorporates medical values into her or his research may become a deliberate or unwitting agent of social control" (1977, 166). The solution, according to Gold, was for the field to take steps to gain greater independence from medical norms and values and to strengthen the identity of medical sociology as a separate and critical framework for analyzing health and health care from a sociological perspective.

These developments signalled a move toward developing a **sociology of medicine** (the "outsider's" viewpoint) that attempts to provide basic explanations for the behaviour of physicians, nurses, and other health-care practitioners, as well as that of their patients. Contrasting this perspective with sociology in medicine, Timmermans (2013, 1) writes,

> The sociology of medicine or, more broadly, health, in contrast, is a sub-specialty of sociology that happens to study the health field. Its purpose is to contribute to a broader scholarly literature with ideas, concepts, methods, and theories drawn from the substantive area of health. The main warrant here is to conduct solid, theoretically driven social science research, paying only secondary attention to the humanitarian subtext of healing and suffering.

The objective of this perspective is to improve our theoretical understanding of social phenomena such as the organizational structure in which patients and practitioners interact. Sociology of medicine attempts to offer a critical analysis of issues involved in both patient compliance and medical dominance of the health-care sector. The social scientist who adopts a sociology of medicine viewpoint typically explores research problems derived from a sociological, rather than a medical, framework. This perspective treats the health-care system basically as an object of investigation, since the main concern of the sociology of medicine is generating sociological understanding rather than applied knowledge.

To illustrate the sociology of medicine perspective, a medical sociologist might decide to study the structure and functioning of a hospital as one example of a large bureaucratic organization. In fact, there have been many studies of the way in which work is organized in modern hospitals (i.e., the way in which nurses, doctors, and hospital administrators interact with each other in their daily efforts to provide patient care). For example, Ducey (2009) examined how pro-market restructuring policies negatively affected frontline health-care workers, making it more difficult for them to do their jobs and thereby compromising patient safety. The results of this type of research might be compared to information about other formal organizations that provide services to the public without being directly concerned about discovering ways to provide more cost-efficient patient care in hospital settings in the way that sociology in medicine would.

The sociology of medicine perspective raises critical questions about health-care workers, their organizations, and their relationships with others (including patients, other health-care professionals, and government officials). For example, studies have explored the working relationships between physicians and other health-care professionals, such as nurses, pharmacists, and chiropractors, as well as the impact of universal government health-care insurance programs (such as medicare) on the practice of medicine. The basic purpose of these types of sociology of medicine studies is to address sociologically informed research questions about health and health care.

Following this period of critical reflection, efforts were initiated, starting in the early 1980s, to transform the field of medical sociology into health sociology. The objective has been to shift the major emphasis of sociological research away from the study of illness and disease at the personal level within a medico-centric framework to a critical examination of the determinants of health and the functioning of the health-care system at both the societal and personal levels of analysis. The primary focus of health sociology is population health behaviour rather than patient illness behaviour (which preoccupied medical sociologists in the past). In other words, health sociology focuses on the health status and health behaviour of members of the general population and not simply those who are already in treatment settings (i.e., patients using medical and hospital services). Health sociology is interested in learning more about the factors that keep people healthy in addition to exploring how they behave when they become sick.

According to Twaddle (1982), sociology has been abandoning its medically dominated approach to the study of health in favour of a perspective that views the medical profession as one aspect of a complex health-care system. In his words, "Sociology is divorcing from the medical perspective and medico-centric perspective to one that takes medicine as one element associated with the health of both individuals and populations" (Twaddle 1982, 349). To a great extent, current sociological inquiry includes not only the study of disease, patient illness behaviour, and the practice of organized medicine but also the study of population health status and health-protective behaviour. In other words, the transition from medical sociology to health sociology means a shift in research focus away from patient illness behaviour and pathways to professional health care to an analysis of the determinants of population health status and self-health management.

Twaddle (1982) identifies several key factors that have contributed to the shift from medical sociology to health sociology. Just as medical sociology originally emerged from developments in both sociology and medicine, Twaddle attributes the emergence of health sociology to changes in the theoretical paradigms and research methods available for the sociological analysis of health as well as changes in the delivery of health-care services. Many of the assumptions about the benefits of modern medicine that were taken for granted in the 1950s began to be challenged in the late 1970s and early 1980s. There was growing criticism on the part of both social scientists and the general public about the extreme emphasis in health care on technologically based, highly specialized institutional medical practice. Growing patient dissatisfaction with the fragmented and impersonal nature of care and perceived deterioration in the quality of health care led to the consumer movement's call for increased protection of patient rights (e.g., a patient's bill of rights) and an increase in alternative approaches to health. At the same time, organized medicine began to experience increased competition and challenges from other health occupations (e.g., chiropractic) and healing systems (e.g., Traditional Chinese Medicine). As a result, serious questions were raised about the effectiveness of medicine in general and its relevance for dealing with the prevalent health problems facing contemporary society (e.g., chronic conditions such as arthritis).

In addition, questions were raised about the extent to which access to medical care was a major determinant of health status. The types of health-care services offered by the medical profession are important and do affect personal health. However, focusing on medical practice and the organization of formal health-care institutions does not tell us why people get sick in the first place or why the distribution of disease differs among diverse social groups in society. The traditional approach of medical sociology also did not tell us much about the "mystery of health" (Antonovsky 1979; 1987; 1996) or how people manage to stay healthy.

The services offered by physicians emphasize disease intervention and treatment. For example, physicians are trained to diagnose and treat diseases and to help us manage our health problems (particularly in treatment settings such as the hospital). While the prevention of disease is also a stated objective of contemporary health professionals, there is growing recognition that disease prevention and health maintenance are significantly different. An annual physical examination and immunization (e.g., a flu shot) may help older adults to prevent the onset of specific conditions such as influenza. At the same time, it is now recognized that personal health practices (e.g., being physically active, eating properly, and getting enough sleep) play a much more crucial role in shaping our everyday health and well-being.

In summary, over the past several decades, health sociology has adopted a more critical approach to studying health and health care and, at the same time, has developed more sophisticated theoretical perspectives and methods for analyzing the social dimensions of health and illness behaviour. There is growing recognition within the subfield that the use of formal health care does not necessarily equate with improved health. Thus, the focus of sociological analysis has changed from patient illness behaviour to population health behaviour to be able to better understand the full range of factors that help to keep people healthy (Blaxter 2000). The major shifts that have occurred over the years in the primary focus of the sociological study of health and health care are summarized in Figure 1.2. The transition from medical sociology to health sociology has involved a number of key changes in the nature of sociological analysis (e.g., changes in the unit of analysis and changes in the underlying conception of health problems and healing roles).

	Unit of Analysis	Health/Health-Care Focus
Sociology in Medicine	Individual and Interaction (Personal Health)	Disease and Illness + Physicians and Patients
Sociology of Medicine	Individual and Social Organizations (Personal Health)	Ilness and Sickness + Health-Care Professionals and Patients
Health Sociology	Society and Social Structures (Population and Personal Health)	Health and Wellness + Self-Health Management (Informal and Formal Health Care)

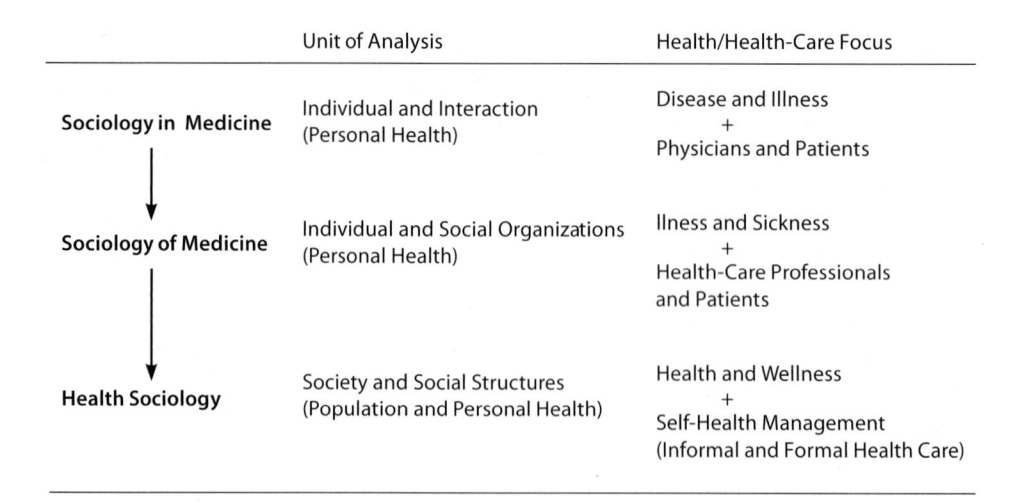

Figure 1.2 From Medical Sociology Toward Health Sociology

The first major shift in emphasis was away from concentrating exclusively on the diseased person (i.e., the biophysical aspects of the organism and disease pathology) that characterized the sociology in medicine approach toward inclusion of psychosocial aspects of the illness experience and organized responses to illness. While the basic unit of analysis was still the individual (i.e., personal health), the sociology of medicine approach was broadened to include psychological dimensions (e.g., health locus of control beliefs) and social roles (e.g., the sick role) that influence the illness experience of the individual. The next major shift in emphasis away from medical sociology and toward health sociology has meant changing the unit of analysis from the individual to society and redirecting research attention to an exploration of the structural determinants of population (and personal) health. In other words, the fundamental research question now is: What societal factors help to keep Canadians healthy?

Health sociology is dedicated to exploring the social structures that shape people's lives as well as their health and well-being. This perspective focuses on good health as well as ill health (i.e., disease and illness) and critically evaluates the link between social status (e.g., income) and health status. In a recent review paper examining the different ways in which we can understand health sociologically, McDaniel (2013, 2) asserts that health sociology provides us with important insights into "the complex roles social factors and structures play in health and well-being of individuals and societies." As we will learn in Chapter 9, the move toward health sociology has also meant a growing recognition that people are primary providers of health care and are not simply consumers of professionally provided health-care services. Health sociology emphasizes the importance of self-health management (i.e., the relationship between our routine everyday activities and our health). Self-health management is examined in detail in Chapter 9 as we explore the hidden depths of health care through a critical analysis of the links between informal care, social support, and the production of good health. Thus, health sociology stresses the importance of the social environment and lifestyle factors (such as physical activity, nutrition, and smoking) as important determinants of our health status. Finally, while medical sociology highlighted disease prevention and illness intervention and treatment, health sociology highlights health promotion and health maintenance (i.e., risk reduction and health-protective behaviour).

Today, the field is typically called health sociology rather than medical sociology. However, it is interesting to note that the section of the American Sociological Association is still called "medical sociology" while the International Sociological Association calls its health research committee "the sociology of health." The editors of the fifth edition of the American Sociological Association's *Handbook of Medical Sociology* stated that while they all believed "that our discipline is better defined as the Sociology of Health and Illness than as Medical Sociology, we have chosen to keep the traditional title" (Bird, Conrad, and Fremont 2000, viii). The *Handbook* is revised once a decade, and the focus continues to be on medical sociology. For example, the editors state in the preface of the latest edition that "we continue here with the sixth edition, reflecting some changes and new vistas in medical sociology, while updating and reconfiguring some perennially important topics" (Bird et al. 2010, viii). Perhaps greater internationalization of the field will ultimately be the factor most responsible for a full transformation of medical sociology into health sociology.

Health Sociology in Canada

The growth of health sociology in Canada mirrors to a great extent the trends occurring in other countries (such as the United States, England, and Australia). Canadian sociologists working in the health-care field have systematically documented the development of health sociology in Canada (Badgley 1976; Kelner and New 1984; Coburn and Eakin 1993). In the initial review, Badgley (1976) notes that although sociology of health in Canada was a recently established field, it was starting to grow rapidly. Typical medical sociology research issues dominated the work of Canadian sociologists at this time. For example, medical sociology in Canada in the 1970s focused on themes such as the complex nature of health-care services; the changing relationships between health-care professionals, including growing challenges by nurses and chiropractors to biomedical dominance of the health-care sector; and, finally, the dynamics of the sick role and patient illness behaviour.

According to Kelner and New (1984), the 1980s witnessed an expansion of health sociology in Canada to include a broader range of topics, such as health promotion and the impact of population aging on health and health care. They argue that by the early 1980s, there was a growing awareness of the value of a social science perspective on health and important Canadian research initiatives intended to address "the social, political and economic structures influencing and constraining developments in health care" (Kelner and New 1984, 189). These early reviews predicted a promising future for the sociological analysis of health in Canada.

In the last of these three published reviews, Coburn and Eakin (1993) comment on the shift from a sociology in medicine perspective to health sociology in Canada but emphasize that research in this field continues to be predominantly applied in nature (i.e., it focuses on issues that have important health-care program and policy implications). Their review of the development of health sociology in Canada is divided into three areas, which will be briefly summarized in the following subsections. They suggest that the dominant themes in Canadian health sociology at the time included (1) the social determinants of health status, (2) health and illness behaviour, and (3) the health-care system. It is important to keep in mind that the three are not mutually exclusive research areas.

The Social Determinants of Health

A great deal of the research in this country in the field of health care has been devoted to investigating the health status of Canadians. This research collects data through large-scale population health surveys such as the ongoing *Canadian Community Health Survey* and the *Canadian Longitudinal Study of Aging*. These surveys provide us with a wealth of information about the health status and health behaviour of Canadians and will be used as sources of data to illustrate a number of critical issues discussed in following chapters. More details about these surveys and other important data sources will be provided when we turn our attention in Chapter 3 to problems of measurement involved in assessing the health status of the Canadian population.

Coburn and Eakin (1993, 86) point out that health surveys typically explore the social etiology (causation) of disease and illness and illustrate the fact that social factors are "the most important determinants of health status." In other words, there is a strong causal link between social status and health status. Social factors such as socioeconomic status (e.g., income and education) as well as gender, age, and ethnicity (e.g., being Native Canadian) all play a vital part in shaping our health status. In addition, population health surveys provide persuasive evidence that there are persistent social inequalities in the health status of Canadians despite nearly half a century of medicare in this country (i.e., publicly financed universal health insurance and access to the formal medical-care system). Some of this evidence will be considered in Part Two when we examine sources of inequality and health disparities.

Coburn and Eakin (1993) also point out that studies of the social determinants of health status have examined the impact of the social environment on health, particularly the workplace. Workplace and health studies (e.g., Eakin 1992) have explored occupational differences in health status related to the nature of work, exposure to hazardous materials, and dangerous working conditions. This research has also investigated the relationship between the organization of work (e.g., shift work, degree of autonomy on the job, and workplace stress) and the health status of Canadians. Another aspect of the social environment that has been examined is family life. Both the negative aspects of family life (e.g., family violence) and its positive aspects (e.g., the health-protective benefits of social support, as discussed in Chapter 9) have received research attention. Overall, these studies highlight the importance of gaining a better understanding of the social determinants of health status.

Health and Illness Behaviour

In the second major research area, Canadian health sociology has been interested in explaining the ways in which people behave to maintain their health and respond to illness. Coburn and Eakin (1993, 92) define health and illness behaviour as "the way in which people perceive, understand, and respond to health and illness related states or events." Once again, the link between social status and health is highlighted, but this body of research concentrates on investigating how one's position in the social structure shapes health and illness behaviour. Social variables include gender, age, socioeconomic status, ethnicity, and rural/urban residential location as correlates of health and illness behaviour. For example, studies have investigated differences between men and women and between socioeconomic groups in lifestyle health practices (health behaviour) and in patterns of health care, including utilization of formal health-care services (illness behaviour). Canadian health sociology research in the area of health and illness behaviour attempts to be less descriptive and more interpretive than studies that focus on assessing the social causes of health status. An excellent example of this type of research is Arthur Frank's provocative account of the experience of life-threatening illness in his 1991 book *At the Will of the Body* (1991a). The objective of such research is to explore the meaning of the lived experience of the individual as he or she attempts to maintain health, prevent illness, overcome sickness, adjust (in some cases) to living with long-term chronic disease and disability, or come to terms with death and dying.

The Health-Care System

According to Coburn and Eakin (1993), this final area of interest has received most of the research attention of Canadian sociologists working in the health-care field. Numerous studies have examined the structure and functioning of health-care institutions (such as hospitals) as well as the role of formal health-care providers (such as physicians, nurses, and chiropractors). Much of this research focuses on questions about access and utilization of the health-care system, such as the following: Who uses what health-care services? When are health services used? Why are health services used?

In addition, beginning in the 1980s, Canadian health sociology research began to reflect a growing recognition that the health-care system consists of both formal and informal care and that informal caregivers (e.g., family members and friends) play an important part in the provision of health care. In fact, an increasing number of studies now investigate the ways in which families care for chronically ill or disabled members. For example, a national study of Canadians living with dementia and their informal caregivers found that about half of the older adults diagnosed with dementia live in the community and are cared for by unpaid family members, friends, or relatives (CSHA 1994). The "hidden depths" of health care will be examined in Chapter 9 when we take a closer look at informal care.

Finally, research on the Canadian health-care system also focuses on health policy issues and the reorganization of health services. For example, health sociologists have contributed to the ongoing debates in this country regarding the process of health-care reform and the reallocation of health-care resources (both human and financial). Efforts to reform the health-care system include shifting the focus from disease prevention to health promotion, transferring care from institutions to the community, enhancing self-health management as a health promotion mechanism, and redefining the role of formal health-care practitioners and health-care facilities (e.g., hospitals). These types of issues receive careful attention in Part Three.

It is interesting to note that the first two reviews of the development of health sociology in Canada (Badgley 1976 and Kelner and New 1984) appeared in an international journal devoted to social science and medicine. During the early stages of the growth of sociological analysis of health in Canada, no Canadian journals were devoted exclusively to this field of inquiry. Yet by 1993, the most recently published review paper (Coburn and Eakin 1993) appeared in the first volume of a Canadian journal focusing on health and Canadian society. Unfortunately, this journal survived only until 2000. Even though there is a Canadian Society for the Sociology of Health, no more recent reviews of developments in this field of study have been published, nor is there a journal devoted exclusively to Canadian health sociology. What does this suggest regarding the current state of sociological analysis of health in Canada? There are a number of possible interpretations. It may signal a decline in the extent of health sociology research being carried out in Canada. Or it may mean that sociological health research has now moved beyond the disciplinary boundaries of sociology into related fields, such as health studies, community health, and nursing.

Chapter Summary

It should now be apparent that the pursuit of health and wellness is a fundamental aspect of everyday life and is consequently an important topic for sociological analysis. As demonstrated in this chapter, we are continually involved in monitoring our health status, assessing and interpreting the condition of our minds and bodies, engaging in a wide variety of health actions on a routine basis, seeking out health-related information and technology, and buying an ever-expanding array of health-care products and services. The sociological study of health in Canada is clearly rooted in the traditional research interests of medical sociology but has a broader focus and covers a wider variety of health-related topics. Sociological analyses provide us with a basis for understanding how social structures and the process of social interaction are related to both population and personal health. To date, developments in the sociology of health have contributed to a growing recognition on the part of the public, health-care providers, and policy analysts that health is not simply a fixed, biological attribute of the person. Instead, health is now generally understood to be a dynamic social process that is shaped by structural factors (such as social class and gender) and is given personal meaning within the socio-cultural context in which we live and work.

There is still a need, however, to expand the focus of sociological analysis to ensure that it includes both the applied study of ill health (sickness) and illness behaviour and the study of good health (wellness) and health behaviour. This type of paradigm change is necessary if we are to gain a greater understanding of the social determinants of good health and the factors that enable Canadians to stay well. A more insightful understanding of the process by which people pursue health and wellness requires a more theoretically oriented sociological approach. Chapter 2 discusses both traditional and contemporary sociological theoretical paradigms that have informed the study of health. The following chapters highlight the importance of adopting a comprehensive theoretical perspective and methodological approach that recognizes health as both an embodied experience and part of an ongoing social process.

Study Questions

1. What is meant by saying that from a sociological perspective, health is a social construction?
2. Define the meaning of the term "health consciousness." How "health-conscious" are you?
3. Do you use the Internet to obtain health-related information? How might this affect your health behaviour?
4. Why would the late twentieth century shift in morbidity patterns stimulate growth in medical sociology?
5. Explain what is meant by the dual focus of medical sociology.
6. What are the major limitations of medical sociology?
7. Summarize the key differences between medical sociology and health sociology.
8. Outline the dominant research themes in Canadian health sociology, providing an example of a Canadian study that highlights this type of health research.
9. Is there a difference between producing population health and consuming health-care products and services?

Recommended Readings

Ali, S.H., and R. Keil, eds. 2008. *Networked Disease: Emerging Infections in the Global City.* Oxford: Wiley-Blackwell.

Coburn, D., and J. Eakin. 1993. "The sociology of health in Canada: First impressions." *Health and Canadian Society* 1: 83–110.

Henderson, S., and A. Petersen, eds. 2002. *Consuming Health: The Commodification of Health Care.* London: Routledge.

McDaniel, S. "Understanding health sociologically." 2013. *Current Sociology Review* 0: 1–16.

Moynihan, R., and A. Cassels. 2005. *Selling Sickness: How the World's Biggest Pharmaceutical Companies Are Turning Us All into Patients.* Toronto: Greystone Press.

Twaddle, A. 1982. "From medical sociology to the sociology of health: Some changing concerns in the sociological study of sickness and treatment." In T. Bottomore, M. Sokolowska, and S. Novak, eds, *Sociology: The State of the Art*, 323–58. Beverly Hills, CA: Sage.

Recommended Websites

Australian Sociological Association Sociology of Health Thematic Group:
www.tasa.org.au/thematic-groups/groups/health

Canadian Society for the Sociology of Health:
www.cssh-scss.ca

European Society for Health and Medical Sociology:
www.eshms.eu

International Sociological Association Research Committee on Sociology of Health:
www.isa-sociology.org/rc15.htm

Medical Sociology Online:
www.medicalsociologyonline.org

Medical Sociology Section of the American Sociological Association home page:
www2.asanet.org/medicalsociology

The "Cost of Living":
www.cost-ofliving.net

Recommended Audiovisual Source

Selling Sickness: An Ill for Every Pill. Directed by Catherine Scott, produced by Pat Fiske, co-written by Ray Moynihan. Brooklyn, NY: Icarus Films, 2004.

Applying the Sociological Imagination to Health and Illness

Learning Objectives

In this chapter, you will be introduced to some of the major theoretical paradigms guiding sociological analysis of health and illness, including

- the structural functionalist paradigm, which understands health and illness as "social roles";
- the conflict paradigm, which understands health and illness as "professional constructs";
- the symbolic interactionist paradigm, which understands health and illness as "interpersonal meanings";
- the feminist paradigm, which understands health and illness as "gendered experiences";
- the sociology of the body paradigm, which understands health and illness as "embodied cultural facts"; and
- the importance of adopting an intersectional life course perspective for understanding health and illness.

Applying Sociological Paradigms to Theorize Health and Illness

In the previous chapter, you were introduced to the idea that health can be understood as a social construction and that this differentiates a sociological understanding of health from medico-centric approaches to health and illness. But how does health sociology avoid a medico-centric bias? According to Cockerham (2013, 2), the answer lies with sociological theory: "sociological theory remains the most important pillar of medical sociology's uniqueness in studies of health and disease. It is the sociological perspective, as exemplified by its theoretical gaze, which gives medical sociology its distinctiveness in comparison to research in public health, health psychology, health services research, and behavioral medicine." Theory is the spark that ignites what was described in the previous chapter by C. Wright Mills (1959) as "the sociological imagination." The idea that society shapes and is shaped by human behaviour lies at the heart of sociological theory, and this is what is unique about health sociology's efforts to understand health and illness. As Turner (1995, 2) suggests, by addressing "the central theoretical problems of sociology," health sociology can move beyond the dichotomy between sociology in medicine and the sociology of medicine described in Chapter 1. The basic motivation behind applying the sociological imagination and sociological theory to understanding health and illness is twofold: First, by better understanding society and culture, we will be better able to understand health and illness. Second, a better understanding of health and illness will, in turn, allow us to more fully understand society and culture. This is the task and the promise of the sociological imagination when applied to the pursuit of health and wellness.

Sociologists study society and culture from a number of different perspectives (or theoretical paradigms). A **theoretical paradigm** is a conceptual framework or school of thought in which interrelated ideas and concepts about an aspect of reality are formulated. Health sociology, like the general discipline of sociology, is characterized by a number of different theoretical paradigms and methodological approaches. Depending on the paradigm that guides their work, sociologists make certain assumptions about how the social world works, focus on specific aspects of social life, formulate selective research questions, and use particular methods to try to answer these questions. The dominant sociological paradigms that have guided the analysis of health and illness have been described in great detail in the literature (e.g., Cockerham 2013; Cockerham and Scambler 2010; De Maio 2010a; Fox 1994; Gerhardt 1989; McDonnell et al. 2009; Scrambler 2012; Shilling 2012; Turner 1995). This chapter will first consider three paradigms that influenced sociological analysis for many years: the structural functionalist paradigm, the conflict paradigm, and the symbolic interactionist paradigm. Then we will turn our attention to an examination of the feminist paradigm and the sociology of the body paradigm that increasingly guide many studies of health and illness.

Each one of these paradigms provides a different conceptual framework for understanding human behaviour that is based on a number of underlying assumptions. For example, each paradigm consists of interrelated assumptions about the nature of the social world, the basic relationship between the individual and society, and the most appropriate methods for investigating human behaviour. Consequently, each theoretical paradigm offers a different understanding of how best to think about health and illness. Further, as Chapter 3 shows, the definition and the measurement of health differ considerably depending on which of these paradigms is guiding the investigation. In reviewing the paradigms, we will cite examples to illustrate the influence each of these conceptual frameworks has had on Canadian health research.

Health and Illness as "Social Roles"—The Structural Functionalist Paradigm

As its name suggests, the basic assumption of the structural functionalist paradigm is that human behaviour is guided by social structure or relatively stable patterns of behaviour that we learn from our society's culture. Structural functionalism contends that the proper level of study is society (as a whole) or the social system. Drawing upon the classical tradition of Émile Durkheim, the **structural functionalist paradigm** views society as a harmonious social system made up of a number of interconnected parts or institutions that function to maintain order and stability. Institutions are a specific kind of social structure that organizes the behaviour of large numbers of people into standardized patterns, such as the family and educational, economic, and political systems as well as the health-care system. Structural functionalism explores how large-scale social structures and institutions work together to pattern human behaviour. When social structure is supported by culture, you get an institution. For example, when patterns of responding to and dealing with illness are supported by cultural values and beliefs about doing so, you get the institution of the health-care system. For structural functionalists, institutions such as the health-care system are explained in terms of the tasks they perform or the functions they serve for some other institution or for the maintenance of society as a whole. In this approach, health care is explained in terms of the contribution it makes to managing the threat illness poses to the overall stability of the social system. As such, structural functionalism is one of the original systems theories.

Social structures exert an influence on individual behaviour because institutions are linked to social roles. A role is simply a behavioural pattern attached to a specific institution (e.g., the roles of professor and student are attached to the educational institution of the university). We all play many different roles throughout our lifetime in different social institutions (e.g., family, school, and work). According to the structural functionalist perspective, being ill also involves occupying a unique social position and performing a special social role (i.e., the sick role). In this way, the structural functionalist paradigm understands health and illness as social roles.

Structural functionalism is associated with a quantitative approach to studying human behaviour (e.g., careful observation and measurement) with the aim of discovering the effects social structure has on behaviour. As we will see in the next chapter, typically this means that sociologists guided by this paradigm rely on methods such as survey research and statistical analysis to collect and analyze quantitative data. Such methodology is intended to provide an objective view of social structures and their effects on human behaviour. This paradigm dominated American and Canadian sociology for many years, including the formative period during which medical sociology first emerged as a subfield within the discipline of sociology (i.e., the 1950s and 1960s). Structural functionalism is making something of a comeback in the form of modern systems theory (Scrambler 2012).

In his 1951 book on the social system, Talcott Parsons used medicine as an illustration of the structural functionalist approach to understanding the importance of the social role as a key concept in the relationship between culture, social structure, institutions, and individual behaviour (see Box 2.1). In a paradigmatic example of the structural functionalist approach to

Box 2.1 Talcott Parsons (1902–1979)

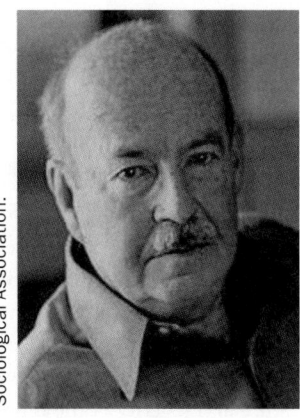

- Leading US sociologist of the mid-twentieth century and chief proponent of structural functionalism
- Developed the concept of "the sick role" in *The Social System* (1951)
- Used medicine to illustrate the importance of the social role in understanding the relationship between culture, social structure, institutions, and behaviour

"Illness incapacitates the effective performance of social roles" (1951, 430).

health and illness, Parsons (1951, 436) described the "four aspects of the institutionalized expectation system relative to the sick role" at a very early stage in the development of medical sociology and, hence, is often credited with establishing medical sociology as a subfield of sociology. With the concept of the **sick role**, Parsons argued that a set of behavioural expectations about how a sick person is supposed to behave (and be treated) is built into our social system (i.e., it has been institutionalized, or become a patterned part of our culture).

Because of the widespread nature of illness, it has been recognized for many years that the sick person occupies a special position in society with an associated behavioural pattern and set of reciprocal role relationships. However, it was not until Parsons (1951) theoretically formulated the behavioural dimensions of this social role that the sick role emerged as a central concept in the sociological analysis of illness behaviour. When it comes to health, the basic assumption of the structural functionalist paradigm is that people learn from their culture how to behave in socially patterned ways in responding to health and illness concerns. In other words, according to structural functionalism, health and illness can be viewed as social roles that are attached to the institution of health care and connected to certain cultural expectations and social behaviours.

The sick role includes a set of cultural expectations regarding the behaviours of both the sick person and those with whom she interacts (e.g., family members, health professionals). Over the past several decades, these interrelated dimensions of the sick role have been the subject of many review papers (e.g., Burnham 2014; Frank 1991c; Segall 1976b; Shilling 2002; Levine and Kozloff 1978; Arluke, Kennedy, and Kessler 1979; Williams 2005). Williams (2005, 123) explains:

> Parsons' analysis of illness as social deviance, and the sick role as a socially prescribed mechanism for channelling and controlling this deviance, is a key point of reference in the history of medical sociology, and a staple part of the diet that students of medical sociology (or sociology of health and illness as it is now more commonly known) are fed, year in year out, on both sides of the Atlantic.

These reviews explain that initially, the concept was widely adopted by medical sociologists. During the transformation to health sociology, however, it was subjected to increasing criticism, resulting in its disuse. More recent reviews, however, suggest a renewed interest in the concept. As we will learn, while there are problems associated with Parsons' original formulation of the sick role, his analysis of illness as a social role highlights the importance of understanding both the social aspects of ill health ("sickness") and the psychological components ("illness"), in addition to the biological components ("disease"). Today, in large part because of his early work, health is generally understood as a multi-dimensional phenomenon consisting of physical, psychological, and social dimensions. Parsons outlined the specific behavioural patterns of the role of the sick person in terms of two major rights and two major duties (See Box 2.2).

According to this theory, the occupant of the sick role has two fundamental rights. First, as Parsons explains, the sick person in our society is typically exempt from responsibility for the illness condition, since it is viewed as beyond the control of the individual. While there are some exceptions (e.g., sexually transmitted diseases), in our culture we typically do not blame people for becoming sick. Second, if the situation is defined as illness (based on medical diagnosis), the sick person is also temporarily exempt from performing normal social role behaviours (e.g., sick leave is a legitimate basis for being excused from work for a specific period of time). To a certain extent, this second right associated with the sick role depends on the nature and severity of the illness and on how well the sick person fulfills her duties. In other words, the sick individual's exemption

Box 2.2 The Behavioural Dimensions of Parsons' Sick Role Concept

The occupant of the sick role

- is exempt from responsibility for being ill (right 1)
- and is also exempt from usual well roles and task obligations (right 2)

- is expected to try to get well and to resume normal social roles as quickly as possible (duty 1)
- and is also expected to seek technically competent help and to comply with the recommended medical treatment (duty 2)

from normal role behaviours depends, in part, on the first duty of recognizing the role expectation that it is inherently undesirable to be ill and, therefore, that this person has a duty to try to get well and resume normal social roles as quickly as possible. For example, family members and friends may take over some of your routine chores as long as they believe you are sick and actively trying to recover.

According to Parsons, the second duty of the sick person is to seek technically competent help (i.e., the services of a physician) and to cooperate in the process of getting well. However, as Chapter 11 discusses, just what counts as technically competent help depends on the cultural context. For example, while a doctor's note will likely excuse your absence from a missed university exam, a note from your witch doctor explaining your absence in terms of "spirit possession" is not likely to be regarded as a legitimate excuse in the cultural context of the university institution. "Thus, sick role occupancy is perceived by others as legitimate only if the sick person clearly demonstrates a desire to get well by seeking medical care and complying with the physician's recommended treatment regimen" (Segall 1997, 290).

Early medical sociology was strongly influenced by the structural functionalist paradigm and devoted much of its research attention to the sick role concept. Based on this paradigm, illness was conceptualized as a form of deviant behaviour and a potential threat to the stability of the social system unless properly managed. To illustrate, adopting the sick role involves an exemption from performing usual well roles (e.g., the sick person has a legitimate reason

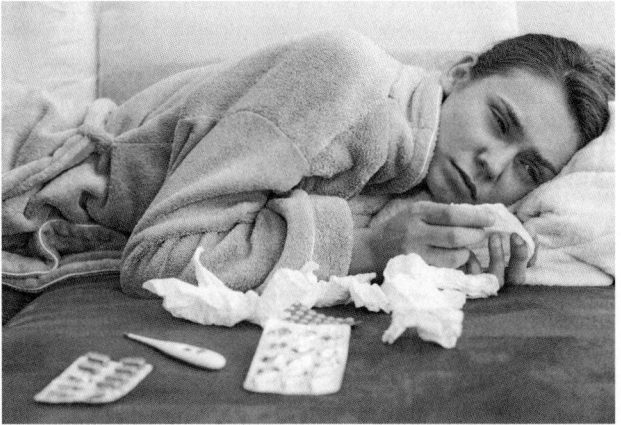

What are some behaviours of a sick person that may be influenced by society's idea of how people should act when they are not feeling well?

for missing an examination or being absent from work). Therefore, the structural functionalist paradigm characterizes medical institutions as agents of social control. This perspective on health and illness closely tied the duties of the sick person (i.e., an obligation to get well) to the power of the physician to regulate entry into this social role. In other words, organized medicine is viewed as the social institution that possesses the knowledge and technical expertise necessary to be responsible for legitimating claims to the sick role (e.g., by issuing a medical certificate), managing illness conditions, and returning the sick person to good health as soon as possible. In the early stages of its development, medical sociology concentrated on the study of illness behaviour and "accepted the legitimate authority of the medical profession and the pre-eminence of physician-centered healing and devoted a great deal of research attention to the social control issues inherent in Parsons' sick role concept" (Segall 1997, 291). Like early medical sociology, the sick role has been criticized as medico-centric in that it focuses on sickness from the perspective of medicine.

Segall (1997) explores the historical link between the sick role concept and the identity of the field of medical sociology. His review summarizes the basic dimensions of the sick role and the early research stimulated by this concept as well as its major limitations (see Box 2.3). First, Parsons' sick role concept has been criticized because it applies only to temporary, acute illness episodes (not chronic illness conditions). The original formulation of the sick role might apply to acute, or short-term, illness behaviour, such as when you catch a flu and go to see a doctor who gives you a sick note to excuse you from work or school, but what about the behaviour of people who suffer from long-term, chronic illness, such as arthritis, or permanent disabilities? Such situations mean that people live with illness and disability for their whole lives. In such cases, illness is not just a temporary disruption to normal social roles but, rather, becomes an important part of the sick individual's subjective self-understanding. The original sick role does not explain chronic conditions and disability very well.

Similarly, while the original sick role might explain certain physical conditions, what about those that are emotional or psychological in nature, such as mental illness? Here again, Parsons' formulation fails to fully explain all of the behavioural expectations surrounding illnesses with a psychological component, such as mental illnesses, that can be accompanied by a high degree of stigma (an extremely powerful, negative social label; Goffman 1963). Again, such sicknesses may have profound and lasting consequences for the person's self-identity rather than simply being a temporary social role.

Furthermore, Segall (1997) contends that Parsons overestimated the therapeutic impact of the physician and formal medical care and, at the same time, underestimated the importance of the caregiving functions performed by members of the individual's informal social network.

Box 2.3 Major Criticisms of Parsons' Sick Role Concept

1. Focused on acute illness rather than chronic illness
2. Limited to selected physical conditions, ignoring psychosocial conditions
3. Medico-centric with a professionalist bias against lay, self-care behaviour
4. Decontextualized, failing to consider the influence of aspects of social location such as culture, class, and gender

Source: Based on Segall 1997.

According to Parsons' original conception, the individual can have the sick role identity bestowed upon her only if the sick person clearly demonstrates a desire to get well by seeking medical care and complying with the physician's recommended treatment regimen. Therefore, the original formulation of the sick role is medico-centric in that it makes the institution of medicine the main player in determining what counts as illness. Patients are seen as essentially passive objects, but, as we will learn in our discussion of medicalization in Chapter 10, they can sometimes be active and willing participants in the medical encounter. Furthermore, people are not simply passive consumers of professional medical services but are often active primary health-care providers. For example, think of all of the times when you get sick but do not see a doctor, instead relying on some form of self-care. As Chapter 9 explains, the vast majority of illnesses are managed not by the medical profession but rather by people acting on their own to maintain or restore their health.

Finally, in keeping with the structural functionalist emphasis on social stability and order, Parsons' original formulation of the sick role tends to offer a universalized account of illness behaviour. Research oriented by the other theoretical paradigms we are going to consider, however, makes it clear that factors such as class, gender, culture, and age all affect how we respond to illness. Chapters 5, 6, and 7 will present some of this research evidence when we consider social class factors, gender, and ethnicity as sources of inequality and health disparities. Overall, these limitations suggest that Parsons' model does not provide an adequate conceptual framework for analyzing the behavioural expectations and role performance of the sick person. Thus, Segall (1997) argues that health sociology requires a redefined, non-medicalized sick role concept for studying everyday health and illness behaviour. This modified sick role concept will be presented in more detail in Chapter 9 when we discuss self-care health beliefs and behaviour.

Guided by the structural functionalist paradigm, Segall (1988) investigated whether systematic socio-cultural differences exist in sick role behavioural expectations. In an effort to validate empirically the rights and duties of the sick role as formulated by Parsons and to assess the extent to which lay expectations are affected by socio-cultural factors, information was collected from a random sample of 524 residents of Winnipeg, Manitoba, who participated in a community survey. To measure sick role expectations, respondents were asked to indicate their level of agreement with a series of statements about the behaviour expected of a sick person.

The findings of Segall's study indicate that there is fairly widespread agreement that the sick person has the right to depend on lay others, particularly for informal consultations (i.e., to discuss her condition with others when she is not feeling well). At the same time, study participants were found to be divided in their views about the right of the sick person to be relieved of usual well role responsibilities. To what extent can the lack of consensus about sick role behavioural expectations be accounted for by socio-cultural factors? It turns out that factors such as age, employment status, education, and income were found to be significantly related to sick role expectations. "In other words, those who believe that the sick person is entitled to role release and dependency tend to be younger respondents who are gainfully employed and enjoy a higher socioeconomic status" (Segall 1988, 257). In contrast, no statistically significant differences were found in terms of a number of other socio-cultural factors (such as ethnicity). Consequently, a good deal of the variance in the behavioural expectations associated with the sick role concept remains unexplained. This study illustrates the type of sociological analysis of health undertaken by Canadian health sociologists guided by the structural functionalist paradigm. Our attention now turns to a theoretical paradigm that, in stark contrast with structural functionalism, sees conflict rather than stability as an enduring feature of social life.

Health and Illness as "Professional Constructs"—The Conflict Paradigm

The conflict paradigm offers a critical alternative to some of the conservative aspects of structural functionalism. Once again, analysis focuses on the societal level, but, according to the **conflict paradigm**, the distinctive feature of capitalist society is that it is composed of a number of competing interest groups. Drawing upon a long tradition of Marxist theory, the conflict paradigm focuses on group power struggles (e.g., social class, gender, ethnic relationships) and interprets social relations primarily in terms of the political and economic dimensions of social inequality. Conflict theorists point out that rather than promoting the stable operation of society as a whole, capitalist social structure benefits some people while depriving others. In keeping with a Marxist commitment to social praxis, the conflict paradigm highlights the possibility of societal change stemming from the ongoing power struggles between these different groups. For conflict sociologists, understanding human behaviour is not sufficient, since knowledge should also serve as the basis for action to change society and to address social injustice. This accounts for the interest that health sociologists, guided by the conflict paradigm, have in participatory research methods that are directed toward addressing social inequalities in health as they are experienced by vulnerable groups and toward reform of the health-care system.

Applying this paradigm to the study of health focuses attention on the political economy of health care and social inequalities in the distribution of illness and access to health-care services. McGibbon and McPherson (2011, 62) explain that "Political economy analyses, grounded in the work of Marx and Engels, continue to focus on social class as a key marker of material and social well being." **Political economy** is an interdisciplinary field of social science that critically analyzes the political, economic, and social relations of the capitalist social system. The conflict paradigm attaches a great deal of importance to power and exploitation as key concepts in understanding society. While structural functionalism concentrates on issues related to patient compliance with the medical institution, conflict theorists argue that the social control features of the medical profession must be understood within the wider political and economic context of capitalist society. The central research question orienting conflict theorists is: How does the medical system serve as an instrument of social control in a capitalist society marked by exploitation and social inequality?

The basic answer offered by the conflict paradigm is that in capitalist society, the profession of medicine possesses the ultimate authority in health-related matters. The conflict paradigm understands health and illness as professional constructs because professional medicine determines what counts as disease (i.e., by developing disease classification schemes) and physicians legitimate sickness claims through diagnostic and treatment procedures. The medical profession controls the diagnostic process (i.e., by making the final decisions regarding who is really sick and what type of health condition the individual is experiencing) as well as access to treatment technology, such as laboratory and screening tests, prescribed medication, and hospitalization. Thus, it is the medical profession that not only defines disease in theory and identifies it in practice but also supervises those in the sick role in their efforts to regain good health. In these ways, professional medicine serves the interests of capitalists and capitalism.

For conflict health sociologists, the medical profession is a powerful instrument of social control by which the ruling capitalist class legitimates capitalism and stays in control of a class-divided and conflict-ridden society. In other words, the conflict approach shifts the focus to the issue of **medical dominance** and how organized medicine attained and maintains its position of dominance in the health-care field. As a paradigmatic example of the conflict approach to the study of health and illness, Eliot Freidson's *Profession of Medicine: A Study of the Sociology of Applied Knowledge* and *Professional Dominance* (both in 1970) together explain how the medical profession gained the legitimate autonomy necessary for exerting power over the health-care system through a complex and lengthy process of political negotiation and public persuasion (see Box 2.4). For example, physicians' exclusive rights to diagnose and treat disease (e.g., to prescribe medication and perform surgery) are codified in law and protected by legislation. These rights were won by the medical profession over time by pre-empting the claims of competing health-care practitioners (e.g., midwives, homeopaths, chiropractors). At the same time, the public was convinced through the influence of **medical ideology** (i.e., the dominant beliefs of organized medicine) that physicians are indeed the ultimate authorities on health matters (as reflected in the familiar deferential phrase often stated by patients when interacting with their physicians—"you're the doctor"). With his exposition of professional dominance, Freidson argues that the medical profession dominates health care because doctors are politically well organized and have a lot of power within capitalist society.

The underlying ideology or belief system that characterizes the practice of modern medicine consists of beliefs that are useful to capitalism, such as the notion that illness is best treated by technically competent physicians using expensive and high-tech medical equipment and pharmaceuticals. Conflict theorists (e.g., Navarro 1976) have argued that the social control features of the medical profession must be analyzed within a broad political and economic context. A full understanding of the ways in which the medical sector of the economy functions requires an examination of the distribution of power in contemporary capitalist societies as well as the nature of the class structure that perpetuates social inequalities in health. For example, Baer (1989, 1103) explains that "with its emphasis upon pathogens as the external cause of the disease, 'scientific medicine' or 'biomedicine' provided the capitalist class with a paradigm that neglected the social roots of illness, but yet could in at least some instances restore workers back to a level of functional health essential to capital accumulation."

Box 2.4 Eliot Freidson (1923–2005)

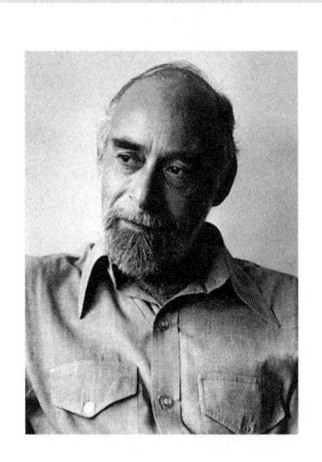

- US sociologist of the professions working within the conflict paradigm
- Documented how organized medicine attained and maintains its position of dominance in the health-care field in *Profession of Medicine* (1970b)
- Explored the effects of medical dominance on health, society, and the healing professions

"Disapproved behaviour is more and more coming to be given the meaning of illness requiring treatment" (1970b, 248).

Since its inception with Friedrich Engels' *The Condition of the Working Class in England* (1845/1999), conflict approaches to understanding health and illness have sought the development of a **social medicine** aimed at addressing social structural determinants of illness. Social medicine takes the view that illness is a consequence of the social structural organization of capitalist society and that addressing social inequalities can improve the health of the population. In other words, social medicine argues that the way to make people healthy is to make society healthier! The emphasis placed by the social medicine approach on social and economic determinants of health can be credited with drawing attention to both the wider social forces shaping the pursuit of health and the connection of the medical profession to capitalism. Working within the conflict paradigm, researchers such as Illich (1976), Navarro (1976), and Waitzkin (2000) have advanced critiques that highlight the interconnections of capitalism and the biomedical profession. For these researchers, ill health is understood primarily as a consequence of the capitalist mode of production that exploits workers, and professional medicine is criticized as an instrument of social control and capitalist accumulation of profit. In this line of thinking, what makes people sick is capitalist society, and the medical profession acts to keep people in line and to add to capitalist profit by treating illness with health-care goods and services produced by capitalists for profit.

In keeping with their commitment to social medicine, researchers influenced by the conflict paradigm advocate socially based therapeutic measures such as welfare programs (Raphael 2001), labour laws (e.g., occupational health and safety regulations; McDonough 2001), and environmental protection standards (Jerrett et al. 2001) as solutions to illness. For example, Canadian sociologists have pointed out the impact of "environmental racism" (Ali 2009) whereby poor air quality in urban centres is more of a problem for socially excluded people who live close to factories and other sources of pollution. Social medicine approaches view environmental pollution as a cause of illness that can be addressed through measures such as regulating industrial pollution and not allowing factories to put toxic chemicals into surrounding neighbourhoods. These are the same neighbourhoods where the working poor tend to live, whereas the capitalist owners of the factories live in areas geographically removed from the sites of production (O'Neill et al. 2003). However, state-sponsored social medicine is expensive and necessitates taxation and other obstacles to corporate profit, such as regulation of industrial activities.

Conversely, a medicalized view of illness that is centred on the individual and constructs illness as something rooted in the individual's biology (caused by either heightened susceptibility to external pathogens or some other individualized problem) serves as ready-made ideological argument against calls for expensive social medicine. (We will return to this issue in Chapter 10 when we discuss the conflict paradigm's approach to understanding medicalization.) According to this belief system, the reason that children in poor families suffer from higher incidence of asthma is not because of capitalist factories emitting pollutants into their environment; rather, it is because they have "genetic susceptibility" to pollution (Yang et al. 2008). This is a form of victim-blaming that individualizes causes of illness.

Further, the highly expensive technological approach to dealing with illness characteristic of biomedicine has been very successful in generating profit for the sector of the capitalist economy described as the "medical-industrial complex" (Relman 1980) and is big business. Why legislate clean air when you can make money selling asthma medication? The **medical-industrial complex** is a term originally coined by Vicente Navarro and colleagues (see Navarro 1998, commenting on his earlier work) and then popularized by Arnold S. Relman (1980), editor of the *New England Journal of Medicine*, to describe the development of a huge, profit-driven health-care industry. (See Box 2.5 for a contemporary illustration of the social consequences of the collusion of the medical profession with the medical-industrial complex.) Thus, according to researchers working within the conflict paradigm, medicine has become a major institution of social control in capitalist society; it has expropriated health from individual control and made people increasingly dependent on professional health-care products and services offered by biomedicine. In other words, thanks to the medical profession, we see health as an individual responsibility, not a societal issue. Such an ideological belief system obviously fits well with what the previous chapter described as "medical consumerism."

Guided by the conflict paradigm, Benoit and colleagues (2010) examine how changes in politics and growing medical consumerism may be challenging medical dominance over maternity care practices in Canada compared with those in Australia. They begin by asking "whether neoliberalisation places countervailing or complementary pressures on the medicalisation of childbirth" (2010, 476). In an approach characteristic of the political economy paradigm, they are interested in the extent to which changing political, economic, and social relations affect the medical control of childbirth. They contend that despite the differing patterns that neo-liberalism takes in both Australia and Canada, medical dominance over childbirth has "intensified." As evidence, they explain that in Canada, the proportion of births attended by obstetricians has increased, the caesarean delivery rate has increased to 26.3 per cent, and less than 5 per cent of births are attended by certified midwives. Benoit and co-authors conclude that "This neoliberal rhetoric of consumerism provides the justification for the continuing hegemony of medicine over maternity care in Canada and Australia" (2010, 480). The focus these researchers place on issues of power and politics in health care is characteristic of conflict approaches within health sociology.

Box 2.5 What's in the Envelope?

What's in the Envelope? Health Authority Makes "Value-Added" Contracts the Way to Do Business By Jen Skerritt

Winnipeg Regional Health Authority has accepted more than $20 million in money, equipment and other gifts from medical suppliers since 2000—money senior officials admit was handed over in brown envelopes from companies who won health contracts in the region.

The funds are part of the Winnipeg Regional Health Authority's "value-added" policy—a practice that some experts say falls in an ethical grey area and which states that WRHA senior management may accept cash and other bonuses given out by medical suppliers awarded contracts.

WRHA CEO Dr. Brian Postl said equipment suppliers, joint suppliers and drug companies have tried to influence health organizations for a long time, and the WRHA's bid system tries to limit that relationship. Postl said they want the best product at the best price, and that keeping any extras sealed in a brown envelope keeps added benefits separate. . . .

Critics slammed the policy, saying the practice is ripe for abuse and creates a perception of impropriety.

"I've never heard of that, where they open it up, and 'Oooh, extra surprises,'" said Rob Warren, director of the Asper School of Business. "If I win the tender and I turn around and give someone unrestricted monies, that to me is definitely not ethical."

Continued

Most public organizations require that any extras a contractor offers are outlined, in detail, as part of the bid proposal.

But WRHA's policy states that these benefits aren't to be disclosed in the bid, and that suppliers that offer them should be informed that "unrestricted" funds that can be used at the discretion of health administrators are preferred.

Documents show the WRHA received more than $2.2 million in unrestricted money from suppliers that was allocated to other accounts as "an extra source of funding"—including the regional corporate department, which accepted more than $1.1 million.

Officials will not provide a detailed breakdown of how the money was spent or the name of the suppliers. Health officials told the *Free Press* to file an access to information request for that information.

Postl said money from suppliers has essentially dried up since the WRHA has moved to limit those relationships—although he thinks some doctors may still be taking money directly from companies.

"The truth is, I still think there's some potential that physicians, without system knowledge, can be having relationships with the companies—certainly that's the experience in the United States," Postl said. . . .

Although the policy states that unrestricted funds are preferred, the WRHA has also accepted more than $17.9 million in other funds put toward research, equipment and hospital programs at the discretion of the medical supply company, including thousands of dollars that went towards equipment and operating costs of critical care, cardiology and surgery.

WRHA chief financial officer Paul Kochan said there isn't anything ethically wrong with the policy, and said what's inside the brown envelope doesn't influence who gets a contract. Officials know if suppliers have included a brown envelope in their bid, but Kochan said the envelope remains sealed until a winning supplier is selected.

"We open a brown envelope after and it could be nothing, it could be cash," Kochan said, adding that taking extra benefits from medical suppliers is commonplace in health care.

Accounting and business critics have never heard of such a practice.

Source: Excerpted from Jen Skerritt, "What's in the envelope? Health authority makes 'value-added' contracts the way to do business," *Winnipeg Free Press* 31 January 2009.

This research exemplifies the type of sociological analysis of health undertaken by Canadian health sociologists working within the conflict paradigm. Benoit and her co-researchers link medical dominance to global economic and political developments. In addition, they characterize the health-care system as a set of relationships among competing interest groups (i.e., government, health occupations, and the general public). The picture becomes even more complicated when we add medical technology, hospital and physician supply, and pharmaceutical industries to the analysis of the health-care sector. Finally, Benoit and colleagues demonstrate that from this perspective, health and illness may indeed be viewed as professional constructs and commodities with important market value.

In these ways, conflict health researchers point out a paradox associated with medicine under capitalism. It not only individualizes the causes of ill health by taking the focus off the way that capitalist society makes people sick but also robs them of control over their health because of the way they are taught to rely on the products and services of biomedical health care in their pursuit of health and wellness. People come to believe that they need doctors and expensive health-care products and services if they want to remain healthy or overcome illness. While this view individualizes responsibility for health and illness, individuals are deprived of autonomy in dealing with their health; instead, they rely on costly medical interventions controlled by the medical profession. Rather than looking at how the structures of our society might contribute to illness, in capitalist society we offer individuals expensive medical treatment focused on biology and make money doing it! In essence, the conflict paradigm argues that health and illness can be understood as professional constructs leading to confusion in capitalist society between the consumption of formal health care and the production of population health.

One criticism of the conflict theoretical approach to health and illness is that it offers somewhat of a caricature of the medical profession. With its focus on social inequality and conflict, the paradigm overlooks, or at least minimizes, the preventive aspects of contemporary medical practice. In caring for their patients, many physicians do indeed emphasize the importance of preventive health behaviour. We now turn our attention to a theoretical paradigm that focuses explicitly on social interaction.

Health and Illness as "Interpersonal Meanings"—The Symbolic Interactionist Paradigm

The perspective that the symbolic interactionist paradigm offers for understanding health and illness stands in contrast with the analysis of broad societal factors offered by the first two paradigms. The key to remembering what this paradigm is all about is the "interaction" part of "symbolic interactionist": the **symbolic interactionist paradigm** views society as the socially constructed product of the everyday interactions of individuals. According to symbolic interactionists, people construct the reality of their lives in society through interactions with others. The level of analysis for the symbolic interactionist paradigm is individual interaction. In fact, according to this perspective, society is made up of selves (i.e., unique individuals) who make their lives meaningful through social interaction.

Drawing upon the classical sociological theory of Max Weber (1947, 88), who said that the goal of sociology should be the development of *verstehen*, or interpretative understanding, the focus of symbolic interactionism is on how people's ideas continually shape and reshape the world. Thus, the paradigm offers an interpretive framework for understanding the process by which individuals attach meaning to social experiences. The basic assumption of the paradigm is that we need to understand the individual's social construction of reality and definition of the situation to be able to understand behaviour. The idea of the social construction of reality is that social phenomena are actively produced through social interaction. Thus, an individual's definition of the situation is a subjective process of assigning meaning to personal social experience. As we will discuss in the next chapter, the focus of the paradigm is on the meaning of health and illness for individuals, and the goal of research is to learn more about how individuals socially construct what "being healthy" means to each of them personally. In this way, the symbolic interactionist paradigm understands health and illness as interpersonal meanings.

The symbolic interactionist paradigm attaches a great deal of importance to key concepts such as subjective meaning and interpretative understanding. As we will learn in the next chapter, this type of sociological analysis is linked with the use of qualitative research methods to examine each individual's definition of the situation. To illustrate, general definitions of good health (i.e., societal standards) may differ significantly from individual definitions of what it means to be healthy (i.e., personal meanings). Presumably, by discovering the subjective meaning of health for individuals, we will be better able to understand their personal health behaviour. In other words, if health behaviour is to be understood in meaningful ways, the goal of health research is to learn more about the complex process of negotiation that we each go through to interpret what "being healthy" means to us. According to the interactionist paradigm, our views about health and illness can be understood as personal meanings that we construct with others in everyday social situations.

A paradigmatic example of the symbolic interactionist approach to understanding health and illness as interpersonal meanings can be found in the work of the famous Canadian-born sociologist Erving Goffman (see Box 2.6). Influenced by his exposure to the ideas of symbolic interactionism while studying at the University of Chicago, Goffman went on to develop an approach called dramaturgical analysis in which behaviour is understood as analogous to theatrical performance. For Goffman, people actively play social roles in everyday life and work to manage the impressions others have of their performance, like an actor playing a dramatic part for the benefit of an audience. The reactions of others, or, in keeping with the definition of the situation, what we believe are the reactions of others, shape an individual's sense of self. In a participant observation study of a mental hospital, Goffman showed how this is the case for mental illness. He (1961) describes the mental hospital as a total institution—that is, a social setting in which the individual is separated from the wider society and behaviour is observed and controlled in accordance with strict and uniform rules of conduct. For example, mental patients are closely observed by nurses and orderlies; they live in standardized wards, are dressed in hospital gowns, are fed the same hospital food, and have a standardized schedule of therapy, medication, and rest enforced on them. Such strict regimentation of behaviour as part of the social context of the hospital has profound effects on the mental patients' self-concept. In this way, Goffman shows us how it is possible to understand mental illness not as a characteristic of the individual

Box 2.6 Erving Goffman (1922–1982)

- World-famous Canadian sociologist and highly influential symbolic interactionist
- Described the effects of total institutions on self-concept in *Asylums* (1961)
- Used participant observation of a mental hospital to study the ways in which the social context affects the behaviour and identity of patients

"To describe the patient's situation faithfully is necessarily to present a partisan view" (1961, x).

patient but, rather, as a response to the social context of the mental hospital and the medicalized treatment of deviant behaviour.

Adopting the symbolic interactionist focus on interpersonal meanings allows health researchers to explore the manner in which medical knowledge, like all forms of understanding the world, is socially constructed in relation to the social context. In keeping with the social construction of reality, symbolic interactionists argue that subjective definitions of social reality are constructed by individuals as part of ongoing daily interaction. Thus, the object of health research, according to this paradigm, is to discover how each individual experiences the reality of health or illness and, in turn, how this relates health behaviour.

In our biologically determinist culture, we tend to think of the body as a biophysical, natural phenomenon. The symbolic interactionist paradigm, however, encourages us to challenge the "taken for granted" (Schutz 1967) aspects of reality. Influenced by this paradigm, health sociologists maintain that medical knowledge is not objective, universal, or unchanging but rather is always influenced by social interactions within particular cultural contexts. The symbolic interactionist paradigm leads us to question our culture's beliefs about what we assume to be natural and self-evident.

As an illustration of the social construction of medical knowledge, consider this excerpt from an interview one of your authors (Fries) conducted with a family physician of Chinese ancestry whose practice in Calgary, Alberta, includes many patients who immigrated to Canada from mainland China and who use both Western biomedicine and Traditional Chinese Medicine (TCM) for health care:

> What occurs is that patients from the mainland come to see me after they have consulted a TCM and there is a problem with two languages. They are diagnosed by the TCM as having "fire in the liver" and they come to me expecting me to run a liver panel. And I don't want to . . . there's no reason. But I give in and run it anyway, and when it comes back normal they don't believe it and go back to another TCM. It's a real problem of communication.

Symbolic interactionism provides a means for understanding the "problem with two languages" this physician describes having with patients who use alternative medicine. The problem is not literally one of two different languages, for this doctor is fluent in both his native Chinese (Mandarin) and English. Rather, such communication problems experienced within the context of multicultural medical encounters originate with two differing medical belief systems.

Within Traditional Chinese Medicine, organs (such as the liver) reflect holistic function rather than the biological structure of the organ itself, as in biomedicine. In the case of the Traditional Chinese Medical diagnosis of "fire in the liver," the idea is that people who are irritable, have a hot temper, or are highly emotional are said to have "a liver problem" even though physiologically there is nothing wrong with the structure of the liver itself. In the language of Western biomedicine, the problem was caused by the patient being either anxious or emotionally distressed, but in the language of TCM, they had "fire in the liver." Symbolic interactionism points out that our understandings of our bodies and health are relative to the situation of different cultural contexts. In effect, two different cultures produce two different symbolic languages for understanding health, illness, and the body. Because the social construction of the medical belief system in China is different from that of Western societies, differing understandings of the body and illness arise (Fries 2005). Medical knowledge of the human body is socially constructed! Thus, the symbolic interactionist paradigm argues that medical knowledge about the body and its illnesses cannot be understood as objective and detached scientific knowledge. Rather, it is based upon each individual's definition of the situation.

Several Canadian health researchers have been influenced by the symbolic interactionist paradigm. For example, Litva and Eyles (1994) examined the distinction between people's definition of good health and their explanation of what "being healthy" means to them personally by exploring how the meaning of healthiness is negotiated by the residents of a southern Ontario town. They report that study participants found it difficult to define health. Many simply could not define it, while others defined health in rather general or abstract terms. Furthermore, Litva and Eyles point out that respondents tended to focus on physical aspects and typically described health in negative terms (i.e., as being free from disease and illness). In contrast, when asked to talk about the personal meaning of being healthy, study participants provided a very different viewpoint. Healthiness (i.e., the negotiated personal meaning) was closely tied to quality of life issues and was typically described in psychological terms "such as the ability to feel happy, enjoy life, and feel good about oneself" (Litva and Eyles 1994, 1085).

More recently, Philips and colleagues (2012) employed a symbolic interactionist approach to investigate the degree to which health-care workers providing health and social services to stigmatized sex workers experience "stigma by association." Citing Goffman to explain "courtesy stigma," Philips et al. note that challenges faced by stigmatized persons spread out in waves of diminishing intensity among those with whom they interact. Based on their mixed-methods analysis of data collected from participant observation, interviews, and a survey of employees of a centre providing frontline services to sex workers in Victoria, British Columbia, Philips and colleagues found that participants "noted a variety of contexts in which they experienced perceived and enacted courtesy stigma, both at home and on the job" (2012, 687). In particular, these researchers found that professionals who provide services to stigmatized populations suffer negative health consequences, such as workplace stress and burnout, attributable to stigma by association. Following on the work of Goffman (1963), Philips et al. further demonstrate how service workers use their professional credentials such as educational degrees as a form of "impression management" "to distinguish themselves from those served—as a strategy to distance themselves from the stigmas associated with their clientele" (2012, 689). This research provides vivid accounts of the ways participants manipulate their social interactions in order to manage stigma. The authors conclude that "it is crucial to not only educate the staff serving vulnerable groups about stigma in service environments, but also to invest in employee wellness strategies" (Philips et al. 2012, 692).

In shifting emphasis to the way in which meanings are subjectively created through individual social interaction, symbolic interactionist approaches to understanding health and illness are open to the criticism that they ignore the manner in which differential power relations among groups structure health outcomes and experiences. The next paradigm we will consider places the effects of power relations on everyday experience at the centre of analysis.

Health and Illness as "Gendered Experiences"—The Feminist Paradigm

Each of the three paradigms we have examined so far has roots in classical sociological theory. Addressing the lack of a feminist perspective in classical sociological theory, Shilling (2012, 27) speculates that "The risks women faced during pregnancy, the high numbers who died during childbirth, and the rates of infant mortality may have been reflected through a greater consideration of the body if Marx, Simmel, Weber and Durkheim had been women." In a telling play on words, O'Brien (1981) describes how mainstream Western social scientific thought has been dominated by "malestream" thinking, or the privileging of masculine perspectives on social life. Just as sociologists warn about the dangers associated with ethnocentric and medico-centric thinking, there is an analogous bias associated with **androcentric** thinking, or the privileging of the masculine perspective when trying to understand social life. The ideas of women thinkers such as Mary Wollstonecraft, Harriet Taylor, Harriet Martineau, and Florence Nightingale have been excluded from the traditional sociology canon and are only recently being reintroduced, thanks to the efforts of feminist scholars (McDonald 2004). Pointing out that our knowledge of the social world is grounded in particular social relations, internationally renowned Canadian feminist sociologist Dorothy Smith (1990, 12) advances a critique of male-dominated social science by asking "how a sociology might look if it began from women's standpoint." Smith explains that adopting a feminist perspective on everyday social life produces "a radical critique of sociology." Following Smith, we might ask how sociology's understanding of health and illness would look if it began from women's standpoint?

The **feminist paradigm** is comprised of many diverse waves of feminist thought that have in common a focus on the historical oppression of women within patriarchy. Patriarchy is a form of social organization in which men dominate women, exercising power in its many different forms (i.e., social, economic, political) over women's lives. Patriarchy is built into the social structures of our "gendered" society and reflected in norms and values that have become part of our culture. Adopting the perspective of women allows feminist sociologists to investigate how society and social relations are "gendered" and produce inequality.

To describe society and social relations as "gendered" recognizes that the socially constructed gender roles of "woman" and "man" contribute to gender inequality that shapes the lives of both women and men and affects the health of each. The inequalities between women and men constitute an important starting point for feminist analyses of society and behaviour. As Marshall (2000, 26) explains, "Feminist sociology has been concerned not simply with documenting gender difference, but with understanding how gender difference is constructed as social inequality. Feminist usages of gender, then, have always been bound up with exposing its relationship to power and status."

In investigating the relationship of gender to power and status, feminist health sociologists use a mix of research methods to study the relationship between gender inequality and health at both the broad societal level and the individual level. In this way, unlike the three paradigms we have thus far reviewed, feminist analyses cross both the societal and the individual levels of analysis. As we will see, this "intersectionality" is a distinctive feature of feminist research methodology. While realizing that women and men do not constitute two homogeneous groups (Rieker, Bird, and Lang 2010), feminist health researchers working at the broad societal level investigate how patriarchy differentially makes women and men sick. At the individual level, feminist health sociologists explore how gender is produced and reproduced in women's everyday relationships with men, with their families and children, with their own bodies, and with the medical profession and other healers. Thus, the relationship between gender and health is extremely complex. Social class, ethnicity, and other aspects of social location, such as age, interact with gender to produce variations in health and illness within groups of women and men. In other words, male social and health advantages associated with patriarchy do not benefit all men, nor do female social and health disadvantages affect all women (Rieker, Bird, and Lang

2010). Health sociologists influenced by the feminist paradigm show that differences in women's and men's health cannot be explained solely by biological sex differences but, rather, are a consequence of patriarchal social construction of gender. Chapter 6 details some of the information produced by feminist health researchers, but for now, a few points are worth highlighting.

There is a growing body of research evidence indicating that there are important gender inequalities in health and illness, as well as gender differences in how women and men understand their bodies and health. It is to these inequalities and differences that we are referring when we state that health and illness are "gendered experiences." Women and men experience health and illness in different ways because of the structural and cultural effects of patriarchy. These health inequalities and differences are sometimes reduced to the cliché "women are sicker, but men die quicker." As we will learn in Chapter 6, while there is some truth to this oversimplification, the whole picture is more complex. We do know that women live longer than men and yet, at the same time, they experience more ill health during their lives and make more extensive use of formal health-care services. However, despite extensive study, there are still many unanswered questions about the relationship between gender and health. In an analysis of the social production of health, Denton and Walters (1999, 1233) conclude that "there are very real differences in the factors that predict women's and men's health." They argue, however, that to be able to adequately explain these differences, we need to more closely examine the part played by structural and behavioural determinants in shaping women's and men's health. We also need to gain a better understanding of the ways in which women and men subjectively experience health and illness. A feminist perspective is appropriate in the search for answers to these questions, since women predominate both as informal health-care providers and as consumers of formal medical goods and services.

Traditional female gender roles burden women with a disproportionate responsibility for both their own health and the health of others, such as husbands and children. In patriarchal societies, women occupy gendered social locations, which have "become favoured territory for medical intervention" (Findlay and Miller 2002, 185). Long the target of medicalization and medical consumerism, women have had a gendered social history created for them (Ehrenreich and English 1979). A major theme in feminist analysis of health has been the medicalization of women's lives. "Much of this analysis has focused on the dominance of the medical care system, medical practitioners, and the medical constructions of knowledge with regard to reproductive issues such as birth control and childbirth, PMS and menopause" (Clarke 2008, 20). Feminist health researchers have demonstrated that women's bodies have been subjected historically to far greater control and regulation by the medical profession than have men's.

While there are many varieties of feminism, most share a critical perspective on the biomedical model of disease. It is argued that this model is reductionist because it does not take the whole person into account (including social, psychological, and spiritual factors) but instead focuses on biological differences between the sexes. Feminists, therefore, view it as insensitive to the social determinants of health, such as gender, social class, ethnicity, employment and working conditions, and family life. The medical-care system is built on and reinforces patriarchy as well as structured inequality between the genders and social classes (Lupton 2012a). Furthermore, the biomedical model promotes and privileges the expertise of physicians while often discounting the feelings, experiential knowledge, and practical wisdom women have of their bodies and health. This is illustrated by paradigmatic feminist health research undertaken by Ann Oakley.

Oakley's health research (see Box 2.7) is motivated by a fascinating question: "Why is culture, in the form of the medical profession and other 'experts,' so apparently intent on defining what motherhood is and how childbirth must happen?" (Oakley 2005, 118). Typical of feminist

> **Box 2.7** Ann Oakley (1944–)
>
> - Internationally renowned UK feminist sociologist and novelist
> - Described the medicalization of women's bodies and childbirth in *The Captured Womb* (1984)
> - Uses feminist research methods to study gender relations in women's everyday lives and health
>
> *"Everyone has a stake in moving towards a more humane society where health and illness are not split off from the rest of experience" (1993, 18).*
>
> By permission of Ann Oakley.

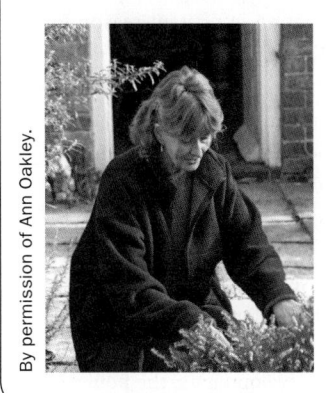

methodology, her research explores mothers' personal experiences of childbirth and becoming mothers (1980; 1981) and also provides a rich historical account of the development of a masculine, assembly-line style, medicalized approach to reproduction and birth (1984). She explains that a transformation occurred in which childbirth moved from being a natural event that happened in the home under the care of other women (i.e., midwives) to a medicalized event that placed men in control of women's bodies in the context of the hospital maternity ward. Oakley challenges the contention that these changes occurred in the interests of health by demonstrating the surprising lack of evidence to prove that medicalized birth is actually safer for mothers or babies. Rather, her research points to a patriarchal drive to control and commodify women's bodies as explaining these developments. As Oakley (2005, 119) explains, "The technologies applied to childbirth and motherhood have another covert function: they suggest that women can only be women with expert (mostly male) professional help." The cultural meaning of childbirth was transformed from a natural process to a medical issue, and doctors gained a great deal of power over women's lives as a result. According to Oakley, because of these gendered social transformations, women became objectified as "captured wombs" (1984) who knew less about their own bodies than did their mostly male physicians. In this way, the medical profession reinforces patriarchal domination of women.

The feminist paradigm has informed Canadian health research directed at understanding how gender relates to health inequalities and differences in how women and men think about their bodies and the pursuit of health and wellness. Some of this information will be presented in Chapter 6 when we explore gender inequality and health disparities. The feminist paradigm attaches unique importance to understanding the "intersectionality" of how gender intersects with other aspects of social location to affect the health outcomes of Canadian women. De Leeuw and Greenwood (2011, 55) state that

> Broadly speaking, intersectionality is a theory that wrestles with, and attempts to explain, how socio-culturally constructed categories (predominately but not exclusively categories such as gender, ethnicity, and sexual orientation) interact with and affect one another to produce differentially lived social inequalities among people.

Developing a Canadian perspective on the determinants of health, Hankivsky and Christoffersen (2008, 271) note that while the country has been a world leader in research on the determinants of health, "significant inequalities in health persist and Canada is losing its reputation as an innovator in the field." Basically, these researchers suggest that an important reason for Canada's falling behind in population health research and promotion is the lack of progress in understanding how aspects of social location (such as gender, social class, ethnicity, and age) intersect to produce overlapping disadvantages in health. Drawing upon the feminist paradigm, Hankivsky and Christoffersen (2008, 276) maintain that "intersectionality challenges dominant analyses of health determinants by revealing how to better conceptualize the cumulative, interlocking dynamics that affect human experiences, including human health." In this way, characteristic of a feminist methodology, intersectional health research crosses both the broad societal level and the individual level of the lived experiences of women. These feminist health researchers conclude that "the explicit focus on power, which is so central in an intersectional paradigm, is essential to the pursuit of social justice in health" (Hankivsky and Christoffersen 2008, 278). Dhanoon and Hankivsky note that "Despite significant theoretical developments, the potential of intersectionality frameworks has not been realized in the context of health research and policy" (2011, 32). If we want to address the sources of disparities in health in Canada, we need to understand the many different and interacting sources of inequality in health together rather than separately. Part Two of this text introduces an intersectional exploration of the factors that combine to shape health and wellness, culminating in the presentation of an intersectional model of health in Chapter 8.

In promoting research into the intersectional relationship between gender inequality and health, there is a danger of reducing "gender and health" to "women and health." Despite increasing evidence that patriarchal gender roles are often bad for men's health as well as women's, Hankivsky and Christoffersen (2008, 273) observe that "the fact is that in the Canadian context, most discussion of men's health amongst feminist health researchers is viewed as an unjustifiable detraction from the agenda of the women's health movement." While the feminist paradigm has informed us about how the bodies of women are socially constructed in line with patriarchal ideologies, feminist approaches are susceptible to overlooking the fact that men also have bodies. The flesh-and-blood nature of human existence makes issues of the body central to health sociology. The final theoretical paradigm we will explore places the embodied dimension of social life at the centre of its analysis of health and illness.

Health and Illness as "Embodied Cultural Facts"—The Sociology of the Body Paradigm

Shilling (2012, 21) describes how the body has historically had "an absent presence" in sociology. That is, the body has always been in the background of sociology's attempts to understand society and culture, although until recently, it has not occupied centre stage in these understandings. As Shilling observes, this "dual status" (2012, 21) of the body in sociology is especially curious given the centrality of the human body to social life:

> Our experience of life is inevitably mediated through our bodies. . . . To put it another way, we have bodies and we act with our bodies. Our daily experiences of living . . . learning in schools, traveling to work, buying and preparing food for a meal, or making love—are

inextricably bound up with experiencing, managing and responding to our own and other people's bodies (2012, 24).

The centrality of the body to human experience makes it clear that understanding issues of embodiment is crucial to the realization of the sociological imagination. **Embodiment** simply means that human perception and experience of society and culture happen through our bodies. As the study of society and culture, sociology is fundamentally the study of bodies acting in and through society. Thus, Turner (1992, 162) suggests that "sociology of the body provides an important, and possibly innovative, bridge between medical sociology and the core components of contemporary sociology." Despite the obvious importance of the body in social life, embodiment is often overlooked in sociology. As Frank (1991b) points out, the reason for this has to do with the philosophy developed by French Enlightenment philosopher René Descartes, which began what can be thought of as an academic turf war between biology and sociology. Descartes' philosophical separation of mind and body set the stage for the modern understanding of what it means to be human in terms of what is known as the nature/nurture controversy.

One side of this controversy argues that if you want to understand human beings, you need to understand our biological nature (i.e., "biological determinism"). The other side of the debate argues that if you want to understand human beings, you have to understand how aspects of our social environment, such as the learning and nurturing we receive from others, shape our behaviour. As part of the modern understanding of humanity, our culture separates the natural (i.e., the body) from the social (i.e., the mind) and assigns particular academic disciplines to specialize in the separate study of each. In other words, both biology and sociology are academic disciplines that promise to tell us something about what it means to be human—but from different perspectives.

As we saw in the previous chapter, the biologically determinist idea that biology can explain human behaviour is extremely popular in our culture. Armstrong (1987, 59) explains the situation this way:

> Biology is directly concerned with living things and in so far as animal behaviour is concerned, would appear to have a virtual monopoly of study and explanation. When it comes to human behaviour, and at least by implication to social phenomena, biologists have always seemed on more shaky ground, but this has not prevented them from laying claims to this domain. Many biologists believe that the difference between animal and human behaviour is a quantitative rather than a qualitative one, simply a question of complexity rather than one of fundamentally different explanatory form.

Thus, from its earliest beginnings as an academic discipline, sociology has had to deal with the dominance of biological explanations. Classical sociologists (such as Durkheim) sought to carve out a niche for the newly emerging discipline of sociology by accepting the nature/society divide of Cartesian dualism, placing the body firmly on the nature side and saying, in effect, that the study of the human body should be left to biologists. Shilling (2012, 21) explains that "It was only when sociology subsequently questioned the nature/society distinction that the body became seen as central to social action and to the sociological enterprise." The past few decades have witnessed an increased interest in the sociology of the body, culminating in some sociologists calling for a serious sociological engagement with issues of biology and the body (Williams, Birke, and Bendelow 2003).

The **sociology of the body paradigm** offers a way of understanding society and social life that seeks to rectify the legacy of the mind–body dualism by putting minds back into bodies. It does this in order to reclaim the body and issues of embodiment as important sociological issues—not leaving them to the biological sciences alone. In this way, the paradigm puts bodies back into society. By understanding our bodies as socially constructed (i.e., more than just biological), the paradigm seeks to put society back into the body. In other words, the sociology of the body paradigm attempts to realize the promise of the sociological imagination by "bringing bodies back in" (Frank 1990; 1991b) to understand the dual process wherein society affects the body and, in return, the body affects society. Turner (1992, 170) explains that "Essentially the argument behind the sociology of the body is, first that sociology is genuinely a sociology of action, and that the social actor is not a Cartesian subject divided into body and mind but an embodied actor whose practicality and knowlegability [sic] involve precisely this embodiment." As such, the paradigm offers a sociological perspective both on and from the body. In this way, the sociology of the body paradigm understands health and illness as embodied cultural facts. The focus of the paradigm is on understanding how society and social relations both shape and are shaped by the human body. As with the feminist paradigm, both the individual and societal levels of analysis are encompassed by the sociology of the body paradigm. Sociologists of the body study such topics as the understanding individuals have of their bodies and bodily experiences and how such understandings inform health behaviour. They also study topics such as how broader cultural changes—for example, the growth in medical consumerism—are related to changing conceptions of the healthy or fit body in society. The next chapter shows how sociologists of the body use qualitative research methods, such as the analysis of people's narratives of their bodily experiences, to understand issues of health and embodiment.

A paradigmatic example of how the sociology of the body can be applied to understanding health and illness emerges from the work of Michel Foucault (see Box 2.8), introduced in the previous chapter. While Foucault was not a sociologist, he can be credited with founding the sociology

Box 2.8 Michel Foucault (1926–1984)

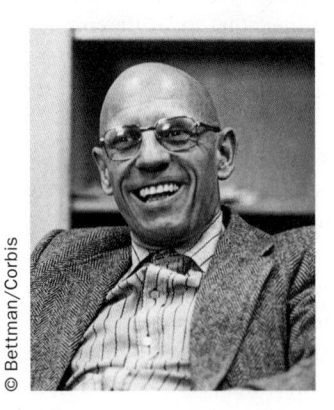

- Highly prolific French philosopher and social historian
- Highlighted the connections between power/knowledge and creation of "subjectivity" within institutions
- Studied the roles of madness, medicine, prisons, and sexuality in the control of the body

"'Health' is a cultural fact in the broadest sense of the word, a fact that is political, economic, and social as well, a fact that is tied to a certain state of individual and collective consciousness" (2000, 379).

of the body as a subfield of the discipline (Cockerham and Scrambler 2010). Petersen (2012, 7) adds that "Of the many social scientists who have contributed to the field of health and health care, few have shaped thought to the extent that the French philosopher and historian Michel Foucault has." He explains that this is due to the "rich 'toolkit' of ideas" that Foucault developed. A mainstay of this toolkit is Foucault's well-known concept of power/knowledge (see the collection edited by Gordon, 1980), which shows us that how we understand aspects of our reality is actually an act of power and control connected with particular institutions. As Foucault demonstrates in *The Birth of the Clinic: An Archaeology of Medical Perception* (1973), this is the case with the human body. In the book, Foucault shows how the development of a modern medical view of the human body as an object (what Foucault referred to as the **medical gaze**) was connected to the institution of the teaching hospital ("the clinic") and led to new ways of understanding and, hence, controlling both individuals and populations. As the subtitle makes clear, Foucault is interested in the origins of the current biomedical way in which we understand the reality of our bodies.

To conduct this "archaeology" of the modern understanding of the body, Foucault studied hospitals in eighteenth-century France. He explored the way that medical discourses of the body, health, and illness have developed and changed over time. Basically, discourses are ways of talking about, representing, and understanding phenomena linked to particular institutions. *The Birth of the Clinic* describes the medical gaze as a specific discourse on the body in which the body is perceived as a physical object capable of being observed, measured, and treated without reference to the person's subjective perceptions. Foucault shows how the practice of the physical dissection of bodies in early teaching hospitals was related to the development of a way of understanding the body as a physical object. To this day, as part of many biology courses at university, students dissect the bodies of animals. We assume that this is done so that students can learn about the inner workings of life, and, in a way, it is. Yet these dissections also serve a more important cultural purpose linked to power/knowledge. After all, realistic computer simulations can show us, with extreme precision, what organisms look like on the inside. For instance, since 1994 the US National Library of Medicine has run The Visible Human Project®, which makes detailed, three-dimensional digital representations of actual cadavers of a man and woman available over the Internet to medical students and researchers (Nettleton 2013). Despite the availability of this technology, having biology students perform dissections is a highly effective way of getting students to model biomedical discourses for understanding life. This is one reason why, even with the availability of technologies such as The Visible Human Project®, students learning about biology still dissect bodies. Thus, we internalize these discourses while failing to see them as a product of our particular culture. In Western culture, this anatomical way of thinking about the body starts early in childhood socialization. As an illustration, what child has not heard the words "The ankle bone's connected to the shin bone . . ."?

Foucault shows how the medical gaze changed cultural understandings of health and illness, locating them within the bodies of sick individuals. Despite the apparent naturalness of the idea of locating sickness within the body, Foucault (2000, 379) explains how it is possible to understand health as a "cultural fact . . . that is tied to a certain state of individual and collective consciousness." As Petersen (2012, 10) explains, "Foucault's work provides something of an antidote to biomedical imperialism, whereby 'health' is viewed as an innate or natural quality of the body, reducible to, for example, genetic makeup, hormones or brain wiring." Following Foucault, the pursuit of health can be understood as a process in which health is socially constructed as a cultural fact. In other words, health is much more than biological; it is a social construction linked to how people understand what it means to be human. Foucault argues that the body, while it now appears as a natural phenomenon to us, is produced through the medical gaze in a way that allows for the objectification of the human body and, hence, human life. This is what he is referring to when he writes "that the body obeys the exclusive laws of physiology and that it escapes the influences of history, but this too is false. The body is moulded by a great many regimes" (1977, 153). The body was produced by biomedicine via the medical gaze: How we talk about and understand the body has changed over time and is not the same across different historical periods or cultures! Following Foucault, sociologists of the body argue that health and illness must be viewed as socially constructed, cultural facts. Foucault is trying to show that the particular, culturally bound way that modern medicine understands bodies is linked to how power is exercised in modern societies.

Foucault's central contribution to the sociological analysis of health comes from highlighting the relationship of medical knowledge to social power and control within society. For Foucault, power/knowledge is always a contested struggle within society. Foucault offers a vision in which power is a productive force circulating through a web of relations involving discourses, institutions, and "individuals [who] are the vehicles of power, not its points of application" (1980, 98). Often when we think of power, we think of "force" and, therefore, something oppressive. In contrast, Foucault offers a vision in which power is a productive force because of the way it produces ways of understanding ourselves when combined with knowledge. In other words, how we "know" things is linked to the power of defining reality. By explaining the relationship of knowledge to social power and control within society, Foucault (1978) highlights the manner in which medical knowledge of human biology provides a basis for a type of social power he calls "**biopower**," a term describing the way that power is exercised in modern societies. This form of power rests on having knowledge of and, thus, power over people's bodies.

As Foucault explains, in traditional society power was based on the threat of death. People obeyed the rule of kings, who were seen as God's representatives on earth, because if they did not, they faced bodily suffering, such as punishment, torture, and even death. But with the birth of the clinic, the medical gaze offered a new way to control individuals and populations as tradition shifted to modernity. More and more, the exercise of power came to be based not on the threat of death but rather on the promise of life and health. The objective knowledge of the body produced by the medical gaze in the institution of the hospital offered people in modern society a means of understanding the health of their bodies. Doctors were able to provide people with information on the causes of sickness and, perhaps more important, how to prevent illness. Box 2.9 provides an illustration of a contemporary public health promotion campaign that can be understood as an exercise of biopower.

In explaining medicine's role in the exercise of biopower, Foucault (2004, 13) notes that "In the twentieth century doctors are in the process of inventing a society, not of law, but of the norm. What governs society is not legal codes but the perpetual distinction between normal and abnormal, a perpetual enterprise of restoring the system of normality. This is one of the characteristics of contemporary medicine." By this he means that in modern society, people are encouraged to engage in healthy bodily practices that are based on normative knowledge produced by medicine. In other words, the pursuit of health and wellness is guided by biopower.

As we will see in our discussion of health behaviour and lifestyles (Chapter 8), another central theorist in the sociology of the body whose ideas have influenced health sociology is Pierre Bourdieu. Bourdieu's approach is central to health sociology because it provides a means of understanding the relationship between bodies, society, and behaviour. In fact, the goal of Bourdieu's sociology is to understand society and behaviour by overcoming the dichotomy

Box 2.9 Biopower in Modern Society

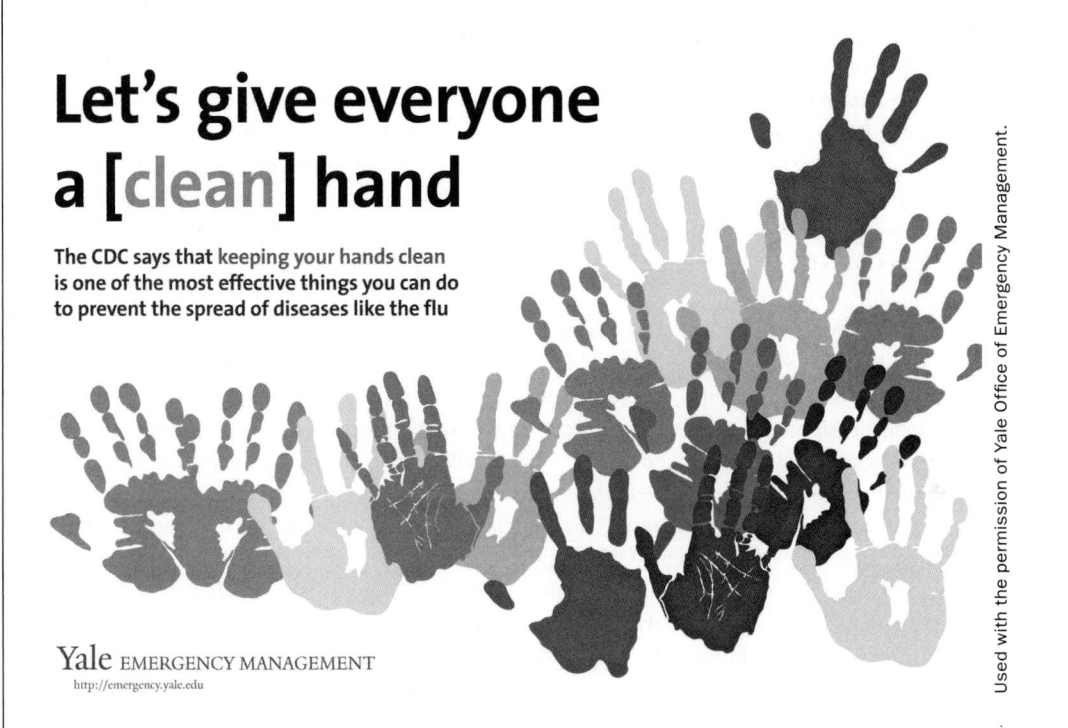

Let's give everyone a [clean] hand

The CDC says that keeping your hands clean is one of the most effective things you can do to prevent the spread of diseases like the flu

Yale EMERGENCY MANAGEMENT
http://emergency.yale.edu

Used with the permission of Yale Office of Emergency Management.

The Centers for Disease Control (CDC) in the United States conducts an ongoing public campaign aimed at making people aware that hand washing is an effective way of reducing the spread of disease. This type of campaign is based on research evidence indicating that proper hand washing, as recommended by the CDC, is not being practiced. In fact, a 2013 article in the *Journal of Environmental Health* reports that only 1 in 20 people (or 5 percent of the more than 3700 people observed in public restrooms) properly wash their hands and concluded that America has a hand washing problem. This form of social control is based on knowledge produced by health care professionals, and that is the essence of biopower.

---

between the two concepts created by the Cartesian separation of mind from body (Fries 2009). To explain the relationship between society and behaviour, Bourdieu developed the concept of "habitus."

To understand habitus, you first need to recognize that Bourdieu offers an approach to explaining human behaviour that is very different from that usually followed within the social sciences, such as sociology and psychology. Based on mind–body dualism, these disciplines typically understand behaviour in terms of a rational mind acting in an objective world. The idea behind such approaches is that humans objectively experience social circumstances and rationally decide on their behaviour. Bourdieu argues that most behaviour does not actually occur in this way. Rather, he suggests that much of our behaviour happens according to a preconscious "logic of practice" (1990) that is embodied within what he calls the **habitus**: the habitus simply refers to the embodiment of social location and culture within human bodies.

With his concept of habitus, which Bourdieu describes as "a structuring structure" (1984), he demonstrates how the human body comes to embody culture. From our location within society, we get our habitus: our beliefs, values, and attitudes about the nature of social reality. Habitus rests upon early socialization and life experiences that become embodied. Bourdieu's (1984) research shows how factors such as where we work, what we eat and how much, and the type of exercise we get affect the size and shape of our bodies. For example, he explains how social class differences are reflected in the different health behaviours of the working class compared to those of the wealthy. With habitus, Bourdieu demonstrates that social structures are actually ingrained in our bodies. All of the patterned ways of acting and behaving that we learn from society become embodied in us as social actors. Our habitus reciprocally informs our position within society. Because these social structures are embodied in us (i.e., in our habitus), we reproduce them unthinkingly in our own social behaviour according to what Bourdieu calls "the logic of practice."

A classic example (Calhoun, Rojek, and Turner 2005) comes to us from a character in George Bernard Shaw's play *Pygmalion* (1913; later recreated as the 1964 movie *My Fair Lady*, starring Audrey Hepburn and Rex Harrison). The play tells the story of Professor Henry Higgins' efforts to train cockney flower girl Eliza Doolittle how to talk and behave like a member of the upper class so that she may pass as a refined society lady. Despite Higgins' and Eliza's best efforts, her habitus reveals her lower-class heritage. She cannot simply unlearn all the culture that became embodied within her habitus as she grew up and developed in a lower social class environment.

Thus, Bourdieu uses the concept of the habitus as a bridge between society and behaviour. Social inequalities are reproduced through the manner in which they are inscribed in people's bodies. As Shilling (2003, 129) explains, "Bourdieu's analysis of the physical bases of social inequalities provides us with a view of the body as an unfinished phenomenon which is in a constant process of becoming while living within society." Drawing upon Bourdieu's research, Shilling (2012, 138) explains that bodies "develop through the interrelation between an individual's social location, habitus, and taste." He explores how people use their bodies in order to construct a sense of themselves as important and worthwhile individuals. As Shilling (2012, 2) remarks, "growing numbers of people are deliberating the health, shape 'purity' or appearance of their own bodies as expressions of individual, group, cultural or religious identities." Shilling uses the term **body projects** to describe the manner by which bodies have become a medium for the expression of identity and social status:

> Treating the body as a project . . . involve[s] individuals being conscious of and actively concerned about the management, maintenance and appearance of their bodies. This involves a practical recognition of the significance of bodies as both as personal resources and social symbols that "give off" messages about identity (2012, 7).

We judge both ourselves and others by what we either do or do not do with our bodies and how we choose to take care of (or neglect) our bodies. For example, consider how you react when you see an obese person eating junk food in public.

Turner (1992, 164) notes that "within consumer culture the emphasis on body-beautiful and body-maintenance provides the conditions for expansions of the market for the sale of a new range of commodities related to the enhancement of individual prestige through bodily displays." In other words, in a health-conscious consumer culture, how we look after the health of our bodies says a lot about how we understand ourselves and how we want others to see us. In our health-conscious culture, the body has become a key site of health maintenance activities that place the body directly into consumer culture. Turner explains how these and other cultural developments (such as the growth of feminism, an aging population, the global emergence of diseases such as AIDS, and new medical technologies) can be usefully understood by the sociology of the body paradigm (see also Shilling 2012). Over the past few decades, the impact of the sociology of the body paradigm on efforts to understand these and other issues has been profound. Since the late 1980s and early 1990s, Canadian sociologists such as O'Neill (1985) and Frank (1990) have played an important part in establishing the sociology of the body as a subfield within sociology. Following their work, many Canadian health researchers have been influenced by the sociology of the body paradigm.

For example, Frank's *The Wounded Storyteller* (1995) is an influential exploration of the embodied nature of illness experience. Frank uses qualitative research to show how people with bodies troubled by serious injuries or illnesses (such as cancer or heart disease) use embodied stories to make sense of what is happening in their lives as they try to "live a good life while being ill" (1995, 165). His 2004 book uses the same narrative approach to consider the stories of physicians and nurses as they try to make sense of working in a profession that presents them with illness as an embodied part of everyday life.

Malacrida (2005) blends the sociological theories of Goffman and Foucault to understand the ways in which a total institution located in Alberta placed the bodies of people stigmatized as "mental defectives" under the surveillance of the medical gaze in order to exert social control over these "institutional survivors." Malacrida's research provides a vivid illustration of medicine's social control functions. Poudrier and Kennedy (2007) have employed the sociology of the body paradigm to understand the perspectives First Nations women living in rural communities have of healthy body weight and body image. This research suggests that in order to address obesity and its associated health risks as experienced by some of Canada's Aboriginal peoples, it is necessary to understand how elder knowledge and traditional First Nations values interact with the everyday experiences of First Nations women as they purchase and prepare food for their families and community. Each of these studies clearly illustrates the importance of the emphasis the sociology of the body paradigm places on understanding issues of embodiment if we are to more fully understand the complex relationship between bodies, society, and behaviour and to realize the promise of the sociological imagination when applied to health and illness.

In each of the four paradigms for understanding health and illness sociologically, we followed a "Health and Illness as . . ." format. It should now be clear to you that each paradigm's basic image of society offers an alternative way of conceptualizing health and illness (as summarized in Table 2.1). It should also be clear that health is a multi-dimensional concept. In other words, each of the paradigms contributes to our understanding of the ways in which health is shaped by intersecting aspects of social location such as social class, gender, ethnicity, and age. However, the picture is even more complex than that! Time itself adds another important dimension to the complexity of health. Health is a dynamic process that changes over the course of our lives in society. In this sense, health is an ongoing process of becoming, which we strive to achieve throughout our lives—something pursued rather than a static state (Twaddle 1974). This means that, whichever paradigm is used to apply the sociological imagination to understanding health and illness, we also need to adopt what is known as a life course perspective.

Table 2.1 Major Theoretical Paradigms Guiding Sociological Analysis of Health and Illness

Theoretical Paradigm	Image of Society	Health and Illness as . . .	Central Research Question	Key Concept	Level of Analysis	Associated Research Methods	Paradigmatic Example
Structural Functionalist	Harmonious social system made up of a number of interconnected parts	"Social Roles"	How is the threat illness poses to the overall stability of the social system managed?	sick role	macro	survey research and statistical analysis	Talcott Parsons
Conflict	Capitalist social system comprised of inequality, competing interest groups, and power struggles	"Professional Constructs"	How does the medical system serve as an instrument of social control in a capitalist society marked by exploitation and social inequality?	medical dominance	macro	participatory action research	Eliot Freidson
Symbolic Interactionist	The socially constructed product of everyday interactions of individuals	"Interpersonal Meanings"	How do individuals socially construct meanings of health and illness?	definition of the situation	micro	participant observation	Erving Goffman

Feminist	A patriarchal form of social organization in which men dominate women by exercising social, economic, and political power	"Gendered Experiences"	What parts are played by structural and behavioural determinants in shaping women's and men's health and their subjective experience of health and illness?	intersectionality	intersectional mixed methods	Ann Oakley
Sociology of the Body	Society and social relations shape and are shaped by human bodies.	"Embodied Cultural Facts"	How have medical discourses of the body shaped understandings of the body and bodily conduct?	medical gaze	intersectional narrative analysis	Michel Foucault
Life Course Perspective	Society as the dynamic intersection of individual biographies and historical events	"Unfolding across Time"	How are current and future health status shaped by past experiences and their timing?	life course	intersectional longitudinal analysis	Glen H. Elder, jr

Health and Illness as "Unfolding across Time"—The Importance of Adopting an Intersectional Life Course Perspective

Think about the last time you caught a cold. How do you think you became ill? Perhaps you were "partying hard" and didn't get enough rest, running down your immune system? Maybe you went outside in winter without a toque and caught a chill? Maybe you forgot to take your vitamins and didn't eat enough fruit and vegetables? Perhaps your beliefs about the common cold are more scientifically based? Maybe you think you caught a cold because someone who already had one sneezed on you and "got you sick" by exposing you to a cold virus? As we will discover in Chapter 9, health researchers (Baer et al. 2008) have shown that lay explanatory models for the common cold tend to integrate both folk and scientific knowledge. As Box 2.11 depicts, an alternative factor in your susceptibility to the common cold has to do with your parents' financial security when you were a child!

As Box 2.10 illustrates, health researchers are beginning to understand that what happens to us earlier in our lives affects our present and future health. This is the case for cardiovascular disease, respiratory disease, stroke, gum disease, and some forms of cancer (Cohen 2005). The events that we experience early in life (for example, during childhood and adolescence) shape individual differences in outcomes measured in adulthood, such as health status and the onset of chronic illnesses later in life. Braveman and Barclay (2009, S164) argue that health disparities actually begin in childhood and present evidence to demonstrate that early-life experiences (particularly those related to social inequality) shape health "across an entire lifetime and potentially across generations." For this reason, regardless of the theoretical paradigm guiding sociological analysis of health and illness, it is important to adopt an intersectional life course perspective to focus attention on the ways in which "early experiences, present circumstances, and the timing of various historical events in lives can all work together to affect health and well-being" (McDaniel 2013, 4). In other words, all theoretical approaches in health sociology benefit from adopting a life course perspective that incorporates the intersection of individual biographies with historical events. Pavalko and Willson (2011, 449) define the life course perspective as "a theoretical framework, concepts, and analytical tools for examining how individual lives unfold in historical and institutional contexts." They go on to explain that by adopting a life course perspective and "focusing on the importance of a dynamic view of individuals and their social contexts," health researchers are better able to realize what we outlined in the previous chapter as the task and the promise of the sociological imagination.

Alwin (2012) points out that the concept of the life course has gained considerable popularity today in the study of population health and aging. In fact, the life course perspective (or framework) "is now in common use across a broad range of disciplines and specialties" (2012, 206). Although the term life course is not always used consistently in the research literature, Alwin contends that it essentially refers to the "processes, events, and experiences that occur in the biographies of individuals" (2012, 207) as biography and history intersect and people's lives and health status unfold across time. Elder (1994, 5) notes that "Overall the life course can be viewed as a multi-level phenomenon, ranging from structured pathways through social institutions and organizations to the social trajectories of individuals and their developmental pathway." The **life course perspective**, then, is the view that past experiences and their timing shape aspects of our current and future lives such as health status. This contention is supported by Canadian researchers who have adopted a life course perspective for the study of age-related health issues such as childhood stress and mental health (Avison 2010) and the illness trajectory of people with

Box 2.10 What Happens to Us Earlier in Our Lives Affects Our Present and Future Health

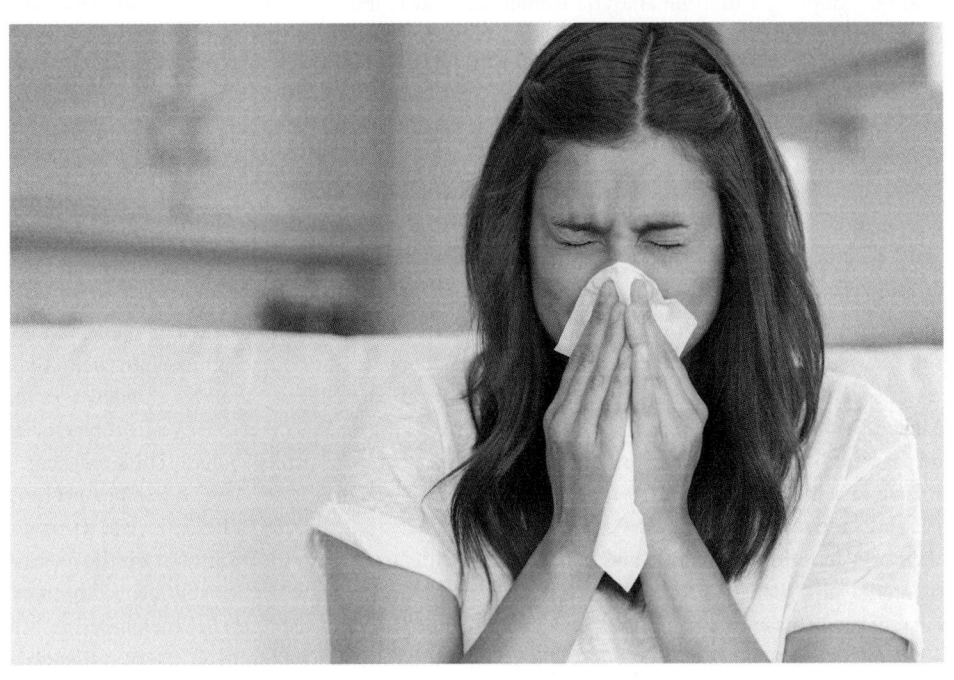

In order to learn about the effects early childhood experiences have on health later in life, Dr Sheldon Cohen and a team of researchers exposed 334 healthy volunteers to two strains of the common cold virus through direct nasal injection and then quarantined them for five days. During the study, the researchers gathered blood samples and clinically assessed the volunteers to see whether they had contracted a cold infection and whether they displayed the signs and symptoms of a cold. Prior to exposure, the volunteers were asked detailed questions about their own and their parents' socioeconomic status and home ownership. The results showed that independent of previous immunity, gender, ethnicity, age, body mass, virus type, and month of exposure, volunteers whose parents owned their homes and had longer home ownership periods were less likely to contract a cold and, when infected, had less severe cold symptoms compared to volunteers whose parents did not own their own home or owned it for shorter periods. Parental home ownership is an important measure of childhood socioeconomic status, leading Cohen and colleagues to conclude that "our data are consistent with childhood SES playing a role in susceptibility to cold viruses in adulthood" (2004, 557). While researchers such as Cohen are still trying to understand the exact mechanisms for such findings, it seems clear that what happens to us earlier in our lives affects our present and future health status. What was your childhood like, and how might it affect your present and future health?

Alzheimer's disease (Carpentier et al. 2010). Box 2.11 presents a paradigmatic example of the life course perspective.

The life course perspective is certainly not new. Many years ago, Elder (1975, 165) described age differentiation as a basic aspect of social structure and commented at length on the importance of adopting a lifetime analytic framework that emphasized "the social timetable of the life course." According to Elder, our lives consist of a series of stages with related roles as we transition from childhood, to adulthood, to later life. Mortimer and Shanahan (2002) state that the **life course** refers to an age-graded sequence of stages or phases and roles embedded in a network of social relationships. In their words, the central premise of the life course perspective is "that no period of life can be understood in isolation from people's prior experiences, as well as their aspirations for the future (2002, xi). For example, as the research by Cohen and colleagues demonstrated (see Box 2.10), our present health is shaped by past experiences. This dynamic way of understanding health focuses attention on social change and the different ways in which people's lives are organized through the passage of time.

As further discussed in Chapter 5, to gain a better understanding of the complex relationship between age and health, researchers have also adopted a life course approach in their studies of social inequalities and adult health disparities (Blane 2006; Holland et al. 2000; van de Mheen, Stronks, and Mackenbach 1998; Wadsworth 1997). In this case, the investigations focus on the ways in which social factors (such as class, gender, and ethnicity) operate at different stages throughout life and contribute to disparities in health. According to a life course perspective, people experience social structures, such as class, gender, and ethnicity, differently depending on their age, and ultimately these long-term determinants have a significant impact on the quality of later health (Blane et al. 2004). According to Blane (2006), adult health is influenced both by current social location and circumstances and by those experienced in earlier life phases. As we will see in the next chapter, life course analyses of longitudinal data (gathered over time as people age) help to clarify the causal linkages between social location and health and the pathways through which social inequalities in health develop across the life course.

Studies adopting the life course perspective show us that what happens to us as children or even before we are born has ramifications for the pursuit of health and wellness throughout our

---

Box 2.11   Glen H. Elder, jr (1934–)

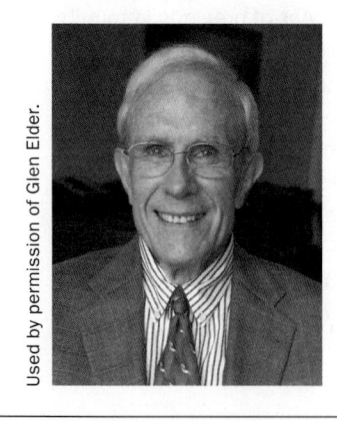

Used by permission of Glen Elder.

- Forerunner of the life course paradigm in his studies of growing up during the Great Depression (1974), veterans of World War II (1987), and adolescence during the farm crisis of the 1980s (1994)
- Interested in how individual lives are linked through a series of stages with related roles as we transition from childhood, to adulthood, to later life

"The later years of aging cannot be understood in depth without knowledge of the prior life course. Role histories clearly matter for health." (1994, 5)

lives! Adopting a life course perspective helps health researchers to realize the promise of the sociological imagination because it draws attention to how social structures are reproduced in the embodied experiences and behaviours of individuals. Reflective of the life course perspective, Wilkinson and Marmot (2003, 14) explain that "a good start in life means supporting mothers and young children: the health impact of early development and education lasts a lifetime." The life course perspective makes it clear that the foundations of health are established early in life and that the pursuit of health and wellness starts before birth and continues until death!

Chapter Summary

All of the theoretical paradigms reviewed in this chapter contribute to our understanding of health and illness in different ways. As the next chapter shows, they each provide unique conceptual and methodological guidelines for applying the sociological imagination to understanding health and illness. Turner (1995, 14) argues that "given the complexity of health and illness in contemporary societies, various theories and methodologies will be necessary for medical sociology to develop an adequate perspective on medical phenomena." In keeping with this necessity, this book adopts an eclectic approach to the analysis of health and wellness in Canada. That means that we have selected key features of each of the theoretical paradigms and integrated them into the discussion of various issues addressed throughout the book. For example, our examination of the sources of inequality and health disparities in Chapter 5 uses the conflict paradigm's emphasis on social inequality to consider how social class factors influence population health. In the same way, the feminist paradigm's intersectional understanding of the gendered nature of health and illness informs Chapter 6's analysis of the relationship between health and gender. Chapter 8 uses insights from Bourdieu's sociology to help solve the intersectional puzzle of health behaviour and lifestyles. Discussion of the hidden depths of health care in Chapter 9 is influenced by the symbolic interactionist paradigm and the need to understand the individual's definition of what it means to be healthy (i.e., notions of healthiness) in order to appreciate the contribution of informal care and social support as key determinants of health. Foucault's ideas concerning the relationship between medical knowledge and social power, as well as the conflict paradigm's understanding of health and illness as professional constructs, are reflected in our assessment in Chapter 10 of the link between population health promotion and biomedical health care. In other words, our analysis of the pursuit of health and wellness is informed by a combination of insights derived from each of the sociological paradigms for understanding health and illness. Since health is a complex, multi-dimensional concept, an eclectic approach combining theoretical paradigms provides the most comprehensive strategy for applying the sociological imagination to the study of health and illness.

Because the issues of health, illness, and the body compel health sociologists to explore difficult questions (such as the relationship between bodies, behaviour, society, and health), health sociology lies at the heart of the sociological imagination. The understandings health sociologists generate about the nature of the relationship between the individual and society are not just central to the social study of health but, rather, speak to all theoretical issues entailed in applying the sociological imagination to the study of society and culture. This means that, in terms of sociology, health sociology is "where it's at"! Simply stated, the way to better understand society and culture is to better understand health, illness, and the human body. This is the task and the promise of the sociological imagination when applied to a critical examination of the pursuit of health and wellness. It is to this task that this textbook is dedicated, continuing with the next chapter's look at how health as a multi-dimensional concept can be defined and measured.

Study Questions

1. How is the theory of Talcott Parsons a paradigmatic example of the structural functionalist approach to understanding health and illness?
2. Explain the major criticisms of Parsons' sick role concept.
3. According to conflict theory, how does the medical system serve as an instrument of social control in a capitalist society?
4. How is the theory of Eliot Freidson a paradigmatic example of the conflict theory approach to understanding health and illness?
5. How is the theory of Erving Goffman a paradigmatic example of the symbolic interactionist approach to understanding health and illness?
6. How is the theory of Ann Oakley a paradigmatic example of the feminist approach to understanding health and illness?
7. How is the theory of Michel Foucault a paradigmatic example of the sociology of the body approach to understanding health and illness?
8. Explain how biopower rests upon having knowledge and control of the human body.
9. How, according to Bourdieu's concept of the habitus, does culture shape the human body, which, in turn, shapes society?
10. Why is it necessary to adopt a life course perspective in analysis of disparities in health?

Recommended Readings

Armstrong, P., H. Armstrong, and D. Coburn. 2001. *Unhealthy Times: Political Economy Perspectives on Health and Care in Canada*. Don Mills, ON: Oxford University Press.

Cockerham, W.C., ed. 2013. *Medical Sociology on the Move: New Directions in Theory*. New York: Springer.

Malacrida, C., and J. Low, eds. 2016. *Sociology of the Body: A Reader*. Second Edition. Toronto: Oxford University Press.

Morrow, M., O. Hankivsky, and C. Varcoe, eds. 2007. *Women's Health in Canada: Critical Perspectives on Theory and Policy*. Toronto: University of Toronto Press.

Pavalko, E.K., and A.E. Willson. 2011. "Life course approaches to health, illness and healing." In B.A. Pescosolido, J.K. Martin, J.D. McLeod, and A. Rogers, eds, *Handbook of the Sociology of Health, Illness, and Healing: A Blueprint for the 21st Century*, 449–64. New York: Springer.

Recommended Website

National Library of Medicine's Visible Human Project:
www.nlm.nih.gov/research/visible/visible_human.html

Recommended Audiovisual Source

The Sterilization of Leilani Muir. National Film Board of Canada, 1996.

Measuring the Dimensions of Health 3

Learning Objectives

In this chapter, you will explore conceptual and methodological challenges encountered in measuring population health and wellness and will gain an understanding of

- the multi-dimensional nature of health and the link between the meaning and measurement of health;
- a sociological perspective on population health and health status indicators;
- the importance of adopting a salutogenic approach for defining and measuring the dimensions of health;
- the process of health status designation;
- the difference between health inputs and health outcomes;
- the difference between the indicators of good health and ill health; and
- the need for a mixed-methods approach to measuring the dimensions of health, using surveys, statistics, and stories.

The Meaning and Measurement of Health

Although "health" and "illness" are common terms that we use regularly in our daily conversations, we know that it is not safe to assume that their meanings are shared by everyone. How would you define good health? Would other members of your family or your friends agree with your definition? Is there a universal conception of good health (i.e., a general definition that applies equally well to women and men and cuts across age groups, ethnic groups, and social class boundaries)? In fact, health is a relational concept, and it is important to recognize that good health is not something that is either completely present or completely absent. The meaning of good health is socially constructed and varies across cultures and social groups. Furthermore, from a life course perspective our personal interpretation of the meaning of good health may change as we age. It must, therefore, be acknowledged that good health is "a concept that can be defined in a number of different ways—all of which have equal validity" (Dines and Cribb 1993, 8). In this chapter, we will take a closer look at the meaning and measurement of good health.

The previous chapter demonstrated that health is a multi-dimensional concept. Each of the theoretical paradigms reviewed in the previous chapter provides guidelines that help to formulate research questions about the types of social factors that have an effect on health and methodological guidelines that influence ideas about the nature of evidence and the selection of appropriate measures to use in unravelling the mystery of health. For example, if we believe that health is an objective state of being that is primarily the outcome of biophysical factors, then we are likely to rely on the type of quantitative methods (e.g., survey research and statistical analysis) recommended by the structural functionalist paradigm to assess the health status of the population. In contrast, if we view health as a part of an ongoing process with socially constructed subjective meanings, as suggested by both the symbolic interactionist and sociology of the body paradigms, then we typically rely on qualitative methods (such as illness narratives and health diaries) to measure health. In other words, the theoretical paradigm adopted focuses attention on different aspects of health and illness, raises specific questions about the types of factors that shape health, and suggests the use of particular methods to gather information needed to understand health from a sociological perspective.

Depending on the theoretical paradigm, health and illness have been characterized as social roles, professional constructs, interpersonal meanings, gendered experiences, and/or embodied cultural facts. In each case, the conceptual representation of health embedded in the paradigm must be operationally defined or transformed into precise indicators before we can actually measure the health of populations. There are a number of interrelated conceptual and methodological challenges that need to be addressed before we can engage in a sociological analysis of the pursuit of health and wellness.

While health and illness appear to be straightforward terms, they are actually difficult to define precisely because health is a multi-dimensional concept that is given meaning through complex social processes. The process of health status designation, along with the challenge of distinguishing between the dimensions of health, will be examined in the following discussion. As we turn our attention to measuring population health, we must realize that the dimensions of health are empirically correlated (i.e., they occur together in our everyday lives). While it is possible to conceptually distinguish between the dimensions of health, it is apparent that, on a day-to-day basis, normal health consists of a combination of aspects of good health and ill health. In other words, **normal health** is a unique blend of feelings of healthiness, physical fitness, and the performance of one's usual well roles, combined with the routine experience of a variety of symptomatic conditions. For some people, particularly in later life, normal health even includes living with daily symptoms (such as pain) and disability associated with chronic illnesses (such as arthritis).

The multi-dimensional nature of health raises methodological challenges when it comes to measurement. In addition, "emerging research on health from a life course perspective is demanding methodologically" (Pavalko and Willson 2011, 453). Exploring the ways in which health unfolds over time requires the availability of longitudinal data sets and statistical innovations enabling us to fully understand changes in health over the life course. In this chapter, we will examine the ways in which health researchers, guided by different theoretical paradigms, have measured health by addressing key questions such as the following:

- Is it possible to develop separate measures of good health and ill health?
- What do disease and death rates tell us about the health of Canadians?
- How can we measure the presence of good health (rather than simply documenting the absence of ill health)?
- To what extent does health change over time?
- What are the best indicators of population health?

Evidence provided by ongoing Canadian health studies will help us to answer these questions.

Differentiating Personal and Population Health

The biomedical approach to measuring health focuses on **personal health status**. This type of assessment generally takes place in the doctor's office or some other formal health-care setting. Measuring personal health directs attention to the individual and primarily concentrates on the biological level of functioning (although, in some cases, psychological functioning may also be considered). Measurement includes taking a medical history (e.g., being interviewed by a doctor, a nurse, or another formal health-care provider) and having a physical examination, plus blood tests, x-rays, ultrasounds, CT scans, and many other forms of diagnostic assessment common in clinical practice. These measures provide health-care professionals with the basic information necessary to assess an individual's personal health.

In contrast, measuring **population health status** is a very different matter. By definition, this approach to measuring health status focuses on general populations (e.g., the health of Canadians) or specific subpopulations, such as university students or Aboriginals. The biomedical approach to personal health measurement focuses on individuals, specifically those who already have a health problem or are at risk of developing one. Cohen and colleagues (2014, 2) note that "Traditionally, healthcare leaders have struggled to move away from the narrow biomedical model, with crisis management and the immediacy of demand for healthcare services leaving little time and resources to incorporate the population health approach into planning and day-to-day management." Population health measurement shifts attention to the health of the overall population, including those who feel healthy, those who feel ill, and those who consider themselves sick (and have become patients). Indeed, a commitment to focusing on health and wellness proactively is a hallmark of the population health approach. Thus, this approach avoids medico-centrism in that it includes those in the community who are managing their health through informal care as well as those who are receiving treatment from the formal health-care system. In other words, all members of society (i.e., those who are healthy or ill, including those who are in the community or formal health-care setting) must be taken into account if we are to gain a sociological understanding of the population health status of Canadians.

In addition, population health assessment involves a multi-dimensional approach to measurement and recognizes that health is multi-faceted and includes a physical dimension (i.e., the experience of signs of disease and symptoms of illness), a psychological dimension (i.e., feelings of well-being), and a social dimension (i.e., the capacity to perform usual well roles). Consequently, population health measurement emphasizes the importance of social and psychological aspects of health (e.g., quality of life issues) as well as physical functioning; it highlights the need to combine positive indicators of good health (wellness) with the usual negative indicators of ill health (sickness).

Finally, population health includes a broad range of personal and structural factors that affect health status, not just traditional risk factors related to the onset of diseases. A population health approach recognizes that there are multiple health determinants, including biology, genetic endowment, personal practices such as diet and level of physical activity, and the availability and accessibility of health-care services, as well as social and economic factors such as living and working conditions. Chapter 4 examines the general determinants of health, but for now it is sufficient to note that a population health approach recognizes that social structures and personal practices interact in shaping health status. In summary, population health measurement requires a multi-level analysis of the ways that community and individual characteristics are linked to good and poor health and involves a societal focus, a multi-dimensional conception of health, and the inclusion of a broad range of health determinants.

Despite growing popularity, the population health perspective is not without its critics. For example, the basic assumptions underlying the model of population health that has become quite influential in Canada have been critiqued (Coburn et al. 2003). Researchers have pointed out that historically there has been a lack of consensus about the meaning of population health (Cohen et al. 2014; Kindig and Stoddart 2003; Raphael and Bryant 2002; Frankish, Veenstra, and Moulton 1999; Dunn and Hayes 1999). Kindig and Stoddart (2003, 382) assert "that the time has come for a clarification of the meaning and scope of the term population health." In a comprehensive discussion of the population health framework, Kindig (2007) contends that the distinction between population health and public health merits particular attention and emphasizes the need to clarify key population health concepts (such as determinants, disparities, and outcomes). There has also been an ongoing debate about the lack of a theoretical foundation for contemporary population health research. Echoing the importance attached to applying the sociological imagination to an improved understanding of health and illness, Carpiano and Daley (2006, 564) argue that "while more research is needed that focuses on the multiple determinants of population health, a solid theoretical basis should underpin this research." Future population health research requires a sound theoretical base and a more rigorous approach to measurement. Selection of the best set of indicators of population health has also been the subject of debate (Etches et al. 2004; Hancock, Labonte, and Edwards 1999).

Even acknowledging these limitations, a population health perspective is valuable for a number of reasons. First, it focuses attention on the need for a sociological framework for understanding why some Canadians are healthier than others. A population health perspective highlights the social production of health and well-being as well as the ways in which social relations contribute to the maintenance of good health and the onset of ill health. Furthermore, it emphasizes the importance of gaining insight into the ways in which social factors affect health. According to McDaniel (2013, 8), "the population health perspective takes the view that social structures, such as socioeconomic inequalities, have an effect on overall health of populations independent of any individual level relation to social hierarchy or pathways." Consequently, this perspective offers the promise of identifying more effective ways of addressing inequalities and improving the health of all members of society.

Adopting a Salutogenic Approach for Understanding the Dimensions of Health

Antonovsky's (1979; 1987) salutogenic model of health was briefly introduced in Chapter 1; it is important to take a closer look at the features of this conceptual framework in the context of population health measurement. Antonovsky formulated a revolutionary model of health (see Box 3.1) that emphasizes the salutary factors that protect and promote good health. Salutary factors may be identified at both the individual (e.g., formal education) and community (e.g., neighbourhood characteristics) levels. He points out that just as health is a complex, multi-dimensional phenomenon, so too are the many overlapping factors that promote health. According to Antonovsky (1996, 12), the critical issue that needs to be addressed is "the question of the creation of appropriate social conditions which underlie or facilitate health-promotive behaviors." His intention was to develop a conceptual model that would provide a guide for population health research and practice. Looking at the dimensions of health through

> **Box 3.1** Aaron Antonovsky (1923–1994)
>
> - Developed the "salutogenic model" of health in *Health, Stress and Coping* (1979) and its sequel, *Unraveling the Mystery of Health* (1987)
> - Developed the sense of coherence scale, which has been used in at least 33 languages in 32 countries with at least 15 different versions of the questionnaire
>
> *"The mystery of health is indeed intriguing"* (1979, 35)

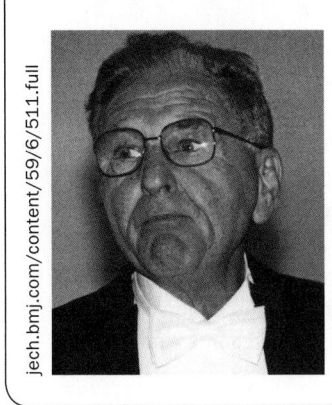

a salutogenic lens allows us to gain a better understanding of the issues involved in measuring population health. Adopting a salutogenic approach focuses attention on the meaning of good health, as well as health-related quality of life, and the diversity of factors that contribute to the pursuit of health and wellness.

Antonovsky's salutogenic approach to health has helped researchers to apply the sociological imagination to understanding the factors that promote population health. For example, Frohlich and Potvin (1999, 212) begin by discussing the importance of theory development in health promotion research, and then, using population health as a sounding board, they state that one of their major objectives is "to bring together the various ways that population health can inform health promotion by creating a conceptual framework, a framework that will later be called the salutogenic setting." In other words, they attempt to integrate aspects of Antonovsky's salutogenic model of health, a population health research agenda, and health promotion policy and practice. In a more recent critical commentary on the salutogenic model of health and health promotion research, Mittelmark and Bull (2013) agree that salutogenesis is an important theory and has a role to play in health promotion research. They argue, however, that Antonovsky's original ideas about the nature of health need to be expanded in order to "help health promotion research operationalise well-being's positive aspects" (2013, 37).

Eriksson and Lindstrom (2010) have also commented on the benefits of linking the salutogenic conceptual framework with population health promotion (see also Lindstrom and Eriksson 2005; 2006). They describe salutogenesis as "a good theory base for health promotion" (Lindstrom and Eriksson 2006, 240) and argue that Antonovsky's ideas are important because they direct our attention to people's resources and assets, or their capacity to create health, rather than limiting our focus to biological risk factors, ill health, and disease. According to the salutogenic model, health involves continuous movement along a continuum between good health (wellness) and ill health (sickness). Antonovsky claims that each individual's unique view of life and capacity to respond to stressful situations helps to explain why some people manage to stay well and even improve their health. We will return to the salutogenic model later in the chapter, but first, keeping this approach to the dimensions of health in mind, let's examine the meanings of good health and ill health more closely.

The Meaning of Ill Health (Sickness) and Good Health (Wellness)

Ill health is typically defined in terms of the experience of illness and the presence of disease, but is there more to good health than the absence of illness and disease? Yes! A health sociology perspective argues that good health consists of feelings of well-being (healthiness) plus adequate performance at the physical, psychological, and social levels of functioning. In other words, in keeping with the World Health Organization (WHO) definition of health introduced in Chapter 1, health is much more than the absence of disease and illness. Therefore, it is important to clarify the distinction between good health (wellness) and ill health (sickness) and to explore the possibility of measuring the positive aspects of good health rather than simply relying on the absence of indicators of disease and illness as the basis for assessing health status. In their discussion of the challenges of measuring population health at the community level, Hancock, Labonte, and Edwards (1999, S22) express "the view that health is much more than the measurement of death, disease and disability, it also encompasses mental and social well-being, quality of life, life satisfaction and happiness." In other words, understanding population health means not only measuring wellness (and sickness) at the individual level but also determining the healthiness of the communities in which we live. Although sickness and wellness are interrelated, they reflect different dimensions of health, and each warrants careful examination.

Sickness: The Presence of Disease and the Experience of Illness

Sickness includes both the presence of disease and the experience of illness. From a sociological perspective, it is important to distinguish between these two components of ill health. Stated in an oversimplified manner, you might be experiencing feelings of illness when you decide to see a physician. Subsequently, after the medical examination is completed, you may learn that you have a disease. People experience illness in informal social contexts, and physicians diagnose and treat disease in formal health-care settings. It is essential, therefore, that we clarify the distinction between the medical profession's conception of disease and the ways members of the lay community experience illness in their everyday lives.

According to the biomedical model, **disease** is an objective, biophysical phenomenon that is characterized by altered functioning of the body as a biological organism. This type of condition is presumably identifiable as a particular clinical syndrome, and diagnosed disease is viewed as objective because it can be directly observed and measured. Judgments regarding the presence of disease are based on an assessment of observable indicators of bodily change known as **signs**. There are many potential signs of disease. Some are directly apparent to the observer (e.g., bleeding, swelling, or a rash), while others require the use of diagnostic instruments (such as a thermometer or stethoscope) to gauge changes within the body. Finally, more sophisticated medical technology is used to assess less readily apparent biophysical changes, such as composition of the blood, the presence of internal tumours, and cellular pathology. Thus, the biomedical approach to ill health focuses on the biological organism and pathological processes that are revealed through a variety of observable indicators (or signs). These indicators serve as the basis for medical practitioners to diagnosis the presence of disease and to provide treatment intervention. While the biomedical approach is valuable, it is important to recognize the difference between disease prevention and health promotion and the fact that this approach does not allow us to unravel the mystery of human health. As stated earlier, medicine does not necessarily equate with health!

Many people suffer from chronic degenerative diseases, such as heart disease and cancer, which pose serious challenges for the biomedical approach and, ultimately, for the pursuit of health and wellness. These widespread diseases cannot be understood or treated solely on the basis of biophysical factors. The challenge is to provide quality care while continuing to try to find a cure. Without minimizing the importance of biophysical components of ill health, it is apparent that a comprehensive approach requires attention to the psychological and social components of health and illness and incorporates the behavioural dimensions of the illness experience. This is because when an individual is sick (i.e., feeling unwell or unhealthy), there are consequences for the whole person and her life, not just a specific biophysical part of the body.

While feelings of illness typically accompany the presence of disease, illness and disease are not the same. Feelings of illness can vary substantially among people with the same diagnosed disease. For example, two people with gallstones may experience very different symptoms. One person may be basically asymptomatic, not even aware that the condition exists. In contrast, the other individual may experience nausea, indigestion, and pain. Consequently, the presence of disease and the experience of ill health must be defined and measured independently. We must keep in mind that a disease can be present in an individual without the person being aware of feelings of illness or without other people knowing about her sickness.

It is also possible for a person to feel ill without any detectable organic manifestations of disease. In some cases, this may mean that the individual feels so sick that she is unable to carry out usual activities at home or at work, or perhaps even get out of bed, although this illness experience occurs in the absence of any determinable disease. As shown by the research of health sociologists influenced by the conflict paradigm, the dominance of the medical profession means that evidence of a state of ill health is generally dependent on biophysical indicators, since these signs can be directly measured. In fact, biomedicine demands objective proof of the presence of disease in order to assess the legitimacy of illness claims. Twaddle (1974, 30) points out that "in the absence of corroborating signs, symptoms are generally not held as in themselves defining health status." In other words, no matter how bad you feel, if there are no detectable signs of disease, you may have a difficult time convincing others that you are really sick! Medicine has a label for this type of sickness—psychosomatic illness (suggesting that the condition may exist in your mind but not in your body).

According to symbolic interactionists, **illness** is a subjective psychosocial phenomenon in which individuals perceive themselves as not feeling well and engage in different types of behaviour in an effort to overcome their ill health (e.g., they may self-medicate or decide to make lifestyle changes, such as altering their diet or getting more rest). Illness is characterized as subjective because it is based on personal perception, evaluation, and response to symptomatic conditions. In assessing the nature of illness, we rely on individuals reporting that they are experiencing **symptoms** such as pain or feelings of nausea and dizziness. These illness indicators or symptoms cannot be directly observed. Instead, they are inferred based on things that people say and do (i.e., they are assumed to exist based on indirect evidence). For example, one of the most prevalent symptoms of illness—pain—is revealed to others in a variety of ways. We will examine the meaning and management of pain in more detail in Chapter 9, but for now it is sufficient to note that we have many different ways of letting others know that we are in pain (e.g., crying, complaining, grimacing). Each of these practices may be presented to other people as evidence that we are experiencing pain. It is important to recognize that individuals must disclose these essentially private sensations (symptoms) in some way for them to become public and for others to learn about their illness experiences.

While the primary focus of sociological analysis, particularly for health researchers working within the symbolic interactionist paradigm, is on the subjective experience of illness (i.e., the ways in which we make sense of sickness and manage our everyday health concerns), sickness has an important biophysical component. Even common symptomatic conditions, such as a headache, are situated within the body. In other words, illness experience is usually accompanied by the identification of specific bodily sites that are affected. At the same time, sickness is also an experience that occurs in a social context and reflects the nature of the sick person's relationships with others in their social network (such as family, friends, and co-workers). Consequently, it is important to remember that "stating that disease and illness are not the same certainly does not argue that they are unrelated" (Lau 1997, 52). Indeed, this cautionary note suggests that a thorough understanding of this dimension of health must be based on a comprehensive approach that reflects the fact that sickness is both an important social event and, according to the sociology of the body paradigm, an embodied cultural fact.

Wellness: More Than the Absence of Disease and Illness

If sickness is defined in terms of the presence of disease and the experience of illness, is wellness then simply the absence of these aspects of ill health? Alternatively, is it possible to define good health or wellness as something more than the absence of disease and illness? Furthermore, can we even recognize good health in ourselves and others? In practice we are better able to recognize the presence of disease (and illness) rather than the presence of good health. Idler (1979) points out that the difficulty stems from the fact that good health is essentially taken for granted. In other words, we typically spend little time thinking about the meaning of good health in our daily lives. Idler contends that it is only when sickness occurs that health loses its taken-for-granted status. To illustrate, think about such basic bodily functions as breathing and swallowing. We generally pay no attention to these activities until the onset of a head cold or a sore throat. Once we are unable (even temporarily) to breathe or swallow easily, we become painfully aware of the change in our physical health. In Idler's words, "A healthy body functions to the full extent of its capacities, free from limitations of pain and illness. It does not demand one's conscious attention; it allows consciousness to focus fully on the external world" (1979, 726). Consequently, good health (as long as we have it) is generally taken for granted while we focus our attention on the social world around us and the demands of everyday life.

This has implications for the definition and measurement of wellness, since it suggests that good health can only be understood in relation to illness and disease. It is time, therefore, to address the fundamental question—is it possible to define good health as more than the mere absence of illness and disease? According to the World Health Organization's definition of good health (see Chapter 1), the answer to this question is yes. More than 60 years ago, the World Health Organization offered a more positive definition of good health as "a state of complete physical, mental and social well-being and not merely the absence of disease or infirmity" (1948, 100). Based on this definition, the indicators of good health include subjective feelings of well-being plus adequate performance at the physical, psychological, and social levels of functioning. The drawback of this definition is that it does not offer clear guidelines for measuring health and well-being. As a result, we need to consider whether concepts such as good health and wellness can be more explicitly defined and measured.

The term "wellness" has been used in the health research literature for many years. For example, Bruhn and colleagues (1977, 209) describe wellness as a continually ongoing process characterized by an integration of all aspects of the individual's "physical, mental, social, and environmental well-being." In another early discussion of health and wellness, Baranowski (1981, 247) reinforces the view that the concept of wellness entails "the capacity of the individual to cope with and successfully master the social and physical environment." Wellness has now become a widely accepted concept in health research and government policy documents outlining strategies for population health promotion (Carlise and Hanlon 2008). According to Kirkland (2014b, 959), the term wellness has become popular today because it "captures the sense that the era of combating diseases has given way to a more complex problem of success in modernity: living well, since so many more of us live long lives, entirely avoiding the diseases and accidents that killed our ancestors." With increasing health consciousness, as described in the first chapter, the marketplace is now crowded with wellness products and services that promise opportunities to achieve success in the pursuit of good health and well-being. Do these developments mean that we now have a better understanding of the meaning of wellness? Although wellness has become a cultural ideal and an important marketing tool, it remains an abstract concept that poses serious conceptual and measurement challenges (Miller and Foster 2010). In a critical synthesis of the ways in which wellness has been conceptualized and measured, Miller and Foster (2010, 20) explain that "The integrative and dynamic nature of wellness makes it difficult to control for variables, resulting in the inadequacy of the existing measures."

It is also important to recognize that the good health dimension of wellness has a number of key components. First, good health includes a psychological component expressed as a **sense of healthiness** or emotional well-being. This component is related to factors such as a sense of coherence and control as well as life satisfaction. In addition, the good health dimension of wellness includes one's level of **fitness**. Being fit refers to the individual's adaptation to life circumstances (i.e., as in survival of the fittest). The term "fitness" is generally used to refer to physical condition (i.e., aspects of physical health such as aerobic capacity and muscle strength). In addition, "fitness" is used in reference to psychological health and social functioning. For example, in the context of mental health law, the courts occasionally assess people's fitness to stand trial. The focus in this case is on the individual's psychological ability to understand legal charges and to participate meaningfully in the criminal justice process. Finally, social fitness is judged in the context of determining whether people are able to adequately perform social roles and meet societal responsibilities (e.g., suitability to become adoptive parents). Thus, wellness includes physical, psychological, and social fitness.

It is important to emphasize that there is a crucial social component to the good health dimension of wellness. As we will discuss in Chapter 9, we generally perform our usual well roles and life tasks as part of an interconnected network of supportive relationships that contribute to our social well-being. This aspect of wellness is described as functional ability or the capability of the individual to meet the demands of everyday life in a particular social and physical environment. Functional ability includes both the social capacity to adequately perform our well roles as family members and participants in the paid labour force and our ability to take care of the activities of daily living. This is a highly significant component, since wellness is often defined in terms of the **optimum capacity** of an individual to fulfill personal goals and to perform socially defined roles in a way that meets cultural expectations.

In summary, social capacity for performing well roles combines with level of fitness and sense of healthiness in defining one's position on the good health dimension of wellness. Wellness has an important behavioural dimension that includes the specific health-promoting and health-protective lifestyle behaviours that are examined in Chapter 8. To conclude the present discussion, it appears that the good health dimension of wellness has a reality that is independent (to some extent) of the ill health dimension of sickness and the presence or absence of disease and illness. Consequently, it is important to try to separate these two health dimensions.

The Process of Health Status Designation: Separating the Dimensions of Health

If we are going to be successful at defining and measuring wellness (good health) and sickness (ill health) as separate entities, we need to conceptualize these two dimensions as different but intersecting aspects of health. Antonovsky (1996, 14) argues that the dichotomous classification of people as healthy or sick is misleading: "A continuum model, which sees each of us, at a given point in time, somewhere along a healthy/dis-ease continuum is, I believe, a more powerful and more accurate conception of reality." Figure 3.1 illustrates that good health and ill health are independent (but related) dimensions and do not define two ends of a single continuum. In other words, wellness and sickness are not opposite ends of the same dimension. Furthermore, it must be recognized that movement (in different directions) along either dimension is possible. According to Antonovsky, if we are to solve the mystery of health, it is just as important to understand the salutary or health-promoting factors that facilitate the pursuit of good health and wellness as it is to understand the risk factors that contribute to the onset of diseases and the experience of illness. The double-sided arrows in the figure are intended to represent the possibility of separate movement in either direction on the good health and ill health dimensions.

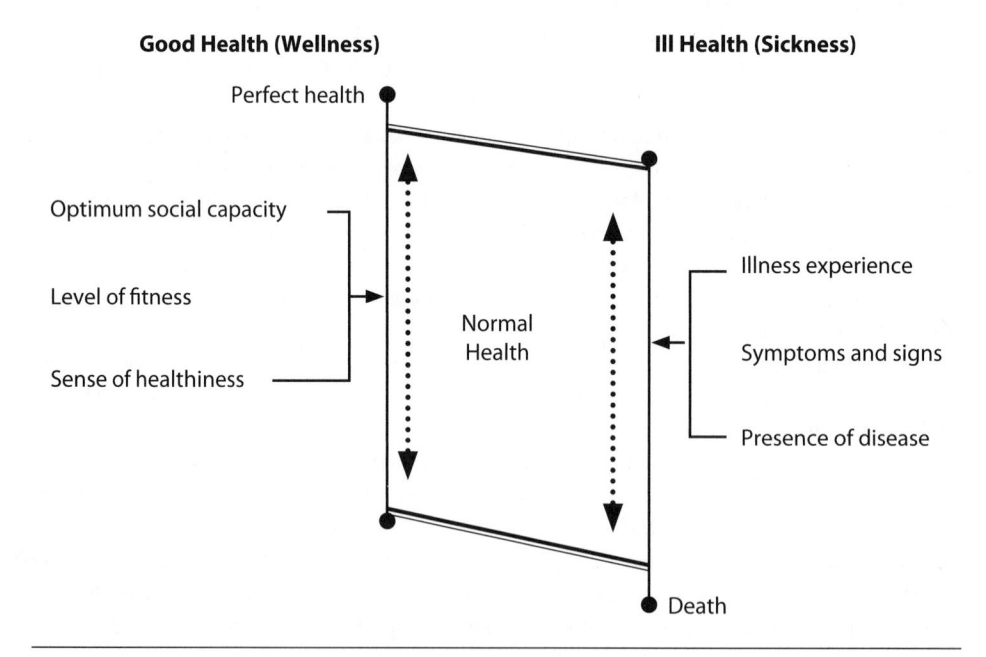

Figure 3.1 The Dimensions of Health

The figure summarizes much of the preceding discussion. For example, the ill health dimension (sickness) consists of the experience of illness and the presence of disease and, in some cases (depending on the nature and severity of disease), may result in death. Position on the ill health continuum depends primarily on biophysical factors and, to some extent, on psychophysical factors (e.g., stress) that are associated with the presence of disease and the experience of illness. While death is the natural limit on the ill health dimension, the absence of clinical evidence of biophysical disease and feelings of illness does not necessarily translate into good health.

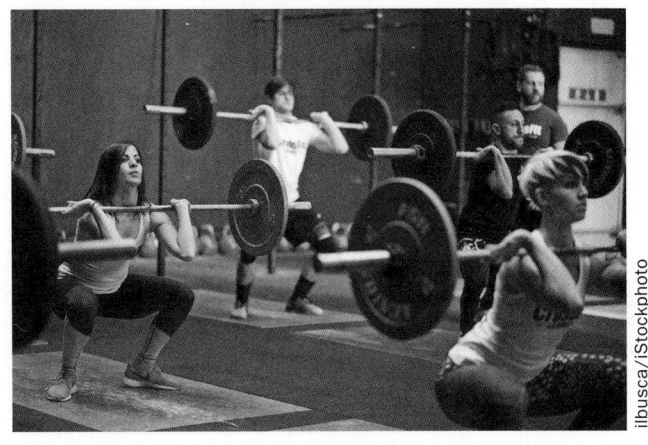

Many people participate in exercise programs as part of a healthy lifestyle.

The good health dimension, by comparison, consists of feeling healthy, being fit, and having the social capacity to achieve one's life goals (i.e., it is a resource for living). A person's position on this continuum is based primarily on psychosocial factors such as a sense of healthiness, level of fitness, and functional capacity. In other words, wellness reflects the existence of positive aspects of health and well-being, not merely the lack of negative aspects of illness and disease. There is no upper limit to the good health dimension other than one's optimum level of personal adaptation (e.g., the ability to adjust successfully to changes in the social and physical environment). Thus, we do not all experience good health or wellness in the same way. In commenting on the pursuit of wellness, Cowen (1991, 404) states that "I see it not as something one has or doesn't have, but rather as an ideal that, in fact, exists along a continuum." Similarly, a number of years earlier Twaddle (1974, 31) argued that "we may conceptualize a state of perfect health as an ideal toward which people are oriented rather than a state they expect to attain." Ideal standards of good health and wellness may help us to set goals and to monitor our personal health practices. At the same time, Twaddle contends that no one ever really attains this ideal state. Instead, we all routinely experience a range of less than perfect health that may be defined as normal. In other words, everyday life consists of a dynamic blend of good health and ill health. We are all very familiar with the experience of having good days and bad days.

Normal health, as depicted in Figure 3.1, consists of a combination of good health and ill health. In fact, it is possible to argue that the experience of illness and, under certain circumstances, even the presence of disease, can be viewed as part of normal health. Starting with familiar everyday symptoms such as a sore throat or a runny nose, these conditions may be characterized as "going around" and recognized as normal if they are associated with the common cold or flu season. In other words, these types of widespread symptomatic conditions may be expected, and therefore accepted, as part of normal health. It is certainly possible to experience this type of sickness and, at the same time, continue to feel generally healthy and perform one's usual well roles.

Additionally, from a life course perspective, there are specific diseases that typically occur at certain stages in the lifespan, and since they are expected, they tend to be viewed as normal. For example, childhood ailments such as ear infections are accepted as part of normal health at this stage of development. And because of their increasing prevalence, certain late-life diseases are now regarded as normal for older adults (e.g., arthritis). In any case, we need to critically examine some of our implicit assumptions about normality and health, recognizing that personal accounts of good health and ill health involve a relative assessment in which we compare our health status not only to abstract standards but also to the perceived health status of others our own age or gender. In addition, this assessment process often involves comparing our current health status to our past health status (e.g., how we felt last year or two years ago). Consequently, Twaddle (1974) argues that health status actually involves a process of becoming rather than a state of being. Or, paraphrasing the lyrics of an Aerosmith song, "Health's a journey, not a destination!" Once we recognize that health involves a process of becoming (i.e., a means of achieving personal potential and a resource for living), then we will be better able to solve the mystery of health.

Twaddle argues that good health and ill health are part of a complex, ongoing social process. He characterizes the process of living and adapting to the changing demands of life (including health concerns) as **health status designation**. As Table 3.1 illustrates, the process of health status designation outlined by Twaddle (1974) involves

- judgments about different levels of functioning (i.e., physical, psychological, and social well-being);
- participation by different sources of evaluation (i.e., status definers such as self versus other and lay versus professional others); and
- an emphasis on different frames of reference for assessing health (i.e., selective attention to the components of the good health and ill health dimensions).

This active process reflects the multi-dimensional nature of health and the fact that there are a number of different people involved in the process of health status designation. There are at least three different sources of evaluation (or health status definers) typically involved in assessing an individual's health and well-being. Obviously, the individual is intimately involved in this process on a daily basis. In addition, other informal (e.g., family and friends) or formal (e.g., healthcare professionals) status definers may be actively involved. The different frames of reference

Table 3.1 The Process of Health Status Designation

Levels of Functioning	Physical	Psychological	Social
Source of Evaluation	Physician	Self	Family/friends
Frame of Reference	Biological changes	Changes in feeling state	Changes in capacity
	(*Signs*)	(*Symptoms*)	(*Task/Role Performance*)

used as a basis for assessing health status are not mutually exclusive. Status definers draw on a variety of indicators in making their health assessments (e.g., biophysical or psychosocial changes) but generally emphasize the importance of certain aspects of health (e.g., physicians' reliance on the presence of biophysical signs as evidence of ill health).

The process of health status designation typically begins when the individual becomes aware that she is not feeling well (i.e., changes occur in one's personal feeling state). This psychological shift (from "I feel healthy" to "I feel ill") may be based on the perception of symptomatic conditions, such as nausea or abdominal pain, as well as the discovery of a physical change, such as a lump or swelling. The next step in the process generally involves disclosing these health concerns to others. You may tell a family member that your stomach hurts or that you feel quite nauseated when you eat. You may make an appointment with your physician to have the lump examined. Depending on your assessment of the meaning of these types of psychophysical changes and the response you receive from other health status definers, the process may lead to changes in role performance (e.g., you may call in sick and miss a few days of work). Alternatively, health professionals may set the process in motion by legitimating your claims to the sick role (as described by the structural functionalist paradigm). For example, a physician may diagnose the nature of the lump based on a physical examination, the results of laboratory tests, and your family health history. Finally, family members may be concerned about your signs and symptoms once they become aware of their existence, but as informal health status definers, they usually focus on noticeable changes in social performance. For instance, family members or friends who know you well might express their concerns about your health status by asking, "Are you okay? You haven't been yourself lately." In other words, they may become aware of a change in your usual behaviour and attempt to assess whether this can be interpreted as an indication of a change in your health status. Overall, then, a number of different participants, using a variety of criteria, are constantly involved in monitoring our health status as part of a dynamic and highly complex process.

Understanding the Difference between Health Inputs and Health Outcomes

Before turning our attention to an examination of the health status indicators used to assess the health of populations, it is important to consider the difference between health inputs and health outcomes. A population health perspective includes the study of both health determinants (inputs or causes) and health consequences (outcomes or effects). In fact, population health research focuses on the impact of multiple determinants of health (such as biology and lifestyle) on specific outcomes (such as life expectancy and health-related quality of life) and emphasizes the importance of precise measurement and the need for standardized health indicators. "To improve the health of populations and increase opportunities for comparability, more valid, comprehensive, transparent, and standardized ways of measuring and reporting on population health are needed" (Etches et al. 2006, 30). A critical first step in improving the measurement of the health of populations (as illustrated by Table 3.2) is to clarify the distinction between health inputs (i.e., determinants or factors that affect our health status) and health outcomes (i.e., direct measures of both our present and estimated future health status).

It is important to distinguish between direct measures of health status and measures that have become popular in health surveys but that do not actually measure health directly. (This topic will be discussed in more detail later in the chapter.) Direct measures of health status include

Table 3.2 Population Health Indicators

Health Inputs (Determinants)	Health Outcomes (Health Status)	
	Present	**Future**
Salutary factors	Self-rated health	Life expectancy
Risk factors	Functional ability	Potential years of life lost
Living and working conditions	Morbidity	Health-adjusted life expectancy
Access to health-care services	Mortality	Quality of life

perceived health (i.e., self-rated or self-reported health) and the usual types of morbidity and mortality data collected (i.e., rates of disease and death). In addition, attributes such as vision, hearing, speech, and mobility (included in the Health Utilities Index) directly reflect functional aspects of health. Present and future estimates of health status are equally important health outcome measures. Future health status is typically gauged by life expectancy (i.e., the number of years from birth to death) as well as health-adjusted life expectancy (i.e., the number of years of good health added to the lifespan). Length of life and quality of life are both key health outcomes!

Although it is common for population health surveys to ask questions, for example, about risk factors such as smoking, this behavioural practice is not a direct measure of health status. Rather, it is a behaviour that has been empirically correlated with health status. To illustrate, since smoking is related to the presence of diseases such as cancer, it is assumed that smoking behaviour may be interpreted as an indirect indicator of ill health. Population health assessments also rely on other proxy measures related to the availability and use of formal health-care services in gauging health status (e.g., the number of doctors in the community or the number of hospital beds available). While access to these types of health resources is important, this information does not provide direct evidence regarding the health status of the population. In order to be able to measure changes in population health status (e.g., to demonstrate that Canadians are getting healthier), we need to clarify these measurement issues and improve our ability to evaluate the indicators of good health and ill health. Unfortunately, some attempts at population health measurement continue to "group outcomes and determinants components together, which can be confusing and misleading to both policymakers and researchers" (Kindig 2007, 146). As a result, there is still room for improvement in measuring the indicators of population health.

Health Status Indicators

It is time to take a closer look at the specific types of health status indicators used in population health surveys. Two general types of health status indicators will be briefly reviewed: single-item measures (global self-rated health) and composite measures (the Health Utilities Index). The following section will then critically examine the indicators of ill health and good health used most frequently in assessing population health. Information from Canadian population health surveys will be used to illustrate each of these health status indicators.

Single-Item Measures: Global Self-Rated Health

Population health surveys typically start with a general question to gauge **self-rated health**, or the individual's perceived health as an indicator of overall health status. Perceived health refers to a person's health in general—not only the absence of disease or illness but also physical, mental, and social well-being. This straightforward question has become a standard measure in health surveys. As illustrated in Figure 3.2, approximately 60 per cent of Canadians rated their health as either excellent or very good in the 2012 *Canadian Community Health Survey*. In other words, most Canadians perceive themselves to be in very good health. There were no significant differences between women and men, but the proportion who reported that they are in very good or excellent health decreased for older age groups.

Two critical measurement questions need to be addressed before we can feel confident that self-rated health is an accurate portrayal of the health status of Canadians. First, we need to ask, is this single-item measure a valid indicator of health status? Validity refers to whether the question really measures what it was intended to evaluate. Do we know what the global self-rated health question really measures? Second, we need to question the reliability of this measure (i.e., does it consistently measure the same thing?). In fact, health researchers are still learning about what self-rated health actually measures and whether it stays the same or changes over time. For example, Layes, Asada, and Kephart (2012, 1) point out that despite the popularity of this measure and its frequent use in population health research, "debates continue as to what exactly self-rated health captures."

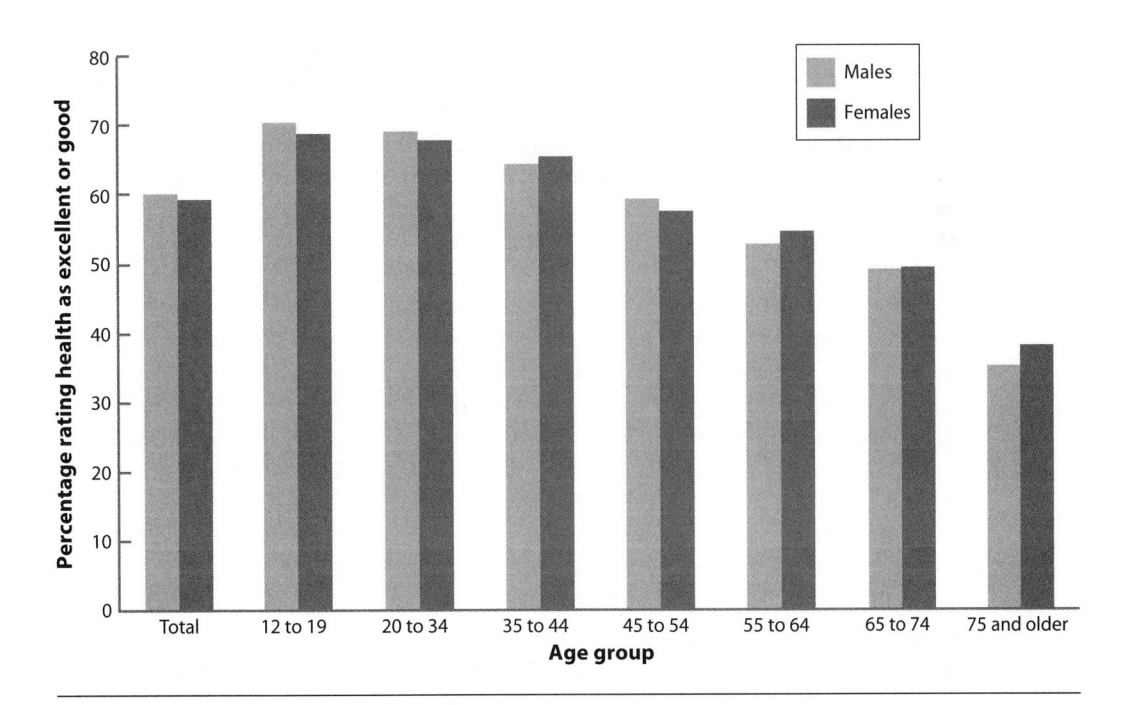

Figure 3.2 Global Self-rated Health of Canadians

Source: *Canadian Community Health Survey*, 2012. This analysis is based on the Statistics Canada Canadian Community Health Survey, 2012. All computations, use, and interpretation of these data are entirely that of the authors.

Measurement is at the heart of sociological research on health and illness. Only by coming up with valid and reliable measures of concepts such as health status can we realize the promise of the sociological imagination when applied to understanding how society contributes to health and illness. As a multi-dimensional concept, health can mean different things to different people. Chapter 2 explained how various sociological paradigms each have a different understanding of the concept of health. The multiple meanings of "health" raise a host of measurement questions for sociologists trying to assess population health. Central among these is: What can we learn about the health status of Canadians by asking questions about self-rated health?

A large body of research has demonstrated that asking people to rate their own health using this single-item measure has some value (e.g., Jyhla 2009, 1994; Fylkesnes and Forde 1992). Self-rated health has proved to be a useful proxy measure for clinically assessed health status. Jyhla (1994, 983) points to the fact that this global measure is frequently "used as a proxy question for more thorough, more complicated and more expensive measurements of health status." For example, studies have shown a correlation between the self-rated health of older adults and more objective indicators such as physical functioning based on clinical assessments. The evidence indicates that there is a persistent, positive relationship between self-rated health and physician assessments (e.g., La Rue et al. 1979; Thorslund and Norstrom 1993). For example, it has been found that physician ratings consistently correlate highly with older adults' judgments about their own health, suggesting that self-rated health is a valid health status indicator.

In addition, Giltay, Vollaard, and Kromhout (2012) found that self-rated and physician-rated health independently predict all-cause mortality. For many years now, studies have used actual life expectancy to validate self-rated health and generally conclude that older adults' self-assessed health is a strong predictor of mortality (i.e., death rates; e.g., Mossey and Shapiro 1982; Kaplan, Barell, and Lusky 1988; Idler and Kasl 1991; Rakowski et al. 1993; Benyamini and Idler 1999). These international studies demonstrate that self-evaluation of health status has a direct and independent effect on mortality. In other words, people who are going to die rate their health as poorer than those who end up living longer. Today, there is general agreement that self-rated health, measured by a single question, is a significant predictor of how long an individual will stay alive (Alfonso et al. 2012; Benyamini 2011; Shooshtari, Menec, and Tate 2007). Overall, there is ample evidence that global self-rated health provides a valuable summary measure of how various aspects of the individual's health are perceived.

Krause and Jay (1994) directly address the question of validity in their paper titled "What do global self-rated health items measure?" This suggestive, but inconclusive, paper reports the results of a study that was carried out in the United States to try to identify the specific referents (i.e., frames of reference) that people use in answering a global question about their self-rated health. Study findings suggest that people do not necessarily think about the same aspects of good health or ill health when rating their overall health status. According to Krause and Jay, some study participants were thinking about specific health problems, such as hypertension, when rating their health (i.e., they focused on the presence of disease and the experience of illness). Other study participants were thinking about either general physical functioning, such as mobility, or health maintenance behaviours, such as a good diet or regular exercise (i.e., they focused on functional ability and personal health practices). Krause and Jay conclude that health researchers have not yet identified all of the referents used by people when they are rating their own health. As Krause and Jay (1994, 931) explain, "Although physical and mental health problems appear to play a major role in shaping global health perceptions, a significant proportion of the variance in this single-item indicator remains unexplained." These findings reflect the multi-dimensional nature of health—the reality that individuals focus on different dimensions when assessing their own health status.

Subsequent studies have explored the subjective meanings of self-rated health (e.g., Idler, Hudson, and Leventhal 1999; Kaplan and Baron-Epel 2003; Mavaddat et al. 2011; Layes, Asada, and Kephart 2012; Dowd 2012; Picard, Juster, and Sabiston 2013). Unfortunately, these studies have not yet provided a clear explanation of what global self-rated health really means to study participants. As a result, we still do not know very much about what people are actually thinking when they rate their health as excellent, good, or poor. We don't know whether responses to this question reflect "true" health or differences in reporting behaviour. Furthermore, we know very little about whether there are subgroup differences in the referents that are used as a basis for self-evaluations of health. For example, does "excellent health" mean the same thing to men and women? Does "poor health" mean the same thing to older and younger adults? It is apparent that health does not mean the same thing to everyone (or, for that matter, to the same individual at different stages in her life course). These types of unresolved issues led Kaplan and Baron-Epel (2003, 1676) to conclude that "the evaluation of subjective health is a complex process that seems to be unique for different groups of individuals" and that more research is needed to improve our understanding of the meaning of self-rated health.

Over the past decade, Canadian health researchers have started to shed light on these issues. For example, Smith, Glazier, and Sibley (2010, 419) analyzed data from the *Canadian Community Health Survey* to examine whether self-rated health is interpreted consistently across socioeconomic groups. Based on their findings, they conclude that this single-item measure of health "assesses a broad variety of factors, including physical health status, mental health status, health utilization, and health behaviours, relatively equally across SES groups." Although his findings are inconclusive, Veenstra (2011b) also used the same national health survey dataset to explore the relationships between a number of intersecting sources of social inequality, such as class (household income, educational attainment), race, and gender, and global self-rated health.

Do subjective evaluations of health remain constant or change across the life course? Unfortunately, very few studies have explored change in self-rated general health status. The limited evidence suggests that changes in self-rated health vary depending on baseline (or usual) health status. For example, self-rated health among older adults at follow-up did not change significantly from baseline ratings (Leinonen, Heikkinen, and Jylha 1998). Bailis, Segall, and Chipperfield (2003) report that when controlling for all other variables, self-rated health at baseline is the best predictor of follow-up ratings. This study used longitudinal data from two successive waves of the *National Population Health Survey* to test a model of change in self-rated health. They found evidence that Canadians' perceived health reflects an assessment of changes in one's health status and involves an enduring self-concept as a healthy or unhealthy person. This conclusion is supported by a number of recent international studies using longitudinal data to assess changes in self-rated health among adults in countries such as Australia (Sargent-Cox et al. 2014) and Britain (Giordano and Lindstrom 2010). Furthermore, it is now possible to find examples of research designed to test a life course model of self-rated health that indicate that perceived health through adolescence and young adulthood is significantly associated with childhood family experiences such as early health challenges and parental health conditions, as well as parental education and income (Bauldry et al. 2012).

Reviewing the reliability and validity of self-rated health, Desesquelles, Egidi, and Salvatore (2009, 1124) conclude not only that this measure is a "good predictor of mortality" and "strongly associated with morbidity and disability" but also that "the perception of health may be influenced by contextual factors, either social, economical, political or cultural." All things considered, we seem to know that people with poor self-rated health are, in fact, more ill and more likely to die sooner than people with better self-rated health. In other words, single-item measures do have some reliability. Health researchers, however, do not yet fully understand precisely how contextual factors, such as gender, social class, ethnicity, and age, relate to self-rated health assessments. This means that the validity of self-rated health measures is still questionable. McHorney (2000, 344) summarizes health status assessment by noting that "In general, the assembly of measures can be described as strong in methodologic rigor but weaker in conceptual underpinnings. In other words, the field of health status assessment is regarded more for how it quantifies and validates health status indicators than for how and why it conceptualizes health." Clearly, self-rated health is an example of a health measure that might be improved through the application of sociological theory. As recommended by both the symbolic interactionist and sociology of the body paradigms, there is a need for an in-depth qualitative analysis to gain a more insightful understanding of the subjective meanings of self-rated health.

Composite Measures: The Health Utilities Index

Health surveys, such as the *National Population Health Survey*, also include composite measures of health status. For example, the Health Utilities Index (HUI) consists of a series of questions intended to measure both quantitative and qualitative aspects of health. It was designed to be a summary measure of overall health status, although most of the items in the index are limited to biophysical aspects of health. The HUI provides a description of an individual's functional health status based on responses to questions about eight health attributes: vision, hearing, speech, mobility (ability to get around), dexterity (use of hands and fingers), cognition (memory and problem-solving), emotion (feelings of happiness), and pain and discomfort. From a biomedical perspective, the "HUI is comprehensive in that it classifies health status in terms of the most important basic attributes or dimensions of health" (Furlong et al. 2001, 375).

These eight self-reported attributes of health serve as the basis for calculating a summary index score. In other words, a single numerical value is assigned to each individual that presumably reflects functional health status on a scale ranging from perfect health (1.00) to dead (0.00). A number of years ago, Erickson and colleagues (1989) compared the relative merits of the HUI and two other similar measures and critically reviewed the usefulness of these types of composite measures for assessing population health. They contend that global measures overestimate the level of health in the general population and suggest that composite measures such as the HUI have considerable potential. Their argument hinges on the fact that health problems are prevalent in the general population and, if they are not included in measurement, the estimate of population health status will be upwardly biased. Researchers (e.g., Manuel, Schultz, and Kopec 2002; Furlong et al. 2001) have documented the widespread use of the Health Utilities Index in a number of different countries and the existence of supporting evidence that this multi-attribute measure has become a useful tool for assessing population health status. More recently, Layes, Asada, and Kephart (2012, 3) point out that the HUI has now "been tested extensively using Canadian populations in terms of its reliability and validity." However, the benefits of this type of composite measure will only be realized with further methodological refinement and the development of more comprehensive measures that also include indicators of health-related quality of life.

Indicators of Ill Health: Limits to the Standard Approach

If we are to be successful at developing better measures for use in population health surveys, we must not only resolve the problem of specifying the best set of indicators to use but also ensure that the assessment includes indicators of both good health (wellness) and ill health (sickness). From a sociological perspective, comprehensive population health assessments must involve measuring both dimensions of health. At the same time, we know that the presence of disease (and the experience of illness) can be recognized more readily than the presence of good health. The point was made earlier that good health is generally taken for granted and only when sickness occurs do we typically pay attention to our health status. Consequently, it is not difficult to understand why the standard approach adopted by most studies to date has been to focus on the measurement of ill health, not good health. At present, most studies attempt to understand health by measuring sickness! In fact, population health surveys have traditionally concentrated on the following indicators of ill health.

Morbidity and Mortality

If it is easier to recognize sickness than wellness, it stands to reason that it would also be easier to measure this dimension of health. The standard approach to assessing health status has been to collect a great deal of data on disease, disability, and death. For example, the presence of disease (i.e., morbidity rates) and the major causes of death (i.e., mortality rates) have been extensively documented. **Morbidity** refers to the distribution of disease in human groups. This type of health status measurement helps us to learn whether a condition such as heart disease is equally common among men and women and whether arthritis occurs at the same rate among younger and older adults.

The occurrence of specific diseases is calculated in terms of prevalence and incidence rates. The proportion of people in the general population who have a diagnosed disease at a given point in time constitutes the **prevalence rate**. This information tells us how widespread the selected condition is. To illustrate, a variety of Canadian studies have demonstrated that arthritis and rheumatism are the most prevalent conditions among those who are over the age of 65. Along with arthritis and rheumatism, morbidity data reveal that heart disease, hypertension, and diabetes are prevalent chronic health problems experienced by older segments of the population.

The **incidence rate** is based on the number of new cases of a specific disease identified over a period of time such as a year. This information tells us whether more people are now affected by a particular condition than in the past. Referring again to arthritis, the incidence rate reflects the number of older adults who were diagnosed with arthritis during the past year (compared to five or ten years ago). In general, morbidity data suggest that in a country with an aging population such as Canada, an increasing number of people will be subject to these types of chronic degenerative diseases.

The *National Population Health Survey* (*NPHS*) collects information about the presence of disease by documenting the types of chronic health conditions that are prevalent in the

Canadian population. For the purposes of this survey, **chronic disease** is defined as a long-term physical health problem that lasts more than six months and has been diagnosed by a health professional. Although the majority of Canadians describe their health in positive terms, more than half (58 per cent) of the NPHS participants reported that they have at least one chronic condition (Schultz and Kopec 2003). In fact, a significant proportion of these people were living with several different chronic health problems (i.e., two or more conditions). The presence of a number of different diseases at the same time is referred to as **co-morbidity**. According to the Canadian Institute for Health Information (CIHI 2013b), the most prevalent chronic diseases in the Canadian population (aged 18 years and older) are high blood pressure (19 per cent), depression (12 per cent), osteoarthritis (11 per cent), diabetes (10 per cent), and asthma (7 per cent). In conclusion, morbidity rates can tell us something about how widespread a specific disease is at a particular point in time and whether the proportion of the population affected by this disease is increasing.

Population health assessments relying on the standard approach to measurement (i.e., collecting information about the indicators of ill health) also devote a great deal of attention to documenting mortality (death) rates. Reflecting our culture's medico-centric understanding of health and illness, we have become accustomed to measuring health in terms of death. For example, Nolte and McKee (2008) measured the health of nations by relying on one indicator—age-standardized death rates. They compared amenable mortality (i.e., deaths from certain causes that could have been prevented by timely and effective health care) in 19 developed countries. Canada falls approximately in the middle of the countries studied, while the United States has one of the highest death rates from causes amenable to health care. In addition to calculating general mortality rates for the overall population, more specific rates are also computed for maternal mortality (i.e., the number of women who die during pregnancy or childbirth) and infant mortality (i.e., the number of deaths of children one year of age or younger per 1000 live births). For many years, the average was just over 5.0 infant deaths for every 1000 live births in Canada, but by 2011 the rate had decreased to 4.8 (Statistics Canada 2012b). Thus, **mortality** rates reflect the number of deaths in a population within a prescribed time, expressed as either crude rates for the overall population or rates specific to diseases or to age, sex, or other attributes. For example, age-specific mortality rates reveal that cancer and heart disease (followed by stroke and respiratory diseases) have become the major causes of death among older segments of the population (Wilkins 2005). In 2011, these four diseases continue to be the leading causes of all deaths in Canada (Statistics Canada 2011b).

It is not surprising that the major causes of death and **life expectancy** (i.e., the estimated number of years that we can expect to live) are frequently measured health status indicators, since they are readily quantifiable. Calculating these types of indicators is straightforward because national, standardized information about births and deaths is collected by government agencies. Canadians can generally expect to live longer lives than their parents and grandparents. According to the Canadian Institute for Health Information (CIHI 2008), overall life expectancy at birth for Canadians was 80.4 years in 2005 and reached 81.1 years by 2009 (Statistics Canada 2009). Does the increase in life expectancy mean that Canadians have become healthier? Alternatively, does it mean that we are living longer and feeling worse (i.e., experiencing more long-term health problems)? On the surface, an increase in longevity appears to be good news; however, we need to be cautious in interpreting lower death rates as a valid indicator of improvement in population health. We will return to this point shortly when we take a critical look at what the indicators of ill health tell us about general health status.

Disability and Utilization of Health Services

Population health surveys also typically use disability days and health-care utilization patterns as indicators of health status. Disability measures focus on the type of restrictions on daily activities that result from long-term health conditions. In the NPHS, for example, information was collected about health limitations on activities at home, school, and work. Approximately 20 per cent of the study participants reported that as a result of disease or injury, they were restricted in the kind or amount of activity that they could perform at home, school, and work or during their leisure time. This type of data can be used to calculate the rate of occurrence of specific types of disability days (such as the number of days a person is confined to bed or absent from work because of sickness). Researchers also compile extensive data on Canadians' health-care utilization patterns (e.g., physician contact and hospital admissions) on the assumption that this is an important indicator of the health of the population. Once again, the interpretation of this type of data and the link between the use of formal health-care services and the health status of Canadians need to be critically examined (as we will see in Chapter 10).

What Can We Learn about Health from Disease and Death Rates?

We can learn a great deal about sickness and its consequences from morbidity and mortality data. However, the standard approach to health status measurement and the reliance on negative indicators tell us little about good health or wellness. In other words, the primarily biophysical indicators of ill health do not give us a complete picture of the health status of the population. We learn little about the mystery of health by studying illness and disease. To illustrate the limitations of the medico-centric approach to assessing population health, it is important to take a brief, but closer, look at some of the indicators of ill health routinely used. Let's start with mortality rates. It has become customary to measure health in terms of death. This type of information is interpreted as an indication of the health of the population, with lower death rates presumably indicating a healthier population. However, this is an oversimplification, since the meaning of death rates is difficult to interpret. Mortality rates reflect not only personal health characteristics (e.g., heart disease) but also lifestyle practices (e.g., smoking) as well as a combination of social and economic factors (e.g., income and employment). Any measurement relying solely on the calculation of mortality rates basically reflects the loss of life and not necessarily the loss of health! "How death in an individual is perceived or interpreted depends highly on its circumstances, causes, and timing, as well as on the evaluators, and thus it may or may not be deemed unhealthy" (Wallace 1994, 450). In other words, death rates alone do not really tell us a great deal about the overall health status of the population.

There is one other issue regarding the use of mortality as a measure of health that warrants comment. Extending the number of years we can all expect to live may be a desirable goal, but the obvious question is: Do the years added to our lifespan necessarily mean years of good health? The answer to this question provided by health sociologists is "no." Indeed, part of the legacy of longevity is an increase in the prevalence of disability in later life associated with chronic degenerative diseases such as arthritis (i.e., the non-fatal diseases of aging). Olshansky and colleagues (1991) provide guidelines for testing the hypothesis that we may indeed be trading off longer life for worsening health. They argue that "if, in the current mortality transition, we are unavoidably trading off a lower risk of death from fatal diseases at older ages for an extension of disabled years, then more attention must be given to ameliorating the nonfatal diseases of aging" (1991, 212).

In other words, we have to pay as much attention to quality of life issues as we do to issues of quantity (or length) of life in the past. Lifespan in most industrialized countries such as Canada has been extended substantially over the years, but if added years of life really mean more years of living with multiple chronic health problems, then we need to seriously question whether longer life means better health. Life expectancy data alone do not indicate how healthy a life is. Comprehensive population health assessments must incorporate both length of life and quality of life measures. Assessing the number of years of good health added to the lifespan seems to be the critical issue. We will return to this point later in the chapter when we discuss health-adjusted life expectancy as an indicator of health status.

Before concluding this section, let's quickly consider the limitations of one other frequently used indicator of ill health (i.e., utilization of formal health-care services). Does the volume of health-care services consumed tell us anything meaningful about the health status of the population? For example, does a higher rate of use of health-care services mean a healthier population? Perhaps it is just the opposite, with a lower rate of use indicating a healthier population. Obviously, the link between health-care utilization patterns and population health status is difficult to interpret. Furthermore, as health research guided by the conflict paradigm has established, rates of physician contact and hospital-based treatment are affected not only by patients' health-care needs but also by professional medical decisions, the availability of health services (e.g., appropriate medical specialists, hospital bed space), and changing government policies on the delivery of health care. Thus, utilization data reveal as much about the allocation of health resources and the current focus of health policies as they do indirectly about the health status of the population. For these reasons, then, the standard approach to health status measurement is limited in its ability to unravel the mystery of health.

Indicators of Good Health: The Challenge of Measuring Wellness

A sociological assessment of population health requires a comprehensive approach that includes all members of society, not just those who use the formal health-care system (i.e., we need to measure the health of all people, not just that of patients). Furthermore, official statistics on disease and death do not adequately reflect population health status. A comprehensive approach would give equal weight to the indicators of good health. In other words, assessing population health means measuring wellness, not just sickness. Millar and Hull (1997, 147) acknowledge that although "measuring human wellness is an inexact and changing science," it is important to attempt to measure positive aspects of health other than the standard health status indicators. For example, they contend that population health assessments must also include indicators of well-being that measure aspects such as sense of control, self-esteem, and job/life satisfaction. Their basic argument is that by focusing on these indicators of good health, we may be able to improve our ability to measure human wellness.

In other words, it is time to adopt an assets model of health (Morgan and Ziglio 2007). The traditional approach to population health assessment has been based on a deficit model. That is, the focus has been on biophysical risk factors, disease, and the utilization of formal health-care services. The deficit model emphasizes the negative aspects of the ill health dimension of sickness and is highly medico-centric, viewing health as the absence of disease. It fosters dependency on professionally provided services. An assets model shifts the focus to the positive aspects of the good health dimension of wellness, such as health creation, the individual's adaptive capacity, and the availability of health-promoting salutogenic resources at both the individual and the community level. This model builds on Antonovsky's ideas about salutogenesis and recommends investigating health assets that contribute to the creation of good health.

According to Morgan and Ziglio (2007), **health assets** can be defined as any factors that enhance the ability of individuals or populations to maintain health and well-being and include social, economic, and environmental resources (e.g., supportive social networks, employment skills, level of education). They argue that developing an assets model as a counterweight to deficit models means "promoting the population as a co-producer of health rather than simply a consumer of health care services" (2007, 18). The assets model of health necessitates a multi-method approach to measurement using a set of quantitative and qualitative salutogenic indicators to assess the positive aspects of population health.

At present, however, we are better at measuring sickness than we are at measuring wellness. Indeed, wellness remains an elusive concept that is difficult to define and even more difficult to measure. Earlier in this chapter, the good health dimension of wellness was defined in terms of subjective feelings of healthiness, along with physical fitness and the capacity to achieve life goals and perform socially determined well roles. Consequently, an assessment of the ways in which Canadians experience good health and well-being requires a comprehensive and more innovative approach to measurement. A number of years ago, Adams, Bezner, and Steinhardt (1997) adopted a salutogenic approach and made one of the few attempts in the research literature to develop a valid and reliable measure of perceived wellness, including

- physical wellness—level of fitness and physical activity;
- psychological wellness—sense of optimism and happiness;
- emotional wellness—sense of self-esteem (i.e., a positive self-identity);
- social wellness—being part of an effective social support network;
- spiritual wellness—sense of purpose and level of life satisfaction; and
- intellectual wellness—feeling challenged and stimulated by life experiences.

These researchers contend that these aspects are interrelated and should be integrated in a measure of wellness. While there is growing agreement about the components of wellness and the importance of incorporating indicators of good health in population health assessments, there is still room for methodological improvement. Consequently, the challenge facing researchers today is the development of measures that accurately reflect the positive health and well-being of the overall population, such as the Wellness Belief Scale developed by Bishop and Yardley (2010) and the effort by Bringsen, Andersson, and Ejlertsson (2009) to design a salutogenic health indicator scale. Kindig (2007, 142) summarizes the situation by stating that "while the general understanding of health often is negative, such as the absence of disease, the modern understanding of health also stresses its positive aspects, like wellness or well-being, and considers health in relation to all aspects of life in the environments in which we live."

Sense of Coherence

An example of a positive indicator of good health and well-being can be found in Antonovsky's analysis of the process of staying well. The salutogenic model of health emphasizes the importance of an orientation to life that Antonovsky refers to as a sense of coherence. He argues that the origins of health can be found in our sense of coherence. Antonovsky (1979, 123) defined a **sense of coherence** as "a global orientation that expresses the extent to which one has a pervasive, enduring though dynamic feeling of confidence that one's internal and external environments are predictable and that there is a high probability that things will work out as well as can reasonably be expected." The concept was redefined in Antonovsky's subsequent publications but basically refers to a way of seeing the world and the course of one's life (dispositional orientation) that consists of three core components:

- Comprehensibility—the extent to which one perceives life events as making sense (i.e., the view that life is ordered, consistent, and predictable)
- Manageability—the expectation that things will work out as well as can reasonably be expected (i.e., the view that one has the resources to deal with life's demands or a sense of confidence in one's ability to cope)
- Meaningfulness—the extent to which one feels that life makes sense emotionally (i.e., the view that there are areas of life that are worthy of commitment)

Antonovsky (1987) also developed a scale to measure sense of coherence and to test the relationship between this way of looking at the world and health status. The scale measures sense of coherence by asking respondents a series of questions with response categories ranging along a seven-point scale from "very often" to "very seldom or never." To gain an understanding of how the components of a sense of coherence are measured, try answering the sample questions in Box 3.2. Two questions have been selected to illustrate each of the three core components. When responding to the questions, think about the relationship between each of these factors and your own self-rated health status.

Antonovsky contends that in combination, these three factors constitute a sense of coherence and play a critical role in shaping our health and well-being. This contention is supported by Canadian research findings. For example, Martel and colleagues (2005, 4) analyzed *NPHS* data and report that the chances of healthy aging are significantly enhanced by "a strong sense of coherence, that is, finding life meaningful, manageable and comprehensible." In other words, a positive outlook on life is associated with staying healthy while we age. In a more recent study in

Box 3.2 Measuring Your Sense of Coherence

How often

- does it happen that you have feelings inside that you would rather not feel?
- do you have the feeling that you are in an unfamiliar situation and don't know what to do? [*comprehensibility*]
- do you have feelings that you're not sure you can keep under control?
- do you have the feeling that you are being treated unfairly? [*manageability*]
- do you have the feeling that you don't really care what goes on around you?
- do you have the feeling that there's little meaning in the things you do in your daily life? [*meaningfulness*]

Germany, Wiesmann and Hannich (2010) carried out a salutogenic analysis of healthy aging and similarly reported that sense of coherence is significantly related to health maintenance in later life. Since this measure of socio-emotional well-being was first introduced by Antonovsky, it has been used in studies carried out in a number of different countries and has been found to be a reliable, valid, and cross-culturally applicable way of assessing how people manage to stay well (Eriksson and Lindstrom 2005). A number of review papers conclude that sense of coherence appears to be a vital health-promoting resource that is strongly related to two important components of wellness—perceived health (Eriksson and Lindstrom 2006) and quality of life (Eriksson and Lindstrom 2007). Efforts are ongoing to improve the measurement properties of the sense of coherence scale (Holmefur et al. 2014).

Antonovsky believes that sense of coherence develops during childhood and adolescence and is relatively stable throughout adulthood. While the relationship between age and well-being remains somewhat ambiguous, a common finding in population-based studies of the development of this positive aspect of health is that level of sense of coherence continuously increases over time. For example, it has been reported that sense of coherence increases over the life course (Feldt et al. 2011; Lindstrom and Eriksson 2010) and seems to generally improve with age group (Nilsson et al. 2010; Lindmark et al. 2010). This evidence strongly suggests that the development of a sense of coherence is a lifelong process and that health-promoting resources may in fact become stronger in later life.

Canadian Index of Wellbeing

According to the researchers who are currently developing this measure, the Canadian Index of Wellbeing (CIW) focuses on quality of life and assesses the things that matter to Canadians. "The CIW was created through the combined efforts of national leaders and organisations, community groups, research experts, indicator users, and importantly, the Canadian public. Through three rounds of public consultations, everyday Canadians across the country candidly expressed what really matters to their wellbeing" (Canadian Index of Wellbeing 2012, 12). The CIW includes a total of 64 indicators within eight interconnected quality of life categories that were identified as playing a vital part in the lives of Canadians. These eight domains are: community vitality, democratic engagement, education, environment, healthy populations, leisure and culture, living standards, and time use. The data are combined into a composite index that provides a picture of overall well-being and is now being used to gauge the quality of life of Canadians.

Health Expectancy: Estimating Future Health Status and Quality of Life

It has been argued that the development of health-related quality of life measures is essential for the assessment of population health (Gold, Franks, and Erickson 1996). In order to accurately estimate the future health status of Canadians, we must continue to develop valid and reliable measures of health-related quality of life. It is evident that comprehensive population health assessments must not only incorporate measures of the physical, psychological, and social components of health but must also pay as much attention to the positive indicators of good health (wellness) as they have to the negative indicators of ill health (sickness). At the same time, there is growing recognition that the measurement of wellness means investigating both quantitative and qualitative aspects of health (i.e., life expectancy, or length of life, and health expectancy, or quality of life). As previously stated, life expectancy data alone do not indicate how healthy or how good a life the individual experiences. Health-adjusted life expectancy, or **health expectancy**, is still a relatively new summary measure of population health, but it is a more comprehensive indicator because it includes both quantity (and length) of life and quality of life and measures the number of years lived in good health. In other words, "health-adjusted life expectancy is a composite measure that captures a more complete estimate of population health than standard (or ordinary) life expectancy" (Public Health Agency of Canada 2012, 1).

Canadian life expectancy is now among the highest in the world and continues to be extended. This achievement should not be minimized, since life expectancy is an important indicator of the health status of the population. The percentage of seniors in the Canadian population is growing and will increase dramatically as individuals from the baby boom generation enter this age group. Furthermore, a closer look at population aging trends reveals that the oldest age groups (i.e., those over the age of 80) have substantially increased. Although it is a controversial issue, scientists are engaged in a debate about whether it is possible to extend average lifespan beyond 120 years to perhaps 150 years. The fundamental question then becomes, would you like to be able to live to be 150 years old?

"While most people view a longer life as desirable, a long life in good health is certainly a more important goal" (Turcotte and Schellenberg 2007, 44). In other words, promoting healthy aging means addressing not just life expectancy but also the quality of life enjoyed by Canadians as they age. Thus, the challenge facing societies that are experiencing this type of change in population age structure is to find ways to extend life expectancy and, at the same time, to improve health-related quality of life. This issue is receiving growing attention in the research literature as investigators debate the best means of achieving "dependence-free life expectancy" (Martel and Belanger 2000), "disability-free life expectancy" (Guralnik 1991), "active life expectancy" (Manton and Stallard 1991), or simply the "compression of morbidity" (Fries 1980). Although the language is inconsistent, the basic objective is the same, and that is to extend healthy life expectancy (i.e., the number of years we can expect to live in the community in good health without serious disability or restrictions on our daily activities). According to Kaplan (1991, 170), "Although the wish to prolong life and reduce disability and suffering to a minimum is shared by all," a more attainable goal is to concentrate on finding ways to lessen the burden of chronic illness and improve the quality of life experienced by older persons.

As depicted in Box 3.3, there are a number of critical differences between life expectancy and health expectancy. First, and foremost, health expectancy at birth is shorter than life expectancy for all Canadians. Extending life expectancy involves finding effective means of preventing premature death and potential years of life lost. If increases in longevity are not accompanied by comparable improvements in health expectancy, then the gap between the two will continue to grow. Gains in health expectancy and the quality of later life are, in fact, not keeping pace with increases in length of life. According to a recent report on health-adjusted life expectancy in Canada, while life expectancy was 83.6 years for women and 78.9 years for men in 2006, health-adjusted life expectancy was still only 72.1 years for women and 69.6 years for men (Public Health Agency of Canada 2012). Extending health-adjusted life expectancy entails postponing the onset of disability and the associated decline in functional ability as well as delaying dependency and deterioration in quality of life in an effort to add more years of good health to the lifelong pursuit of wellness.

From a sociological perspective, the challenge is to continue efforts to refine measures of population health so that we can accurately assess present levels of both good health and ill health and estimate the future health status of Canadians. Current studies of health expectancy

> **Box 3.3** "Make Death Wait" (Life Expectancy) or "Make Health Last" (Health Expectancy)
>
> The Heart and Stroke Foundation's 2011 "Make Death Wait" campaign reflects a cultural preoccupation with life expectancy. The controversial advertisements featured a voice-over of the personification of death stalking victims. In 2013, the foundation changed the discourse of its health promotion campaign to focus on more positive messaging concerning health expectancy. Which health promotion campaign do you think is most effective for the Heart and Stroke Foundation?

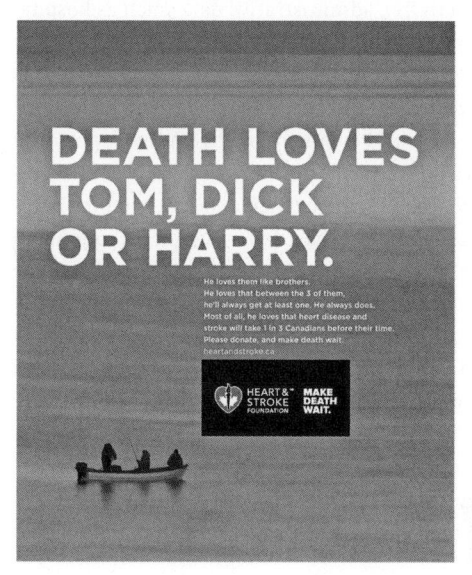

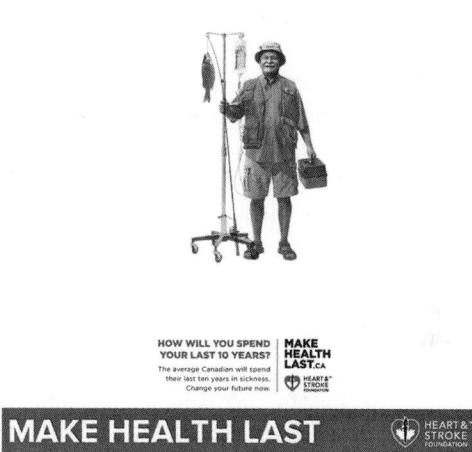

combine quantitative factors, such as the number of years lived, with qualitative factors, such as the quality of life enjoyed in the years added to the lifespan (i.e., life satisfaction). Health expectancy is a construct that has the potential to make a significant contribution to advances in the sociological measurement of population health and may help us to gain a better understanding of the factors that shape the health and well-being of the population.

The Need for a Mixed-Methods Approach to Measuring Health: Surveys, Statistics, and Stories

Etches and colleagues (2006, 31) point out that "current concepts of population health recognize that many interconnected aspects of society, the environment, and individuals all contribute to health." Therefore, a sociological understanding of population health requires a mixed-methods approach drawing on various types of information and incorporating multi-level analyses. In other words, health needs to be measured in multiple ways to gain a complete picture. In their review of population health indicators, Etches and colleagues comment on various sources of information that reflect the health of the population, including health survey data (regarding personal practices such as smoking and physical activity), administrative data (such as hospital and medical use statistics), census and vital statistics (such as birth and death rates), and data on economic factors (such as income and housing quality and the use of social services). This approach suggests that health and non-health sector data need to be combined to create comprehensive measures of population health. Etches et al. also comment briefly on the importance of including qualitative data in population health assessments. Consistent with the symbolic interactionist paradigm, they argue that by giving "voice" to study participants and listening carefully to their narrative histories, it is possible to learn about the lived experience of the individual and the social context within which health and wellness are given meaning. In their words, "The loss of contextual information in quantitative data increases the risk of misinterpretation of meanings" (Etches et al. 2006, 40). For example, quantitative surveys provide us with a wealth of data about the way that people rate their health, but qualitative studies are required to gain an understanding of the subjective meanings of self-rated health. Consequently, in concluding our discussion of the challenges we face in measuring the dimensions of health, we need to consider the relative merits of quantitative and qualitative studies and the ways in which diverse sources of population health information, such as surveys, statistics, and stories, can be integrated to give us a more complete understanding of the complex factors involved in the pursuit of health and wellness.

Population Health Surveys: The Canadian Experience

Let's take a quick look at the history of health surveys in Canada and consider the extent to which assessments of population health status in this country have incorporated measures of good health along with traditional measures of ill health. Although the Canadian experience of measuring the health of the population is lengthy, it is also uneven (Kendall, Lipskie, and MacEachern 1997). The first national household health survey, the *Canadian Sickness Survey*, was carried out in 1950–1. As the title of the survey suggests, the major focus was on the indicators of ill health, such as morbidity patterns and health-care utilization. Over the next 25-year period, little effort was made to assess the health status of Canadians at the national level, with the exception of the occasional survey of smoking habits or nutritional practices.

The next major national health survey, the *Canada Health Survey*, was not carried out until 1978–9. Despite the name change, the previous emphasis on measuring disease, disability, and utilization of formal health services remained. It should be noted, however, that the *Canada Health Survey* also collected information on emotional health and lifestyle practices, such as tobacco and alcohol use, daily activities, and preventive health behaviours. This study is important because it influenced the increasing number of health surveys that were subsequently carried out in Canada. A number of these population health assessments continued to focus on sickness (e.g., the nature, severity, and impact of disability), such as the *Canadian Health and Disabilities Survey* (1983) and the *Health and Activity Limitations Survey* (1986; 1991). Other surveys departed from the standard approach to health measurement and attempted to assess the positive aspects of population health. Examples include the *Canada Fitness Survey* (1981) and the follow-up to this study, the *Campbell Survey on Well-Being in Canada* (1988) as well as the *Health Promotion*

Survey (1985; 1990). In addition to the usual health status indicators and lifestyle practices, these studies explored attitudes and beliefs regarding health maintenance, barriers to health, and the influence of social relationships on health.

The National Population Health Survey (NPHS)

Building on this shift in research focus, the *National Population Health Survey* was explicitly designed to measure the health of Canadians and to monitor changes in health status and health behaviours over time. The first wave of data collection for this longitudinal survey was carried out in 1994. The goal of the NPHS was to collect longitudinal health-related information every two years on an ongoing basis from a panel of respondents drawn from a national sample of Canadians. The most recent data collection phase for which findings are available is Cycle 9, which was carried out in 2010–11.

The NPHS contains measures of both good health and ill health, including several measures that assess positive indicators of the good health dimension of wellness. For example, the NPHS assesses Antonovsky's sense of coherence as well as physical wellness—leisure-time physical activity and fitness levels; psychological wellness—sense of personal mastery, or the extent to which people believe that their life chances are under their control; emotional wellness—and self-esteem, or the positive feelings that an individual has about herself; and social wellness—levels of social support and social involvement. The NPHS made a concerted effort to measure the positive aspects of health and wellness (in addition to the usual negative indicators of sickness—e.g., chronic conditions, activity limitations, and the use of health-care services). The objective of the NPHS was to draw a sample that was sufficiently representative of the total population to permit generalizations, since it was impossible to include all Canadians in the study. Tambay and Catlin (1995) provide a detailed description of the NPHS two-stage sample design. In summary, the first step in the data collection process was to select the most knowledgeable member of the household and then to interview that person to obtain basic demographic and health-related information about all members of the household. The next step was to randomly select one individual (12 years of age or older) in each of the households to be a member of the longitudinal panel. This respondent was then interviewed in depth about her health in 1994 (and again in each of the subsequent waves of data collection). The sample of 17,276 Canadians included in the 1994 NPHS constitutes the longitudinal panel that was followed over time. Response rates varied from a high of 92.8 per cent in Cycle 2 to a low of 69.7 per cent in Cycle 9. Unfortunately, after nine cycles of data collection, the *National Population Health Survey* was discontinued.

The Canadian Community Health Survey (CCHS)

The first three cycles of the *National Population Health Survey* (i.e., 1994, 1996, and 1998) were both cross-sectional and longitudinal in design. Starting in 2000 (Cycle 4), the NPHS became strictly longitudinal—collecting standardized health information from the same individuals each cycle. The *Canadian Community Health Survey* was introduced in 2000 to replace the cross-sectional component of the NPHS and to collect data on Canadians' health status, risk factors, and health-care use. The target population for the CCHS once again included household residents aged 12 and over with the same exclusion criteria (e.g., Indian reserves and some remote areas). Each two-year collection cycle is composed of two distinct components, a health regional-level survey followed by a province-wide survey. The focus of the CCHS changes with each cycle and includes different respondents. For example, in 2013 the survey focused on access to health-care services and wait times and also collected supplementary information on food preparation skills to gather information about the types of ingredients used and the ways recipes are adjusted to prepare healthier meals. The ongoing objective of the CCHS is to provide cross-sectional health data at the sub-provincial level to assist regions in evaluating health services delivery and planning health promotion campaigns.

The Canadian Health Measures Survey (CHMS)

In 2007, the *Canadian Health Measures Survey* began to collect data and carried out the third cycle between January 2012 and December 2013. At this point, you may be wondering whether another national population health survey is really necessary. According to the proponents of the CHMS, a direct health measures survey is required for several reasons. The rationale for the survey is based on the argument that certain kinds of data, such as blood pressure and level of physical fitness, cannot be accurately determined by interviewing respondents; they require direct physical measurement. Furthermore, self-reported information, it is argued, may be biased and therefore unreliable for health-care planning and health promotion programs that require more accurate data. For example, when asked about their body weight, individuals may under-report their actual weight. The CHMS collects information about the health of Canadians through direct physical measurement of height and weight, waist circumference, resting heart rate, blood pressure, urine composition, and physical fitness (as well as questionnaires covering the usual topics of nutrition, smoking, alcohol use, and current health status). The data collection process begins with an in-home interview with each respondent, followed by a visit to a CHMS mobile examination centre specifically designed for this survey where the physical measures are carried out by health professionals. The information is intended to evaluate the relationship between disease risk factors and the types of health problems associated with prevalent diseases such as cardiovascular disease, hypertension, and diabetes, as well as obesity.

Although this continuing survey includes direct physical measures of health and "aims to overcome important data gaps in Canada's health information system through the collection of direct measures of health and wellness" (Tremblay, Wolfson, and Gorber 2007, 19), the CHMS fails to adequately address the psychosocial aspects of health and illness. The survey faces many challenges, not least of which is that the measures used do not adequately assess wellness! Physical fitness is clearly important, but it is equally imperative to gauge people's sense of healthiness and their social capacity to perform well roles in order to gain a complete understanding of the health and well-being of Canadians.

The Canadian Longitudinal Study of Aging (CLSA)

Finally, the most ambitious survey of population health conducted in Canada is currently underway. The *Canadian Longitudinal Study of Aging* was launched in 2009 and is unique in a number of respects. For example, this national survey explicitly reflects the importance of adopting a life course perspective for measuring health and wellness. The design of the study clearly acknowledges the fact that the effects of complex interactions among biological, psychological, and social factors, which change during an individual's lifetime, can take years to become evident in that individual's health and well-being. The longitudinal study design and extended follow-up are intended to provide a means of examining health trajectories and transitions over time. Furthermore, the study includes a combination of psychosocial and physical measures of health and illness.

The *CLSA* consists of a national, stratified random sample of 50,000 Canadian women and men between the ages of 45 and 85 (at the time of recruitment). Data collection will occur at three-year intervals, and the plan is to follow participants for at least 20 years. A short questionnaire is administered annually to maintain contact and minimize losses to follow-up. All study participants are asked to provide a great deal of information about demographic, social, psychological, and physical factors relevant to health and aging. In addition, 30,000 of the participants are asked to provide in-depth information through physical examinations and biological specimen collection (blood and urine).

Study participants were recruited from Statistics Canada's *Canadian Community Health Survey* and from provincial health registration databases. *CLSA* data will be linked to health administration databases such as publically funded drug plans, medical services plans, hospitalization, and continuing care/long-term care. By August 2013, the first 30,000 participants had been successfully recruited, and data collection is ongoing. The ultimate objectives of the *CLSA* are:

- to gain a better understanding of the complex interplay over time of multiple determinants of health;
- to learn more about the impact of non-medical factors (such as the social and economic changes that people experience as they age); and
- to contribute to improvements in the health and quality of life of Canadians.

In concluding this discussion, it should be acknowledged that health surveys have produced a great deal of statistical information about the health status of the Canadian population. Counting the prevalence and incidence of disease and calculating morbidity and mortality rates, however, is not the same as giving people the opportunity to account for their health and illness experiences and to explain how they manage ill health and maintain good health. Current trends in population health surveys suggest that there is still a way to go before we will be adequately prepared to design a survey that is based on a clear conceptualization of good health and positive indicators of wellness. Population health surveys provide little insight into the subjective meaning of good health or the processes involved in the pursuit of health and wellness. In other words, statistics don't tell the whole story!

Health Diary Studies and Illness Narrative Accounts: The Importance of Digging Deeper

In addition to collecting statistical information from interviews, direct physical health measures, or administrative data, health researchers need to give people a chance to describe, in their own words, what good health means to them. We also need to give them an opportunity to explain the activities they undertake in the pursuit of health and wellness and the way in which they make sense of sickness and manage illness experiences in their daily lives. In other words, we need to dig deeper if we hope to be able to unravel the mystery of health. Radley and Billig (1996) suggest that people's views about health and illness are best understood as accounts that they give to others and that there is an important difference in the type of health information that they disclose in public versus what they might disclose in private. They contend that public statements about our health (such as the information that we might provide an interviewer in a health survey or a health-care professional in a clinical setting) differ significantly from private stories about our health (such as what we might tell a close personal friend). In other words, there is an important distinction between the public statements we make about our physical condition or sense of well-being in response to questions raised by people who are perceived as experts and the health information we share with a close confidant in a private conversation that might start with "Have I got a story to tell you." According to Radley and Billig, it is vitally important that we listen closely when people talk about their health and tell their personal stories and that we recognize that public and private accounts of health and illness reflect the nature of social relationships in which they are embedded and the social context within which the information exchange occurs. With these points in mind, the following discussion briefly summarizes two qualitative methods that have been used to gather more in-depth health information: health diary studies, which allow people to provide information about their health and illness behaviour, and narrative accounts, which enable people to tell personal stories about their health and illness.

Health Diaries

Although health diaries have been used as a data collection method for many years, this approach to measurement remains underutilized. Verbrugge (1980) provides a good summary of the advantages and disadvantages of health diaries as a prospective method for collecting health information. She begins by pointing out that personal interviews and medical records allow a limited view of population health because "many health problems are self-treated or receive no treatment, and many health activities taken by individuals are preventive rather than curative in purpose" (Verbrugge 1980, 73). In her opinion, a **health diary**, or a daily record, is well suited for gathering information about transient symptomatic conditions that do not restrict daily activities or prompt medical care and for gaining a more complete picture of population health. The health diary is a data collection instrument used to gather detailed information about ongoing health and illness behaviours. While the health diary may be similar in format to the type of questionnaire used in survey research, the critical difference is that survey questionnaires are completed retrospectively and usually only once while the health diary is filled out each day during the period of the study. According to Verbrugge, the health diary has several advantages, including reduced recall error, increased validity, and higher levels of reporting. At the same time, she notes possible disadvantages, such as increased respondent burden, conditioning effects, and the complexity of data collection and analysis, but concludes that these limitations are not supported by the evidence and that diaries provide a more comprehensive and accurate view of people's health than retrospective interviews.

Over the years, health diaries have been used for studying the types of self-care practices people employ to deal with everyday health problems (Freer 1980) as well as older adults' self-care responses to symptoms (Stoller, Forster, and Portugal 1993). In fact, daily health diaries have been used in a number of different studies of older adults to investigate the process of health-care decision-making (Hickey, Akiyama, and Rakowski 1991), the interpretation of symptoms (Stoller 1993), and general health and well-being (Milligan, Bingley, and Gatrell 2005). These studies highlight the importance of the social context within which people interpret the seriousness of their symptoms and decide on a course of action (i.e., whether to self-treat or seek professional health care). Other diary studies have used daily health records to investigate gender differences in illness behaviour (Gijsbers van Wijk, Huisman, and Kolk 1999) and more recently to explore the links between family functioning, stressful daily family experiences, and long-term health problems (Robles et al. 2013). This last study concluded that "intensive diary designs have great promise for unpacking the mechanisms that explain how family settings impact emotions and health" (2013, 186).

Overall, health diary studies provide unique insights into the nature of health and illness behaviour. This approach to measuring the dimensions of population health has contributed significantly to the body of knowledge about the process by which people interpret the meaning of daily symptoms and manage their illness experiences and, to a lesser extent, the ways in which they attempt to maintain good health. For example, Hickey et al. (1991, 183) conclude that "the health diary method provides a useful way to identify the number and type of illness symptoms that tend to occur daily and to examine the process of making treatment decisions." At the same time, it should be noted that the diary method has the potential to collect valuable information (that is not captured by population health surveys) about people's routine preventive practices and the types of daily behaviours in which they engage to maintain and enhance their health. Milligan, Bingley, and Gatrell (2005) agree that health diaries provide valuable insights into the often hidden (or taken-for-granted) aspects of our daily lives and our health status. They describe diaries as "an underused method in the health researcher's toolbox" even though evidence indicates that they "can offer unique insights and increased opportunities to understand the context in which health and illness is experienced, needs expressed and accounts given" (Milligan et al. 2005, 1891). The question that remains, then, is: Why have social scientists been so slow to adopt this promising health research method?

Illness Narrative Accounts

To conclude this discussion, let's take a quick look at a qualitative approach that focuses explicitly on the way in which people attempt to make sense out of sickness. **Illness narrative accounts** enable people and patients, particularly those living with chronic illness, to recount their stories and to describe the factors that they believe influenced the onset of their condition, the seriousness of their symptoms, and personal strategies for managing the condition, as well as present and anticipated future effects of the condition on their body, self-identity, and social relationships. Narrative accounts have been described as a "means by which the links between body, self and society are articulated" (Bury 2001, 281) and as way to gain a better understanding of the lived experience of illness and disability (Garden 2010).

A number of studies have used narrative methods. For example, Kleinman (1988) highlights the importance of the illness narrative as a method for gaining a more meaningful understanding of the suffering that typically accompanies serious, disabling chronic illness. Similarly, Frank (1995) characterizes people in ill health as "wounded storytellers" and points out that while medical records may contain the official account of the illness, the embodied stories that people tell reveal the personal and social significance of their illness. According to Bury (2001), there is a renewed interest in illness narratives as a research method, in part as a result of the increasingly common experience of learning to live with chronic illnesses. Some of the recent studies using this approach to measuring health focus on the consequences of serious illness and disability for self-identity (Medved and Brockmeier 2008). Others emphasize the importance of listening to the voice of experience (not just the voice of the expert) and recognizing the power of stories over statistics (Hurwitz, Greenhalgh, and Skultans 2004). Similarly, Pederson (2013) advocates the use of a technique she calls "narrative interviewing" in illness contexts as a way of getting the "whole story." In any case, the common message of this research is that we need to acknowledge that illness is an important occasion for storytelling. At the same time, even Verbrugge (1980, 94), after extolling the advantages of diary studies, concludes that "no single procedure for collecting health data is superior in all respects." There is no one methodology able to completely unravel the mystery of health! Clearly, then, what is called for is a mixed-methods approach to measuring the dimensions of health.

Chapter Summary

It is generally acknowledged today that health is a multi-dimensional concept that includes three interrelated components: physical—the presence or absence of signs of disease and symptoms of illness; psychological—feelings of well-being; and social—the capacity to perform usual well roles. This is certainly not a new idea and can be traced back to the 1948 World Health Organization's definition of health, which recognized that health is multi-dimensional. Furthermore, there is now widespread agreement that good health means more than just being relatively free of disease and illness; it means being fit (physically), feeling healthy (psychologically), and effectively performing well roles (socially).

Good health (wellness) and ill health (sickness) can be viewed as two separate but related dimensions. The meanings of wellness and sickness are socially constructed through a complex ongoing process of health status designation and are therefore subject to change. While meanings may be renegotiated, the good health dimension of wellness refers to "the ability of the person to adapt to continuing physical, social, and personal change" (Baranowski 1981, 247). In social terms, the adaptive capacity of the individual is reflected in our ability to carry out routine tasks associated with our well roles (e.g., familial and occupational roles). In turn, the other components of wellness (i.e., fitness and feelings of healthiness) may vary with the rights and duties of our usual well roles. For example, mild bronchitis may be a serious health problem for a professional singer but only a minor inconvenience for an office worker. Similarly, an older university professor might be able to continue to view herself as healthy despite having arthritis, in contrast to an undergraduate student who is a competitive athlete. Thus, although health may be viewed as a crucial resource for living, it is evident that we do not all experience wellness or sickness in the same way.

Furthermore, we typically take good health for granted until it becomes ill health and demands our attention. Consequently, we are better at recognizing ill health and tend to rely on standardized indicators of sickness (e.g., morbidity and mortality rates) to assess population health status. Good health is more difficult to define precisely and to recognize in ourselves and in others. This has important implications for our ability to measure wellness and the positive aspects of good health, such as sense of coherence and life satisfaction. Adopting a salutogenic model of health to guide population health research can help us to discover the meaning of good health and to gain a better understanding of the ways in which salutary factors protect and promote good health and social factors contribute to the pursuit of health and wellness.

It should be apparent from this discussion that population health assessment requires a comprehensive, inclusive approach to measurement and multi-level analyses. This means conducting innovative research on the health of Canadians that combines

- measures of risk factors that increase our susceptibility to disease and illness;
- measures of salutary factors that protect and enhance our health and well-being;
- positive indicators of good health (wellness);

- standard negative indicators of ill health (sickness);
- social and psychological aspects of health (quality of life and health expectancy); and
- physical functioning and length of life.

To gain a more complete picture of the health of Canadians, we have to do a better job of integrating quantitative and qualitative approaches to measurement, such as population health surveys and health diary studies, and synthesizing health-related information from diverse sources, such as narrative accounts and personal stories, survey interviews, administrative databases, and official government statistics. By integrating surveys, statistics, and stories, we can improve our ability to effectively assess population health to both count and account for health and illness and, ultimately, advance our understanding of the complex factors involved in the pursuit of health and wellness.

It is time to conclude our discussion of the theoretical and methodological issues involved in studying health and turn our attention to the factors that shape our health and wellness. After an overview of the general determinants of health, we will systematically examine both structural (e.g., social class, gender, ethnicity, and age) and personal (e.g., lifestyle behavioural practices) determinants of health. The next section of the book will explore the link between sources of social inequality and health disparities and review Canadian and international evidence that clearly demonstrates that social location creates a set of life chances that, in turn, influence our health choices and ultimately our health status.

Study Questions

1. Explain the major differences between measuring personal health and population health status.
2. Summarize the key features of the salutogenic model of health.
3. Describe the process of health status designation.
4. Explain the difference between the presence of disease and the experience of illness.
5. Comment on the validity of global self-rated health as an indicator of health status.
6. Summarize the limitations of health status assessments that rely entirely on the indicators of ill health.
7. Describe the advantages and disadvantages of using health diaries in assessing population health.
8. Comment critically on our current ability to measure the positive indicators of good health and wellness.

Recommended Readings

Antonovsky, A. 1996. "The salutogenic model as a theory to guide health promotion." *Health Promotion International* 11(1): 11–18.

Etches, V., J. Frank, E. Di Ruggiero, and D. Manuel. 2006. "Measuring population health: A review of indicators." *Annual Review of Public Health* 27: 29–55.

Frankish, J., G. Veenstra, and G. Moulton. 1999. "Population health in Canada: Issues and challenges for policy, practice and research." *Canadian Journal of Public Health* 90: S71–5.

Kaplan, G., and O. Baron-Epel. 2003. "What lies behind the subjective evaluation of health status?" *Social Science and Medicine* 56: 1669–76.

Kindig, D., and G. Stoddart. 2003. "What is population health?" *American Journal of Public Health* 93: 380–3.

Lindstrom, B., and M. Eriksson. 2005. "Salutogenesis." *Journal of Epidemiology and Community Health* 59: 440–2.

Millar, J., and C. Hull. 1997. "Measuring human wellness." *Social Indicators Research* 40: 147–58.

Milligan, C., A. Bingley, and A. Gatrell. 2005. "Digging deep: Using diary techniques to explore the place of health and well-being amongst older people." *Social Science and Medicine* 61: 1882–92.

Recommended Websites

Canadian Community Health Survey (CCHS):
www.statcan.gc.ca/imdb-bmdi/3226-eng.htm

Canadian Index of Wellbeing:
https://uwaterloo.ca/canadian-index-wellbeing

Canadian Institute for Health Information:
www.cihi.ca

Canadian Longitudinal Study on Aging:
www.clsa-elcv.ca

Center on Salutogenesis: The Resource Center on Salutogenesis at the University West:
www.salutogenesis.hv.se/eng/Home.2.html

Health in Canada:
www.statcan.gc.ca/health-sante/index-eng.htm

Health Indicators:
www.statcan.gc.ca/pub/82-221-x/01201/4149364-eng.htm

Health Utilities Group/Health Utilities Index:
fhs.mcmaster.ca/hug

Institute of Population Health:
www.iph.uottawa.ca/eng/index.html

International Union for Health Promotion and Education (IUHPE) Global Working Group on Salutogenesis:
www.iuhpe.org/index.php/en/global-working-groups-gwgs/gwg-on-salutogenesis

National Population Health Survey (NPHS):
www.statcan.gc.ca/eng/survey/household/3225

Public Health Agency of Canada—Population Health Approach:
www.phac-aspc.gc.ca/ph-sp/approach-approche/index-eng.php

Part Two

Exploring the Factors That Shape Health and Wellness

Part Two, Exploring the Factors That Shape Health and Wellness, contains five chapters that provide a comprehensive critical sociological analysis of structural and behavioural factors that influence health status. Chapter 4 starts with an overview of the factors that are recognized as major determinants of population health (i.e., human biology, lifestyle, environment, and the use of formal health-care services) and highlights the important part played by social determinants in the pursuit of health and wellness. This introductory review is followed by a discussion of the relative importance of health determinants and the need to clarify the distinction between the determinants of good health and ill health. The chapter concludes by emphasizing the fact that if we hope to learn more about what makes people healthy, we need to adopt an intersectional life course approach in order to gain a better understanding of the cumulative effect of health determinants.

The next three chapters address sources of social inequality that are associated with disparities in population health. Chapter 5 begins with a discussion of the meaning of social inequality and then examines the link between socioeconomic circumstances and health status. The chapter summarizes Canadian and international evidence that clearly demonstrates that income, occupation, and education are closely related to position on the social gradient of health. Alternative explanations for persistent class-based disparities in population health are explored. Chapter 6 continues to critically assess the relationship between social location and health and well-being by examining the gendered nature of health disparities. The chapter summarizes research evidence indicating that there are significant differences between women and men in life expectancy, major causes of death, health and illness experiences, and the use of formal health-care services. In addition, gender differences in the social determinants of health are discussed, and the chapter ends with a review of alternative explanations for gender differences in health and illness. Chapter 7 extends the analysis of structural factors that shape health by considering the relationship between ethnicity and health. The chapter examines the links among minority status, social exclusion, and migration and health by selectively reviewing ethnic group differences in health and illness. Aboriginal health issues are highlighted. Each of the three preceding chapters in this part of the book considers the importance of adopting an intersectional life course perspective to gain a greater understanding of the ways in which social factors operate at different stages in the lifecycle, interact with one another, and together contribute to the creation of health disparities.

The last chapter in Part Two shifts the focus to personal determinants of health and wellness. Chapter 8 tackles the unresolved debate about what constitutes a health lifestyle. The discussion addresses the structure–agency question and makes the case that a better understanding of the ways in which lifestyle behaviours contribute to good health requires a more systematic effort to identify the relative contributions of social context (chance) and personal conduct (choice) to the production of health. The chapter concludes with a theoretical discussion of the ways in which structural and behavioural determinants interact with one another and the multiple pathways through which they influence our health across the life course. An intersectional model of health across the life course is outlined to provide a conceptual framework for guiding future research on the combined intersecting effects of social locations, such as class, gender, and ethnicity, and personal factors, such as lifestyle behavioural practices, in shaping population health and wellness.

Making People Healthy: General Determinants of Health and Wellness

Learning Objectives

In this chapter, you will examine a variety of factors that shape health status and gain a greater understanding of the general determinants of population health by considering

- the distinction between personal and structural determinants of health;
- the major determinants of health status;
- the relative importance of health determinants; and
- the need to address the determinants of both good health and ill health.

What Makes People Healthy? Two Different Answers

This is not an easy question to answer. Although we have learned a great deal over the years about the general determinants of health status, we still know much more about what makes people sick than we know about what makes them healthy. Due to the dominance of the biomedical approach to health care, the primary emphasis traditionally has been on searching for the causes of disease and illness. To illustrate this point, let's briefly consider two different ways to answer the question: What makes people healthy?

The traditional health promotion answer to this question emphasizes the importance of disease prevention and personal practices such as smoking and physical activity. The health promotion message typically conveyed to the public is directed at raising the health consciousness of individuals and is based on the assumption that people can control the major factors that influence their health (i.e., modifiable risk factors). As we will see in Chapter 8, this message highlights the importance of individual responsibility for engaging in health-protective behaviours and reflects the type of ideas about what makes people healthy that have dominated the thinking and actions of most health-care professionals and public health officials for many years. For example, traditional tips for better health include:

- Don't smoke. If you can, quit. If you can't quit, cut down.
- Keep physically active.
- Follow a balanced diet with plenty of fruit and vegetables.
- If you drink alcohol, do so in moderation.
- Manage stress by, for example, taking time to relax.

This list is a condensed version of the 10 traditional tips for better health discussed by Raphael and colleagues (2006, 119). Health sociologists point out that while these types of health-protective activities are a necessary component of health promotion, they are not sufficient to significantly improve the health and well-being of Canadians. The individualized approach to health promotion has had limited success (e.g., the majority of Canadians are still not physically active), in part because it omits critical social determinants of population health.

The alternative health promotion answer to the question "what makes people healthy?" emphasizes the social determinants of health. The World Health Organization (2014b) defines the **social determinants of health** as "the conditions in which people are born, grow, live, work and age, including the health system. These circumstances are shaped by the distribution of money, power and resources at global, national and local levels, which are themselves influenced by policy choices." As previously described, a population health perspective focuses on societal factors that affect our health (such as the living and working conditions of Canadians) and is based on the assumption that the most important health determinants are beyond the control of the individual. Alternative tips for better health from a social determinants perspective might include:

- Don't be poor. If you can, stop. If you can't, try not to be poor for long.
- Practise not losing your job, and don't become unemployed.
- Don't live in a neighbourhood with high rates of crime and low rates of civic participation.
- Don't belong to a visible minority that makes you a target of discrimination and social exclusion.
- Don't live in a society characterized by social inequality, or, if you must, be rich and powerful.

Once again, this list was influenced by Raphael's 10 social determinants tips for better health (Raphael 2006, 119). In this case, however, the list was revised to emphasize the impact of the social environment and societal factors such as the distribution of income and wealth, employment, and housing on our health. The basic idea underlying the population health approach is that, without minimizing the importance of discovering the causes of prevalent conditions such as cancer and heart disease, it is equally important to learn more about the causes of good health and the contribution of factors that are health-protective. Finding more effective ways to keep Canadians healthy and to promote population health requires a better understanding of the determinants of good health and wellness.

The population health promotion message reflects Antonovsky's (1979) salutogenic model of health discussed previously. For example, it highlights the importance of improving the living and working conditions of Canadians to provide a more health-protective environment that enhances the health and wellness of the population. As well, this approach recognizes that health is shaped by societal factors that are beyond the control of the individual. In contrast, the traditional health promotion message reflects a pathogenic approach to personal determinants of health and highlights the importance of encouraging individual Canadians to change their behavioural practices in an effort to reduce risk factors that contribute to ill health. It should be apparent that a complete explanation of why some Canadians are healthier than others requires a critical examination of a broad range of health determinants, including both individual routine practices and the social context within which health-related behaviours occur.

In an effort to explain how people manage to stay healthy, Antonovsky (1979) made an important distinction between pathogenesis and salutogenesis. The first term is much more familiar to us than the second one. **Pathogenesis** refers to the origins of disease. The biomedical model that guides contemporary health care emphasizes the importance of gaining a greater understanding of the etiology (causes) of major diseases and the nature of the pathology (signs and symptoms) associated with these conditions. The search for an explanation of disease causation is driven by the hope that this will lead to the discovery of effective means of treatment and, ultimately, cures for prevalent diseases. While these are obviously worthwhile and highly desirable objectives, it is evident that as diseases that were widespread in the past have been brought under control in most countries (e.g., diphtheria) or essentially eliminated (e.g., smallpox), other, equally threatening diseases have taken their place (e.g., cancer, cardiovascular disease). Consequently, Antonovsky challenged us to consider whether conquering one disease at a time will eventually lead us to a healthier life.

To reach the goal of improving population health, we also need to gain an understanding of the determinants of good health. Antonovsky introduced the term **salutogenesis** to encourage researchers to explore the factors that protect and enhance good health (versus those that contribute to ill health). The concept of salutogenesis is based on the Latin term for health (*salus*) and refers to the origins (or genesis) of positive health. To reinforce the importance of this alternative approach, Antonovsky devoted a great deal of attention to the significance of studying health instead of disease. In his opinion, the following are crucial questions that need to be answered:

- Why do people stay healthy (rather than asking why people get sick)?
- What types of salutary factors help us to maintain good health (rather than asking what types of risk factors increase our susceptibility to illness and disease)?

Antonovsky provides a thought-provoking analysis of how we manage to stay well and characterizes salutogenesis as a great mystery waiting to be solved. In his words, "It should, then, be clear that the mystery of health is indeed intriguing" (1979, 35). More than three and a half decades have passed since Antonovsky made this statement, and we are still trying to unravel the mystery of health and wellness!

The salutogenic model is valuable because it demands that we learn more about the determinants of good health. It should be obvious that the development of effective population health promotion strategies requires a thorough understanding of what makes people healthy. Despite Antonovsky's advice, however, attention continues to be focused primarily on pathogenesis and disease prevention. It is time once again to echo Antonovsky's call for a shift to a salutogenic model of health. In addition to addressing the causes of ill health (sickness), we must make a concerted effort to discover the sources of good health (wellness). Haflon, Larson, and Russ (2010, 17) agree that we need to pay more attention to positive health-promoting social factors and state that "not all social determinants are negative, and a greater understanding of positive determinants could inform the design of effective health promotion interventions."

We need to learn more about the salutary factors that contribute to the maintenance of good health and enhance individuals' hardiness and health-protective behaviours, as well as people's resistance to adverse social and physical conditions related to the onset of ill health. In addition, we need to learn more about the types of factors that foster a sense of healthiness, physical fitness, and general social capacity for the performance of well roles and, ultimately, contribute to improvements in the level of population health. While we still do not have all the answers, at least questions about how some people, and not others, manage to stay well have been receiving growing prominence over the past few decades in the research literature addressing the social determinants of population health (e.g., Evans, Barer, and Marmor 1994; Eyles et al. 2001; Mahamoud, Roche, and Homer 2013; Marmot and Wilkinson 2006; Mikkonen and Raphael 2010; National Forum on Health 1996; Prus 2011; Raphael 2009).

For example, Evans (1994, 4) argues that there are important unanswered questions about the determinants of health for both individuals and populations. In his opinion, "Many of the conventional explanations of the determinants of health—of why some people are healthy and others not—are at best seriously incomplete if not simply wrong." He further states that "This is unfortunate, because modern societies devote a very large share of their wealth, effort, and attention to trying to maintain or improve the health of the individuals that make up their populations." This highlights two important points that need to be addressed today regarding population health promotion strategies. First, conventional explanations of disparities of health are incomplete and need to be expanded to gain a more comprehensive understanding of the social determinants of both good health and ill health. Second, we need to incorporate both individual and societal factors in our search for a causal explanation of differences in health status if we are going to be able to keep Canadians healthy and make significant improvements in population health.

Personal and Structural Health Determinants

Studies of health determinants and their contribution to improvements in the health of the population typically distinguish between personal (or individual) factors and structural (or collective) factors. For example, Gunning-Schepers and Hagen (1987) suggest that the major determinants of health can be divided into two broad categories: determinants that are endogenous in nature, or specific to the individual, and determinants that are exogenous, or exert an external influence on health. **Personal determinants** are evident at the individual level and include factors such as genetic makeup as well as beliefs, attitudes, and personal health practices. **Structural determinants** are evident at the societal level and include aspects of the social and economic environment such as income distribution, rates of unemployment, living and working conditions, and the changing age structure of society, as well as the way in which health-care services are organized and delivered.

While we can distinguish between personal and structural health determinants, it is important to recognize that "the social determinants of health operate in a complex and dynamic manner at various nested levels of influence" (Haflon, Larson, and Russ 2010, 18). The basic assumption underlying this distinction is that while these interrelated determinants operate at different levels, they also interact with each other, and, together, the intersections of history and biography have combined effects on population health. To illustrate, it is typically assumed that structural or collective factors (such as supportive social environments and available health services) provide the societal context within which personal or individual factors (such as lifestyle health and self-care practices) take place. For example, the decision to engage in specific health-protective behaviours (e.g., to make a change in dietary practice or level of physical activity) may be affected by the socioeconomic resources available to the individual, encouragement from family members, and/or the advice of a health-care professional. Consequently, a thorough understanding of what makes people healthy requires a sociological analysis of both structural and personal health determinants.

Figure 4.1 summarizes the major social determinants of population health that will be considered in this book. The arrows in Figure 4.1 illustrate the fact that both structural and personal factors have direct effects on our health. They also influence each other and, ultimately, have

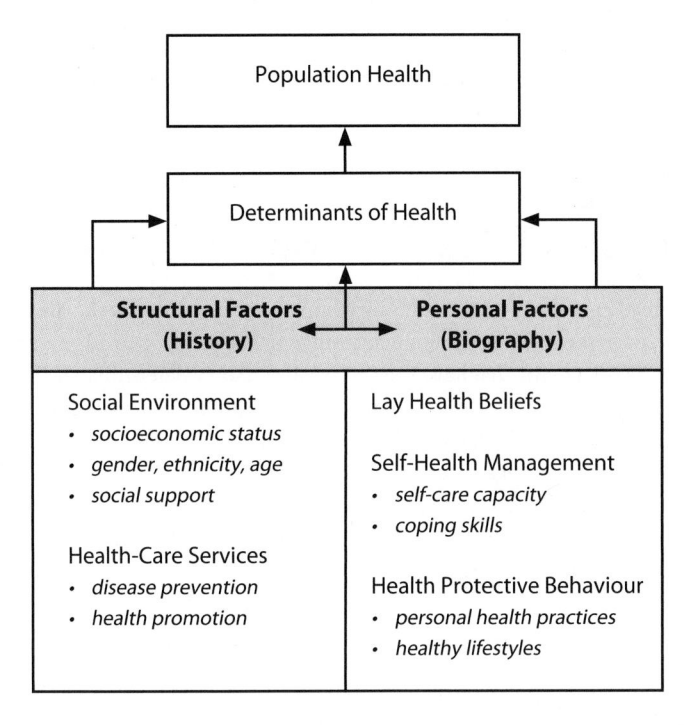

Figure 4.1 Social Determinants of Population Health in a Sociological Perspective

```
                    Population Health
                           ↑
                  Determinants of Health
                           ↑
    ┌──────────────────────┬──────────────────────┐
    │  Structural Factors  │   Personal Factors   │
    │      (History)       │     (Biography)      │
    ├──────────────────────┼──────────────────────┤
    │ Social Environment   │ Lay Health Beliefs   │
    │  • socioeconomic     │                      │
    │    status            │ Self-Health          │
    │  • gender, ethnicity,│   Management         │
    │    age               │  • self-care capacity│
    │  • social support    │  • coping skills     │
    │                      │                      │
    │ Health-Care Services │ Health Protective    │
    │  • disease prevention│   Behaviour          │
    │  • health promotion  │  • personal health   │
    │                      │    practices         │
    │                      │  • healthy lifestyles│
    └──────────────────────┴──────────────────────┘
```

a combined effect on our health (i.e., the three-headed arrow). This interaction effect makes it challenging to identify the unique contribution of structural and personal factors to population health, as we will discuss shortly when we consider the relative importance of health determinants. At the same time, it clearly demonstrates the need to use the sociological imagination to incorporate both history and biography in our explanation of what makes people healthy.

To explore the factors that shape our health in more detail, we will examine both structural and personal determinants. A critical analysis of structural health determinants begins in Chapter 5 with an investigation of the link between health disparities and sources of social inequality such as socioeconomic status. Chapters 6 and 7 then examine the impact that gender and ethnicity have on population health. The analysis of structural determinants also includes a discussion of the relationships between informal care, social support, and health (Chapter 9) as well as formal medical care and population health (Chapter 10). Our systematic examination of the determinants of health also considers the influence of personal factors such as health lifestyle behavioural practices (Chapter 8). The personal determinants that receive closer attention include lay beliefs about health maintenance and illness management and routine health behaviours such as participation in leisure-time physical activity.

The purpose of this critical examination of the social determinants of health is to learn more about the salutary factors that enable Canadians to stay well. Adopting a population health perspective (as described in Chapter 3) means that we have accepted the sociological view that good health is a dynamic social product that is shaped by structural factors and is given personal meaning within the context of people's lived experience. This perspective also means that the objective of analysis is to advance our understanding of how societal factors and social interaction are related to population health.

The Major Determinants of Population Health: An Overview of the Four Key Factors

There is widespread agreement that the many complex, interacting factors affecting our health can be summarized in terms of four major determinants. The purpose of this discussion is to provide an overview of the factors that have been recognized as key determinants of health, ranging from human biology to the social environment. A number of the issues raised in this section will be pursued in more detail in the chapters that follow.

As research attention slowly shifts from disease and illness to health and wellness, the search for causal factors becomes progressively broader and more complex. According to Raphael, "Canadian and international interest in the social determinants of health has led to a refocusing upon the non-medical and non-behavioural precursors of health and illness" (Raphael 2006, 116). Researchers continue to argue that "the primary factors that shape the health of Canadians are not medical treatments or lifestyle choices but rather the living conditions they experience" (Mikkonen and Raphael 2010, 7). Canadian ministers of health have played a leading role in the development of population health initiatives at national and global levels. A critical turning point in thinking about the determinants of health was the publication in 1974 by Lalonde (as federal minister of health) of a new perspective on the health of Canadians. This policy document explicitly acknowledged that health status is not simply the direct result of access to formal health-care services and that a variety of other factors are more important in determining the health of the population. Lalonde identified four key determinants of health: human biology, lifestyle, environment, and health care. This broad approach to the investigation of health determinants has proven to be quite influential.

A number of years later, another federal minister of health (Epp 1986) developed a framework for health promotion that builds on this earlier approach to health determinants. In this policy document, health is characterized as an essential part of everyday living. Based on this viewpoint, it is argued that health cannot be understood as simply the result or outcome of the treatment—or even the cure—of disease and illness. Furthermore, the health of the population cannot be adequately measured in terms of sickness and death (as discussed in the previous chapter). Health is portrayed as a resource for living! As such, "It is a basic and dynamic force in our daily lives, influenced by our circumstances, our beliefs, our culture and our social, economic and physical environments" (Epp 1986, 3). In other words, health is influenced by a broad range of factors that, once again, are categorized as human biology, lifestyle, the organization of health care, and the social and physical environments in which people live. Let's take a closer look at these four key factors.

Biology

The starting point for discussions of health determinants is typically biology. As the sociology of the body paradigm makes clear, because we are embodied beings, human biology plays an important part in shaping our health status. This includes factors such as individual genetic endowment (or genotype) and the functioning of various body systems (e.g., the immune and hormonal systems). Each person inherits a combination of genes from their parents that influences many of their physical characteristics and personality traits as well as (in some cases) certain diseases, or susceptibility to diseases, that may run in the family. In fact, many diseases have a genetic basis (such as cystic fibrosis, muscular dystrophy, and hemophilia).

There is no question that biology is a fundamental health determinant. The genetic endowment of the individual and biology in general contribute directly, in many different ways, to our health. In addition, biological factors interact with other personal and structural determinants (i.e., social, cultural, and psychological factors) and therefore also indirectly shape our health. It is now understood that the combined effect of hereditary factors (e.g., a particular genetic defect or chromosomal abnormality) and environmental factors contributes to the causation of most diseases (Burdon 2003). For example, heredity is a major factor in the development of some forms of asthma along with exposure to air pollutants such as dust and tobacco smoke. In other words, heredity may make us susceptible, but environmental and lifestyle factors (e.g., smoking) may influence the onset of the disease. Our genetic makeup, along with our personal health practices, the environment in which we live, and the developmental and aging processes that our bodies undergo, affect the types of diseases that we experience across the life course.

It is important to keep these points in mind as we proceed. It has been argued, however, that biological factors are of limited relevance to population health. For example, Millar and Hull (1997, 148) contend that "biological influences do not appear to explain the large differences which exist in population health." They point to the significant differences that exist in the health status of various groups of Canadians (e.g., Aboriginal people) and suggest that the search for explanatory factors should focus on the social environment, particularly living and working conditions. More specifically, they highlight the importance of factors such as unemployment, underemployment (i.e., low-paying but demanding work), and lack of social support from family, friends, and communities as key health determinants.

Consequently, we need to gain a better understanding of the ways in which social determinants affect population health if we are going to be able to better explain inequalities in health status among Canadians. In addition, we need to identify health promotion strategies that might be more effective at improving the health of all Canadians. It has been recognized for some time that in achieving health for all (Epp 1986, 4), "the first challenge we face is to find ways of reducing inequities in the health of low- versus high-income groups in Canada." While this is an extremely challenging task, it is possible to develop community interventions aimed at changing the social circumstances that affect people's health. In contrast, most biophysical aspects of health cannot be easily modified, since biology and genetics are not (at this time) readily amenable to significant interventions without considerable controversy (e.g., genetic engineering and cloning). Therefore, without disregarding the importance of biology and its impact on personal health, the following discussion will focus primarily on social determinants and their impact on population health. As we turn our attention to the remaining key determinants of health, it is important to remember that there is a complex relationship between biology and the other major social factors that shape our health status.

Lifestyle Behaviour

It has been claimed for some time that health behaviours may be understood as a part of a complex lifestyle that affects our health status. The relationship between lifestyle behaviour and health has received considerable research attention over the past several decades (e.g., Abel 1991;

Blaxter 1990; Bruhn 1988; Cockerham 2005; Kickbusch 1986). Many studies have documented the fact that routine personal practices aimed at protecting health and preventing illness (i.e., healthy lifestyle behaviours) contribute to good health, while other personal practices contribute to ill health. The ways in which lifestyle behaviours contribute to the social production of health will be examined in Chapter 8 when we consider the unresolved debate about what constitutes a healthy lifestyle. For now, it is sufficient to acknowledge two important points concerning the sociological understanding of health lifestyles.

The first is that personal practices such as smoking, drinking alcohol, eating habits, and physical activity affect our health and well-being. In fact, "personal health practices have an important influence on health at any age" (Statistics Canada 1999, 83). It has been argued that many of Canada's most common health problems today are linked to these practices (Arnett 2006). For example, smoking is the leading cause of lung cancer and a major risk factor for cardiovascular disease, while alcohol misuse is associated with premature death resulting from accidents and injuries. In the same way, unhealthy eating habits and poor nutrition are associated with conditions such as cardiovascular disease and diabetes.

A study by Mokdad and colleagues (2004; 2005) attempted to clarify the major causes of death. These health researchers employed a sophisticated methodology to compare and rank causes of death as designated by the US Centers for Disease Control (CDC) with the "actual" causes of death. The data reported in Table 4.1 clearly illustrate the important role that lifestyle behaviours play in morbidity and mortality. A large proportion of deaths each year result from modifiable lifestyle-related behaviours. The data show that "tobacco use and poor diet and physical inactivity contributed to the largest number of deaths, and the number of deaths related to poor diet and physical inactivity is increasing" (Mokdad et al. 2005, 293).

Reviewing these data prompted Arnett (2006, 28) to raise a critical question: "Since knowledge about behavioural risk factors for a variety of serious illnesses that lead to significant morbidity, mortality, as well as to enormous cost, has been so well established, one might wonder if health care systems have taken the initiative to implement effective programs to achieve and

Table 4.1 What Causes Death?

Rank	CDC Designated Causes of Death	Rank	"Actual" Causes of Death
1	Heart disease	1	Tobacco use
2	Cancer	2	Diet/physical inactivity
3	Cerebrovascular disease	3	Alcohol consumption
4	Chronic lung disease	4	Microbial agents
5	Unintentional injuries	5	Toxic agents
6	Diabetes	6	Motor vehicle accidents
7	Flu/pneumonia	7	Firearms
8	Alzheimer's disease	8	Risky sexual behaviour
9	Kidney disease	9	Illicit drug use

Source: Arnett 2006.

maintain behavioural change to improve health." Unfortunately, as Arnett goes on to point out, the focus of the existing health-care system on the biological determinants of health has taken up resources that might well be better directed at social determinants of population health. This conclusion is supported by recent data showing the powerful relationship between lifestyle behaviours and morbidity and mortality. For example, Murray and Lopez (2013) review international evidence that clearly demonstrates that lifestyle behaviours such as tobacco and alcohol use, dietary practices, and physical inactivity are among the leading risk factors that contribute to the "global burden of disease." Similarly, Ford and colleagues (2012) examined the links between these fundamentally important lifestyle behaviours and all-cause mortality in a national sample of adults in the United States and conclude that people who do not smoke, engage in adequate physical activity, and eat a healthy diet can substantially reduce their risk of early death. Their results show conclusively that these lifestyle behaviours have "an enormous impact on mortality" (2012, 26).

The second important point concerning health lifestyles that arises from a sociological analysis is that while we usually consider these types of behavioural practices to be based on individual choice, health sociologists point out that our position in the social structure patterns health lifestyles among different groups of people within society. We will explore this point in more detail in the following chapters, but for now it should be noted that those living in poverty (or who are in some other way socially excluded) have higher rates of risky lifestyle behaviours such as smoking, high-fat diets, and substance abuse.

Environment

Commenting on the environment as a major determinant of health, Brown (2000, 143) contends that "it would be impossible to consider thinking or writing about medical sociology, public health, or social medicine without placing the environment in a central position." Brown (2013) uses the term "environmentally induced diseases" to describe environmental health problems that are caused, at least in part, by toxic substances in people's immediate surroundings (such as air, water, soil, food, and household goods). Most discussions of the determinants of health distinguish between the impact of the physical environment and the social environment on our health and well-being. Following this distinction, we will first consider the physical environment as a major determinant of population health before moving on to consider the social environment and health.

The Physical Environment

Although widespread recognition of the negative impact of industrialization on the environment is a fairly recent development, we have known for a long time that population health depends to a great extent on the water we drink, the air we breathe, and our ability to avoid exposure to hazardous waste. For example, Taylor and Rieger (1984) point out that in 1848 the Prussian government sent Dr Rudolf Virchow to investigate an outbreak of typhus in what is now part of Poland. Virchow, a physician recognized today as the founder of modern cellular pathology, caused huge political turmoil among government officials in Berlin when he suggested that the epidemic was the result of problems in the physical and social environments. Much to the displeasure of his political masters, Virchow proposed health reforms that focused not on biological determinants but on the physical and social environmental factors that had contributed to the typhus outbreak.

Following the example of early health researchers like Virchow, public health initiatives have traditionally stressed the importance of ensuring that people have a safe, clean supply of drinking water and an effective sanitation system. In fact, McKeown (1976) has argued that it was environmental interventions such as these during the nineteenth century, rather than investments in biomedical science and technology, that produced the most dramatic increases in life expectancy. These aspects of the physical environment are directly linked to the prevalence of infectious diseases such as cholera. While we have made progress in developed countries in reducing the risk of contracting this type of disease (e.g., through chlorination of drinking water and widespread immunization), infectious disease linked to environmental pollution is still a major health concern in developing countries. Shamefully, in Canada three-quarters of drinking water systems in First Nations communities continue to pose significant risks to the health of on-reserve Aboriginal populations (Senate of Canada 2007).

In countries such as Canada and the United States, there is growing awareness of the types of health problems related to air and water pollution that accompany increasing industrialization and urbanization. For example, there is evidence that air pollution associated with exposure to second-hand tobacco smoke as well as industrial emissions has a significant impact on our health, often resulting in respiratory illness and increasing the risk of lung cancer. According to Hofrichter (2000, 1), "We live in a toxic culture that degrades human and environmental health. In workplace, home, communities, and recreational areas, exposure to an expanding array of toxic conditions in the air, water, and soil poses an increasing long-term threat to public health." Perhaps the clearest evidence of the profound negative effects environmental pollution has on our pursuit of health and wellness comes from the finding that each of us carries a "body burden" of toxic chemicals (stored in our bodily tissues) because of exposure to environmental contaminants (Steingraber 1997)!

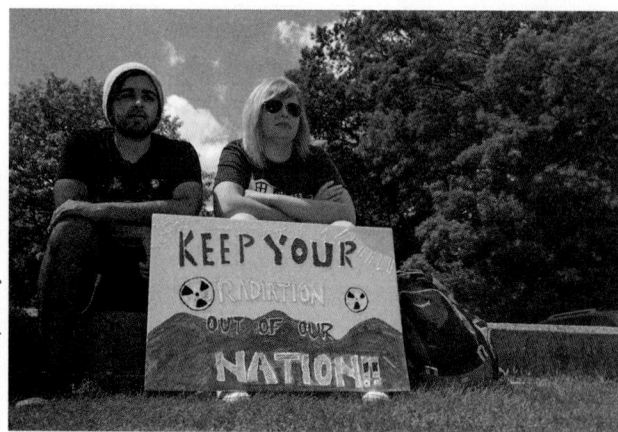

The physical environment in which we live has an effect on our health. Here, Canadians and Americans protest the Ontario Power Generation's plan to store nuclear waste under Lake Huron. A federal panel approved this plan in early 2015. Opponents of the plan have expressed concern about the potential for radioactivity to eventually leak into the main source of drinking water for millions of people.

The physical environment consists not only of factors such as air and water quality (i.e., the **natural environment**) but also of the type of housing in which we live, the type of workplace in which we spend a significant portion of our lives, and the planning and design of our cities (i.e., the **built environment**). It is clear that housing is an important aspect of the physical environment that contributes to population health Those living in substandard housing, along with the growing number of homeless people in major Canadian cities, can be viewed from a health (as well as a social and economic) perspective. According to Mikkonen and Raphael (2010, 29), "housing is an absolute necessity for living a healthy life . . . and living in unsafe, unaffordable or insecure housing increases the risk of many health problems." In addition, we now acknowledge that office buildings and work settings can be unhealthy (e.g., due to recirculated air, asbestos insulation) and that we must pay more attention to promoting workplace wellness. According to Savitch (2003, 600), "Not only do we construct our built environment, but after that construction our built environment constructs us." In other words, a sociological imagination helps us to understand that the built environment has important consequences for health and well-being.

Much of the health research on the built environment has shown that those who live in urban centres have worse health than those who live in less urbanized areas, a disparity sometimes called the **urban health penalty** (Galea, Freudenberg, and Vlahov 2005). At the same time, a study by the Canadian Institute for Health Information (CIHI 2006) found that health decreases the farther a person lives from an urban centre. After reviewing the somewhat contradictory evidence, health researchers have concluded that some features of urban life, such as increased access to health and social services as well as the availability of social support, benefit the health of those who live in cities. For example, Vlahov, Galea, and Freudenberg (2005, 4) conclude that "all cities have characteristics that both promote and harm health. The ultimate health status can be viewed as the sum of the urban advantages minus the sum of the penalties." This means that there are both advantages and disadvantages to living in cities in terms of health and wellness.

One aspect of the built environment that has conclusively been shown to be bad for health is the increasing trend toward living in sprawling suburban neighbourhoods. For example, there is growing evidence that urban sprawl and population density are related to levels of obesity in both Canada (Seliske, Pickett, and Janssen 2012) and the United States (Ewing et al. 2014; Zhao and Kaestner 2010). This trend is a peculiarly North American phenomenon stemming from the way in which we have chosen to construct our built environment (Frumkin, Frank, and Jackson 2004; Dannenberg, Frumkin, and Jackson 2011). In Europe, settlement is much more compact, with communities clustered around central railway terminals. In contrast, there has been an increasing trend in North America since the end of World War II to develop sprawling suburban neighbourhoods surrounding urban centres. Urban sprawl is "a form of urbanization distinguished by leapfrog patterns of development, commercial strips, low density, separated land uses, automobile dominance, and a minimum of public open space" (Gillham 2002, 8) and is characterized by four main factors that generally occur together (Abelsohn et al. 2005). The first factor is low residential density, which refers to the number of people living on a given area of land. As an illustration, the urban boundary of the city of Calgary exceeds 700 square kilometres, making it approximately the size of New York City's five boroughs, and yet Calgary is home to only one-tenth the number of people who live in New York City (Gurin 2003). This means that Calgary has a much lower residential density than New York. Like most Canadian cities, as Winnipeg develops and its suburbs grow, it is also losing residential density. For example, in the 20-year period between 1971 and 1992, Winnipeg's population doubled, but its urban boundary quadrupled in size (Gurin 2003). In each of these cases, fewer people living in more space creates a serious drain on infrastructure and transportation resources.

Second, areas of urban sprawl are characterized by a rigid zoning separation of residential areas from commercial and industrial areas of the city. This means that many people live considerable distances from where they work, shop, or find services. This design feature of the built environment necessitates a third characteristic of the sprawl environment, which is extensive automobile use complete with a widespread network of expressways and roads with limited access into and out of residential areas. The migration of people from the central core areas of cities into the suburbs leads to the fourth characteristic of urban sprawl—low-activity town centres.

As people move to the suburbs, less and less commercial activity takes place in downtown areas of major cities, which often appear deserted after the close of commercial business or on weekends. These four characteristics together define the urban sprawl environment and, when taken together, have serious consequences for population health and wellness.

Quite simply, a built environment characterized by urban sprawl is an unhealthy one. This is in no small part a result of the close connection between sprawl, automobiles, pollution, and illness and injury. According to a recent policy document released by the Canadian Medical Association, "the built environment affects every one of us every day, and mounting evidence suggests that it can play a significant role in our state of health and well-being" (2013, 2). Research indicates that the built environment is associated with decreased physical activity, increased prevalence of obesity, increased prevalence of asthma and other respiratory diseases, and an increase in injuries and unintended fatalities. For example, urban sprawl along with access to recreation and fitness facilities and neighbourhood walkability all have an impact on physical activities levels. There is Canadian evidence that people who live in the suburbs tend to drive more, walk less, and suffer from higher rates of obesity than those who live in higher density, walkable neighbourhoods that promote physical activity (Frank et al. 2007). The decline in physical activity among Canadians, in turn, has contributed to the rate of obesity almost doubling over the past three decades. The measured obesity rate was 13.8 per cent in 1978 and increased to 25.4 per cent by 2008 (Canadian Medical Association 2013). The increased prevalence of obesity has extremely important consequences for population health, since obesity is associated with high blood pressure, stroke, and heart disease, which are among the leading causes of death and disability.

Urban sprawl has also been linked to higher vehicle miles travelled per person and longer commute times. The use of private automobiles necessitated by urban sprawl is a major source of pollution, which is harmful to health. As Frumkin (2002, 203) explains, "Sprawl is associated with high levels of driving, driving contributes to air pollution, and air pollution causes morbidity and mortality." The Canadian Medical Association released a report in 2008 estimating that the effects of air pollution would result in 11,000 hospital admissions and 21,000 deaths Canada-wide, totalling a financial cost of close to $8 billion. In addition to pollution, sprawl is related to a series of vehicular and traffic issues that impose enormous costs on physical and emotional well-being. Savitch (2003, 598) comments that "built astride major highways, guided by clover-leaf construction patterns, and lacking in pedestrian walkways or dedicated bicycle paths, these suburbs can be a hazard for anyone not shielded by an automobile." Even those travelling by automobile are at increased risk because of sprawl. Describing automobile accident statistics, Abelsohn and colleagues (2005, 25–6) conclude that

> the statistics are staggering in themselves, approaching a million deaths each year worldwide, tens to hundreds of millions injured, and many incapacitated for life. It is the leading cause of death in the U.S. between the ages of 4 to 35, and third after cancer and heart disease in terms of years of life lost prematurely in the entire population. The economic and social costs are simply incalculable. If this was an infectious disease, it would be called an epidemic.

In the Canadian context, transportation-related injuries and fatalities resulting from motor vehicle, cycling, and pedestrian accidents "accounted for a total of $3.7 billion dollars in healthcare costs in Canada in 2009" (Canadian Medical Association 2013).

In summary, sprawl means that people must drive greater annual distances, make more automobile trips, and navigate complex, high-speed roadways. Not only does this increase the risk of traffic accidents, but studies have also shown that the long and stressful commutes associated with sprawl have negative mental health effects (Frumkin, Frank, and Jackson 2004). Research has demonstrated that the sprawl environment undermines sense of community, lessens social capital, and threatens sources of social support. All these factors, when taken together, show that urban sprawl is bad for population health and underscore the importance of the built environment for health and wellness.

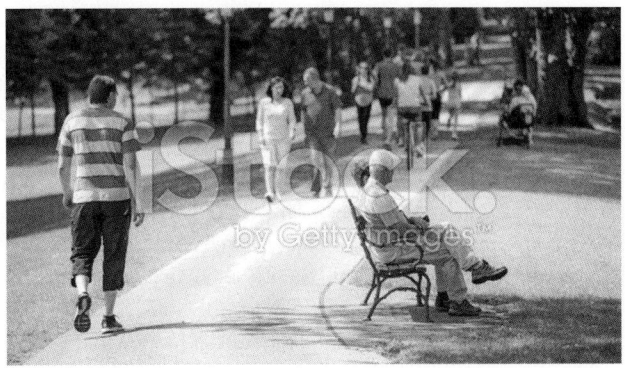

Walkable neighbourhoods are an important part of a healthy built environment.

One way in which cities have tried to address urban sprawl is through the redevelopment of land that was formerly the site of industrial or commercial activity and has been abandoned. Such sites are referred to as brownfields—"abandoned, idled, or under-used industrial and commercial facilities where expansion or redevelopment is complicated by real or perceived environmental contamination" (DeSousa 2006, 393). For example, in Calgary, when an Imperial Oil refinery was decommissioned, the land was transformed into a residential neighbourhood. However, as the experience of the Calgary neighbourhood illustrated, this type of redevelopment is not without environmental and health risks. The toxic contamination associated with the oil refinery resulted in neighbourhood residents experiencing numerous negative health effects and eventually prompted the displacement of the community.

While the extent of such contamination is not known, it is estimated that as much as 25 per cent of the Canadian urban landscape is contaminated because of previous industrial activities and the number of brownfield sites in Canada may be as high as 30,000 (De Sousa 2006). Edelstein (1988) studied the effects that "contaminated communities" have on their residents and found that in addition to negative physical health consequences, people also suffer from a profound loss of sense of coherence. For example, cherished personal beliefs, such as that home is a safe place to raise children, are undermined by the type of events experienced by residents of contaminated communities. There is no doubt that physical aspects of the natural and built environment have a major impact on population health and that we still face many serious challenges in creating healthy environments in which to live and work.

The Social Environment

As slow as we have been in addressing the effects of the physical environment on health, we have been even slower in recognizing the significant impact of the social environment on population health. Indeed, we are still discovering the ways in which aspects of the social structure influence our health status. Williams (2003) notes that despite the fact that sociological analysis of health and illness frequently makes use of this basic concept to frame the interpretation of health inequalities, the precise meaning of social structure requires further elaboration. There is now increasing evidence that there is an important link between social status and health status. The structural determinants that have received the most research attention are aspects of our socioeconomic status (one's position in the social hierarchy as indicated by income, occupation, and education) along with general living and working conditions. Chapter 5 provides a thorough discussion of the effects of societal factors such as income inequality on population health.

At this point in our discussion of the general determinants of health, it is sufficient to note that there is extensive empirical verification that higher socioeconomic status is associated with better health. For example, research has documented the link between income and the health of Canadians. Studies consistently show that people at each step on the income ladder are healthier than those on the step below. To fully understand this finding, it is important to realize that it is not simply a matter of the amount of money that you have but, rather, it is the relative distribution of income and wealth in society that is a key factor in determining population health. "More equal income distribution has proven to be one of the best predictors of better overall health of a society" (Mikkonen and Raphael 2010, 12).

The type of position that we have in the workplace is another component of our socioeconomic status. To begin with, being unemployed definitely puts health at risk. The stress of unemployment and the lack of a stable income may lead to a variety of health problems and substantially increase the risk of premature death (Bartley, Ferrie, and Montgomery 2006; Mikkonen and Raphael 2010; Wilkinson and Marmot 2003). Early Canadian studies (e.g., D'Arcy 1986; D'Arcy and Siddique 1985) demonstrated that unemployed people tend to experience significantly more psychological distress, greater short- and long-term disability, and more activity limitations because of ill health. They report more health problems, including serious conditions such as heart disease and high blood pressure. Furthermore, unemployed people visit physicians more often and are hospitalized more frequently than employed people. The evidence clearly indicates that unemployment has a substantial negative effect on health and well-being.

A final aspect of socioeconomic status that affects our health is the level of formal education that we have attained. Health status improves with level of education (just as it does with income level). In fact, education is highly correlated with other social determinants of health such as level of income and occupation. Education contributes to health by providing people with knowledge and skills that are required for successful daily living. It enhances their ability to pursue employment opportunities and to participate in a range of community activities and is generally associated with higher standards of living. "This in turn improves opportunities to obtain the prerequisites for health—nutritious food, safe housing, a good working environment and social participation" (Bambra et al. 2010, 289). Greater educational attainment is also associated with level of perceived personal control, which has been linked to health-related behaviours and health status (Braveman, Egerter, and Williams 2011).

Furthermore, education is an important health determinant because it improves people's ability to access and understand complex health-related information about effective self-care health practices and the availability of formal health-care services. Education increases our understanding of how to promote our own health and to evaluate which behavioural practices may be harmful or beneficial. "It is widely recognized that education can lead to improved health by increasing health knowledge and healthy behaviors" (Braveman, Egerter, and Williams 2011, 386). These researchers argue that this may be explained in part by literacy, since people with higher levels of education (and greater occupational and income security) are better able to make informed decisions regarding self-health management and the selection of appropriate medical care for both themselves and their family members. The term **health literacy** is used to refer to

Canadians' "ability to access, understand, evaluate and communicate information as a way to promote, maintain and improve health in a variety of settings across the life-course" (Rootman and Gordon-El-Bihbety 2008). In describing the importance of health literacy, these researchers contend that all Canadians should have the opportunities and support they need to obtain and use health information effectively, since this contributes to their capacity to act as informed participants in the process of self-care, their interaction with formal health-care providers, and, ultimately, their health and well-being. There is reason to believe that the impact of this factor on population health will become even more significant in the future with the rapid changes occurring today in information technology. Indeed, given the amount of health information available on the Internet, Hoffman-Goetz, Donelle, and Ahmed (2014) recently described health literacy as an increasingly important determinant of health!

In the following chapter, we will take a more detailed look at the part played by these aspects of socioeconomic status as health determinants, but at this point it is time to turn our attention to another aspect of the social environment that has an impact on population health—the changing age structure of society. Age and stage in the life course intersect with other social determinants such as socioeconomic status in shaping population health. Basically, age is important because it defines many of the rights and privileges that people experience at different times in their lives. To illustrate, children typically begin their formal education at age five, and attendance is mandatory until they reach 16. At that age, you can also get a driver's licence and legally operate a motor vehicle, but you have to wait until you are 65 to be eligible for Old Age Security. In other words, certain privileges are distributed on the basis of age group location. This type of age grading and the typical age group distinctions made in our society (i.e., young, middle-aged, and old) contribute to social inequality. For example, some people are denied the right to vote in elections because they are too young, and eventually individuals are no longer able to participate in the paid labour force when mandatory retirement is enforced (based on the assumption that they are in an age group that is too old to continue working). "Labour-force entries and exits are allocated by age, both directly through labour laws and indirectly by educational criteria, for job entry, and by perceived age-related performance abilities, for job exit" (McMullin 2010, 93). This illustrates that age is a socially constructed criterion for categorizing people that has significant implications for creating and perpetuating structures of inequality, including health disparities. Despite the existence of deep-rooted age-based differences in the distribution of status and power in society, this source of social inequality has not received the same level of research attention as that devoted to class, gender, and ethnicity. However, as a result of the dramatic aging of the population currently taking place, there is growing interest, on the part of both researchers and policy analysts, in addressing age-based inequalities in society.

There is extensive evidence of the changes that are occurring in the rate at which Canada's population is aging. The data in Figure 4.2 demonstrate that in the past, the percentage of Canadians aged 65 and older did not vary significantly (e.g., it was constant between 1951 and 1971). Over the next 20-year period (from 1971 to 1991), the rate of increase was slow but steady. By 2011, older adults accounted for a record high of 14.8 per cent of the Canadian population, up from 13.7 per cent just five years earlier (Statistics Canada 2012d). According to the 2011 census, this rate of growth was more than double the increase for the Canadian population as a whole. **Population aging** is a trend that is expected to accelerate in the future. In contrast to the slow rate of growth in the past, it has been estimated that the proportion of Canadians over the age of 65 will increase dramatically in the decades ahead. In fact, it is

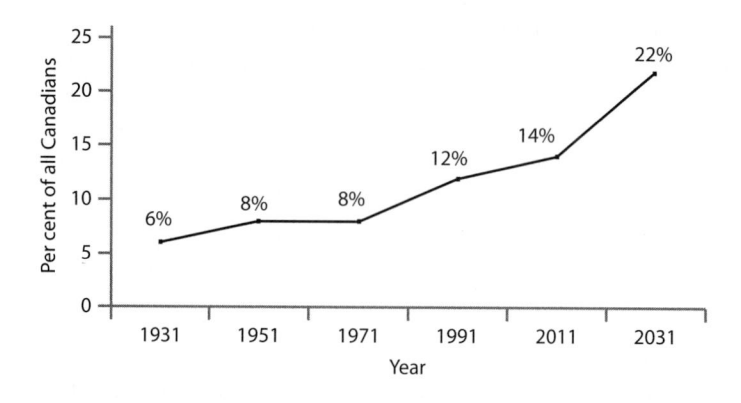

Figure 4.2 Percentage of Canadian Population Aged 65 or Older: Past, Present, and Projected

Source: Statistics Canada 1994, Chart 1.1.

predicted that the figure will almost double by the year 2036, reaching 24.5 per cent (Turcotte and Schellenberg 2007).

Increasing life expectancy combined with lower fertility rates means that we are witnessing a fundamental change in the shape of the **age structure** of Canadian society. Throughout most of the twentieth century, a fairly small proportion of the Canadian population was comprised of people aged 65 and older. In the years ahead, the situation will be quite different. The population pyramid in Figure 4.3 illustrates the aging of Canada's population by comparing the age and sex structure of the population on 1 July 1982 and 2012 (Statistics Canada 2012a). In 1982, the largest age group in the Canadian population was people (both men and women) between the ages of 20 and 35 years. By 2012, the largest age group was people between the ages of 50 and 65. According to the 2011 Canadian census, the 60-to-64 age group experienced the fastest increase (29 per cent) compared to all other age groups (Statistics Canada 2012a). This is essentially the result of the fact that the so-called baby-boom generation (those born between 1946 and 1965) are now in or approaching their 60s. In fact, the first baby boomers reached the age of 65 by 2011, which means that population aging will accelerate in Canada in the coming years. The figure also clearly shows that the base of the population pyramid is shrinking (i.e., the number of Canadians under the age of 35 is getting smaller) while at the same time the middle and upper levels of the pyramid are expanding (i.e., the number of older adults is getting substantially larger). In 2011, census data showed that for the first time there were more Canadians between the ages of 55 and 64 than those aged 15 to 24. It is also worth noting that centenarians (people over the age of 100) were the second most rapidly growing age group in Canada (following those aged 60 to 64)! Overall, this means that Canadians can generally expect to live longer lives than their parents and grandparents.

This is certainly good news, but we need to ask whether past patterns of **age stratification** (i.e., the unequal distribution of wealth, power, and privilege among people at different stages in the life course) are changing as the number and proportion of older adults in the population increases. Even though the population age structure is being radically

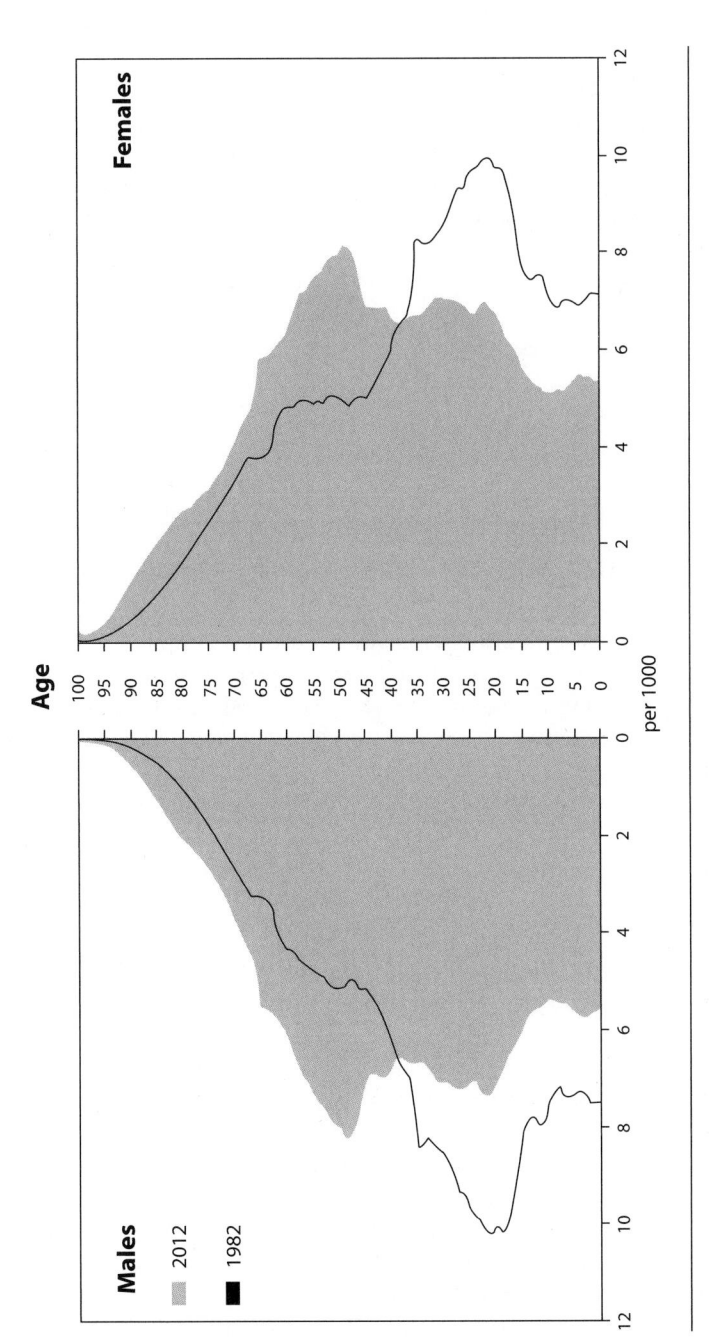

Figure 4.3 Age Pyramid of the Canadian Population as of 1 July 1982 and 2012

Source: Statistics Canada 2012a.

reshaped, age-based inequalities tend to persist despite older Canadians representing an ever-increasing share of the population. McMullin (2010, 101) suggests that "the social construction of old age is especially fuelled by the medical profession, which has transformed aged bodies into sick bodies." In other words, later life is stereotyped as a time of decline, dependency, and diminished capacity to effectively perform meaningful roles in society. This raises a key question—what are the implications of the changing age structure in society for the health of the population?

The World Health Organization (2011b, 1) describes population aging as "a powerful and transforming demographic force" and points out that as length of life and the proportion of older people increases throughout the world, there is a rise in the prevalence of chronic diseases such as heart disease, cancer, and diabetes. Furthermore, the prevalence of dementia (especially Alzheimer's disease) rises sharply with age. These trends have important implications for the health of the population as well as for informal and formal health care, since demographic and family changes mean that older adults will have fewer family members to care for them and difficulties accessing appropriate professional health care. Together, these factors seriously challenge the likelihood of people experiencing a healthy, active old age.

In concluding our examination of the impact of the social environment on population health, let's take a quick look at a salutary factor that contributes to the pursuit of health and wellness and is now recognized as an important health determinant—social support. The health benefit of belonging to a supportive social network has become an important research topic. Supportive social relationships may contribute to feelings of being cared for and valued (**emotional support**) and provide people with vital practical assistance with the activities of daily living (**instrumental support**). In addition, they are a source of information (**informational support**) and can convey a wealth of knowledge about health-related matters. Finally, supportive social relationships help people to feel that they are part of a meaningful network or group of people. An increasing number of studies have examined the direct and indirect effects of these different types of social support on health. It has been demonstrated, for example, that belonging to a supportive social network may be positively linked to a variety of health outcomes, such as self-rated health as well as morbidity and mortality rates (Cheng and Chan 2006). Research has shown that there is a clear link between social relationships and health outcomes in the general population, and we now know that "adults who are more socially connected live healthier and longer lives than their more isolated peers" (Rosich and Hankin 2010, S3). It is also important to recognize that social relationships have both short- and long-term effects on health and that the impact of the social environment people experience during childhood and their formative years accumulates over the life course and has a continuing impact on their health.

People who receive social support from family members, friends, co-workers, and others in the community tend to be in better health. The type of social contacts that they have and the extent of the practical and emotional support that they receive from others influence their health status. Family and friends provide basic support in dealing with the problems of everyday life and help individuals to maintain a sense of control over life circumstances. There is growing evidence (which we will examine in Chapter 9) that social support networks contribute to well-being and life satisfaction and, at the same time, act as a buffer against health problems. "Social support from caring persons in one's life is beneficial to health. It alleviates stress, reduces mortality, strengthens the immune system and decreases the likelihood of serious illness" (National Forum on Health 1996, 74). In fact, it has been argued that the effects of positive social relationships may be as important in determining good health as known risk factors, such as smoking, high blood pressure, and obesity, are in causing ill health. We will return to this topic in Chapter 9 when we take a closer look at the hidden depths of health care, including the complex relationship between social support and self-care practices for maintaining good health and managing ill health.

Use of Formal Health-Care Services

The relationship between the use of health-care services and health status has received considerable research attention. The majority of formal health-care services (e.g., those provided by physicians and hospitals) were designed to provide illness intervention and treatment. In other words, they focus on individual health needs in terms of clinical risk factors and disease management. At best, formal health services have a (personal) disease-avoidance focus rather than a (population) health maintenance emphasis. While these types of services are important and we all want ready access to doctors and hospitals when we are seriously ill, the extent to which medical services contribute to improvements in population health (versus personal health) is not clear.

It is widely assumed that access to medical care was largely responsible for improvements in the health of populations in countries such as Canada and the United States throughout the twentieth century (e.g., as reflected by dramatic increases in life expectancy). Although it is difficult to quantify the extent to which the production of health is the direct result of the consumption of health-care services, "best estimates are that only 10–15 percent of increased longevity since 1900 is due to improved health care" (Raphael 2009, 8). While this estimate is now widely accepted, it has not been universally supported. Poland and colleagues (1998) contend that the contribution of formal health care to health and well-being has been underestimated. Others argue that health-care services have historically not been an important determinant of health and that a variety of social and economic factors have played a more critical part in shaping the health of the population (e.g., CIHI 2007; Rachlis 2004; Evans and Stoddart 1990). Unfortunately, it is difficult to verify the extent to which improvements in population health result from the use of formal health-care services.

There is growing evidence, however, that the current health-care system is not well equipped to deal effectively with major health challenges facing Canadians today (e.g., preventing the occurrence of disease, particularly chronic illness, and enhancing health-promoting behaviour across the life course). In fact, it has been suggested that "the contribution of medicine and health care is quite limited, and that spending more on health care will not result in further improvements in population health" (Health Canada 1994, 12). This is an extremely important issue and will be pursued further in Chapter 10 when we assess the link between formal care and population health. We still have a lot to learn about the effectiveness of formal health-care services and the ways in which these various determinants collectively shape the health of Canadians.

While we have discussed each of the key determinants separately, it is important to keep in mind that they interact with one another in complex ways. Biology, daily personal health practices, the social and physical environments in which we live, and the types of health-care services that we utilize ultimately have combined effects on population health. There may now be general agreement that these four factors are key health determinants, but we still do not adequately understand how they intersect to shape our health status.

The Relative Importance of Health Determinants

The accumulated body of knowledge clearly demonstrates that population health is shaped by many different factors, including a number of crucial social determinants. At the same time, however, there are many unanswered questions about what makes people healthy. For example, we do not know how much each of these factors contributes to health. Is it safe to assume that all of the influences on our health are equally important? Alternatively, are some determinants more important than others? Are some determinants more important in specific circumstances (e.g., for those living in different socioeconomic circumstances) or at different stages in the life course? Finally, we might even question whether it is possible to precisely gauge the impact of each of these factors on our health status.

Upstream and Downstream Health Determinants: Jason's Story

As a way of addressing the relative importance of the health determinants we have been discussing, let's consider a deceptively simple story included in a report on the health of Canadians by the Public Health Agency of Canada (1999). To illustrate what makes Canadians healthy or unhealthy, the report tells the story of Jason's health (see Box 4.1). This account of one individual's health status provides insightful information about the complex sequence of life events and underlying social conditions that ultimately shape our present and future health.

A careful examination of this series of questions and answers reveals a good deal about the connections between Jason's current health status, the neighbourhood in which he lives, his parents' income level, their participation in the paid labour force, and their educational background. In other words, in searching for a causal explanation, the story links Jason's present health status (he is a hospital patient) to his family's socioeconomic status (their living and working conditions). There are a number of important lessons to be learned from a critical analysis of the details in Jason's story (see Box 4.2).

Starting with the obvious cause of his health status, Jason was hospitalized for treatment of an infection in his leg. This tells us the proximal cause (i.e., the downstream factor that is situated closest to the health outcome) of his current health status. This is, however, not a complete explanation of Jason's health condition. The story demonstrates the importance of moving upstream for a more complete clarification of the factors that collectively shape our health status (i.e., by continuing to ask why). We next learn that personal behaviour played a part in this process, since the infection is the result of an injury that occurred while Jason was outside playing in his neighbourhood. What does the story tell us about Jason's neighbourhood? First, it highlights the importance of situating our personal behaviour in the physical environment in which it takes place. Second, the fact that children in Jason's neighbourhood routinely play in a junkyard indicates that there are apparently no safe playgrounds or recreational facilities near their homes.

Despite the lack of such resources, Jason and his family continue to live in this neighbourhood because his parents can't afford alternative housing. This, in turn, reflects the fact that Jason's dad is unemployed and that his lack of formal education makes it difficult for him to find work. On top of that, Jason's mother is sick and presumably also unemployed. The story illustrates the interaction between personal and structural determinants of health and emphasizes the importance of factors in the social environment such as our living and working conditions. Jason's health status is ultimately traced upstream to his family's socioeconomic status. In other words, the social and

Box 4.1 What Makes Canadians Healthy or Unhealthy?

Why is Jason in the hospital?
Because he has a bad infection in his leg.
But why does he have an infection?
Because he has a cut on his leg and it got infected.
But why does he have a cut on his leg?
Because he was playing in the junkyard next to his apartment building and there was some sharp, jagged steel there that he fell on.
But why was he playing in a junkyard?
Because his neighbourhood is kind of rundown. A lot of kids play there and there is no one to supervise them.
But why does he live in that neighbourhood?
Because his parents can't afford a nicer place to live.
But why can't his parents afford a nicer place to live?
Because his Dad is unemployed and his Mom is sick.
But why is his Dad unemployed?
Because he doesn't have much education and he can't find a job.
But why . . . ?

Source: Public Health Agency of Canada 1999.

economic circumstances in which Jason and his family live are identified as the distal causes (i.e., causal factors that are quite distant or far removed from the outcome) of his sickness and his present need for hospitalization. This interpretation is consistent with the fact that "numerous studies indicate that various social determinants of health have far greater influence upon health and the incidence of illness than traditional biomedical and behavioural risk factors" (Raphael 2009, 2).

Primary and Secondary Determinants: Moving Upstream

It has been suggested that one way of capturing the difference in the relative importance of health determinants is by distinguishing between primary and secondary determinants (Kosteniuk and Dickinson 2003). According to this approach, socioeconomic factors, such as household income, education level, and employment status, are characterized as **primary determinants**. That is, they have a direct effect on our health and also influence secondary health determinants. In other words, **secondary determinants**, such as our daily behavioural practices (e.g., smoking) and our psychosocial well-being (e.g., sense of coherence, self-esteem), reflect our living and working conditions and also play an important intervening role in the relationship between social status and health status. Regardless of whether we label the factors that influence Jason's health as structural versus personal determinants or primary versus secondary determinants, we are left with an important unanswered question.

Does the information in Box 4.2 provide us with a complete account of the factors that contributed to Jason's health? As you may recall, the story ends with an unanswered question ("But why . . . ?"). Obviously, we could continue the search for a causal explanation. In other words, we

> **Box 4.2   Interpreting the Causes of Jason's Health Status**
>
> Health status—Jason is a hospital patient (health outcome)
> ↑
> Disease, illness, or injury—Jason has an infection in his leg (proximal cause)   **Downstream Determinants**
> ↑
> Behaviour—Jason was playing in a junkyard and fell down **(personal determinant)**
> ↑
> Living and working conditions—Neighbourhood in which his parents can afford to live **(structural determinant)**
> ↑
> Employment, education, and income—Jason's dad is unemployed and is having a difficult time finding work because of his level of formal education **(structural determinant)**
> ↑
> Social status—The family's socioeconomic status (distal cause)   **Upstream Determinants**

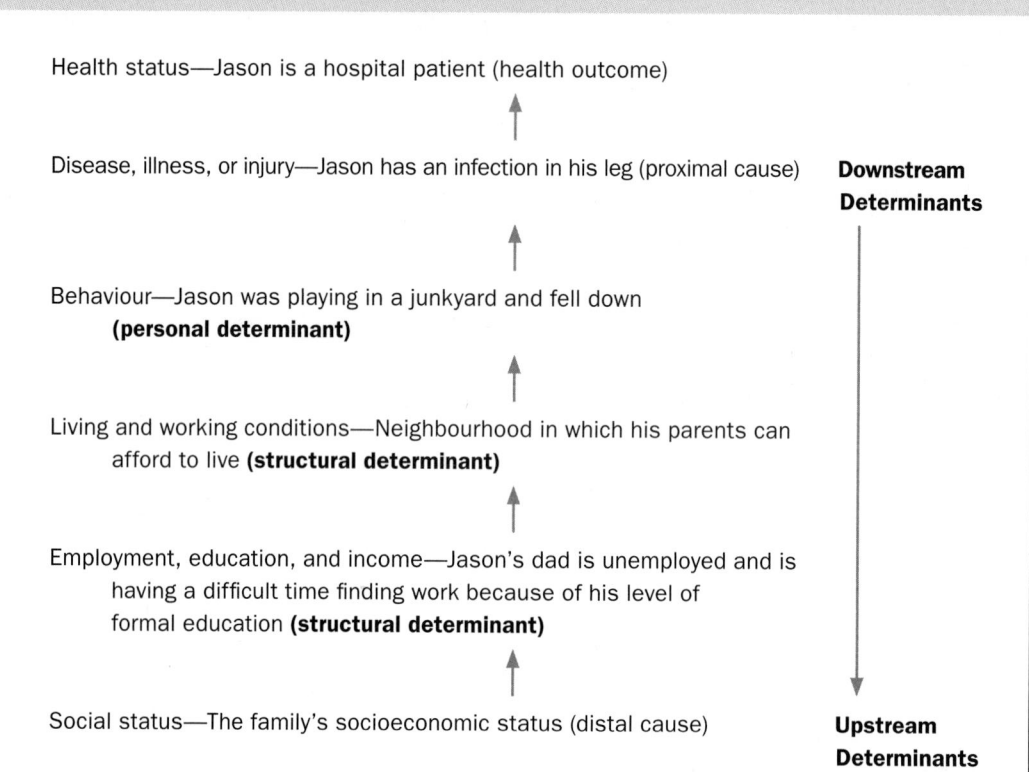

could keep moving further upstream to try to find what Marmot (2006, 2) refers to as "the causes of the causes" of population health. Where would that ultimately lead us? Raphael (Raphael et al. 2006) suggests that in the process of exploring the structural aspects of society that influence our health, we should distinguish between horizontal and vertical structures. According to Raphael, **horizontal structures** are the more immediate factors that shape health and well-being (as illustrated by Jason's story). For example, family environment, the nature of work and workplace conditions, quality of housing, and availability of neighbourhood resources (e.g., recreational facilities) all have a direct impact on our health.

In contrast, **vertical structures** are more distant, macro-level factors that indirectly influence health and well-being. For example, social, political, and economic policies regarding social welfare or taxation (e.g., child tax benefits) "determine in large part the quality of the horizontal structures" (Raphael 2006, 124) and eventually influence population health. This approach contends that the structural aspects of society (e.g., the conditions under which people live and work) that are more directly linked to health status are shaped, in turn, by the types of public policies that are in place in society. For example, public policies related to employment insurance, minimum wage, educational and training programs, child care, and low-income housing all influence the distribution of social and economic resources in society and, ultimately, population health. If this is the case, then these types of structural factors need to be added to Jason's story.

Despite the variation in the terms used, all of these researchers seem to agree that there is an important difference between downstream social determinants, or those factors that are close to the health outcome (i.e., proximal, secondary, horizontal), and upstream social determinants that are further removed (i.e., distal, primary, vertical). There is also agreement that the search for causal explanations needs to continue moving upstream. This is certainly not a new idea. Many years ago, McKinlay (1979) called for a refocusing upstream. Travelling against the current and moving upstream, however, can be a slow and difficult voyage. But it is important to keep moving in this direction, since there is an expanding body of research evidence indicating that upstream social determinants of health are "the factors that play a more fundamental causal role and represent the most important opportunities for improving health and reducing health disparities" (Braveman, Egerter, and Williams 2011, 383).

Understanding the Cumulative Effects of Health Determinants: A Life Course Approach

It could be argued that a life course approach is required to fully comprehend the relative importance of the determinants of population health. For example, in Jason's case we could also consider the extent to which his childhood experiences described in the story have an impact on his future health status as an adult—asking, in effect, how what happened earlier in Jason's life might affect his future health. "Adopting a life-course perspective directs attention to how social determinants of health operate at every level of development—early childhood, childhood, adolescence, and adulthood—to both immediately influence health as well as provide the basis for health or illness during following stages of the life course" (Raphael 2009, 16). As noted earlier, health outcomes can be traced back to both proximal (downstream) and distal (upstream) causal factors. We would be well advised to adopt a life course perspective in our research if we hope to be able to gauge the time lag that occurs between cause and effect and to identify the causal factors that result in both immediate and long-term health effects. For example, sedentary behaviour and smoking during adolescence or as a young adult may not have immediate negative impacts on your health but may be related to chronic health problems in later life, such as adult-onset diabetes or cardiovascular disease. According to Haflon, Larson, and Russ (2010, 10),

> Because early life events are now understood to exert particularly strong influences on immediate health status and health in later life, most scholars now include a broad range of early life exposures as potential social determinants (e.g., the quality of parenting and caregiving, exposure to domestic violence, maternal depression, home organization and neighbourhood safety).

As an illustration, they point to the expanding body of research guided by a life course perspective that clearly demonstrates the ways in which early social influences continue to have an impact on health into mid-life and beyond. For example, Hertzman and Power (2003) state that it is now well understood that life course factors affect a range of health outcomes, including general well-being. They point out that many of the illnesses that emerge in later life have their roots in early childhood experiences. As a result, they conclude that "the health status of populations cannot, therefore, be adequately understood without recognizing health-determining influences across the life course" (Hertzman and Power 2003, 720). More recently, Braveman, Egerter, and Williams (2011, 388–9) reach the same conclusion based on their analysis of the social determinants of health, stating that many of the studies conducted over the past two decades provide compelling evidence that "differences in social advantage can influence health both over lifetimes and across generations." Consequently, they argue, we need more life course research and more longitudinal studies conducted over time periods long enough for health consequences of early childhood experiences to be assessed. A life course approach adds an important dimension to our research on the connections between social structure and health and facilitates a more thorough understanding of the cumulative effect and the multiple pathways through which various social determinants influence population health over time. Indeed, adopting a life course perspective "can enlighten our understanding of wider social determinants of health" (Nicolau and Marcenes 2012, 33).

Estimating the Health Benefits of Major Determinants

Given what we have learned about the major determinants of health, you might wonder which of these factors is most important. Quantifying the relative importance of health determinants turns out to be an extremely difficult task that very few researchers have attempted. One exception can be found in the work of Gunning-Schepers and Hagen (1987). These researchers addressed the question: How much can prevention contribute to health? To answer this question, we obviously must be capable of estimating the health benefits that are attributable to each of the major determinants. For example, we would need to learn whether access to preventive health services plays a more important part in shaping population health than routine everyday self-care practices. Similarly, we would need to know whether life circumstances (e.g., income, occupation) are more important than lifestyle practices (e.g., diet, exercise) in determining our health status. In other words, we must first be able to measure the contribution of each factor and then incorporate this information in an intersectional analysis to assess the significance of the relationship between key determinants and appropriate health outcome indicators (e.g., improvements in population health).

While we still do not have a great deal of solid evidence regarding the relative importance of the social determinants of health, there are increasing indications that structural factors such as living and working conditions are crucially important for a healthy population. In fact, Millar and Hull (1997, 148) assert that "these are the most powerful factors affecting health." Although this assertion could be challenged, there is growing empirical support (as we will see in Chapter 5) indicating that factors such as adequacy of income, availability of jobs, and type of employment are closely linked to population health.

It is also apparent that personal factors such as routine behavioural practices contribute to our health status. For example, it has been demonstrated in the United States that lifestyle behaviours need to be recognized as leading causes of death (Mokdad et al. 2004). While it is possible to establish a link between negative lifestyle practices, such as smoking, and the indicators of ill health (e.g., morbidity, mortality), it is extremely difficult to demonstrate the health benefits of positive lifestyle practices, such as physical activity. Stated another way, it is easier to demonstrate that there is an association between harmful behaviour and ill health than it is to document the relationship between healthful behaviour and good health. Despite our current limited ability to accurately quantify the relative impact of various health determinants, there appears to be an undeniable relationship between lifestyle behaviour and health status.

Gunning-Schepers and Hagen (1987) highlight a number of conceptual and empirical problems involved in assigning a relative weight to health determinants such as social circumstances and lifestyle practices. For example, they contend that while the broad categories we use for summarizing health determinants provide guidelines for research, they oversimplify the complex nature of the interrelationships that exist between the many individual and societal factors that shape population health. In reality, these factors all intersect, and it is difficult to separate their effects on health. To illustrate the point, Gunning-Schepers and Hagen raise questions about the extent to which the link between occupational factors and health status can be interpreted as part of the social environment or, alternatively, as elements of personal lifestyle. In addition, they question whether smoking is simply a lifestyle choice made by an individual or whether smoking behaviour is better understood as a correlate of socioeconomic factors.

In either case, they argue, the problem of classification is further compounded by the problem of interdependency. We know that the major determinants have both direct and interaction effects on our health status. In other words, personal and structural factors not only influence health, they also influence each other! Consequently, these individual and societal factors may have a combined effect on population health that differs substantially from the impact that each factor has separately. Furthermore, Blaxter (1990) suggests that lifestyle practices may play a more important part in shaping health for those in better social circumstances (i.e., people with higher socioeconomic status). For example, the health benefits associated with quitting smoking may be greater for a person who has a well-paid, rewarding job and lives in an affluent neighbourhood than for someone who is unemployed and living in poverty. We will critically assess this point in Chapter 8 when we take a closer look at the benefits of healthy lifestyle behaviour.

It should be obvious from this discussion that understanding the relative importance of health determinants is a complex matter and that we still do not really know the precise benefits associated with each of the factors that determine our health. We will return to this issue in the final chapter when we consider the public policy initiatives that might help us to achieve healthy futures. One thing that is clear is that to be effective, healthy public policy and strategies for promoting population health must be based on a better understanding of the intersection of determinants of good health (wellness) and ill health (sickness).

The Determinants of Good Health and Ill Health

Mackenbach and colleagues (1994) raise an interesting question, which is only recently receiving research attention: Do the determinants of good health differ from the determinants of ill health? They (1994, 1273) suggest that "the distribution and determinants of positive health have not been studied extensively by epidemiologists, perhaps because they feel more comfortable with disease as an outcome measure." This raises, once again, the familiar problem (discussed in Chapter 3) that it is easier to measure the indicators of ill health than the indicators of good health. Researchers tend to be comfortable with established health status indicators, such as disease (morbidity) and death (mortality) rates, and rely on these factors as outcome measures in studying the impact of health determinants. As previously stated, we are much better at assessing the determinants and outcomes of sickness than we are at assessing the positive aspects of health and wellness. As a result, most research to date focuses on the determinants of ill health.

In fact, even Mackenbach and colleagues (1994) fall into this trap! They set out to do an exploratory study of the determinants of positive health and state that their specific research objective is "to assess to what extent the determinants of excellent health are different from those of ill-health" (1994, 1274). Health status was defined and measured in terms of the standard indicators (e.g., self-assessed health and the number of chronic conditions and health complaints reported). These factors were then used to categorize respondents as being in "excellent health" or "ill health" (i.e., the major outcome variables). A problem arises, however, in the selection of the independent variables for this analysis and the types of measures used. These researchers selected two broad groups of determinants: sociodemographic factors and specific "risk factors." Sociodemographic determinants included social environmental factors such as employment status and level of education. Under certain circumstances, these factors might contribute to good health. In contrast, risk factors focused on the negative aspects of life events and practices such as smoking, alcohol intake, coffee consumption, and leisure exercise. While these aspects are obviously components of lifestyle behaviour, actual measurement concentrated on the negative dimensions of these personal practices and the associated health risks. By focusing on the measurement of harmful behaviour, the study was bound to be more successful at assessing the determinants of ill health rather than the determinants of good health.

Does it make sense to try to identify the determinants of excellent health by measuring risk factors? Are there risks associated with enhancing positive health or achieving wellness? Obviously not, since the term "risk" typically refers to the probability of experiencing ill health or sickness (i.e., disease and illness). This analytic problem betrays the fact that many researchers studying the social determinants of population health are constrained by the concepts and methods of the medico-centric illness model (i.e., the pathogenic approach to the search for the causes of disease). In other words, while they may intend to explore the positive factors that determine good health (or, in this case, excellent health), they end up studying the negative factors that contribute to ill health. An investigation of the determinants of good health must include measures of the salutary factors that help to keep people healthy (such as a supportive social network and a sense of coherence).

Another example can be found in the work of Gunning-Schepers and Hagen (1987). They set out to examine the extent to which prevention can contribute to health and yet conclude by suggesting that the broad determinants of health should be divided into different types of known risk factors to facilitate an analysis of the relationships between risk factors and disease. Indeed, they assert that major health determinant categories "are nothing but a grouping of known epidemiologic risk factors" (1987, 949). This statement discloses the fact that the dominance of the biomedical model influences the way that researchers think about and design their studies of health determinants. Learning more about the "avoidable burden of illness" (i.e., the risk factors that make us sick) is important, but it certainly is not the same as learning more about the determinants of good health (i.e., the salutary factors that help to make people healthy).

While Mackenbach and colleagues (1994) raise an important question concerning the difference between good and ill health, they unfortunately fail to provide a clear answer. Basically, they found similar associations between the determinants examined and both excellent health and ill health, although the researchers conclude that these factors are better at explaining variance in ill health. This is not a surprising finding. For the most part, the determinants measured in this study (particularly the risk factors) are known to be associated with ill health. As a result, it could be argued that the findings basically reflect the study design. In other words, the measures selected predominantly gauge the determinants of ill health rather than the determinants of good health. Mackenbach and colleagues acknowledge this limitation in their concluding discussion. They admit that if we want to gain a greater understanding of the variation in positive health, we will need to identify a set of determinants different from the ones included in their study. This means not only recognizing the factors that make people healthy (versus illness risk factors) but also developing better independent measures of the determinants of good health. Mackenbach and colleagues suggest that future research in this area might benefit from Antonovsky's distinction between a pathogenic and a salutogenic approach to health. In their words, "The determinants included in the present study all stem from the pathogenic approach, which aims at finding risk factors for disease and premature death. The salutogenic approach focuses on the protective and health promoting factors which help people stay or become healthy" (Mackenbach et al. 1994, 1280). As previously noted, more researchers are now adopting a salutogenic approach to gain a greater understanding of the differences between the determinants of good health and ill health.

These issues are summarized in Figure 4.4, which attempts to clarify the situation and facilitate the development of a more effective approach for studying the determinants of good health (wellness) as distinct from the determinants of ill health (sickness). Antonovsky's (1979; 1987) salutogenic model of health was used as the basis for organizing the information presented regarding positive health determinants and the dimensions of health-promoting behaviour. The

General Orientation

| Salutogenic | Pathogenic |

Major Determinants

Salutary Factors	Risk Factors
Sense of coherence Coping skills Supportive social environment	Microorganisms Viruses Infectious disease

Behavioural Dimensions

Health Maintenance	Illness Avoidance
Health resource management Enhanced self-care capacity	Preventive medical care Risk reduction

| **Good Health** | **Ill Health** |

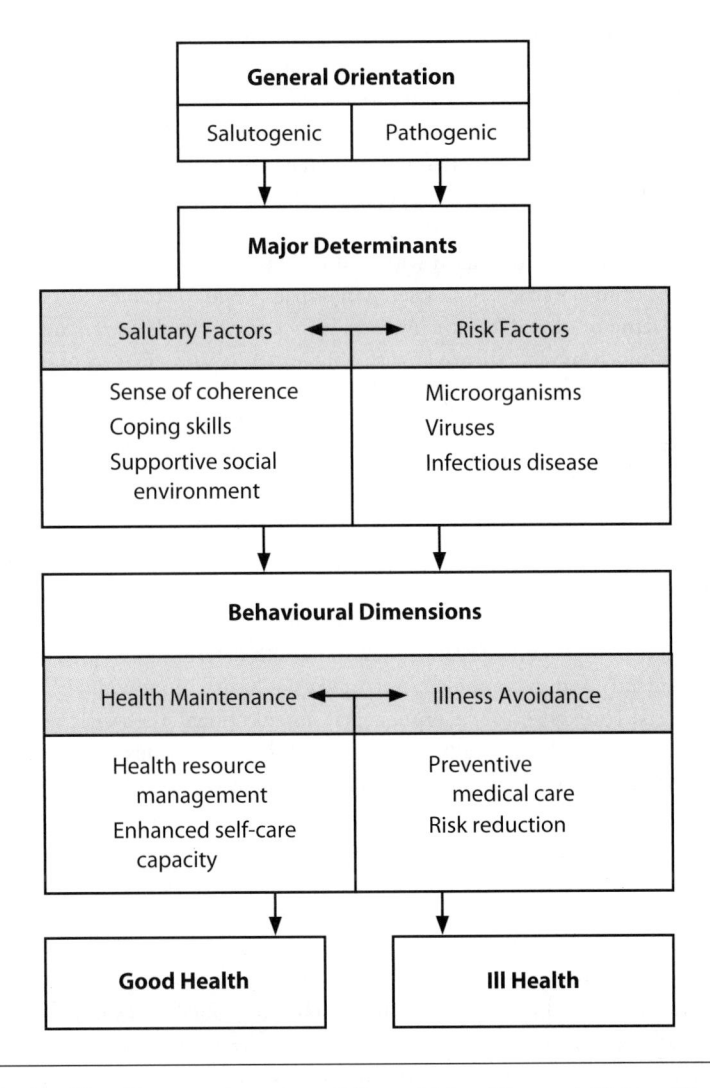

Figure 4.4 The Determinants of Good Health and Ill Health

double-ended arrows reflect the fact that the major health determinants and behavioural dimensions involved in maintaining good health and avoiding ill health are interrelated and do not exist in isolation from each other.

The pathogenic approach emphasizes the biophysical aspects of health status and concentrates its search for the causes of disease on risk factors such as pathogenic micro-organisms and viruses. The goal is to discover the origin and nature of disease in order to devise effective means of treating prevalent conditions. Intervention is at the level of personal health and is aimed at both treatment and prevention through risk reduction. The pathogenic approach has an illness-avoidance orientation, and, consequently, the behavioural activities emphasized in this model are primarily concerned with addressing the determinants of ill health (e.g., germs and infectious disease).

In contrast, the salutogenic approach emphasizes the psychosocial aspects of health status and searches for the sources of good health in the individual's social environment and lifestyle practices. In other words, this approach assigns greater importance to structural determinants of health. The goal is to discover the origin and nature of good health in order to promote health-protective behaviour and to enhance wellness (i.e., a sense of healthiness, physical fitness, and optimal social capacity to perform one's usual well roles). The determinants of good health are characterized as salutary factors that help to make people well, such as having a sense of coherence, effective coping skills, and a supportive social environment. The salutogenic approach has a health maintenance orientation, and, consequently, the behavioural activities emphasized in this model are primarily concerned with addressing the determinants of good health. This means finding ways to enhance people's self-care capacity and to enable them to better manage their health. Because of the salutogenic model's emphasis on the determinants of good health, this approach is much more compatible with contemporary strategies to promote population health.

Chapter Summary

In summary, we know that population health is shaped by a number of different factors, including biology and genetic endowment, individual skills and choices, living and working conditions, the social and physical environments, access to supportive relationships, and the formal health-care system. Each of these factors is important in its own right, but we also know that they intersect. It is now generally accepted that the health determinants discussed in this chapter "act independently and in combination to affect the health of individuals and of the population" (Millar and Hull 1997, 147). Consequently, intersectional analysis is required to gain a greater understanding of the mutually reinforcing effects that various structural and personal determinants have on population health. Chapter 8 presents an intersectional model of health incorporating these factors.

The purpose of this chapter was to review the general determinants of health and to highlight the important part played by social determinants in shaping health and wellness. Today there is a well-established and growing body of research demonstrating that population health is shaped by key social factors, including social status, gender roles, and cultural context, as well as by more specific factors, such as income distribution and income inequality; education and literacy; employment, working conditions, and job security; social environments; social support networks; social inclusion/exclusion; health-care services; personal self-care practices and life choices; and healthy child development. Wilkinson and Marmot (2003) characterize these research findings as "solid facts" that demonstrate the lifelong importance of social determinants and the remarkable sensitivity of our health to the social environment. Raphael (2003a, 36) concludes that the weight of the evidence indicates that social determinants of health

1) have a direct impact on health of individuals and populations,
2) are the best predictors of individual and population health,
3) structure lifestyle choices, and
4) interact with each other to produce health.

Overall, we have made significant progress in gaining a greater understanding of the central role played by social factors in determining the general health status of Canadians.

At the same time, it is important to acknowledge that although we may be better informed about the general determinants of ill health, we still have unanswered questions about *what makes people healthy* (i.e., the major determinants of good health). In addition, we still do not have a full understanding of the exact way in which these factors actually affect our health (i.e., *how they make us healthy*). We have a good deal to learn about how the social determinants are related to our health and how they interact with each other over time to determine why some Canadians are healthier than others. In other words, we cannot yet identify the exact health benefits associated with specific salutary factors (or combinations of factors) that contribute to good health across the life course. As a result, good health remains somewhat of a mystery.

Most discussions of health determinants are based on the underlying assumption that there is a causal relationship between these factors and the health of the population. In other words, we assume that personal and structural determinants directly affect our health. Is this a safe assumption? Does the available research evidence really permit us to conclude that we have identified cause-and-effect relationships between health determinants and health outcomes? The answer to both of these questions is a qualified no. At present, the best that we can claim is that we have identified important aspects of the social environment and lifestyle behaviour that are correlated with health status. Stated another way, they consistently occur together, but our research methods and the quality of available longitudinal data have to improve substantially before we can conclude that we have established causality.

Furthermore, most discussions of health determinants present complex interactions in an oversimplified manner. For example, the claim that lifestyle behaviours account for a significant proportion of the variance in certain health status indicators can lead to false expectations that promoting behavioural changes, such as smoking cessation, might directly result in significant improvements in population health. As we will see in Chapter 8, these behaviours are intimately tied to the social context in which they occur (i.e., the types of lives we lead at home, at work, and in the community) and to our personal beliefs about health (i.e., our ideas about the nature and origin of good health and what we should do to stay healthy). Williams (2003, 148) argues that advances in our understanding of the determinants of health and, more specifically, the links between social structure and health and well-being require "a deeper and more fine-grained understanding of the relationship between the individual and his or her social context." The following chapters in this part of the book are devoted to a closer examination of the ways in which health status is shaped by selected structural factors (e.g., socioeconomic status), the combined intersecting effects of social location (e.g., class, gender, and ethnicity), and personal factors such as lifestyle behaviours. By analyzing healthy life choices within the context of the chances provided by healthy social environments, we may ultimately gain a better understanding of the determinants of good health and the process by which Canadians pursue health and wellness.

Study Questions

1. Summarize the major determinants of population health.
2. Explain the difference between personal and structural determinants of health.
3. Comment critically on our ability to assess the relative importance of health determinants.
4. Is it possible to distinguish between the determinants of good health and the determinants of ill health?
5. Outline an approach for assessing the benefits of the determinants of good health.

Recommended Readings

Burdon, R. 2003. *The Suffering Gene: Environmental Threats to Our Health*. Montreal: McGill-Queen's University Press.

Evans, R., M. Barer, and T. Marmor, eds. 1994. *Why Are Some People Healthy and Others Not?* New York: Aldine de Gruyter.

Frumkin, H., L. Frank, and R. Jackson. 2004. *Urban Sprawl and Public Health: Designing, Planning and Building for Healthy Communities*. Washington: Island Press.

Hoffman-Goetz, L., L. Donelle, and R. Ahmed. 2014. *Health Literacy in Canada*. Toronto: Canadian Scholars Press.

Marmot, M., and R. Wilkinson, eds. 2006. *Social Determinants of Health*. 2nd edn. Oxford: Oxford University Press.

Mikkonen, J., and D. Raphael. 2010. *Social Determinants of Health: The Canadian Facts*. Toronto: York University School of Health Policy and Management.

Raphael, D., ed. 2009. *Social Determinants of Health: Canadian Perspectives*. 2nd edn. Toronto: Canadian Scholars Press.

Recommended Websites

Canadian Council on Social Determinants of Health:
www.ccsdh.ca

Canadian Network for Human Health and the Environment:
www.cnhhe-rcshe.ca

Canadian Public Health Association—Frontline Health: Beyond Health Care:
www.frontlinehealth.cpha.ca

Global Age Watch Index 2014:
www.helpage.org

Health Literacy:
http://healthliteracy.ca

National Collaborating Centre for Determinants of Health:
http://nccdh.ca

Public Health Agency of Canada—What Determines Health?:
www.phac-aspc.gc.ca/ph-sp/determinants/index-eng.php

Social Determinants of Health: The Canadian Facts:
www.thecanadianfacts.org

The Last Straw! A Board Game on the Social Determinants of Health:
www.thelaststraw.ca

World Health Organization—Social Determinants of Health:
www.who.int/social_determinants/en/index.html

Recommended Audiovisual Sources

Manufactured Landscapes. Documentary film directed by Jennifer Baichwal, 2006.

Rx for Survival: A Global Health Challenge. Co-production of WGBH Educational Foundation and Vulcan Productions, Inc., 2005.

5

Addressing Sources of Inequality and Health Disparities: Socioeconomic Status

Learning Objectives

In this chapter, you will explore the relationship between social inequality and population health and gain a greater understanding of one of the key social determinants of health disparities—socioeconomic circumstances. The chapter examines

- the meaning of social inequality;
- the link between social status and health status;
- the social gradient and health;
- explanations of the social gradient in health;
- income inequality and population health;
- socioeconomic status and health outcomes across the life course;
- whether it is possible to reduce class-based disparities in health; and
- the importance of an intersectional theory of health and socioeconomic status across the life course.

Understanding Social Inequality

The International Classification of Diseases (*ICD*) developed by the World Health Organization is an exhaustive attempt to classify the global population's experience of disease and illness. According to the *World Health Report*, condition Z59.5 is the world's most ruthless killer and the greatest cause of ill health and suffering across the globe. What is condition Z59.5, and why does it have such a dramatic impact on health? Furthermore, what can be done to address the effects of the world's leading cause of death? In this chapter, we will take a look at the way in which condition Z59.5, which is listed in the *ICD*-10 as "extreme poverty," along with other socioeconomic sources of inequality, influence health.

Our society is an unequal society. Sociologists understand that social inequality (i.e., unequal life conditions) exists because opportunities are differentially distributed in society based on factors such as social class, gender, ethnicity, and age (McMullin 2010). As a result, material resources, such as income and wealth, as well as cultural resources, such as knowledge and education, are not equally distributed among the members of modern society. Thus, **social inequality** refers to the relatively stable differences between individuals and groups of people in the societal distribution of power and privilege. **Structures of inequality** such as class, gender, ethnicity, and age are associated with enduring patterns of advantage (and disadvantage) that shape the ways people interact on a daily basis. "There is evidence to indicate that social groupings that are distinguishable from others on these dimensions have often been able to maintain significant advantages within the system of social inequality in Canada, and have done so largely because of superior access to economic, political, and ideological power" (Grabb 2009, 12). Consequently, social inequality has important implications for people's lives, including disparities in health.

According to Marmot (2004a), applying sociological theory can help to address the link between sources of inequality and health disparities. He explains that

> features of the organization of society are as crucial to the researcher who wishes to understand reasons for social variation in disease as they are to the sociologist, economist, or political scientist who wishes to understand society. Indeed, the insights of these other disciplines are of vital importance for the student of social determinants of health. One can go further . . . we start with studying health and conclude with fundamental observations about the nature of the good society.

In other words, the sociological imagination is necessary for understanding the links between healthy societies and healthy people.

In this chapter, we are going to concentrate on the ways in which socioeconomic status influences our health and well-being. In the following chapters, we will explore a number of other intersecting sources of social inequality (such as gender and ethnicity) that are also associated with health disparities. The common denominator in each of these cases is that living in poverty or experiencing sexism or racism results in **social exclusion**, a process of marginalization reflecting unequal power relationships between groups in society and involving unequal access to social, cultural, political, and economic resources. In Canada, the groups that have been identified as being at high risk of experiencing social exclusion are women, racialized groups, Aboriginal peoples, and immigrants (Galabuzi 2012). Other marginalized groups include older adults, people with disabilities, and LGBTQ people. Social exclusion consists of four dimensions:

1. exclusion from civil society—limitations due to legal constraints, institutional mechanisms, or systemic discrimination based on factors such as gender, race, or ethnicity;
2. exclusion from social goods—limited access to resources and services such as housing for the homeless and persons with disabilities or support services for seniors;
3. exclusion from social production—limited opportunities to contribute through employment as well as limited access to other key societal institutions (e.g., higher education); and
4. economic exclusion—limited opportunities for acquiring adequate material conditions (e.g., living in substandard housing or high-crime neighbourhoods).

"International and Canadian research shows that groups experiencing various forms of oppression and social marginalization tend to sustain higher health risks and lower health status" (Galabuzi 2012, 97). In other words, social exclusion has a significant impact on the pursuit of health and wellness.

Lynam and Cowley (2007) argue that we need to understand marginalization as a crucial social determinant of health. Drawing on Bourdieu's theoretical perspective, they studied the life experiences of immigrant women in Canada and Britain to illustrate the ways in which the social and material disadvantages that accompany social exclusion are associated with poor mental and physical health. Stewart and colleagues (2008) offer additional insights into the ways in which social inclusion and exclusion are experienced by various groups of Canadians and the implications for health. This study used mixed methods to assess the ways in which low- and high-income residents in Toronto and Edmonton experience social inclusion or exclusion based on their participation in community and civic activities. The researchers (2008, 87) found that "almost all participants living on low-incomes reported on the detrimental impacts of exclusion on their social and emotional well-being, and eventually on their physical well-being." They concluded that a higher level of participation in community life (social inclusion) is related to positive health outcomes.

Social exclusion exposes people to inequality and limits their options in daily life, resulting in feelings of powerlessness, which are ultimately harmful to health. It has been argued that social exclusion is a threat to the cohesiveness of society as well as to individual, community, and population health (Galabuzi 2012; Mikkonen and Raphael 2010). To a great extent, good health is fundamentally a matter of equality of opportunity. In other words, the pursuit of health and wellness depends on being able to live and work in circumstances that are beneficial to well-being. Unfortunately, this is not the case for all members of society. Structured inequality means that good health is not equally distributed throughout the population because opportunities to achieve health are not equally distributed! McMullin (2010, 253) points out that researchers "have long struggled to discover why there are inequalities in health."

In a discussion of the important part played by social factors in health inequalities, House (2001) traced the ways in which explanations for disparities in health have changed over the years. For example, in the middle of the past century, studies analyzing inequalities were influenced by the dominance of the biomedical paradigm. Over the next couple of decades, research on the contribution of lifestyle behavioural practices and a growing recognition that a variety of psychosocial factors (such as stress and social support) influence health added to our understanding but have not adequately explained inequalities in health. House contends that to gain an understanding of the sources of inequality, we need an integrated (or intersectional) theory that incorporates social factors with behavioural, psychosocial, and environmental factors.

In addition, he argues that to discover the "fundamental causes" of disparities in population health, we need to focus on social factors such as socioeconomic position, gender, ethnicity, and race, which act as upstream determinants of health. This argument is consistent with the discussion in Chapter 4 of the importance of focusing on upstream social determinants of health. House concludes by highlighting the fact that there are persistent, and perhaps even increasing, socioeconomic differences in health and challenges researchers to provide more evidence of the ways in which these types of macro-social factors account for disparities in health. In his words, "Understanding and ultimately alleviating social inequalities in health provides a major opportunity for improving population health" (2001, 138).

Social Determinants of Health Disparities: Income, Occupation, and Education

The "fundamental cause" of health disparities that has received the most research attention is socioeconomic status (SES) (Willson 2009). **Socioeconomic status** refers to an individual's relative social and economic position in society based on personal factors such as income, occupation, and education. Position in the social structure is typically analyzed in terms of socioeconomic status and social class standing. **Social class** refers to social groupings based on socioeconomic factors such as income, occupation, and education. These factors are used individually, or in combination, as indicators of social and economic circumstances at the individual, family, neighbourhood, and societal levels. The critical point is that each of these factors has a significant impact on health. Stated simply, higher social status typically means better health! "One of the most consistent findings in health research is that 'social class' is strongly related to health status however measured" (Muntaner et al. 2006, 139). The link between social status and health is also evident regardless of the health status indicator used.

Furthermore, evidence suggests that this is an extremely durable relationship. For example, social class differences in mortality persist over time even though the major causes of death have changed from primarily acute, infectious diseases to chronic, degenerative diseases. In other words, the causes of death may have changed, but the relationship between SES and death has remained essentially the same. Marmot (2005) points out that there are dramatic differences in life expectancy both between and within countries. For example, in the United States there are significant disparities such as "a 20-year gap in life expectancy between the most and least advantaged populations" (Marmot 2005, 1099). According to the *World Health Statistics 2014* published by the WHO (2014b), people everywhere are now living longer. While low-income countries have made the greatest progress over the past decade, there is still a significant gap in life expectancy between rich and poor countries. Life expectancy at birth currently ranges from 47.5 years in Sierra Leone to 84.6 years in Japan. To further illustrate this major rich–poor divide, a boy born in 2012 in a high-income country can expect to live 16 years longer than one born in a low-income country. For girls, the difference is even greater (there is a gap of 19 years in life expectancy between girls in high- and low-income countries). Wilkinson (1996) effectively captured the critical importance of this health determinant when he described the link between social class position and health as social structure's power of life and death over us.

A large body of international research has examined the effects of socioeconomic status on population health. Humphries and van Doorslaer (2000) point out that the link between SES and health status has been found in every country in which the relationship has been examined. For example, "health disparities associated with SES have been documented in both Canada and the US for decades" (Willson 2009, 95). Since it is not possible to review all of these studies, the present discussion will summarize key findings regarding the connection between health disparities and social determinants such as income, occupation, and education.

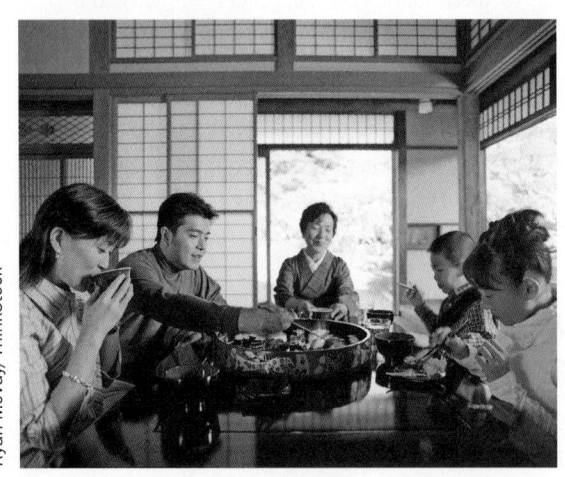

What factors do you think might contribute to Japan having the longest life expectancy in the world?

Income

Income is the most common indicator of socioeconomic status used in studies of social inequality and health, especially those carried out in industrialized societies where economic success and materialism are highly valued. Income is important because it shapes life experiences in many ways and, therefore, influences health. For example, income is related to the quality of early life, educational and employment opportunities, housing, and transportation, as well as the need to use the social safety net and the experience of social exclusion. As Wilkinson and Pickett (2010, 27) explain, "Where income differences are bigger, social distances are bigger and social stratification more important." According to Mikkonen and Raphael (2010, 12),

> Income is perhaps the most important social determinant of health. Level of income shapes overall living conditions, affects psychological functioning, and influences health-related behaviours such as quality of diet, extent of physical activity, tobacco use, and excessive alcohol use. In Canada, income determines the quality of other social determinants of health such as food security, housing, and other basic prerequisites of health.

Both absolute and relative levels of income are critical social determinants of health and health disparities. Studies assessing the relationship between income and health have focused on both the individual level (e.g., absolute income) and the aggregate level, or the relative distribution of income in society (e.g., income inequality). First, we're going to examine research findings on the link between income and personal health, and then, later in the chapter, we will turn our attention to the relationship between income inequality and population health.

"A veritable mountain of evidence links SES and its various indicators to individual health outcomes" (Babones 2010, 130). The association between level of income and health has been extensively investigated in a number of European countries, including the United Kingdom. For example, Ecob and Davey Smith (1999) report that the effect of income on health measures such as self-reported symptoms and long-term illness conditions is comparable to that of the other socioeconomic variables in combination (i.e., level of education and employment status). As is typically the case, they conclude that increasing income is associated with better health but make the interesting observation that there are diminishing returns at higher income levels.

Canadian studies also consistently report that there is a strong association between income and health (e.g., Auger and Alix 2009; Humphries and van Doorslaer 2000; Wilkins, Berthelot, and Ng 2002). Evidence of this relationship has been found for a number of different health status indicators, such as self-assessed health, overall functional health (as measured by the Health Utility Index), general mortality rates (life expectancy), infant mortality, and morbidity rates (e.g., cardiovascular disease). "The most common Canadian approach to studying the income-health relationship is to group individuals on the basis of absolute income into sets of a whole such as deciles, quintiles, or quartiles or other such measures (e.g., high versus low income)" (Raphael et al. 2005, 222). In all cases, higher income is related to better health. In the example presented in Figure 5.1, you can see that maternal socioeconomic status is an important determinant of differences in birth outcomes in Quebec. Mothers living in successively lower-income neighbourhoods experience increased rates of adverse outcomes, including more preterm births, lower birth weight babies, and higher infant mortality. Similarly, infant mortality rates also vary by income quintile in Winnipeg, Manitoba. According to the Winnipeg Regional Health Authority (2013), the infant mortality rate is 4.7 for those in the highest income quintile in contrast to 9.5 (per 1000 live births) for those in the lowest income quintile. Based on the evidence that rates of infant mortality and low birth weight correlate closely with income, Denburg and Daneman (2010, 22) conclude that "inequalities in child health outcomes trace an impressively linear socio-economic gradient."

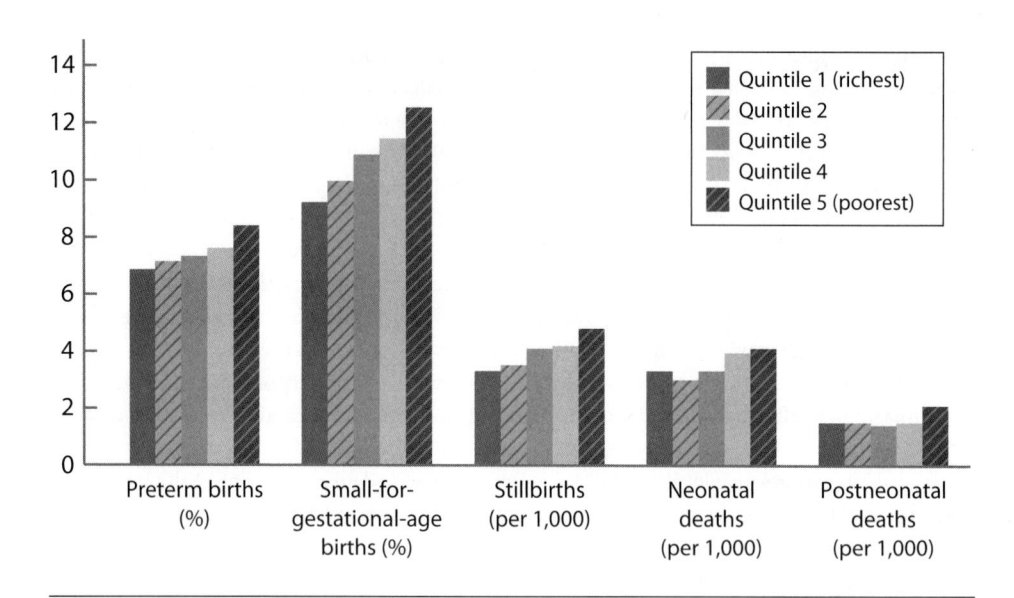

Figure 5.1 Rates of Adverse Birth Outcomes Higher Among Mothers Living in Lower-Income Neighbourhoods, Quebec, 1991 to 2000

Source: Statistics Canada, Socioeconomic status and birth outcomes in Quebec, ...au Courant, 82-005-XIE2006002, September 2006. http://www.statcan.gc.ca/bsolc/olc-cel/olc-cel?catno=82-005-XIE&lang=eng#formatdisp

Based on a review of Canadian research on income and income distribution as determinants of health, Raphael et al. (2010) suggest that a number of conceptual and methodological improvements are needed to gain a better understanding of the influence of income on health. The areas of improvement they identify include: the need for better theoretical models and greater conceptual clarity; more interdisciplinary work on the pathways involved in the income–health relationship; more studies using longitudinal research designs to capture life course effects, as well as qualitative and mixed-method designs, to facilitate the type of complex analyses required to specify the interacting mechanisms by which income contributes to health and well-being over the life course; and, finally, more attention to the policy implications of research findings.

Occupation

Occupation is a second aspect of socioeconomic status. Siegrist and Theorell (2006, 73) point out that "work and employment are of critical importance for health." People who participate in the paid labour force generally report better health than those who are retired, participate only in unpaid domestic labour, or are unemployed. Rosenthal and colleagues (2012) argue that it is not just employment but full-time employment that is particularly important for health and well-being. They assert that the connection between unemployment and underemployment and negative health outcomes is well established. As discussed in the previous chapter, being unemployed definitely puts health at risk. Furthermore, health typically deteriorates as the duration of unemployment increases. Extensive research evidence shows that unemployment and precarious employment are negatively associated with mental and physical health and general well-being (Puig-Barrachina et al. 2011; Rosenthal et al. 2012). The stress associated with unemployment and income insecurity lead not only to a variety of health problems but also to an increase in the risk of premature death (Bartley, Ferrie, and Montgomery 2006; Wilkinson and Marmot 2003). For example, "lack of employment is associated with physical and mental health problems that include depression, anxiety and increased suicide rates" (Mikkonen and Raphael 2010, 17).

Although research has repeatedly shown that there are higher rates of mortality, morbidity, and poor self-rated health among women and men who are unemployed, Bartley, Ferrie, and Montgomery (2006) caution that it is not safe to simply interpret these data as evidence of a causal relationship between unemployment and health. For example, Bartley and Ferrie (2010, 5) suggest that the apparent association between unemployment and mortality may be "due to over-representation among the unemployed of people with diseases that are going to shorten their lives regardless." If this is indeed the case, then it is equally plausible that health-related restrictions may affect participation in the paid labour force. In other words, those who are sick may be unable to work. McDonough and Amick (2001) used US longitudinal data to examine the effects of health on labour force participation and report that a variety of factors affect the risk of unemployment, including gender, age, history of unemployment, and hazardous working conditions. They conclude that social position matters when analyzing health and labour force activity, but it is noteworthy that it is the disadvantaged (i.e., those with limited access to social and economic resources) who, despite experiencing health problems, may continue to participate in the labour market! These studies exemplify the large body of research that has demonstrated that there is a complex relationship between factors such as employment, job security, working conditions, occupational prestige, economic stability, and population health.

It is important to note that while employment typically protects and fosters health, as depicted in Box 5.1, participating in the paid labour force does not necessarily translate directly into better health. "In general, having a job is better for health than having no job. But the social organization of work, management styles and social relationships in the workplace all matter for health" (Wilkinson and Marmot 2003, 18). Muntaner and colleagues (2010) highlight the importance of "employment relations," or the social relationships between workers, supervisors, managers, and owners, in understanding the link between social class and health. It is apparent that stress-related demands associated with being employed might have adverse effects on health and well-being. For example, those in precarious employment situations—who lack job security or work in part-time or temporary positions, as well as those who work long or irregular hours or do shift work—may experience negative health outcomes. In addition, the pace and repetitive nature of work, the frequency of deadlines and reporting requirements, the level of control we have over our daily work activities, and our decision-making authority may create stressful conditions that have harmful health consequences. Finally, physically demanding work and safety issues, such as exposure to chemical hazards in the workplace, have been shown to adversely affect health. Consequently, Warren and colleagues (2004) emphasize the important mediating role that psychosocial and physical job characteristics play in the relationship between socioeconomic status and health.

> **Box 5.1** Employment Stress and Ill Health
>
> In a now classic study, a team of researchers (Winkleby et al. 1988) studied the effects of job stress on the health of urban transit operators. It turns out that driving a bus for a living is a typical example of a job that is bad for your health. Bus drivers endure a highly stressful employment environment complete with the demands of keeping a tight schedule, sometimes unruly passengers, and factors such as traffic and weather conditions. In other words, "bus drivers must respond to multiple demands over which they have little control" (Bhatt and Seema 2012, 201). Research has shown that as a result of their stressful employment conditions and exposure to occupational health hazards, bus drivers experience a host of negative outcomes, including high blood pressure, peptic ulcers, digestive problems, and musculoskeletal problems such as back and neck pain. Studies of bus drivers carried out in a number of countries are similar in their conclusion that the high demands and low control associated with driving a bus lead to the development over time of a range of occupational health problems (Kompier and Di Martino 1995). Something to keep in mind the next time you ride a bus.
>
> Mike Dabell/iStockphoto

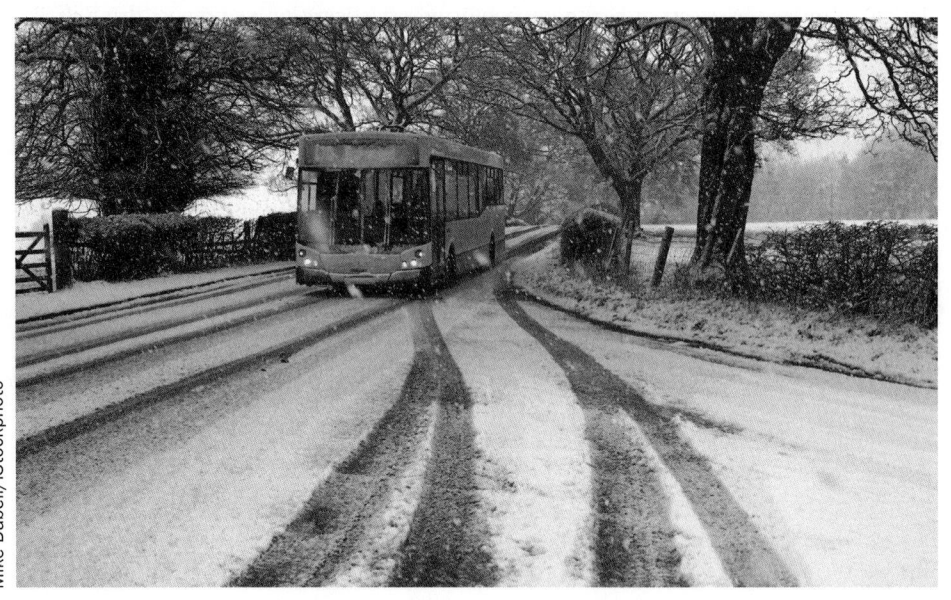

In describing the unhealthy Canadian workplace, Jackson (2009, 99) points out that "high psychological demands at work combined with a low degree of control of the work process . . . has been linked to an increased risk of physical injuries at work, high blood pressure, cardiovascular disease, depression, and other mental health conditions and increased lifestyle risks to health." In contrast, people who have more control over their work circumstances and higher levels of job satisfaction tend to be healthier. Job satisfaction, which is an important aspect of quality of life, is also a reflection of meaningful employment, opportunities to acquire knowledge and skills, adequacy of income, economic stability, and rewarding relationships with co-workers. These types of working conditions and a suitable balance between work and home life are associated with good health.

Mustard, Vermeulen, and Lavis (2003) examined the extent to which position in the occupational hierarchy, characteristics of the psychosocial work environment (e.g., decision authority, skill discretion), and health-related behaviours (e.g., smoking and alcohol consumption) can explain declining self-rated health in a representative sample of the Canadian labour force. Their findings indicate that the probability of a decline in perceived health status is associated with decline in occupational prestige (particularly for male labour force participants in lower-status occupations). According to Mustard, Lavis, and Ostry (2006, 174), "we now know that common diseases such as coronary heart disease, mental illness, and degenerative musculoskeletal disease may be initiated or accelerated by chronically adverse work experiences." Although they go on to state that the "established causes of work-attributable morbidity represent only the tip of the iceberg of health consequences of work" (2006, 174), it is evident that work experiences have pervasive consequences for the health of populations.

Two conceptual models have been developed to try to account for the ways in which stressful job characteristics result in adverse health effects. The first has been characterized as the demand–control model and the second as the effort–reward imbalance model (Siegrist and Theorell 2006). The **demand–control model** focuses on two dimensions of work: (1) the psychological demands on the working person and (2) the degree of control the person has over work schedules and job conditions. A low level of control and decision authority over one's required tasks at work combined with high job strain and continued pressure negatively affect health. The **effort–reward imbalance model** emphasizes the importance of social reciprocity in our work lives. According to this model, health is adversely affected if the time and effort devoted to work are not matched by adequate rewards, such as income, career advancement opportunities, and job security. Both models have been extensively tested and are supported by empirical evidence. In many respects, the two models complement each other, and it is likely "that simultaneously experienced low control and low reward in demanding jobs may increase the probability of ill health above and beyond the risk associated with separate exposure to these conditions" (Siegrist and Theorell 2006, 77). All factors considered, one of the best things you can do for your own pursuit of health and wellness is to find and keep a good job!

Education

Level of formal education is also used as an indicator of socioeconomic status in studies of health inequalities. According to Eide and Showalter (2011, 778), "the correlation between education and health is well established and highly studied." As indicated in the previous chapter, more years of education translate into longer and healthier lives. Numerous studies have documented the link between higher levels of education and better health throughout the life course, although Kawachi, Adler, and Dow (2010) caution that there is still a lot that we need to learn about what type of education matters for health. The health outcomes associated with level of education include: self-reported health, the prevalence of chronic diseases such as diabetes and hypertension, hospitalization, and mortality rates (Eide and Showalter 2011; Goldman and Smith 2011; Albert and Davia 2010). In other words, the higher the level of formal education you have, the better your health is likely to be and the longer you are likely to live. You may want to bear this in mind the next time you wonder why you're studying so hard at university! Marmot (2005) presents international evidence that adult mortality rates vary inversely with level of education, and it appears that this difference in life expectancy is persistent over time and may even be increasing (Cutler and Lleras-Muney 2010).

Explanations of the differences in health outcomes associated with level of formal education typically focus on the relationship between education and health-related behaviours. As discussed in Chapter 4, Mokdad and colleagues (2004) estimate that nearly half of all deaths in the United States are attributable to behavioural factors such as smoking, excessive weight, and heavy alcohol consumption. Individuals with higher levels of education are less likely to smoke or to be obese and consequently may experience better health outcomes (Cutler and Lleras-Muney 2010). This finding is supported by research conducted in a number of countries. For example, the main conclusion of a Swedish study conducted by Brannlund, Hammarstrom, and Strandh (2013) is that education reduces the probability of unhealthy behaviour over the life course. Ross and Mirowsky (2011) adopt a life course perspective to guide their exploration of the connection between personal and parental education, unhealthy lifestyle behaviours, and health. Their basic contention is that education improves health more for people whose parents were also well educated. They state that in contrast,

> if an individual's parents were poorly educated and the individual is also poorly educated, the health disadvantages are amplified, each making the other worse. Furthermore, because one's own level of education is highly structured by that of one's parents, individuals from disadvantaged family backgrounds are likely to be disadvantaged themselves (2011, 591).

They call this "**structural amplification**," since parental education (as well as occupation and income) precede and structure many of our life experiences, including health. According to Ross and Mirowsky, the reason that parental education matters is that lifestyle behaviours have a cumulative effect on health across the life course. Goldman and Smith (2011, 1733) not only agree that lifestyle behaviours contribute to growing health disparities but also stress the fact that "compared to 30 years ago, the probability of having major chronic conditions increased sharply for the least educated compared to the more educated."

A related approach to explaining the connection between education and health concentrates on the ways in which level of formal education improves our ability to understand complex health information—that is, the individual's level of health literacy (Berkman, Davis, and McCormack 2010; Rootman and Ronson 2005; Kickbusch 2001). For example, poor literacy skills may mean difficulties in reading and understanding medication instructions or health and safety educational material. Although education and literacy are not perfectly correlated, "there is a strong relationship between educational level and literacy," which "itself is a strong predictor of health" (Rootman and Ronson 2005, S68). The basic idea is that some health disparities associated with education may be due to differences in factual knowledge (not just the number of years of school completed). Education is an important social determinant because it increases our understanding of which behavioural practices may be harmful or beneficial and how to protect and promote our health. It is important to recognize that improving the level of health literacy in a population means more than the simple provision of health-related information; it also means helping people to develop the capacity both to understand and to act appropriately based on that knowledge. According to Baker and colleagues (2007, 1503), higher levels of education "have direct effects on health through greater health knowledge acquired during schooling and greater personal empowerment and self-efficacy." This means that health literacy is associated not only with increased access to health information but also with better informed decision-making and the skills required to engage in health-protective behaviours and ultimately to improved population health and wellness.

Sophisticated literacy skills are increasingly necessary for individuals to be able to function effectively in contemporary society, including pursuing health and wellness. The relationship between poor literacy skills and health has been well documented (Berkman et al. 2011; Wolf et al. 2010; Baker 2006; Wolf, Gazmararian, and Baker 2005). Studies consistently find that "low literacy in a population is associated both directly and indirectly with a range of poor health outcomes" (Nutbeam 2008, 2072). For example, among older adults, low health literacy is associated with poor self-care of chronic diseases, less frequent use of preventive health services, excessive use of emergency services, and increased risk of mortality (Kobayashi, Wardle, and von Wagner 2014). This is particularly problematic, since health literacy skills tend to decline over the life course. According to recent research evidence, however, Internet use and social engagement (particularly in cultural activities such as visiting museums and art galleries) may offset age-related cognitive changes and health literacy decline. The findings of this longitudinal study of older English adults led Kobayashi, Wardle, and von Wagner (2014, 5) to conclude that "our results indicate that internet use and social engagement may help older adults to maintain the functional literacy skills required to manage health." It seems that the adage "use it or lose it" applies to health literacy!

Health literacy can be viewed as an asset to be developed as a vital component of population health promotion initiatives. According to Baur (2010), a number of issues need to be addressed if we are to gain a better understanding of the link between improvements in health literacy and population health. For example, there is ongoing debate about the evolving meaning of health literacy (Berkman, Davis, and McCormack 2010; Peerson and Saunders 2009; Nutbeam 2008) and the causal pathways linking it to health outcomes (Osborn et al. 2011; Paasche-Orlow and Wolf 2007). In contrast, there is widespread agreement about the benefits of living in a literate society. The Expert Panel on Health Literacy established by the Canadian Public Health Association offers a vision of what a health literate Canada would look like. Achieving societal health literacy would mean that "all people in Canada have the capacity, opportunities and support they need to obtain and use health information effectively, to act as informed partners in the care of themselves, their families and communities, and to manage interactions in a variety of settings that affect health and well-being" (Rootman and Gordon-el-Bihbety 2008). Health and learning are inextricably connected, and while literacy may be associated with level of education, it is also a vital determinant of disparities in health. In fact, it has been suggested that factors such as health literacy and reading fluency may be more powerful predictors than education in explaining the relationship between socioeconomic status and health (Baker et al. 2007). Thus, health literacy is a crucial component of a fair and democratic, healthy society!

"On balance the evidence suggests that income, education, and occupational class all affect health independently of each other" (Babones 2010, 137). While each of these SES measures may be independently associated with health, it is important to note that they intersect and, therefore, also have a combined impact on health status. Education, for example, is highly correlated with income; those with higher levels of formal education tend to have higher levels of income. Furthermore, occupation and employment are related to education and income. Consequently, interpreting the nature of the relationship between SES and health is complicated by the fact that income, occupation, and education are themselves intersectional concepts.

In addition, not only are these social class factors important determinants of health, but they also intersect with other structural factors. For example, findings indicate that age and gender may moderate the impact of unemployment on physical and emotional health (Puig-Barrachina et al. 2011). In other words, life events such as unemployment may be experienced differently by men and women depending on their work history and personal and family circumstances (i.e., supportive social networks). Beland, Birch, and Stoddart (2002, 2034) argue that "unemployment may affect the health of different subgroups of the population differently." According to these researchers, the association between unemployment and health status may be influenced by a number of contextual-level factors, such as the rate of unemployment in the community, labour force participation rates, and the proportion of the population who are immigrants, as well as gender and age-group distributions. To gain a better understanding of the multiple determinants of population health, we need an intersectional model to guide our examination of the ways in which other structural factors and contextual characteristics moderate the effects of socioeconomic status on health and well-being across the life course.

The Social Gradient and Health

Imagine a parade. Everyone in society is ranked according to his or her social position. The unemployed come first, followed by the unskilled manual labourers, then the semi-skilled, the skilled, the clerks and shop assistants, after them the teachers and middle managers, and then the senior managers, the lawyers, doctors and judges. With few exceptions, this ranking by social position has produced a ranking according to life expectancy.

With this thought exercise, Marmot (2004a) introduces one of the most fascinating concepts in health research: the social gradient. According to McDaniel (2013, 8), the discovery of the social gradient in health forced us to reconsider

> the relationship of social inequalities and social hierarchy to health outcomes. If social hierarchy gets under our skins so profoundly, then social factors and policies may matter more deeply to health than was previously imagined. This insight led to the realization of the sensitivity of us all, not only those who are disadvantaged, to our social environments. The result has been nothing short of a quest to understand better the social determinants of health.

Regardless of how we measure socioeconomic status and health status, a gradient consistently appears. In other words, the relationship between social status and health status holds despite the socioeconomic indicator used (e.g., income, education, employment) or the dimension of health analyzed (e.g., mortality or morbidity rates, functional ability, or self-rated health status). In each case, there is evidence of a **social gradient** in health, or a graded association between the indicators of SES and population health. Marmot (2004b, 1) refers to this gradient as the "status syndrome" and asserts that "where you stand in the social hierarchy is intimately related to your chances of getting ill, and your length of life." In other words, your position on the social gradient (relative to others in the hierarchy) will affect your pursuit of health and wellness.

Denburg and Daneman (2010, 23) note that "Evidence of a gradient in health across all social strata is well documented." Indeed, researchers have known about the social gradient in health for quite some time (e.g., Marmot et al. 1997). The ongoing longitudinal Whitehall Studies in

England, which started in 1967 by studying 18,000 men in the civil service, was one of the first to describe the social gradient in health. The original Whitehall study showed that men in the lowest employment grades were three times more likely to die prematurely than men in the highest grades of the British civil service. Since all of the study participants were civil servants, they all essentially had the same socioeconomic status. The difference in mortality rates was therefore attributed to rank within the civil service hierarchy. The second Whitehall study tried to learn more about the factors that explain the social gradient in health among both men and women. According to the findings of these studies, factors such as diet, smoking, and exercise explain only one-third of the variation in morbidity and mortality rates between the different grades of the British civil service. The critical point that the Whitehall Studies demonstrated is that the social gradient in health cannot be adequately explained by lifestyle factors or personal practices and that it is aspects of the social structure, such as our position in the social hierarchy, that have a profound influence on our health.

The gradient has been observed for both physical and mental health and well-being and reflects differences in occupational and educational status as well as income. According to researchers, "lower social position not only increases the likelihood of ill health, but it decreases one's chances for well-being" (Marmot et al. 1997, 906). This means that the social gradient in health is associated with positive indicators of subjective psychosocial well-being (such as self-esteem and sense of coherence) as well as with the negative indicators of physical illness (such as morbidity and mortality). According to Sir Michael Marmot, "the social gradient has shown us how sensitive health is to social and economic factors, and so enabled us to identify the determinants of health among the population as a whole" (2006, 2).

Marmot (see Box 5.2) has written extensively on the subject of social inequality and health and argues that it is autonomy (i.e., how much control you have over life circumstances) and opportunities for social engagement associated with social status that produce the social gradient in health. According to Marmot, the causes of the social gradient in health can be found in our living and working circumstances. In his words, "I am arguing that an important cause of the social gradient in health is that people in different social groups are exposed to different social

Box 5.2   Michael Marmot (1945–)

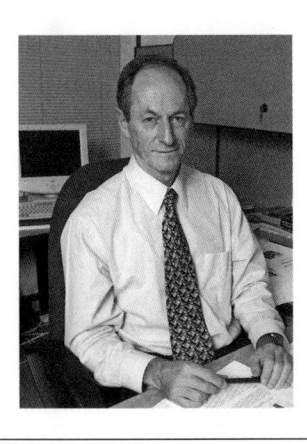

- British epidemiologist and noted researcher of the social gradient
- Principal investigator of the Whitehall Studies
- Analyzed the chain of disease causation from the social environment, through psychosocial influences, biological pathways, to risk of disease in *The Status Syndrome: How Our Position on the Social Gradient Affects Longevity and Health* (2004)

"A way to understand this link between status and health is to think of three fundamental human needs: health, autonomy and opportunity for full social participation" (2005).

and economic conditions. It is these differences in the social environment that are responsible for the gradient" (Marmot 2004b, 33).

The link between position in the social hierarchy and health status appears to be a very robust relationship that persists over time and across countries (Wilkinson and Pickett 2010). Marmot describes the social gradient in health as a remarkably widespread phenomenon. The diseases with the steepest gradients (strongest relationships with SES) may vary from one country to another; however, international evidence indicates that in both rich and poor countries it is relative position within the social hierarchy that is associated with differences in health status. In fact, "even in the most affluent countries, people who are less well off have substantially shorter life expectancies and more illnesses than the rich" (Wilkinson and Marmot 2003, 7).

Research on mortality and morbidity demonstrates that health improves with each incremental increase in socioeconomic position. As illustrated by Figure 5.2, people at each step up

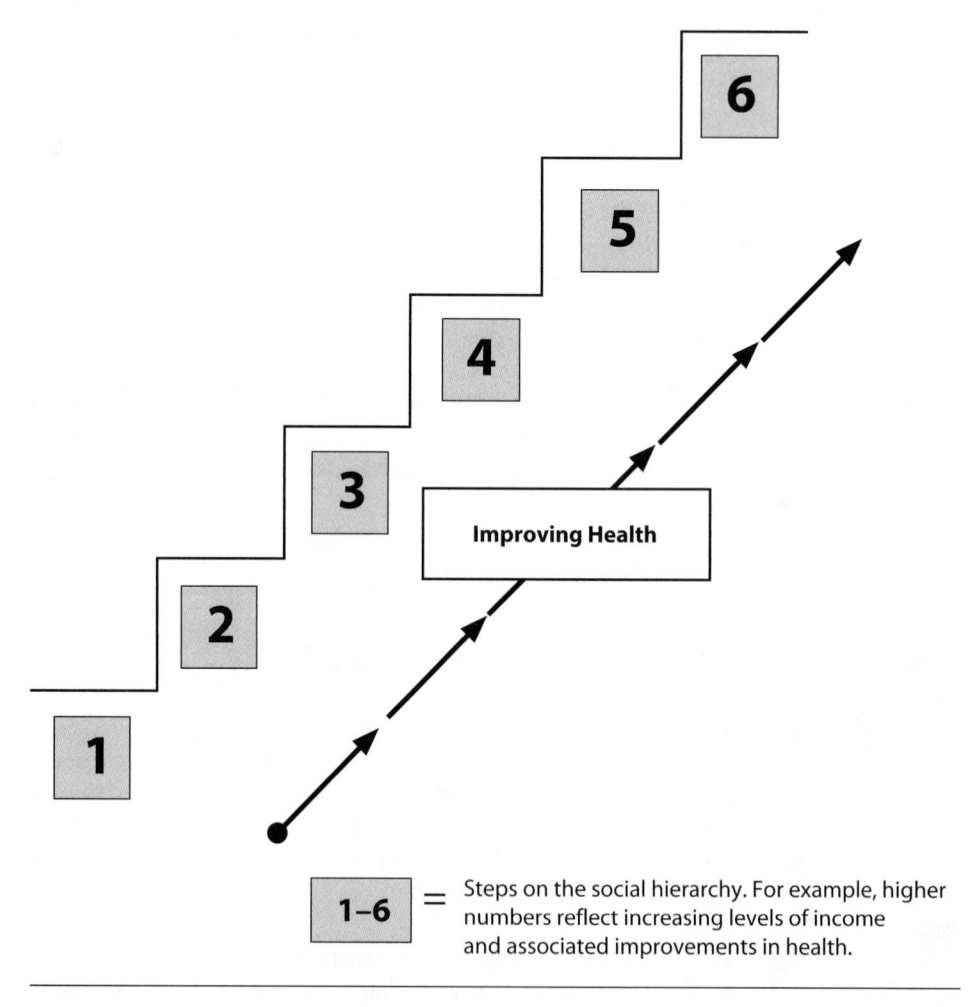

Figure 5.2 Social Gradient in Health

the social hierarchy live longer and healthier lives than those on the step below. This means that those at the top (Step 6) are in better health than those on Step 5, who, in turn, are in better health than those on Step 4, and so on. "With regard to mortality, mean difference in life expectancy between those at the top and at the bottom of a society's social structure (as defined by education, income, employment status) are anywhere from four to ten years" (Siegrist and Marmot 2006, 1). In the Canadian context, Tjepkema and Wilkins (2011) studied trends in mortality and report that the probability of survival to age 75 varies by level of income adequacy. For men, the probability was 73 per cent for those in the highest quintile compared to 50 per cent for those in the lowest. The pattern was similar for women, although the gradient was not as steep. The probability of surviving to age 75 was 83 per cent for women in the highest quintile and 70 per cent for those in the lowest.

The results of a 16-year follow-up study of Canadian mortality rates suggests that while area-based studies have demonstrated gradients in mortality by neighbourhood income, they "fail to reveal the full extent of differences in mortality by income that are evident at the individual level" (Tjepkema, Wilkins, and Long 2013, 14). This study examined age-standardized mortality rates by income adequacy quintile, which was calculated based on all sources of income for all members of each family. An analysis of the data collected from a large, population-based sample of Canadian adults aged 25 and older appears to confirm the existence of a consistent gradient in all-cause mortality by level of income adequacy. In addition, the study examined cause-specific mortality rates by income adequacy and found that "gradients in mortality by income for most causes of deaths demonstrated that the association was not confined to those at the lowest end of the income distribution. Each successively lower level of income had a higher mortality rate" (Tjepkema, Wilkins, and Long 2013, 17). These findings clearly demonstrate that the risk of death is socially graded!

It is also important to note that the gradient is continuous and there is apparently no threshold level at which the connection between SES and health completely disappears. Although "the health effects of inequality are most apparent among those living in poverty," it is not just being at the bottom of the social gradient that affects our health (Raphael 2001, 225). While we need to be aware of differences between poor and wealthy people, it is equally essential to recognize the existence of graded health differences that correspond to everyone's socioeconomic life circumstances. In an early discussion of the SES–health gradient, Adler and colleagues (1994) concluded, based on their review of evidence, that there is an association between socioeconomic status and health at every level of the social hierarchy. For example, studies in a number of different countries (including Canada, the United Kingdom, and the United States) consistently show that people at each step on the income scale are healthier than those on the step below. "This suggests that it is not only being poor or disadvantaged that is a health risk, but that the experience of having less than someone else also has negative health implications" (McMullin 2004, 241).

As illustrated in Box 5.3, the problem of inequality in health is not confined to the poorest members of society; the existence of a social gradient in mortality and morbidity means that there are systematic differences in the health and well-being of all members of society. In other words, it isn't poverty alone that makes people sick! While poverty is undeniably bad for health, so too is social inequality. Even in societies that have done a good job of tackling poverty through social and welfare programs, the social gradient is still an issue. Whenever you have social stratification and inequality, you have a social gradient.

Box 5.3 The Social Gradient in the Health of Academy Award Nominees

While it might be an "honour just to be nominated" for an Academy Award, Canadian health researchers have shown that, on average, Oscar winners live four years longer than nominees who don't win (Redelmeier and Singh 2001). A subsequent reanalysis of the data using different statistical methods suggests that the survival advantage associated with winning an Oscar may not be quite as significant (Sylvestre, Huszti, and Hanley 2006). In any case, unsuccessful Oscar nominees are certainly not poor, but winners have higher positions in the social hierarchy. Link, Carpiano, and Weden (2013) studied the mortality experiences of people who had won a variety of awards (e.g., Emmy Award winners) in an effort to gain a better understanding of the connection between socioeconomic status and mortality. They conclude that social status matters for longevity and that their results provide important insights into the SES gradient in mortality. While the findings of this study failed to show consistent advantages in life expectancy for winners, Link and colleagues (2013, 209) argue that their results highlight the importance of understanding that "it is not just relative position in a status hierarchy that matters for health, but the life circumstances that status differences create that have health consequences." Overall, this research provides further evidence that there is a social gradient in health that runs from the top to the bottom of society and that the status syndrome affects the pursuit of health and wellness of us all!

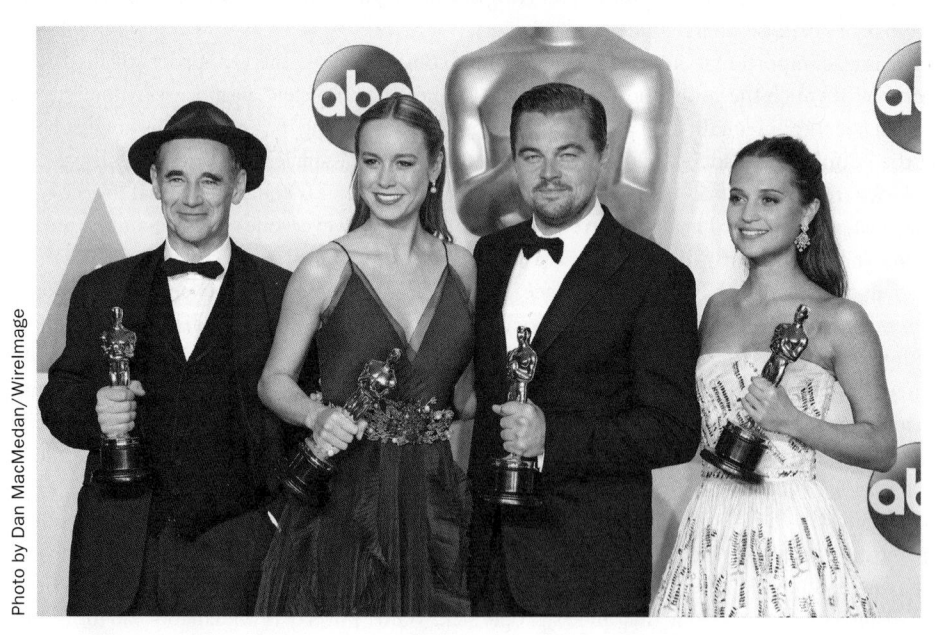

Mark Rylance, Brie Larson, Leonardo DiCaprio, and Alicia Vikander celebrate their 2016 Academy Award wins.

The social gradient in health can also be illustrated by looking at another SES indicator—employment status. For example, research carried out in Denmark by Borg and Kristensen (2000) shows that aspects of the work environment such as low influence, low skill discretion, repetitive tasks, and high job insecurity (often experienced by lower-SES workers) play a significant role in the social gradient with regard to negative changes in self-rated health over time. Although unemployment is generally related to ill health, studies carried out in areas that have high local unemployment rates usually find that there is a weaker relationship between unemployment and health status indicators. If you are unemployed and living in an area where that is the norm (i.e., many of your friends and neighbours are also unemployed), then not having a job may not be as strongly related to your health status. It should be noted, however, that contradictory findings have been reported by Canadian researchers based on a Quebec study of unemployment and health. Beland, Birch, and Stoddart (2002, 2046) state that their research results "did not provide evidence to support the hypothesis that the association of unemployment with health status depends upon whether the experience of unemployment is shared with people living in the same environment." They suggest that contextual factors, such as having a supportive social network, may account for the international difference in findings. The important point to remember about the social gradient in health is that it is not simply being employed or unemployed (or having high versus low income) that is the critical issue; it is your relative position within a particular social context that seems to affect health.

While there is no doubt that a social gradient in health exists, there is some debate about the reasons for the existence of this gradient. According to Kosteniuk and Dickenson (2003, 275), the debate continues "because of the reluctance to challenge society's culture of inequality through changes to our socioeconomic hierarchy." In other words, it is not just a matter of having more income or higher occupational prestige than others; rather, persistent social inequality and the uneven distribution of opportunities and resources in society are the significant factors that produce health disparities. In a hierarchical society marked by profound social inequalities, the social gradient raises not only health concerns but also sociological, political, economic, and indeed ethical issues!

Explanations of the Social Gradient in Health

A number of explanations (listed in Box 5.4) have been offered to account for the continued influence of social determinants (such as socioeconomic status) on population health. Despite improvements in life expectancy and general well-being, significant disparities in health persist in developed countries (including Canada). Commenting on the United States and Britain, Marmot et al. (1997, 901) state that "despite overall decline in death rates, socio-economic disparities in mortality rates have been increasing." There are three alternative approaches to explaining the persistence of these types of health inequalities: materialist and neo-materialist explanations, cultural behavioural explanations, and psychosocial explanations.

Box 5.4 Explanations of the Social Gradient in Health

- Materialist and neo-materialist explanations
- Cultural behavioural explanations
- Psychosocial explanations

Materialist and Neo-materialist Explanations

Influenced by the political economy perspective of the conflict paradigm, this approach emphasizes the material conditions under which people live and characterizes aspects of the social structure, such as differences in socioeconomic status, as powerful determinants of health. These explanations maintain that "lower SES individuals are exposed to more harmful environments and have less access to health care and other health promoting material resources" (Orpana and Lemrye 2004, 143). This is often discussed in terms of a **differential exposure hypothesis**, which argues that the higher number of health problems among lower-SES groups is explained by their greater exposure to psychosocial stressors resulting from financial problems, neighbourhood issues (such as crime), and social isolation. According to this explanation, social inequality leads to more stressful life experiences and, as a consequence of this exposure, to worse health.

The health outcome that has been identified as the most sensitive to the effects of absolute material deprivation is child mortality. According to WHO data, "Under-5 mortality varies from 316 per 1000 livebirths in Sierra Leone to 3 per 1000 livebirths in Iceland, 4 per 1000 livebirths in Finland, and 5 per 1000 livebirths in Japan" (Marmot 2005, 1099). Canada ranks twenty-fourth among industrialized nations in rates of infant mortality. While the overall rate for the country is 5.4 per 1000 live births, it should be noted that major differences exist between provinces, with the rate "ranging from as low as zero and 2.2 in the Yukon and Prince Edward Island, respectively, to as high as 8.3 in Saskatchewan and 10 in Nunavut" (Denburg and Daneman 2010, 22). Standards of living, quality of housing, neighbourhood conditions, employment status, and work environment are all linked to income and contribute to material advantages (or disadvantages), which accumulate over a person's lifetime and produce positive or negative health outcomes. Explaining the materialist approach to understanding the social gradient, Raphael (2010, 156–7) states that "material conditions of life determine health by influencing the quality of individual development, family life and interaction, and community environments." According to this approach, material deprivation leads to psychosocial stress, which in turn weakens the immune system and results in differing likelihood of physical disease as well as delayed or impaired cognitive and social development.

The neo-materialist approach contends not only that differential access to social and economic resources and the life experiences of the individual have a cumulative effect on health outcomes but that the level of funding invested in social infrastructure is also a critical determinant of health. In other words, differences between cities and countries in the quality of public infrastructure available (such as the educational system, libraries, and social services for the unemployed, people with disabilities, and older adults) have important implications for population health. According to this approach, it is societal factors that shape material aspects of living and working conditions, which, in turn, contribute to the perpetuation of health inequalities. Based on a review of more than 200 Canadian studies of income and health carried out between 1995 and 2002, Raphael et al. (2005) found that materialist and neo-materialist approaches were the most common explanatory models guiding research on the social gradient in health in Canada.

Cultural Behavioural Explanations

Cultural behavioural explanations suggest that lower-SES individuals are less healthy as a result of engaging in health-related behaviours such as smoking or poor eating habits (Orpana and Lemrye 2004). This is sometimes described in terms of a **differential vulnerability hypothesis**, which argues that we all have stressors in our daily lives that our position on the social gradient can help to alleviate or make worse. According to these explanations, lower-SES individuals do not cope very well with environmental stressors (i.e., they are more likely to engage in harmful lifestyle behaviours such as smoking or alcohol consumption) and, consequently, experience worse health. The two alternative hypotheses (differential exposure and differential vulnerability) explaining the relationships between SES, stressful life events, and health are summarized in Figure 5.3. It is important to note that they are not mutually exclusive. Both might be in effect in some circumstances, or differential exposure could apply in certain circumstances and differential vulnerability in others.

The cultural behavioural approach argues that the health-related lifestyle practices in which we routinely engage are a result of the type of socialization process (or family upbringing) that we receive. The socialization process, in turn, is shaped by broader societal factors. Singh-Manoux and Marmot (2005) explored the role of socialization in explaining social inequalities in health and suggest that Bourdieu's concept of "habitus" is helpful in understanding the ways in which individual health behaviours are patterned by the socio-cultural context. According to Bourdieu, structural opportunities or constraints are closely tied to the practices of everyday life. It is through the process of socialization that these practices become embodied as patterns of thinking, feeling, and acting and give rise to certain types of behavioural dispositions. In other words, the socio-cultural and socioeconomic environments in which we grow up, and the type of socialization that we experience, are linked to the behaviours that we learn. In terms of health, this may translate into internalizing and repeating healthful or harmful behavioural practices. This may help us to understand why "poor diet, smoking, alcohol consumption, lack of physical exercise and overweight are more prevalent in lower socio-economic status groups" (Siegrist and Marmot 2006, 6). In fact, such behaviours follow a social gradient in health. This is because socialization provides individuals with a framework for dealing with life events (e.g., stress) that are linked to

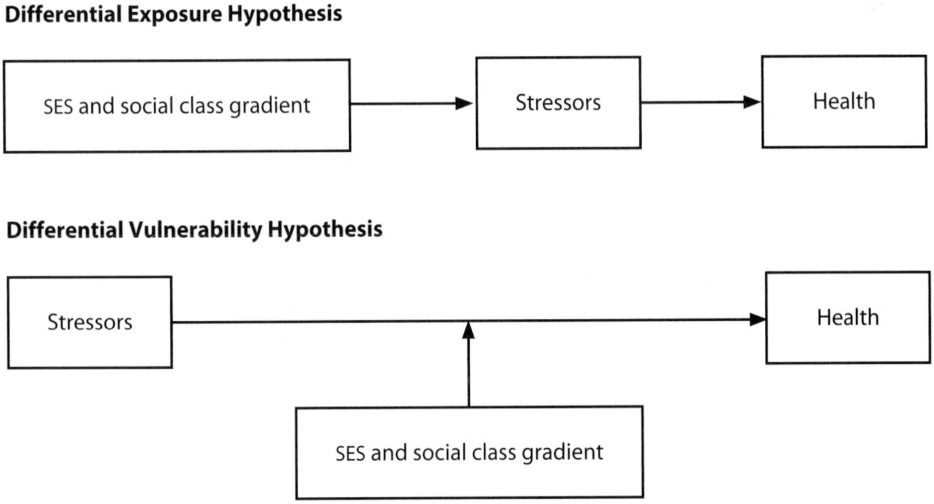

Differential Exposure Hypothesis

SES and social class gradient → Stressors → Health

Differential Vulnerability Hypothesis

Stressors → Health
↑
SES and social class gradient

Figure 5.3 Hypotheses Explaining the Relationships Between Socioeconomic Status (SES), Stressors, and Health

their position in the social hierarchy and may result in negative health outcomes. In addition, at the societal level the process of socialization plays a critical role in reproducing existing social structures. Thus, there is a complex relationship between individual behaviour and society.

According to Abel (2008), we know a great deal more about the ways in which economic capital (such as level of income) and social capital (such as membership in supportive social networks) are associated with health than we know about the link between cultural capital (such as beliefs and values) and health inequality. For example, Ahnquist, Wamala, and Lindstrom (2012, 935) analyzed the impact of social and economic capital on various outcomes such as self-rated health and psychological health and report that both low social and low economic capital are independently associated with poor health but when they occur together "they seem to contribute to an increased burden of poor health." While Abel acknowledges the fact that economic and social resources contribute to the unequal distribution of health outcomes, he makes a strong case for also considering the impact of cultural resources. In addition, he suggests that future research needs to focus on the complex interaction between economic, social, and cultural resources if we hope to gain a better understanding of the multi-dimensional effects of social inequality on health. While "cultural capital is inherently multifaceted," researchers such as Veenstra and Patterson (2012, 278) are trying to clarify the distinct and interconnected effects of cultural, economic, and social capitals on health outcomes (such as mortality).

Drawing on Bourdieu's sociological theory, Abel and colleagues define **cultural capital** as symbolic and informational resources for action, including values, normative beliefs, knowledge, and skills that are acquired through socialization in a particular socio-cultural context (Abel and Frolich 2012; Abel 2008). In his words, "cultural capital refers to the operational skills, linguistic styles, values and norms that one accrues through education and life-long socialisation" (Abel 2008). Wilkinson and Pickett (2010, 164) explain Bourdieu's concept of cultural capital by noting that in addition to the economy of material wealth, there is an "economy of cultural goods" and state that "inequalities in that economy affect people almost as profoundly as inequalities in income."

Health-related cultural capital consists of any cultural resources that affect health and well-being, such as the value people attach to the pursuit of wellness, their beliefs about the causes of health and illness, and their knowledge about informal and formal health-care practices. Linked as it is to social status, cultural capital is an important element of social class disparities. The basic argument is that cultural resources (such as beliefs and values) shape our health and illness behaviour, guide our health lifestyle choices, and contribute significantly to social class differences in population health. For example, members of lower social classes have different understandings of the health consequences of behaviours such as smoking. Abel (2008) concludes that cultural capital is a key factor in explaining the link between social status and the behavioural aspects of health inequality and that cultural behavioural explanations can help health inequalities research "to elucidate the translation of social disadvantage into poor health."

In this way, the cultural behavioural approach attempts to explain the transformation of social inequality into health disparities. While health-damaging behaviours are important, there is mounting evidence that behavioural risk factors account for a relatively small proportion of the variation in population health status. Furthermore, we have compelling support for the argument that these behavioural practices are structured or patterned not just by socio-cultural environment but also by material conditions of life (e.g., where you live and work). We will return to these issues in Chapter 8 when we take a closer look at collective lifestyle patterns and the behavioural dimensions of health-promoting lifestyles, but now it's time to move on to the third explanation of the social gradient in health.

Psychosocial Explanations

According to psychosocial explanations, the persistence of health inequalities is due primarily to people's interpretation of their standing in the social hierarchy rather than to factors associated with material disadvantage or class-based differences in lifestyle practices. These explanations argue that psychosocial processes involved in the experience of inequality have an important impact on factors such as our self-esteem, sense of coherence, and perceived control of our lives and lead to health problems. Wilkinson and Pickett (2010, 44) explain this approach by noting:

> Greater inequality is likely to be accompanied by increased status competition and increased status anxiety. It is not simply that where the stakes are higher each of us worries more about where he or she comes. It is also that we are likely to pay more attention to social status in how we assess each other.

At the individual level, people compare their status, their possessions, and their general life circumstances to those of others, and it is their sense of relative deprivation that leads to feelings of worthlessness, lower self-esteem, shame, or envy. According to Abbott (2007), the greater the inequalities within societies, the stronger the negative feelings experienced by socially disadvantaged people. In turn, these types of feelings are associated with biochemical processes within the body, such as increases in the stress hormone cortisol. As Wilkinson and Pickett (2010, 85) point out, "The psyche affects the neural system and in turn the immune system—when we're stressed or depressed or feeling hostile, we are far more likely to develop a host of bodily ills, including heart disease, infections and more rapid ageing." It has also been argued that there may be a connection between social comparisons (particularly if you compare yourself with people in better socioeconomic circumstances) and the adoption of certain behavioural practices as coping mechanisms, such as overeating and excessive alcohol consumption, that are harmful to health. This approach suggests that "when individuals strive and fail to meet the standard of living that is customary in their community, there are adverse health effects" (Abbott 2007, 153). Summing up psychosocial explanations for the social gradient in health and how inequality is hypothesized to get under our skin, Wilkinson and Pickett (2010, 87) explain, "The biology of chronic stress is a plausible pathway which helps us to understand why unequal societies are almost always unhealthy societies."

Although Abbott (2007) argues that the psychosocial approach has considerable explanatory power regarding socioeconomic inequalities in health, he acknowledges that there are a number of critical unanswered questions, such as the following: How do people assess their own social status? What do they believe are the reasons for their disadvantaged position in society? Whom do they include in their comparative reference group? Finally, how do social comparisons have an impact on health? In other words, what are the causal pathways through which SES determines health? While the impact of psychosocial determinants may be less obvious, Denburg and Daneman (2010, 23) contend that it is important to learn more about "the effects of relative social or socio-economic inequality on individual and population health, and the causal mechanisms that relate them." An increasing number of studies are attempting to answer these questions so that we can be better equipped to address the link between social inequality and health disparities.

Blaxter has written extensively about lay conceptions of health and illness, and we will consider some of her research findings regarding people's ideas about health and their beliefs about the causes of illness in Chapter 9. For now, we are going to focus on one study in which she explored people's beliefs about the reasons for health inequalities. Blaxter (1997) acknowledges that there is extensive evidence of socioeconomic inequalities in health but asks, how do people themselves think about inequalities in health? Whose fault is it? She quickly points out that few studies have tried to answer such questions. Since there has been little research, we still don't know a great deal about how the general public perceives health inequalities or their beliefs about why there are persistent disparities in health. Blaxter points out that in qualitative studies, lay people rarely talk about inequalities in health and "there is, in fact, no evidence that inequality in health is an issue of great concern among the lay public in Western industrialized societies" (1997, 747). Furthermore, she suggests that, paradoxically, this is particularly the case for people who are in the most socially disadvantaged positions and are the most likely to experience adverse health effects. Macintyre, McKay, and Ellaway (2005) used quantitative methods to explore this apparent paradox, and their findings confirm earlier observations that those in lower social classes who are most at risk of experiencing ill health may be less likely to acknowledge the existence of a social gradient in health.

Demakakos and colleagues (2008) attempted to assess the role of subjective social status, or the individual's perception of her position in the social hierarchy, in the relationship between SES and health. This study investigated the extent to which subjective social status mediates the associations between objective indicators of socioeconomic status (such as level of education) and health outcome measures (such as self-rated health). Subjective social status was measured by asking study participants to place themselves on a rung of a ladder that best reflects their social standing in society. The ladder had 10 rungs (similar to the steps in the social gradient in Figure 5.2), ranging from people at the bottom, who have the least amount of money, the least education, and the worst jobs or no jobs, to those at the top of the ladder, who have the most money, the most education, and the best jobs. For both men and women, age-adjusted analyses revealed that subjective social status is significantly related to many health measures, even after adjusting for covariates such as education and occupational class. Overall, the results of this study suggest that people's own assessments of their experiences of deprivation and their perceived social standing in society are important correlates of health.

In another study that explored social comparisons and health, Pham-Kanter (2009) tried to answer the question: Can having richer friends and neighbours make you sick? Using a US national dataset, this research examined the association between relative position in self-defined social networks and a broad range of measures of health and well-being. In brief, the study did find a relationship between relative position (or step on the social gradient) and health status but suggests that it may be extreme differences in relative position that really matter. In other words, it is the people at the very bottom or at the very top of the gradient who are likely to experience the most significant health effects.

Social psychological research "shows that people prefer to compare themselves with those who are worse off than themselves, if they can, thus minimizing negative effects on their sense of self worth" (Abbott 2007, 154). Thinking of the social gradient in Figure 5.2 again, this means that people on Step 6 benefit from the fact that they are at the top. Their reference group, for comparative purposes, may be either others on the same step or on any of the lower steps on the social gradient. People on the middle steps (2 to 5) have the same opportunities. It is only those at the bottom of the social gradient who are unable to compare themselves to others worse off than they are in terms of social status and, therefore, may experience more negative health outcomes. According to Pham-Kanter (2009, 335), "Poor people have worse health not only because they are less able to afford health-promoting goods, but also because they experience health deficits related to the gap between their own circumstances and those of others. These health deficits are thought to stem from the psychosocial effect of finding oneself less worthy in social comparisons." While there may be increasing evidence that perceived social status is an important component of SES that has an impact on health across the life course, further research is necessary to clarify the nature of the causal relationship (Garbarski 2010). Writing from a psychosocial perspective on social inequality, Wilkinson and Pickett (2010, 39) explain, "Insecurities which can come from a stressful early life have similarities with the insecurities which can come from low social status, and each can exacerbate the effects of the other." For a better understanding of the link between social inequality and health across the life course, we need more information about individuals' socioeconomic life circumstances, along with their relative position in society and their comparative reference group. However, it does appear that "keeping up with the Joneses" is bad for individual and population health.

Income Inequality and Population Health: More to the Story

Although Canadians now live longer and are apparently healthier than ever before, it is important to realize that these gains have not been shared equally by all members of society (see Box 5.5). Significant socioeconomic differences still exist in mortality and morbidity rates and in other health status indicators. For example, evidence shows that those at the top of the social gradient with the highest income (e.g., Step 6 in Figure 5.2) not only live longer but they also lead healthier lives (i.e.,

Box 5.5 Income Inequality: The Gap between the Rich and the Poor

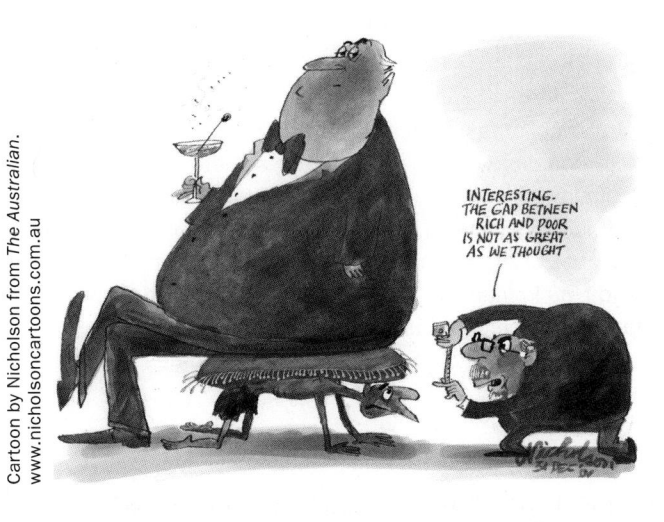

In a report on social and economic inequality in Canada, the Broadbent Institute, a left-wing think tank named after a former leader of the federal New Democratic Party, explains that "Economic inequality is about differences between the top, the middle, and the bottom of society in terms of their share of economic resources, usually measured in terms of income or wealth. In an extremely unequal society, a tiny elite control a huge share of resources, there is a small middle class, and many at the bottom lack the ability to meet even their basic needs" (2012, 3a).

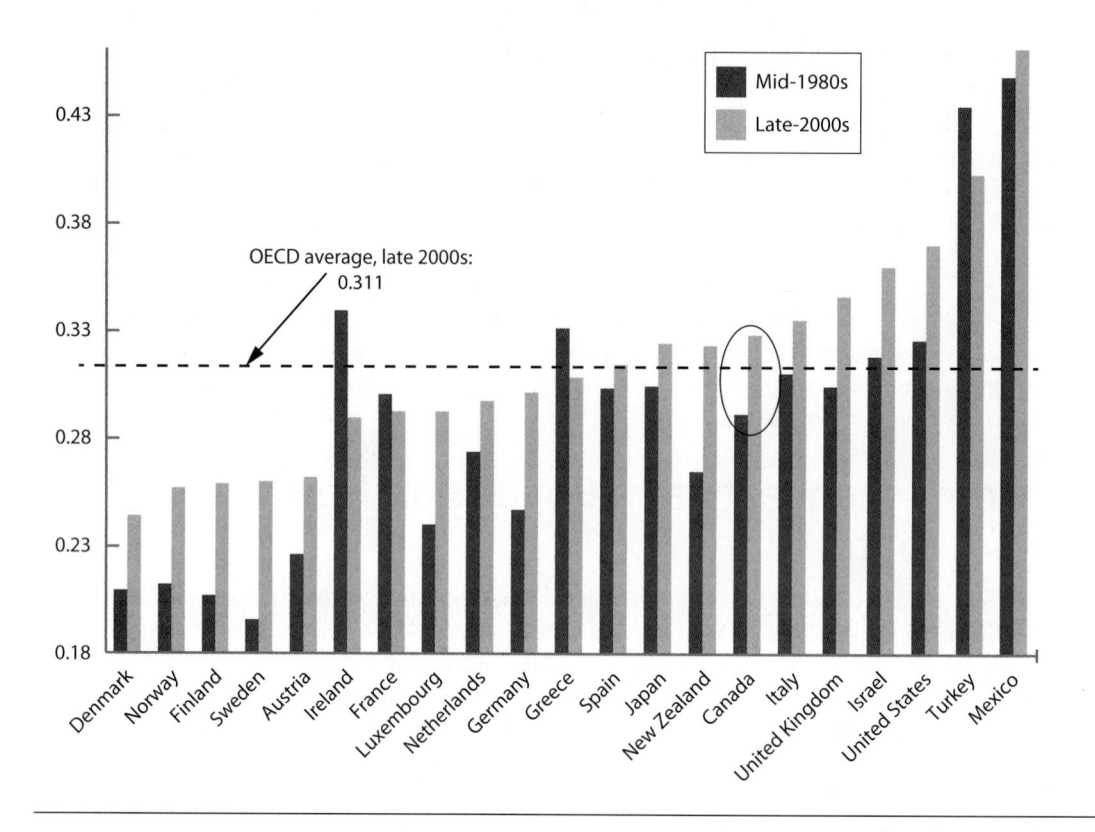

Figure 5.4 Income Inequality as Measured by the Gini Coefficient for Disposable Income, Population Aged 18 to 65 Years, Selected Organisation for Economic Co-operation and Development Countries, Mid-1980s and Late-2000s.

Source: Parliament of Canada 2013, 6.

The Gini coefficient is a commonly used statistical measure of income inequality. Gini coefficients can range between 0 (hypothetical perfect equality wherein everyone in society has the same income) and 1 (hypothetical maximum inequality wherein one person has all the income). A report by the Standing Committee on Finance of the Parliament of Canada (2013, 6) notes that "in the late 2000s—the Gini coefficient for Canada, at 0.324, was higher than the average for oecd countries, at 0.311." Income inequality in Canada, as in many of the richer countries around the world, is growing, and in the late 2000s Canada was among the most unequal of the richer countries. In fact, the Conference Board of Canada (2013) gives Canada a "C" grade when it comes to income inequality for its twelfth-place ranking out of 17 peer countries.

they experience greater health expectancy). As we have just learned, the higher your social status (or the step you occupy on the social gradient), the better your health status is likely to be. While a persistent finding in international research is that higher income is related to better personal health, this is not the whole story when it comes to the relationship between social status and health.

It is now important to turn our attention to the relationship between health disparities and the extent of inequality in society (i.e., the number of steps on the social gradient between the top and bottom) by examining the link between population health and **income inequality**, or the uneven distribution of income within a society or community. In capitalist economies such as Canada's, income is an important indicator of socioeconomic status (as is wealth, or accumulated financial resources). As depicted in Figure 5.4, there is evidence that many developed countries, including Canada, have experienced a substantial increase in income inequality since the 1980s (Alexander and Fong 2014; Cingano 2014; Wilkinson and Pickett 2010). According to Statistics Canada (2014a), the top 1 per cent of earners in 2012 received 10.3 per cent of all income, up from the early 1980s when the 1-percenters accounted for 7 per cent of all income. To be a member of this elite group in Canadian society, comprised of about 261,365 individuals, you needed a 2012 annual income of more than $215,700. In Canada, the 1 per cent in 2012 included Prime Minister Steven Harper, who made $327,400, and the Leader of the Opposition in the House of Commons, Thomas Mulclair, who made $242,000. The median income of the top 1 per cent was $283,400 in 2010, about 10 times higher than the median income of $28,400 for the other 99 per cent of Canadians (Statistics Canada 2013b)! Macdonald (2014) argues that with the wealthiest 20 per cent of families holding almost 70 per cent of Canadian net worth, wealth inequality is an even bigger problem than income inequality. In fact, using Statistics Canada data and a list of Canada's wealthiest people compiled by *Canadian Business*, he points out that the richest 86 people in Canada, while making up only about 0.002 per cent of the Canadian population, have a combined net worth of $178 billion, which is equivalent to that of the poorest 11.4 million Canadians, or 34 per cent of the population. In Alberta, the top 10 per cent of earners have an income share of 50.4 percent (Statistics Canada 2014a), making the wild rose province the most unequal of all Canadian provinces and the only province to have higher levels of inequality than the United States. Taken together, this means that despite the cynical claim depicted in the cartoon in Box 5.5, the gap between the rich and poor is getting wider and income inequality is getting worse because there continues to be substantial growth in income and wealth at the top along with stagnation at the bottom of the income hierarchy. After reviewing Canadian income inequality data, Fortin and colleagues (2012, 127) caution that "Such an uneven distribution of income has not been seen since the dark days of the Great Depression." This raises many questions about the effect of rising income inequality on population health.

In examining the social gradient in health, it is important to recognize that while personal health reflects the individual's position (or step) on the social hierarchy, population health is a reflection of the distance between the top and bottom of the social hierarchy and where people are concentrated on the steps. As Nowatzki (2011, 36) explains, "Income inequality therefore is a characteristic of a group or a place (aggregate level), rather than an individual attribute such as income." Analyses of the link between income distribution in society and population health indicate that both **income adequacy** (i.e., having sufficient income to meet one's needs) and relative position on the social gradient are important determinants of health. As Wilkinson and Pickett (2010, 286) argue, "the relationships between inequality and various health and social problems are not reducible to the direct effects of people's material living standards independent of inequality." This highlights the fact that not only is poverty bad for population health but so too is inequality.

A provocative paper written by Wilkinson (1992) was one of the first to draw widespread research attention to the fact that in developed countries there is a significant association between income distribution and overall population health (as measured by life expectancy). Put simply, Wilkinson found that people live longer in more equal countries. Figure 5.5 depicts Wilkinson

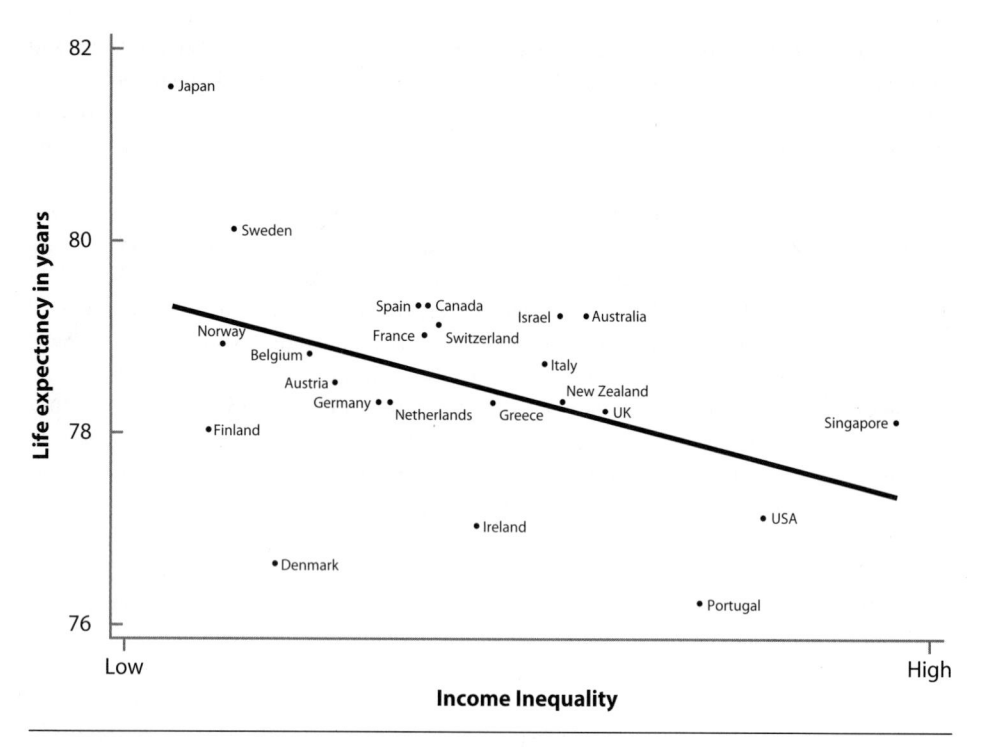

Figure 5.5 Life Expectancy is Longer in More Equal Rich Countries
Source: Wilkinson and Pickett 2010.

and Pickett's analysis of the relationship between life expectancy and income inequality in their 2010 book *The Spirit Level: Why Equality Is Better for Everyone*.

Wilkinson's **income inequality hypothesis** suggests that greater inequality in income distribution within a population increases social problems, including a social gradient in health. He continues to be a major proponent of this viewpoint (e.g., Lobmayer and Wilkinson 2000; Pickett and Wilkinson 2014; Wilkinson and Pickett 2006, 2010). It is interesting to note that Wilkinson's original article was published in a section of the *British Medical Journal* titled "For Debate," and it was certainly successful in stimulating debate! Since then, an extensive body of research has examined income inequality as a determinant of population health. De Maio (2012a, 39) claims that "More than 200 statistical studies have examined the relationship between income inequality and population health." The underlying premise is that income inequality is an important measure of socioeconomic inequality in society and that its extent affects population health. While there remain conceptual and methodological challenges associated with fully understanding the complex nature of the causal relationship between income inequality and health, researchers now generally recognize that the societal distribution of income, not just poverty, matters for population health (De Maio 2012a; Kawachi and Subramanian 2014; Pickett and Wilkinson 2014).

At the same time, however, it must be noted that "the cross-country relationship between income inequality and health outcomes—especially in industrial countries—is not robust" (Kawachi and Subramanian 2014, 144). While researchers have established the correlation between income inequality and aggregate population health within rich countries (i.e., people are healthier and live longer in more equal societies), they have not yet demonstrated that income inequality is a health risk at the individual level. Yes, it is bad for population health measured at the aggregate level (i.e., average life expectancy), but does income inequality pose an individual-level health risk the way lack of adequate income does? Reviewing 79 published studies looking at income inequality and mortality up to 2008, Zheng (2012) argues that multi-level research designs, which can control for individual-level characteristics, such as SES, are needed to establish the individual health risk posed by income inequality. According to this review, the 16 studies that used multi-level design and investigated the impact of income inequality on individual mortality have produced ambiguous results. Based on a meta-analysis of 23 studies, Kondo and colleagues (2011) similarly conclude that studies that measure larger population areas, such as entire countries, are more likely to establish the negative health effects of income inequality. There is also a question as to whether income inequality harms the health of all but the 1 per cent (i.e., a contextual effect) or whether it is only those who are disadvantaged in the invidious game of social comparison who are harmed by income inequality and relative deprivation (Kawachi and Subramanian 2014).

Another issue is the extent to which within-country or community-area policies can act to mitigate the harmful effects of income inequality. An international comparative study of metropolitan-area income inequality in the US, the UK, Australia, Sweden, and Canada conducted by Ross and colleagues (2005) found that within-country income inequality was correlated with mortality only in the US and the UK. This led the researchers to speculate that national health and social policies may act as an important buffer between income inequality and negative health effects. According to Karlsson and colleagues (2010), there is also reason to believe that the relationship between income inequality and health may differ depending on the average income level of the country being considered. Additionally, researchers are still trying to understand issues surrounding the relationship between the timing of income inequality and the onset of particular health effects (Zheng 2012). Here again, multi-level designs are needed to untangle the effects of individual SES and group-level income inequality on health. To this end, Zheng employed a multi-level design that analyzed the level of income inequality at discrete time periods to assess how shifts in inequality over time related to changing mortality risk. He found that "income inequality has long-term effects on individual mortality risk from 5 years later to 12 years. A 0.01-unit increase in the Gini coefficient increases the cumulative odds of death by 122% throughout the 12 years," leading him to conclude that "income inequality is a public health concern" (2012, 45). Finally, researchers are still trying to discover the mechanisms whereby income inequality translates into specific health impacts (Kawachi and Subramanian 2014).

Canadian studies of the impact of income inequality on population health have produced mixed findings. Early studies that focused on the link between population health and the distribution of income based on measuring average income at the provincial level and in metropolitan areas with populations greater than 50,000 people (Ross et al. 2000), in metropolitan areas only (McLeod et al. 2003), in coastal communities in the province of British Columbia (Veenstra 2002a), and in neighbourhoods derived from census tracts in urban areas with a population of at least 100,000 people (Hou and Myles 2005) concluded that income inequality is not significantly associated with the health of the Canadian population. One exception is Veenstra's (2002b) study of income inequality and health carried out in regional health districts in Saskatchewan. Veenstra (2002b, 865) argues that "the inclusion of rural areas and attention to a smaller (with respect to population size) unit of analysis brings the relevance of income inequality as a predictor of a population's health back on stage in Canada."

More recent studies have also not conclusively established that the relative distribution of income is an important determinant of Canadian population health. Unfortunately, many of these studies are characterized by the same conceptual and methodological limitations as earlier research. Auger and colleagues (2012) explain that "Canadian studies are limited by cross-sectional ecological designs and multilevel prospective designs are preferred for evaluating income inequality and health." As illustration, Auger, Zang, and Daniel's (2009) Quebec-based study actually found an inverse relationship between income inequality and all-cause mortality. Another study by Vafaei, Rosenberg, and Pickett (2010) used cross-sectional data from the *Canadian Community Health Survey* to conduct an ecological (i.e., aggregate-level) analysis of income inequality and self-rated health status in Canadian health regions. These researchers concluded that "Across Canadian health regions, health status in populations was a function of absolute income but not relative income" (2010, 2). However, like earlier Canadian studies, this research was limited to aggregate-level data analysis of smaller geographic areas with smaller population sizes. Auger and colleagues (2012) used a cohort of 2 million Canadians followed for mortality from 1991 to 2001. Unlike earlier studies, this research had the advantages of representing the overall Canadian population and using a multi-level design, which controlled for individual-level covariates such as income, education, employment, immigrant status, and age. The researchers (2012) found that income inequality was indeed associated with mortality risk for non-immigrant (but not immigrant) Canadians, leading them to warn, "Canada, so far considered insulated from such effects, is indeed influenced by the extremes of wealth and poverty."

In summary, factors such as the selection of countries (i.e., Western industrialized); the number of countries compared; the size of the area considered or the level of aggregation (i.e., large-scale analyses—international comparisons or within-country studies of states or regions—versus small-scale analyses—studies focused on census tracts, postal codes, neighbourhoods, or individual-level data); the quality of the income data collected; and the types of controls for intervening variables such as gender, ethnic group composition, age, and education all need to be considered when assessing the relationship between income inequality and health. (See De Maio 2012a for a useful review of conceptual and methodological challenges involved in the study of income inequality and health.) Finally, Subramanian and Kawachi (2004, 89) remind us that, most important of all, "income-based inequality is, at best, simply one dimension that could be relevant to population health. Other axes of stratification (or hierarchy), such as the unequal distribution of wealth, political power, cultural assets, social assets, honorific status, human capital (to name a few), could also be important determinants of health outcomes." The Public Health Agency of Canada summarizes the relationship between income inequality and health by noting that "Studies suggest that the distribution of income in a given society may be a more important determinant of health than the total amount of income earned by society members. Large gaps in income distribution lead to increases in social problems and poorer health among the population as a whole" (2013). In other words, the wider the gap in income distribution between the wealthiest and the poorest members of a society, the greater the potential disparities in population health! What remains to be understood is how elements of global political economy, such as neo-liberalism, global trade and monetary policies, and health and social policies, relate to observed health disparities (Coburn 2000, 2004; De Maio 2012a).

Reducing Socioeconomic Differences in Health: Is It Possible to Close the Gap?

Before we conclude our discussion of the relationship between socioeconomic status and health, we need to consider two final issues. First, does the available evidence indicate that the social gradient in health is changing over time (i.e., is it increasing and getting steeper)? We also need to think about whether it is possible to reduce health disparities based on socioeconomic status. In other words, is there reason to be hopeful that we can close (if not eliminate) the gap in social class disparities in health?

Marmot (2004b; 2005) points out that over the past generation, the differences between the top and the bottom of the social gradient have actually been getting bigger. There is now a large body of international evidence demonstrating that inequalities in health have been increasing in the United States and the UK as well as in several European countries. For example, data show that differences in adult mortality rates are not only large—they are also growing. Danish researchers Borg and Kristensen (2000, 1019), commenting on international epidemiological research, state that "in spite of the falling mortality rates in most Western countries and in spite of increasing resources spent on health care, there seems to be a tendency toward increasing social differences in health." Rosich and Hankin (2010, S3) basically agree with this point but go even further by asserting that "despite radical changes in our knowledge of prevention and treatment of disease, inequalities in health and mortality are large and well established, and persist at levels similar to those since the early nineteenth century." In other words, the gap appears to be getting larger and the social gradient in health steeper.

Is this also the case in Canada, and, if so, what are the implications for the health of the population? Curry-Stevens (2009) contends that data clearly show that inequality in Canada is growing and that the economic (as well as the social) gap between rich and poor is getting wider. According to Curry-Stevens, this is occurring because incomes at the top of the social hierarchy are improving dramatically while there is considerable volatility (and increasing insecurity) at the bottom of the income scale. This means that many Canadians, including the working poor, have income levels that are inadequate to meet their daily needs and to give them a chance to lead healthy lives. This is vitally important, since there is growing evidence that "more equal income distribution has proven to be one of the best predictors of better overall health of a society" (Mikkonen and Raphael 2010, 12).

According to Kirkpatrick and McIntyre (2009), this profile of the health of Canadians is reinforced by the first annual report released by the chief public health officer. The report provides evidence of widespread health inequalities in Canada. For example, it highlights persistent and significant gaps in life expectancy, infant mortality, self-reported health, and other health status indicators between high- and low-income Canadians as well as extensive health disadvantages experienced by Canada's Aboriginal peoples. There is no disputing the fact that extreme poverty and absolute material deprivation are related to poor health. While the chief public health officer's report draws attention to health inequalities in Canada, Kirkpatrick and McIntyre point out in their critical commentary that it fails to offer a strategic approach for addressing the situation. In their words, "What is missing is a call for governments to act" (2009, 94).

Is it possible to reduce these types of social inequalities in health? Ridde, Guichard, and Houeto (2007) offer a critical, but not pessimistic, response to this question. They begin by pointing out that the term "social inequalities in health" refers to "the systematic, avoidable, and unjust differences in health between individuals and population sub-groups" (2007, 12). Although social class differences in health may be systemic (i.e., structures of inequality inherent in society systematically reproduce health disparities), if they are indeed avoidable, then change is possible. Ridde and colleagues argue that taking action against social inequalities in health means more than tackling poverty; it means intervening in meaningful ways to create equality of opportunity! While the goal is an admirable one (and has been included in policy documents for many years), the implementation of a strategic framework to actually achieve the objective by taking action to reduce health disparities has been problematic. They conclude that while there may not be agreement on the best practices to redress health inequalities, there are reasons to continue to believe that positive action is still possible.

A number of policy initiatives strongly emphasize the importance of making the ongoing struggle against health inequalities a higher priority. These calls for collective action recommend a comprehensive, integrated approach that combines the implementation of public policies, private-sector responsibility, and the active participation of civil society if we are to achieve greater health equity. The most prominent global health policy documents include two reports by the WHO's Commission on Social Determinants of Health, *Closing the Gap in a Generation: Health Equity through Action on the Social Determinants of Health: Final Report of the Commission on Social Determinants of Health* (2008) and *Closing the Gap: Policy into Practice on Social Determinants of Health* (2011b). The WHO established the commission to investigate what can be done to improve health equity. According to the commission, the social gradient in health and avoidable health inequalities exist nationally and globally because of the unequal distribution of power, income, and goods and services. The commission argues that if disparities in health can get worse, they can get better and that it is time for urgent and sustained action. The 2008 report calls on all governments to lead global action on the social determinants of health in order to achieve greater health equity.

The commission's overarching recommendations include improving daily life by emphasizing the importance of early childhood development and education, planning healthy places to live, creating fair employment and decent work, introducing universal social protection systems across the life course, and tackling the inequitable distribution of power, money, and resources. The commission calls for closing the gap in health disparities in a generation but acknowledges that this is only possible if the political will exists to make major changes in economic arrangements and the ways in which societies are organized. In addition, the authors of the final report recognize that the existing disparities in health are so great that it may not be feasible to close the gap in one generation. Despite this, however, they end on an optimistic note, asserting that greater "health equity within a generation is achievable, it is the right thing to do, and now is the right time to do it" (2008, ii).

The 2011 discussion paper focuses on the implementation of the recommendations of the commission and once again stresses the need for government action to tackle the root causes of health inequities, although the discussion seems less optimistic this time. To illustrate, the authors of the paper begin by stating at the outset that "poor progress in the implementation of a social determinants approach reflects in part the inadequacy of governance at the local, national, and global levels to address the key problems of the 21st century" (2011b, 2). Whether the plan of action proposed by the Commission on Social Determinants of Health results in significant improvements in health equity remains to be seen, but one of the strengths of this policy document is the way in which it illustrates the importance of taking into account the political context of social inequalities and health. This is not a new point of view but one that Navarro and Shi (2001) suggest is rarely included in studies of the impact of social inequalities on health. According to Navarro and Shi (2001, 481), "political forces (such as political movements and parties) and the public policies they follow when in government" play a key role in determining the level of inequality in societies. They contend that social inequalities and health are influenced by government policies—for example, regarding the redistributive efforts of the welfare state (including the level of public health-care coverage and support services for families such as child care).

Coburn (2000; 2004) echoes this standpoint and advocates a political economy perspective that focuses on "the causes of the causes." He argues that not enough attention has been paid to the socio-political causes of inequality and, consequently, it is not possible to comprehend the effects of inequality on population health. He highlights the rise of the neo-liberal political ideology, the decline of the welfare state, and the changing class structure of advanced capitalist societies as the underlying causes of inequality. Lynch (2000, 1001) characterizes Coburn's perspective as "a welcome addition to the debate over interpretations of the link between income inequality and health" and agrees that we need to examine the socio-political background factors that shape unequal distribution of income and contribute to increasing inequalities in society, including health disparities.

Recently, a number of researchers have examined the role of politics by focusing on social democratic countries and more specifically the impact of welfare state characteristics and egalitarian political traditions on the social determinants of population health (Muntaner et al. 2011; Brennenstuhl, Quesnel-Vallée, and McDonough 2012). For example, based on an extensive review of the literature, informed by a political economy perspective, Muntaner and colleagues (2011) argue that welfare regimes are the most salutary and have the most positive health outcomes (e.g., life expectancy and infant and child mortality rates). Consequently, they state that "the main conclusion of our review is that politics appears to have a positive effect on population health with left and egalitarian political traditions producing the most affirmative results" (2011, 954). Brennenstuhl, Quesnel-Vallée, and McDonough (2012) also carried out a systematic review of empirical studies of the social determinants of health that explicitly explored the impact of welfare state policies on population health and social inequalities in health. These researchers critically assessed the basic assumption that population health is better and disparities in health are lower in welfare states with well-established social democratic regimes. While their findings confirm once again that population health is better in social democratic countries, they report that there is little consistent evidence that disparities in health based on socioeconomic status are indeed smaller. They conclude that "studies that find evidence of the salutary health effects of the social democratic welfare regime, compared with others, are more likely to examine population health, rather than socioeconomic inequalities in health" (2012, 407).

Forget (2011) analyzed the health effects of a limited Canadian field experiment carried out in the 1970s designed to provide people with a guaranteed annual income and thereby reduce social and economic inequality. According to Forget, Canada has had a "long flirtation" with the idea of a guaranteed annual income, and the idea is once again receiving attention from policy-makers in the public health field. The purpose of this "upstream" intervention was to address poverty, which is strongly associated with poor health. Box 5.6 provides a summary of the details of this experiment and Forget's analysis. She found that a guaranteed annual income provided stability and predictability for the families involved and that income security is an important determinant of health. The participants experienced a reduction in hospitalization rates and physician contacts, particularly for mental health issues. Based on the findings, Forget (2011, 300) concluded that a guaranteed annual income, "implemented broadly in society, may improve health and social outcomes at the community level" and that even a relatively modest minimum level of income support can improve population health.

The basic point of this discussion is that without a better understanding of structural conditions that give rise to social and economic inequality, we are not going to be able to adequately address the relationship between socioeconomic inequalities and population health. A serious effort to reduce social inequalities in health requires political leadership and involves fundamental changes in the distribution of power and economic resources within society. It seems appropriate to give the last word in this discussion of social inequality and health to Marmot and colleagues. They state, "Wishing for health equity is one thing. Making it reality is another" (Friel et al. 2009, 11).

> **Box 5.6** The Town with No Poverty: A Forgotten Canadian Experiment
>
> The idea of a universal minimum level of income support for all Canadians was first recommended in a 1971 report submitted to the federal government. In 1973, the Manitoba and Canadian governments signed an agreement to carry out a guaranteed annual income experiment. The experiment was known as Mincome and was conducted in Dauphin, Manitoba, between 1974 and 1979. Dauphin was referred to as a saturation site because everyone in the community was eligible to participate in the experiment. A number of small rural communities were selected to serve as controls for the Dauphin residents. Every family in Dauphin that participated in the project received the same offer. Families with no income from other sources received 60 per cent of the Statistics Canada low-income cut-off, which varied by family size. The experiment ran for four years, and Mincome came to an end in 1979 with a change in government at the federal and provincial levels and with essentially no analysis of the information collected. "The Dauphin data, collected at great expense and some controversy from participants in the first large-scale social experiment ever conducted in Canada, were never examined" (Forget 2011, 290).
>
> Forget took advantage of this "historical accident" to re-examine the impact of a guaranteed annual income and to explore the health and social benefits of participating in the Mincome experiment. She gained access to the Dauphin data and information from the provincial health administrative database for people who were residents of the community during the years the experiment was in the field. A quasi-experimental design was used "to determine whether contacts with the health care system declined among subjects who lived in the experimental community relative to a comparison group matched by age, sex, geography, family type, and family size" (Forget 2011, 299). The outcome measures available for her study were limited to health-care utilization data, including hospital discharges and physician claims. The results of the analysis revealed that overall hospitalization rates, particularly for accidents and injuries, and physician contact for mental health issues declined for Mincome participants relative to the comparison group. In its submission to the House of Commons Standing Committee on Finance's hearings on income inequality (2013), the Canadian Medical Association cited Mincome as illustrative of the sort of policy intervention that can challenge the adverse health effects of income inequality.
>
> **Source**: Forget 2011.

Toward an Intersectional Theory of Health and Socioeconomic Status across the Life Course

Orpana and Lemrye (2004, 143) advise that although the three explanations of the social gradient that were reviewed earlier "are often presented as competing hypotheses, there is considerable overlap and potential synergy between them as the effects of one source of health liability may compound the effects of another." As an example, they point out that exposure to environmental stressors such as unemployment might be associated with the onset of depression and an inability to pay for the services of a psychologist could prolong the healing period, leading the individual to smoke more and further harm her health. Singh-Manoux and Marmot (2005) similarly argue that in order to understand the social determinants of health, the different explanations of social inequalities need to be integrated.

A review of Canadian research carried out by Raphael et al. (2005), however, suggests that this type of integration has yet to occur. They found that only 4 per cent of studies had a conceptualization of the relationship between economic inequality and health that combined the different approaches. Together, these explanatory models highlight the fact that social structure and individual behaviour interact with one another, within a cultural context, and collectively contribute to continuing inequalities in health. In addition, they illustrate the fact that both objective and subjective aspects of our position in the social hierarchy can have significant health consequences. "It is not simply that poor material circumstances are harmful to health; the social meaning of being poor, unemployed, socially excluded, or otherwise stigmatized also matters" (Wilkinson and Marmot 2003, 9). There is a complex web of causation comprised of the ways in which intersecting sources of inequality, such as socioeconomic status, socio-cultural factors, and psychosocial factors, interact with biology to shape population health and contribute to the persistence of health disparities both within and between societies.

Many of the studies of the link between SES and health reviewed in this chapter come to the conclusion that we need an intersectional model to understand the complex, interacting determinants of population health and health disparities. For example, Judge, Mulligan, and Benzeval (1998, 578) acknowledged a number of years ago that while low income is clearly associated with poor personal health, population health "is likely to be the product of a wide range of cultural, economic and social factors, many of which are not easily measured and most of which might interact with each other." Similarly, McDonough and Amick (2001, 143) conclude that "the complex patterns observed in our data underscore the need to consider the intersection of gender, age, race and socioeconomic position as multiple sites of experience." Finally, according to the Public Health Agency of Canada (2004), all research must be sensitive to the fact that socioeconomic differences in health are related to gender, ethnicity, age, and geographic location.

Consequently, we need an intersectional theory of health to be able to adequately understand the multiple pathways through which determinants such as position in the social hierarchy, social exclusion, and the distribution of economic and political power in society affect health status over time and contribute to the perpetuation of health disparities. This means changing the central research question from "what is the relative importance of individual social determinants of health, such as income, occupation, or education?" to "what are the relational effects of social factors such as class, gender, ethnicity, and age as determinants of population health and health disparities?" This change in research focus may help us to appreciate the ways in which "deep and entrenched inequities in the wealth, power and prestige of different people and communities" (Friel et al. 2009, 11) ranging across a number of intersecting social categories, such as class, gender, and ethnicity, collectively influence population health across the life course. Future studies of the link between social location and health need to critically examine the interrelationships between health status and structures of inequality as well as the social, economic, and political environments that create inequalities in society. In other words, we need a more comprehensive and better integrated theoretical approach, and a more sophisticated research strategy, if we are going to advance our understanding of social inequality and health disparities across the life course. Liu, Jones, and Glymour (2010, 490) contend that it is critically important to understand the life course antecedents of diseases associated with aging, since this "can provide essential insight into selecting the timing and structure of interventions in order to successfully improve population health."

In a very thorough review of socioeconomic-based health disparities and the fundamental principles of a life course approach, Seabrook and Avison (2012, 63) make a compelling argument that there is a need "to study the relationship among socioeconomic status, cumulative disadvantage processes and health outcomes from a life course perspective." The key point is that health disparities associated with SES increase over time because of differential exposure to risk factors and access to protective resources. Blane (2006) characterizes the life course perspective as a way of capturing the process of selective accumulation of social experiences that shape our health. He explains how a "chain of disadvantage" (2006, 56) associated with different structures of inequality has important health consequences. To illustrate the chain of disadvantage and ongoing, lifelong production of health inequities, long-term health disparities might begin at the earliest stages of life with low birth weight (because of mothers living in poverty at the time of conception and birth). This early social disadvantage may lead to increased chances of poor nutrition and greater risk of childhood infection and disease. Limitations on childhood physical and cognitive development and educational opportunities as well as exposure to a range of health-damaging environmental hazards (e.g., overcrowded housing and polluted neighbourhoods) may eventually be followed by unemployment or job and income insecurity later in life. The consequence of such lifelong social accumulation of disadvantage may be adult health disparities. "This approach suggests that throughout the life course exposure to disadvantageous experiences and environments accumulate, increasing the risk of adult morbidity and premature death" (Holland et al. 2000, 1285). In contrast, being born into a family with high socioeconomic status typically means a lifetime of social advantages that result in health benefits (including both longer life and greater health expectancy). "The health status of populations cannot, therefore, be adequately understood without recognizing health-determining influences across the life course" (Hertzman and Power 2006, 83). This is because what happens to us throughout our lives affects our present and future health status.

"A common tenet among researchers studying the relationship between socioeconomic status and health outcomes is that health inequalities are influenced by circumstances in early life" (Seabrook and Avison 2012, 52). For example, in a discussion of the life course development of health disparities, Power and Kuh (2006) examine the extent to which the social gradient evident in adult health can be explained by factors that occurred during earlier life stages (e.g., socially patterned environmental exposure and emotional and physical development during childhood and adolescence). Based on their analysis, they contend that there is an important "link between childhood disadvantage and poor adult health" because of the many ways in which adverse socioeconomic circumstances early in life can affect health in later life (2006, 36). As we saw in Chapter 2 with the example of Cohen's (Cohen et al. 2004) cold virus study, there is growing evidence that childhood experiences affect health status later in life. Factors such as the type of community or neighbourhood people grew up in, along with their parents' education and occupation, have important implications for health that may not become apparent until they have an impact on adult health, including morbidity and mortality rates (Clarke et al. 2014; Johnson, Schoeni, and Rogowski 2012; Johnson and Schoeni 2011; Conroy, Sandel, and Zuckerman 2010). In fact, Cohen and colleagues (2010, 49) conclude their study of childhood socioeconomic status and adult health by stating that "SES exposures during childhood are powerful predictors of adult cardiovascular morbidity, cardiovascular mortality, all-cause mortality, and mortality due to a range of specific causes."

Studies have also examined the ways in which socioeconomic status is linked to disability trajectories in later life (Bowen and Gonzalez 2010; Taylor 2010, 2011). Taylor's research suggests that higher levels of education and income have an impact on health over the life course that protects individuals from disability onset and progression in later life. Finally, taking a somewhat broader approach, Brandt, Deindl, and Hank (2012) explored the influence of childhood conditions (e.g., parental SES) and social inequality on the individual's chances of successfully aging well (e.g., no major diseases or limitations on activities of daily living as well as high cognitive and physical functioning). Overall, the research evidence indicates that childhood experiences such as overcrowded homes, large family size, exposure to second-hand smoke, and other forms of environmental pollution are both socially patterned (i.e., they are linked to SES) and related to disparities in a variety of adult health outcomes. This information led Hertzman and Boyce (2010, 330) to assert that

> Social environments and experiences get under the skin early in life, and do so in ways that affect the course of human development. Heart disease, diabetes, obesity, depression, substance abuse, school success, premature mortality, disability at retirement, and accelerated aging and memory loss all have social determinants in early life.

It should be apparent by now that "good beginnings early in life have profound effects on health and wellness throughout the life course" (Winnipeg Regional Health Authority 2013, 15). Adopting a life course perspective is essential, therefore, if we hope to gain a fuller understanding of the cumulative effects of a lifetime of deprivation or privilege on health status. Such a perspective directs our attention to the manner in which earlier life events influence the subsequent pursuit of health and wellness.

While research consistently shows that social inequalities in health persist over time, the extent of SES disparities in health apparently differs as individuals move through the life course (Pavalko and Caputo 2013; Wickrama et al. 2013). In other words, the social gradient in health varies across the life course. It is steepest in early to mid-adulthood and then levels off in later life. Although there is some indication that the strength of the association between socioeconomic status and health may decrease with age, it seems that the social gradient in mortality and morbidity persists across the life course. For example, supporting evidence comes from Huisman and colleagues' (2004) comprehensive examination of socioeconomic inequalities in mortality among older women and men in 11 European countries. They state that their research indicates "that not only absolute, but also relative socioeconomic inequalities in mortality among the elderly population persisted into old age and were considerable" (Huisman et al. 2004, 471). These findings suggest that negative health outcomes experienced in later life may be associated with a lifetime of social inequality.

McMunn et al. (2006) agree that SES health disparities continue into old age, although there are reductions in the size of the differences with increasing age. They argue that socioeconomic inequalities in health persist among older adults because the benefits derived from declining morbidity rates and increasing life expectancy are not enjoyed equally by all. In other words, there are greater health benefits for those of all ages who occupy higher status positions on the social gradient. In addition, Prus (2007) contends that the strength of the relationship between SES and health changes over the life course as a result of the fact that the health of higher and lower SES groups declines at different rates. Baeten, Van Ourti, and van Doorslaer (2013) extend this argument by suggesting that factors such as selective mortality and institutionalization rates may help to explain why the social gradient in health appears to level off in later life. To illustrate, they point to the well-known socioeconomic differences in mortality rates and the fact that higher-SES individuals are more likely to survive to older ages as an explanation for the "converging SES health gradient after late-middle age" (2013, 66). Furthermore, they state that this trend is also influenced by the fact that low-SES unhealthy people are more likely to move to institutions such as nursing homes than those who are equally unhealthy but high-SES and are therefore typically excluded from surveys of older adults. In general, it can be concluded that "there is a consensus that more educated and wealthier individuals fare better than their lower SES counterparts on most broad measures of health status and that these patterns persist at the older ages, although the differentials are generally smaller than at younger ages" (Goldman et al. 2011, 308).

In concluding this discussion, it is important to point out that an intersectional life course perspective encompasses both individuals and societies. At the individual level, advantages and disadvantages accumulate over time and have both short- and long-term effects on our health. "Exposure to stressors varies across social groups and the burden accumulates over time" (Hankin and Wright 2010, S11). For example, being born into a family with lower socioeconomic status, living in substandard housing, or working at a poorly paid job may lead to lowered expectations, limited opportunities, and a lack of control over one's life that eventually may result in poorer health outcomes later in life. At a societal level, an intersectional life course perspective directs our attention to factors such as structural change, growing social inequality, and changing social policies that in turn may have implications for population health. McDaniel (2013, 9) concludes that the development of improved theoretical frameworks will benefit future sociological studies of health and illness and that "reliance on life course perspectives of both individuals and societies, particularly of social policies over time, can deeply enhance understandings and ramp up explanatory power."

Chapter Summary

This chapter has demonstrated that health disparities linked to socioeconomic status have been documented worldwide. Overwhelming research evidence from a variety of countries, including Canada, indicates that income, occupation, and education are all related to health status. For example, "the poor are at increased risk for chronic disease, communicable diseases, injuries, social isolation, malnutrition, and stress" (Hankin and Wright 2010, S11). Socioeconomic status has a dramatic impact on morbidity patterns, mortality rates, and the number of years people can expect to live. There can be little doubt that social and economic inequalities create life circumstances that are harmful to population health. It should also be evident that the relationship between social inequality and health is extremely complex and warrants a more in-depth analysis.

Schofield (2007) argues that a critical sociological perspective has a great deal to offer and should be applied to the study of social inequality and health. He uses the term **health inequities** to refer to avoidable health inequalities that are unnecessary and unjust. His basic argument is that an improved understanding of the upstream social determinants of health will help to make the problem of health inequities "real and actionable." In other words, inequalities in health are not inevitable, and action, as well as change, is possible. The sociological imagination and a critical comparative approach, combined with a sound theoretical understanding of the social processes by which structures of inequality are created and, in turn, intersect to produce (and reproduce) health disparities, as well as rigorously conducted analyses have the potential to foster more effective policy interventions aimed at advancing global health equity. According to

Braveman (2006), pursuing health equity means implementing successful strategies for eliminating health disparities and inequalities.

We will return to these issues in the last chapter of the book in our concluding discussion of personal, professional, and public responsibility for health and the types of policy initiatives required for achieving healthy futures. It is now time to consider some of the other social determinants that shape our health. The next two chapters explore the ways in which other sources of social inequality, such as gender and ethnicity, intersect with each other (and socioeconomic status) to influence population health.

Study Questions

5. How does social exclusion affect health?
6. Comment on the relationship between socioeconomic status and health. Provide specific examples to support your answer.
7. Critically evaluate the evidence that the relationship between position in the social hierarchy and health involves a gradient.
8. Critically assess the link between income inequality and population health. Use the available Canadian research evidence to support your answer.
9. Comment on the changes in the social gradient in health across the life course.
10. Review the alternative explanations for the persistence of inequalities in health.

Recommended Readings

De Maio, F. 2012a. "Advancing the income inequality–health hypothesis." *Critical Public Health* 22: 39–46.

Demakakos, P., J. Nazroo, E. Breeze, and M. Marmot. 2008. "Socioeconomic status and health: The role of subjective social status." *Social Science and Medicine* 67: 330–40.

House, J. 2001. "Understanding social factors and inequalities in health: 20th century progress and 21st century prospects." *Journal of Health and Social Behavior* 43: 125–42.

Marmot, M. 2004. *The Status Syndrome: How Social Standing Affects Our Health and Longevity.* New York: Times Books.

Schofield, T. 2007. "Health inequity and its social determinants: A sociological commentary." *Health Sociology Review* 16: 105–14.

Seabrook, J., and W. Avison. 2012. "Socioeconomic status and cumulative disadvantage processes across the life course: Implications for health outcomes." *Canadian Review of Sociology* 49: 50–68.

Wilkinson, R., and K. Pickett. 2010. *The Spirit Level: Why Equality Is Better for Everyone.* New York: Bloomsbury Press.

Willson, A. 2009. "'Fundamental causes' of health disparities: A comparative analysis of Canada and the United States." *International Sociology* 24: 93–113.

Recommended Websites

European Portal for Action on Health Equity:
www.health-inequalities.org

Institute for Work and Health:
www.iwh.on.ca

Oxfam:
http://policy-practice.oxfam.org.uk/our-work/inequality

The Equality Trust:
www.equalitytrust.org

The Globe and Mail **Interactive: How Income Inequality Hurts Every Canadian's Chance of Building a Better Life:**
www.theglobeandmail.com/news/national/time-to-lead/our-time-to-lead-income-inequality/article15316231

The Health Effects of Income Inequality:
www.thinkupstream.net/health_effects_of_income_inequality

Unnatural Causes: Is Inequality Making Us Sick?:
www.unnaturalcauses.org

WHO—Commission on the Social Determinants of Health:
www.who.int/social_determinants/en

WHO—World Health Report:
www.who.int/whr/en

Recommended Audiovisual Sources

Canada's Growing Gap Explained. Produced by the Canadian Centre for Policy Alternatives 2009.

"Sick People or Sick Societies," "Ideas." Two-part CBC radio broadcast, 2008. www.cbc.ca/ideas/podcasts.

Unnatural Causes: Is Inequality Making Us Sick? PBS documentary series, 2008.

Addressing Sources of Inequality and Health Disparities: Gender

Learning Objectives

This chapter expands our examination of sources of inequality and disparities in health beyond socioeconomic status by considering the relationship between health and gender, including

- the importance of sex- and gender-based analysis in health research;
- gender differences in life expectancy and in causes of death;
- gender differences in the experience of health and illness as well as health care, including the medicalization of women's lives and bodies;
- gender differences in the social determinants of health;
- explanations of gender differences in health and illness; and
- the importance of an intersectional theory of health and gender across the life course.

Health and Gender

If you suffer a heart attack, what factors will affect your chances of survival? Factors such as the severity of the heart attack, how quickly you receive emergency medical care, your previous health status and physical condition, and your age all come to mind as important determinants of the odds of making a recovery from a potentially fatal heart attack. However, as depicted in Figure 6.1, your gender also has a major effect on your chances of surviving a heart attack. Research shows that, compared to men, women have a higher risk of dying following a cardiovascular event such as a heart attack or stroke. Women are also less likely to be treated by a specialist, to be transferred to another facility for treatment, or to undergo cardiac catheterization or revascularization to repair their damaged hearts (Pilote et al. 2007). You will remember from Chapter 2 that according to researchers informed by the feminist paradigm, health and illness can be understood as "gendered." Health sociologists recognize that social structures act upon women and men differently and pattern behaviours, including health and health-care behaviours, differently according to socially constructed gender roles associated with being a woman or a man. Owing to the efforts of researchers informed by the feminist paradigm, gender differences in health and wellness have gained increasing popularity as a research topic among health sociologists. The different treatment responses of physicians to women's and men's heart conditions provide clear examples of the gendered nature of health (McKinlay 1996) and the need for further investigation.

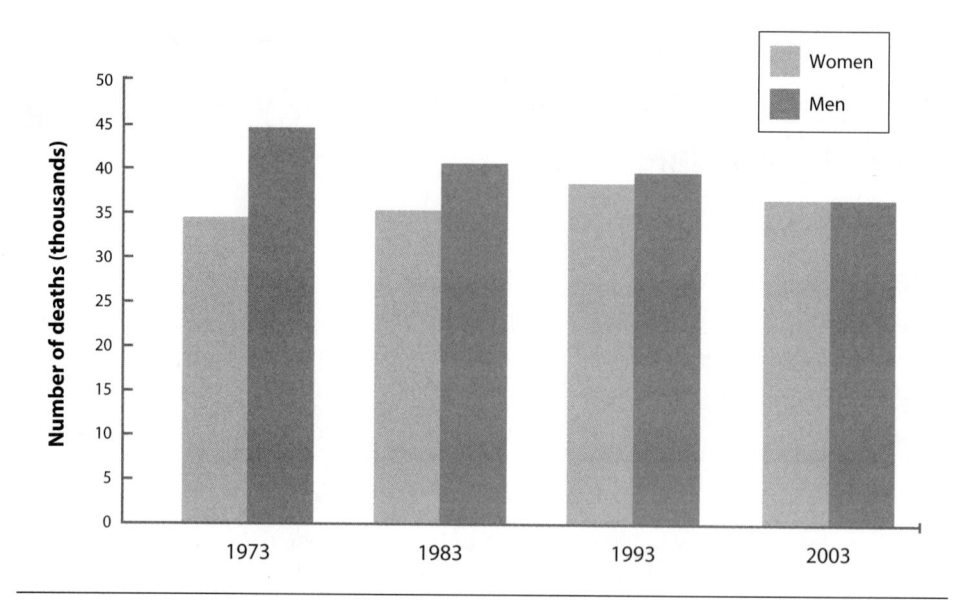

Figure 6.1 Number of Deaths from Cardiovascular Disease

Source: Heart and Stroke Foundation, based on data from Statistics Canada: www.heartandstroke.on.ca/site/c.pvI3IeNWJwE/b.3582053/k.7B9D/2007_Report_Card__Time_to_bridge_the_gender_gap.htm.

When it comes to heart disease and stroke, Canadian women's progress has not kept pace with men's, according to the *2007 Heart and Stroke Foundation Annual Report on Canadians' Health*. In the press release of the report, Dr Beth Abramson, cardiologist and spokesperson for the Heart and Stroke Foundation, says, "We also need to look at access to care through a gender lens."

Knowing that social structures have different consequences for the health of women and men, health sociologists argue that health and illness are "gendered." "Consequently, men's and women's health is the product not only of their biology but also of their social experiences in a stratified society and the gender roles that they enact" (Rieker and Bird 2000, 101). While Annadale (1998, 158) cautions that "research on gender inequalities in health defies the easy summaries that often appear in the literature," an extensive body of evidence has been accumulated that consistently demonstrates that there are significant gender differences in health and illness. For example, health sociologists know that there are gender differences in life expectancy and in the major causes of death. In addition, we know that there are gender differences in the experience of health and illness (e.g., women experience more ill health than men) and in health and illness behaviour (e.g., women make more frequent use of formal health-care services than men). Research also suggests that there are gender differences in the social determinants of health (e.g., having social support is a more important predictor of good health for women than for men).

The adage "women are sicker, but men die quicker" used to be commonly applied to summarize gender disparities in health. While there remains some truth to this generalization, health researchers now know that the adage obscures more than it reveals about how women and men differentially experience health and wellness. Reviewing Canadian data on health and gender led Walters (2003, 5) to conclude that "The general measures of health status as well as the specific measures of mental and physical health problems used in the *National Population Health Survey* [discussed in Chapter 3] indicate different patterns with respect to gender: in some cases no differences between women and men; in others, small or inconsistent differences." As Benoit and colleagues (2009, 8) explain, "Failing to examine sex and gender as fundamental health determinants that intersect with other mitigating factors homogenizes the experiences of women (and men), reifying existing inequities while at the same time overlooking important sources of within-group variation." For example, Cooper (2002) conducted research that shows that socioeconomic inequality accounts for most, but not all, of the health disadvantage experienced by minority ethnic men and women but gender inequality in minority ethnic health remains after adjusting for socioeconomic characteristics. This shows that not all women experience health inequalities in the same way, nor is the health of all men better than that of all women. You should keep this point in mind as we review gender differences in health. In the following sections, examples from research findings are cited to summarize the available information on gender differences in health. The discussion will then shift to a review of the major explanations that have been offered to account for health differences between women and men. First, though, it is necessary to consider the relationship between sex and gender in health research.

The Importance of Sex- and Gender-Based Analysis in Health Research

"Is it a boy or a girl?" This question, asked of expecting and new parents, reveals the importance our culture places on being able to classify individuals into one of two mutually distinct sexes. In fact, sex is the first and most basic means by which humans categorize other humans throughout our lives (Zimbardo 2001). Several decades ago, Garfinkel (1967), an influential sociologist, observed that Western societies operate on the basis of a dimorphic model of sex in which male and female are understood as opposites (Howson 2013). Garfinkel described this model as comprising the "natural attitude" toward gender in Western societies. According to Howson (2013), the natural attitude toward sex and gender has three main characteristics: First, the human body is categorized into the distinct sexes of either male or female. Second, this categorization is believed to be based on fixed scientific standards. Third, sex corresponds to sexuality wherein males are, by nature, sexually attracted to females and vice versa. Feminist analysis has shown that despite its apparent naturalness, the dimorphic model is a social construct associated with patriarchy.

An important early focus for feminist sociologists was to challenge this approach by drawing a clear distinction between sex and gender (West and Zimmerman 1987). According to this distinction, **sex** refers to physiological attributes of the person (e.g., being female), while **gender** represents the socio-cultural expression of sex in terms of personal identity and role performance (e.g., being feminine). Influenced by the feminist paradigm, health sociologists "challenge the implicit assumption in biomedical research that differences in men's and women's health are primarily attributable to underlying sex differences in physiology; rather they have theorized that gender inequality has consequences for men's and women's lives in terms of their physical and psychological well-being" (Rieker and Bird 2000, 101).

However, a drawback with the sex/gender distinction is that it portrays sex as "physical, stable, natural and immutable" (Howson 2013, 51). This oversimplification belies the scientific complexity of sex wherein "absolute dimorphism disintegrates even at the level of basic biology. Chromosomes, hormones, the internal sex structures, the gonads and the external genitalia all vary more than most people realize" (Fausto-Sterling 2000, 20). In reality, life is not as simple as the two sexes and two genders of the dimorphic model! Health researchers need to be sensitive to the diversity of sex and sexuality. While there are biological differences between males and females, such as differences in chromosomal makeup, secondary sexual characteristics, and hormones, "such differences are ordinal rather than dichotomous" (Howson 2013, 51). In describing the diversity of sex categories, using the intersexed (those persons with ambiguous genitalia; a mixture of both male and female body parts) as illustration, Fausto-Sterling (1993, 21) contends that "biologically speaking, there are many gradations running from female to male; and depending on how one calls the shots, one can argue that along that spectrum lie at least five sexes—and perhaps even more. . . . I would argue further that sex is a vast, infinitely malleable continuum that defies the constraints of even five categories." Thus, both sex and gender differences fall along a range of possible human characteristics. As Hankivsky (2012a, 1713) argues, the problem with the dimorphic approach is that it leaves "little space either conceptually or practically for moving beyond two definable sexes and genders, even though intersex and transgendered persons and practices directly destabilize such binary classifications." Reviewing the latest scientific evidence concerning the biology of sex differences led Benoit and colleagues (2009, 2.5) to ask, "is it possible to accurately measure sex as a biological category, distinct from gender?" Despite the challenges associated with scientific efforts to disentangle sex and gender in health research, these authors conclude that "Sex should thus be considered as a basic variable in health research and such studies should consider sex differences beginning in the womb and over what sociologists refer to as the 'life course'" (2009, 2.5).

There is no doubt that sex is an important biological determinant of health. For example, "research has found that estrogen reduces circulatory levels of harmful cholesterol and thereby reduces women's chances of heart disease; for men, the opposite occurs: testosterone increases low density lipoprotein and thus increases their chances of heart disease. Men also tend to have weaker immune systems than women because testosterone causes immunosuppression" (Read and Gorman 2011, 417). The importance of both sex and gender affecting health, sometimes separately but more often in combination, has led to the development of sex- and gender-based analysis in health and medical research.

The chief public health officer of Canada defines **sex- and gender-based analysis (SGBA)** as "a systematic approach to research, policies and programs that explores biological (sex-based) and sociocultural (gender-based) similarities and differences between women and men, boys and girls," adding that this approach to health and medical research "helps to ensure that interventions are effective and inclusive" (Butler-Jones 2012, 2). Since 2009, SGBA has been mandated by Health Canada in that researchers are expected to integrate sex and gender into the research process where possible. The idea behind SGBA is that the conduct of health and medical research needs to be sensitive to the diversity of sex, gender, and sexuality. As Clow and her co-researchers (2009, 1) explain, "Rather than assuming that 'one size fits all,' SGBA reminds us to ask questions about similarities and differences between and among women and men." Noting the compatibility of SGBA with an intersectional perspective on health, Pederson and her co-authors (2013, 8) contend that "Emerging theory and practice in SGBA emphasize the importance of paying attention to the intersection of multiple aspects of identity and experience when it comes to explaining health, illness and care." This means that the process of SGBA helps to avoid the homogenization of populations and subpopulations, realizing that men and women, male and female, are diverse social groups made up of unique individuals. There are many femininities and masculinities (Connell 1995), and sex is ordinal rather than dichotomous (i.e., running along a range of possible categories). These complex aspects of identity overlap with other dimensions of social location across the life course. This intersectional approach means that SGBA places special emphasis on understanding and addressing overlapping sources of health disparities (Clow et al. 2009).

SGBA also draws attention to how the diversity of sexuality intersects with health. As Clow and colleagues (2009, 14) remind us, "diversity also includes differences that are not always evident, such as sexual orientation." Introducing a special issue on lesbian, gay, bisexual, and transgender (LGBT) health in the *Journal of Homosexuality*, Harcourt describes the "dearth" of information pertaining to health and diverse sexualities: "although we know a lot about some health issues such as HIV/AIDS among gay and bisexual men, we know little about other health issues effecting LGBT populations" (2006, 1). Challenges facing researchers interested in LGBT health include the under-representation of LGBT individuals in population health research and the difficulty associated with operationalizing sexual orientation (Bauer 2012; Harcourt 2006). Harcourt (2006) stresses the need to move beyond small-scale, descriptive studies by incorporating mixed-method approaches for a better understanding of the health issues facing LGBT persons. He notes that "Clearly, discrimination based upon sexual orientation or gender identity has an impact on the well-being of LGBT persons, and may have an impact on the health of these populations" (2006, 4). More recently, Mulé and Smith (2014) note that despite greater legal protections and an increasing emphasis on diversity, LGBT communities constitute an "invisible population" in Canadian health policy.

Overall, SGBA demonstrates that while health may be shaped by aspects of biology such as sex, at the same time it is mediated through culture and occurs in a social context. Further, biological development is influenced by the environment. As Chapter 4 made clear, it is apparent that biology and social environment combine to produce health outcomes. Consequently, biology and the social environment are best conceptualized as interacting factors that influence our health and health-care behaviour across the life course. In keeping with this, sex and gender are best understood as interacting to shape the gender differences in health, which we now review.

Gender Differences in Health

Box 6.1 highlights major gender differences in health identified by researchers.

Box 6.1 Gender Differences in Health

- Women live longer than men.
- The genders differ in the major causes of death.
- Women are diagnosed as suffering from more ill health than men.
- Women make more frequent use of formal health care than men.
- There are gender differences in the social determinants of health.

Women Live Longer Than Men

To begin with, as Figure 6.2 shows, while life expectancy has been increasing for all Canadians since 1920, a gender gap remains in length of life. Women consistently outlive men. According to Statistics Canada (2013a), women live, on average, approximately four years longer than men (83.60 years versus 79.33 years), although the gender gap in life expectancy is decreasing because of men's greater gains in life expectancy (Butler-Jones 2012). Turcotte (2011, 40) reports that "Even though women have a higher life expectancy, men made the greatest gains in the last decade." Despite this narrowing of the gap in life expectancy, Nelson and Robinson (1999, 434) point out that "examinations of successive editions of the *Guinness Book of Records* reveal that accurately documented and verified holders of the title as the world's oldest living human being have been, and continue to be, women." While the gender gap has decreased slightly in recent years (likely because of converging lifestyles), women continue to live longer than men. This was not always the case. Andreev (2000) reports that gender mortality rates are variable. Until the 1940s, the rates for Canadian women aged 20 to 49 were actually higher than those for men in the same age group. Since biology alone cannot explain shifting patterns in life expectancy, the question for health sociologists is: How do socio-cultural factors account for the differences between the genders?

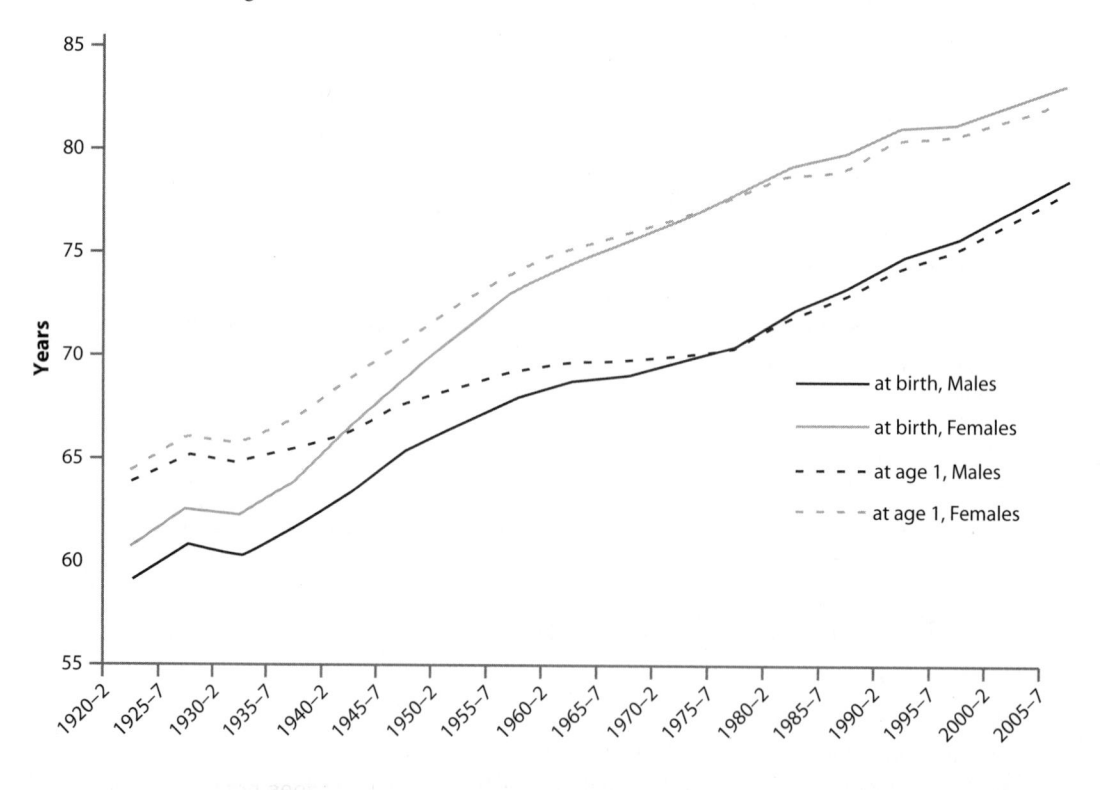

Figure 6.2 Life Expectancy at Birth and at Age 1, by Sex, Canada, 1920–2 to 2005–7

Source: Statistics Canada 2011b.

Although life expectancy is a key indicator of population health status, it is not necessarily the best measure. Research (Mandich and Margolis 2014) indicates that life expectancy is a measure of population health status that perhaps lacks sensitivity to important gender differences in the lived experience of health and illness. For this reason, health researchers have begun to consider gender differences in health using alternative indicators such as the Health Utilities Index and health-adjusted life expectancy (discussed in Chapter 3). Table 6.1 depicts a comparison of life expectancy and health-adjusted life expectancy, 2005 to 2007, for women and men. Chapter 3 made the important point that such health-adjusted life expectancy indicators are more comprehensive measures of population health status than life expectancy because they attempt to include both quantity (or length) of life and quality of life by measuring the number of years lived in good health. If women as a group suffer from more debilitating chronic illness as they age than men do, this is an important source of disparity in health. When DesMeules, Manuel, and Cho (2003) compared women's and men's health-adjusted life expectancy, they found that while women still have longer health expectancy than men (70.0 years compared to 66.7 years), this gap, like the gap in life expectancy, also appears to be narrowing. These researchers conclude that "Although mortality and life expectancy have been well described in the Canadian population, there is a paucity of information concerning the sex and gender gaps in mortality and life expectancy, in particular the factors contributing to the sex gaps observed, and how gender-relevant determinants affect the mortality of subgroups of Canadian women" (2003b, 2). Future intersectional research employing SGBA and gender-sensitive indictors is needed to understand the relationship between gender and both health and life expectancy.

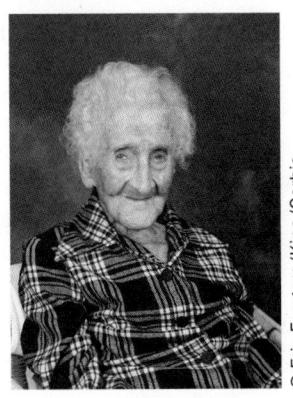

Jeanne Calment holds the record for the oldest recorded person in history. She was born on 21 February 1876 and died at 122 years old on 4 August 1997.

Table 6.1 Life Expectancy and Health-Adjusted Life Expectancy, 2005 to 2007

	Life Expectancy	Health-Adjusted Life Expectancy	Difference	
	Years	Years	Years	%
Male	78.3	68.9	9.4	12
Female	83.0	71.2	11.8	14

Estimates of health-adjusted life expectancy for 2005–7 indicate that women could expect to live almost 12 years, or 14 per cent of their lives, in poor health compared to 9 years (12 per cent) for men. Women's longer overall life expectancy does not mean that they have an equivalent advantage in health-adjusted life expectancy.

Source: Statistics Canada. Death—Shifting Trends. *Health Reports* 12(3): 41–46. Ottawa: Statistics Canada (2001): Cat. No. 82-003-XIE2000003.

The Genders Differ in Major Causes of Death

In part, the difference between women's and men's life expectancy is related to gender differences in role behaviours identified as major causes of death. For example, as shown in Figure 6.3, unintentional injuries resulting from motor vehicle accidents and suicides account for significantly more deaths among men than among women in Canada, particularly younger men. While women still have an advantage in life expectancy, the gender gap is getting smaller because of changes occurring in the types of diseases experienced by women and men. To illustrate, for many years female lung cancer rates increased while male lung cancer rates were decreasing (Canadian Cancer Society Advisory Committee on Cancer Statistics 2014). In fact, smoking rates for young women now exceed those for young men (Greaves and Jategaonkar 2006), and lung cancer has now surpassed breast cancer in terms of premature death among Canadian women (Canadian Cancer Society Advisory Committee on Cancer Statistics 2014). However, preventable deaths (those caused by accidents, amenable to health-care treatment, or avoidable through lifestyle changes) continue to disproportionately end men's lives. In fact, an analysis found that "by excluding these causes preventable through primary prevention, the resulting life expectancy

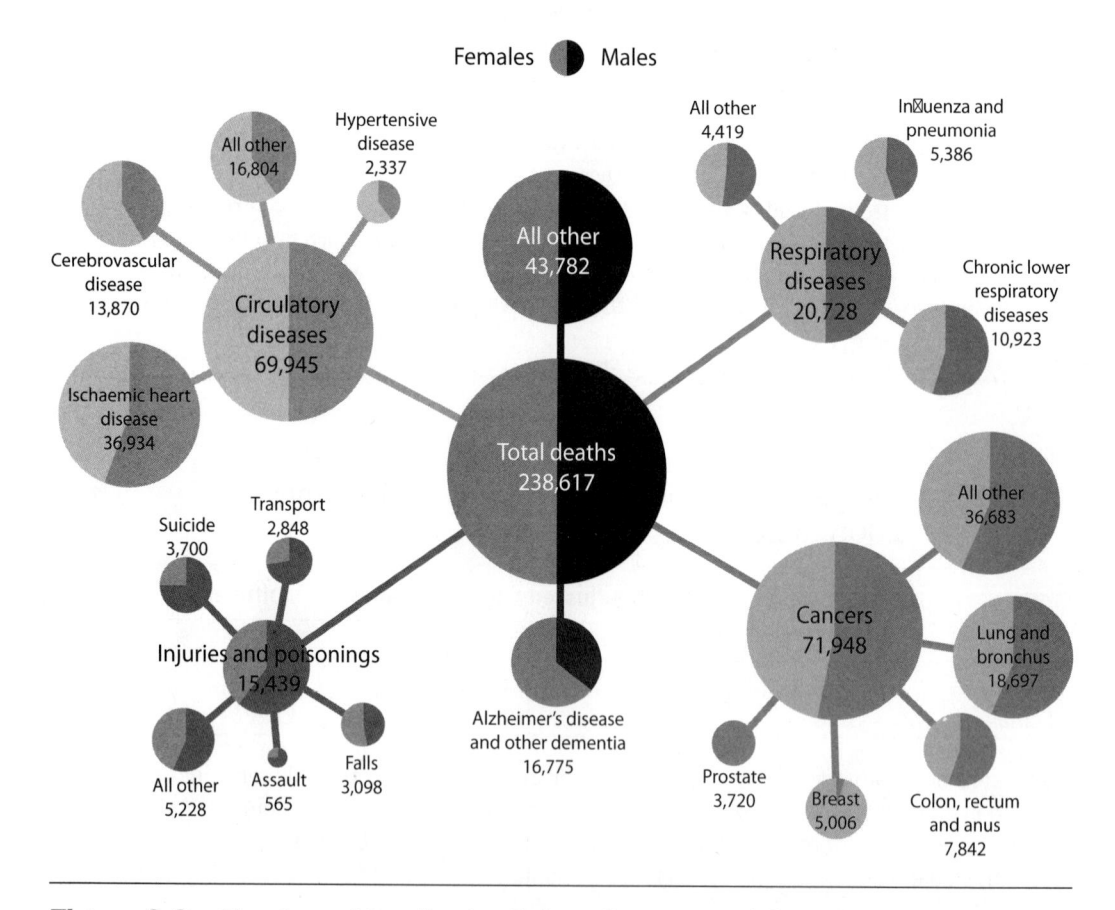

Figure 6.3 Number of Deaths by Select Causes and Sex, Canada, 2008

Source: Butler-Jones 2012, using data from Canadian Vital Statistics, Death Database, Statistics Canada.

was 84.9 and 82.7 for women and men, respectively (a difference of 2.2 years)" (DesMeules, Manuel, and Cho 2003, 5). This finding led these researchers to conclude that "clearly, the factors having the strongest impact on the sex gap are smoking and external causes of death such as accidents and suicide. As smoking-related deaths and disability continue to increase among women and decrease among men, this sex gap is expected to continue to narrow" (2003b, 7). These differences in the causes of death suggest that there is a complex relationship between behavioural practices, types of illness experienced, and life expectancy of women and men. In order to better understand this relationship, research is needed that examines the intersections of these factors over time with other aspects of social location, such as socioeconomic status, ethnicity, and age.

Women Are Diagnosed as Suffering from More Ill Health Than Men

Denton, Prus, and Walters (2004, 2586) summarize current research on gender inequalities in health by noting that "While women generally experience poorer health than men, the pattern of gender differences in health is varied. Women have lower rates of mortality but, paradoxically, report higher levels of depression, psychiatric disorders, distress, and a variety of chronic illnesses than men." In a report prepared for the Canadian Institute for Health Information in 2003, a team of researchers documented important differences in health outcomes and behaviours of women and men. The report provides evidence on physical health indicating that women, across all age groups, are more likely than men to experience chronic conditions such as arthritis/rheumatism, high blood pressure, and allergies, as well as higher incidence of comorbidity (i.e., the presence of two or more chronic conditions). Men have similar or slightly higher rates than women for potentially fatal chronic conditions, such as coronary heart disease and cancer. The report also states that women suffer from severe and moderate disability more than men, noting that "13.3% of women and 11.5% of men (all ages combined) report a disability" (DesMeules, Turner, and Cho 2003, 2). Such findings prompted Read and Gorman (2011, 414) to conclude that "Several systematic examinations of multiple health outcomes at different stages of the life cycle found that the paradox of women's poorer health but longer life expectancy was not really so paradoxical when one considers that men experience more life-threatening illnesses—such as heart disease—that result in death at younger ages, while women experience less serious, chronic illnesses—such as arthritis—that result in longer years spent in poor health." Given men's and women's differing patterns of illness across the life course, it is not surprising that "women are sicker, but men die quicker."

In terms of mental health and emotional well-being, women have a significantly higher prevalence of mood disorders, while men appear to embody the mental health effects of stress through alcohol and substance abuse (Turcotte 2011). Bird and Rieker (2008, 30) summarize gender differences in mental health by noting that "men's and women's overall incidence of mental health problems is similar. However, women experience substantially higher rates of depression than men, whereas men experience higher rates of substance abuse, antisocial behavior, and suicides." This means that both women's and men's health are affected by stress but the genders differ in the manner in which these differences become embodied and are expressed: "Men appear to embody stress-related angst in substance abuse disorders that express anger and hostility, while women do so in affective or anxiety disorders indicative of depression" (McDonough and Walters 2001, 548). The exact causes of these gender differences in the experience of health and illness cannot be understood through statistical analysis of population health data alone.

In an effort to better understand gender differences in physical symptoms and illness behaviour, Gijsbers van Wilk, Huisman, and Kolk (1999) utilized health diaries (described in Chapter 3) as a data collection method. These researchers hoped that the use of health diaries would allow them to investigate the relationship between mood states and gender differences in physical symptoms and illness behaviour on a daily basis. They report that "gender differences in physical symptoms and illness behavior appear smaller when assessed in daily health records with standardized instruments, than has generally been reported in studies which are either cross-sectional or rely on less solid measures" (1999, 1072). While they found a gender difference in the frequency and severity of physical symptoms, with women reporting more frequent and more serious symptoms, Gijsbers van Wilk and colleagues did not find a gender difference in illness behaviour. In their words, Gijsbers van Wilk, Huisman, and Kolk (1999, 1072) conclude that "Gender differences in symptom reporting are attributable to psychological differences between men and women instead of being caused by biology." Future application of intersectional research designs that make use of both quantitative and qualitative methods is needed to unravel this mystery and understand the interacting causes of gender differences in health and illness across the life course.

Women Make More Frequent Use of Formal Health Care Than Men

Gender differences have also been identified in the ways in which women and men deal with their health concerns and use formal health care. For example, Payne and colleagues (2003) report that women were more likely than men to have taken some form of medication in the month prior to participating in the *National Population Health Survey*. The gender difference in medication activities holds when birth control and menopause-related drugs are excluded. Women also visit physicians more frequently (see Figure 6.4) and submit to higher levels of medical screening in the form of laboratory tests, blood pressure monitoring, and the like (Kazanjian, Morettin, and Cho 2003). Data from the *Canadian Community Health Survey* show that men are less likely to have a regular family physician than women, with 19 per cent of the men versus 11 per cent of the women reporting having no regular doctor (Turcotte 2011). As shown in Figure 6.5, when the hospitalization rates for men and women are compared within age groups, women under the age of 20 and those between 45 and 64 years of age are hospitalized less frequently than men. However, considerably more women than men between the ages of 20 and 44 are hospitalized, whether or not hospitalizations for maternity care are included.

Explaining the connection between patriarchal culture and the use of health care, Rieker and Bird (2000, 100) state that "Assumptions about men and women enter into conceptions of health and illness and affect medical research, doctor-patient encounters, and treatment protocols." As illustration, a now-classic study in the United States by Verbrugge and Steiner (1981) of women and men who presented with the same complaints or medical diagnoses found that women were given prescriptions more often than men were. Subsequent studies have confirmed that men and women are treated differently by physicians (Hajjaj et al. 2010). For instance, feminist health researchers (e.g., Munch 2004) have demonstrated a bias in which physicians are more likely to label women's health problems as psychosomatic, whereby "female illness is socially constructed as erroneously or disproportionately embracing psychiatric or sociocultural contributors" (Richman et al. 2000, 178). This type of gender bias in formal health care can obviously lead to women's illnesses being misdiagnosed, with serious health consequences. A personal illustration of this comes from the experiences of the mother of one of your authors (Fries). After

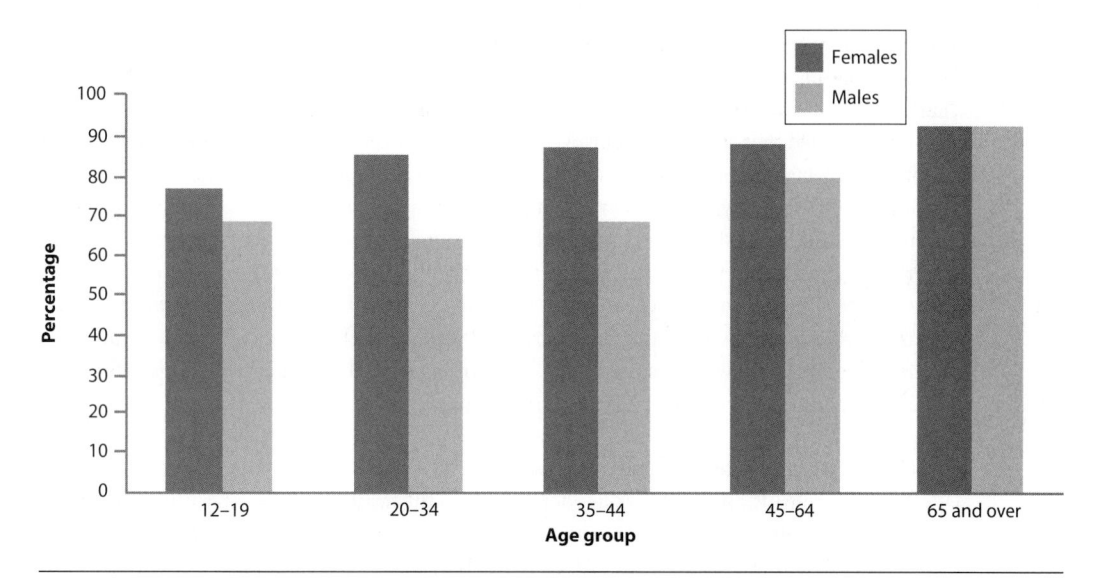

Figure 6.4 Persons Who Saw or Talked to a Doctor in the Previous Year, by Sex and Age Group, Canada, 2009

Note: The term "doctor" includes family or general practitioners as well as specialists such as surgeons, allergists, orthopaedists, gynaecologists or psychiatrists. For the population aged 12 to 17, pediatricians are included.

Source: Turcotte 2011.

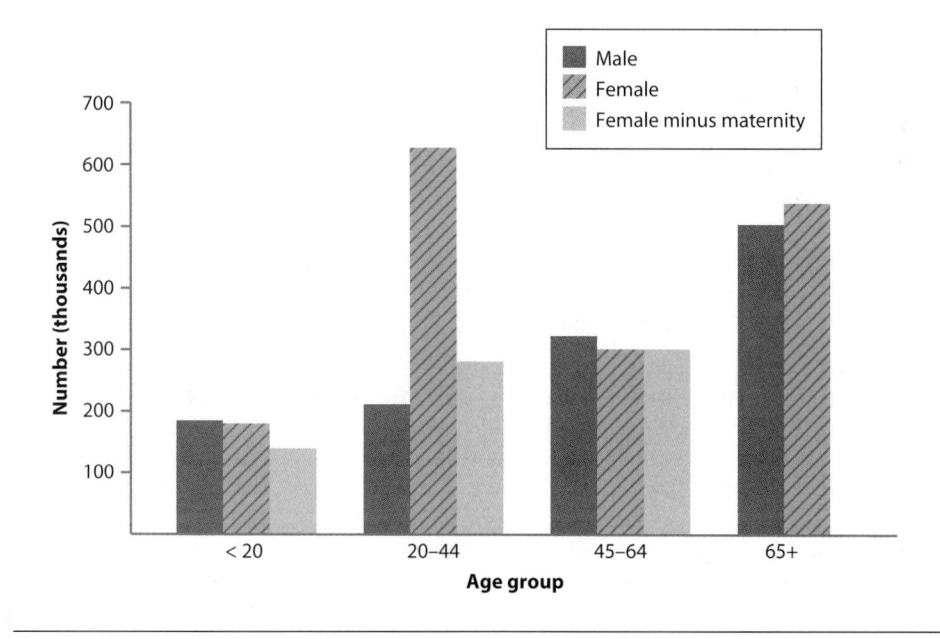

Figure 6.5 Number of Hospitalizations in Acute Care Hospitals, 2000–1, Canada—Age Groups by Gender

Source: DesMeules et al. 2003.

complaining for a number of months to her family physician that she was experiencing severe abdominal pains, rather than pursuing further clinical investigation this doctor inquired as to whether she was a victim of past sexual abuse! Two years later, tests ordered by a new family physician revealed that she had advanced stage ovarian cancer. Abdominal pain is a well-known symptom of ovarian cancer, and, as with most cancers, early detection can improve treatment outcomes. Unfortunately, this woman's first physician may have allowed his patient's gender to bias his clinical decision-making, delaying diagnosis and treatment. This demonstrates the manner in which the health-care system and health-care professionals provide differential access and treatment for different groups. Clearly, research on gender differences in health and illness, as well as health-care behaviour, must be interpreted in light of the realization made clear by the feminist paradigm that women's bodies and women's lives have long been the target of medical consumerism and medicalization. Kazanjian and colleagues (2003, 2) offer this warning:

> There is a much greater expectation for women than men to present themselves for medical care or consultation. Women are dependent on the health care system to ensure, control or terminate their fertility; healthy women are expected to have a Pap test if sexually active and a mammogram if aged 50 or older; they talk to their doctor about the risk of osteoporosis at age 50 and obtain a bone density test if aged 65 and older. The risk of perpetuating the view that women are not only over-users of the system relative to men but also "sicker" than men is high without a thorough analysis of the "gendered" body for the use of health care resources.

While medicalization will be explored further in Chapter 10 when we consider gender differences in health-care behaviour, you should keep in mind that the institution of medicine has been one of the main means by which control and oppression have been exercised over women within patriarchy. Benoit et al. (2009, 2.9) remind us that "Explanations for this kind of sex/gender disparity have been noted by some as the result of biases in diagnostic processes as well as the diagnostic criteria themselves. This argument suggests that men and women are equally as likely to suffer morbidity due to illness and disease, but that health is interpreted differently based on gender, with women more likely to be diagnosed as being sick or ill." An unresolved question is the extent to which the higher morbidity and health-care utilization of women is a result of interacting social and biological factors associated with womanhood or attributable to forces of medicalization within patriarchal culture.

Gender Differences in the Social Determinants of Health

Numerous studies (e.g., Benoit et al. 2009; Denton and Walters 1999; Denton, Prus, and Walters 2004; Luchenski, Quesnel-Vallée, and Lynch 2007; Matthews, Manor, and Power 1999; McDonough et al. 1999; McGibbon and McPherson 2011; Spitzer 2005; Walters, McDonough, and Strohschein 2002) have examined gender differences in major social determinants of health (e.g., socioeconomic position, labour force participation, and earned income). Walters' (2003, 1) introduction to a government-sponsored report on women's health makes clear the gendered difference in the social determinants of health:

> Gender matters. Being born a boy or a girl has a profound influence on the shape of an infant's future life. Compared with men, women are less likely to be employed full time,

more likely to be attuned to caring roles, and more likely to have their working life interrupted by pregnancy and caring responsibilities. Women generally work in lower-paid jobs, and they exercise less control in those jobs. Research also tells us that women's views are more likely to be devalued, women are less likely to occupy top positions in society, and women are more likely to be seen as irrational, emotional and unsuited for responsible positions. Even though women have entered the labour force in greater numbers, they still assume most of the responsibility for household chores. Women's economic dependence on men is signified by the dramatic change in their lives after divorce or separation. It is not surprising that women also have lower self-esteem and are more likely to be concerned about body image.

The previous chapter demonstrated just how important social class factors are to health. Social scientific research has established the clear existence of gendered inequalities in socioeconomic status. For example, using a conservative measure of the wage gap between women and men, a report prepared for Statistics Canada notes that in 2011 the average hourly wage for women working full-time was 87 per cent of that of men (Morissette, Picot, and Lu 2013). This means that for every dollar earned by men, women earned 87 cents. This type of **gender stratification**, or the unequal distribution of wealth, power, and privilege between men and women, has both direct and indirect effects on health (Denton, Prus, and Walters 2004). Studies of the social gradient in health that consider gender generally find less steep gradients for women as opposed to those among men. However, research shows that such gender differences vary by age in addition to the measures of health status and inequality used (Matthews, Manor, and Power 1999). Spitzer (2005, 84) summarizes the existing evidence by suggesting that "economic inequities, evidenced by income, employment and the demands of domestic labour, appear to underpin gendered health disparities most broadly." Research has shown that these are some of the most important determinants of women's health. However, despite numerous policy commitments such as the 1981 Canadian signing of the *United Nations Convention on the Elimination of All Forms of Discrimination against Women*, the 1995 adoption of the *Federal Plan on Gender Equality*, the 2009 adoption of SGBA within Health Canada, and the funding of the Canadian Institutes of Health Research—Institute of Gender and Health (see the recommended websites at the end of this chapter), there continue to be marked disparities in the social determinants of health of Canadian women and men.

Denton and Walters (1999) explored the social determinants of health by examining the extent to which health is shaped by structures of inequality and behavioural practices. The structural determinants investigated included age group, family structure (e.g., marital status, number of children), years of education, occupational status, income adequacy (e.g., household income and size), main activity (i.e., a combined measure of employment status and work hours), and social support. The behavioural determinants included lifestyle practices such as smoking, drinking, and physical activity. Echoing the findings of an earlier British study (Blaxter 1990), Denton and Walters found that structural factors are the most important determinants of health, acting both directly and indirectly through their influence on behavioural determinants of health. In their words, "These analyses suggest that the structural determinants of health play a greater role than the behavioral or lifestyle determinants in shaping the health status of Canadians" (Denton and Walters 1999, 1229). In terms of gender differences in social determinants of health, it is noteworthy that Denton and Walters' findings indicate that there are significant differences in the factors that influence women's and men's health. For women, social structural factors, such as being in a high-income category, working full-time and caring for a family, and having social support, are the most important determinants of health. In contrast, behavioural practices, such as smoking and alcohol consumption, are more important determinants of health for men. Denton and Walters conclude by recommending that future research should be guided by intersectional models that include a broad range of structural and behavioural factors if we are to learn more about the social production of health and illness for both women and men.

Finally, looking at differences in health through a gendered lens reveals that social determinants of health are themselves gender-based constructs that influence women's health in unique ways. For example, McDonough and colleagues (1999) contend that the findings of their study suggest that labour market rewards have divergent meanings for women and men and, therefore, they have different implications for their health (e.g., their death rates). They argue that to be able to understand the link between gender, education, income, and health, we need to consider more carefully "the ways in which socioeconomic position is constituted from individuals' experiences in the labor market and in the family" (McDonough et al. 1999, 27). In other words, structural determinants such as socioeconomic status, employment, and working conditions are experienced differently by women and men and, consequently, have unique effects on health and illness behaviour.

Explanations of Gender Differences in Health and Illness

To date, no single explanation can account for all of these gender differences in health and illness. We have a lot of descriptive information documenting what types of specific gender differences exist, but we still do not have an adequate explanation of why there are such pronounced differences between women and men in the area of health and illness. Nor do we fully understand how gender intersects over time with other factors, such as socioeconomic status and ethnicity, to produce specific patterns in health outcomes. At present, a number of competing hypotheses have been offered as possible explanations for gender differences in health and illness (see Box 6.2). According to Nelson and Robinson (1999, 445), "Each hypothesis has supporters and critics and none has yet emerged as the most compelling" explanation of this complex relationship.

While some of the explanations of women's health in the sociological literature focus on structural inequalities (e.g., gender differences in income levels), other explanations focus primarily on the link between social roles and the gendered experience of health and illness. Such studies argue that rather than biology, it is differences in the social roles occupied by women and

Box 6.2 Explanations of Gender Differences in Health and Illness

- The role accumulation hypothesis
- The role strain hypothesis
- The social acceptability hypothesis
- The risk-taking hypothesis

men that explain differences in health status. For example, Waldron, Weiss, and Hughes (1998) examined the interacting effects of multiple roles on women's health by testing a number of different hypotheses about the effects of employment, marriage, and motherhood on women's general physical health. The major hypotheses include the role accumulation hypothesis and the role strain hypothesis. Waldron, Weiss, and Hughes (1998, 216) point out that "there is general agreement that women's roles can have both beneficial and harmful effects on their physical health, but it remains uncertain whether various combinations of multiple roles have a net beneficial or net harmful effect."

The Role Accumulation Hypothesis

Simply stated, the **role accumulation hypothesis** suggests that more roles result in better health. This hypothesis proposes that multiple roles contribute to better health because they provide a variety of benefits, such as greater self-esteem, life satisfaction, more sources of social support, and improved financial resources. The basic assumption is that these salutogenic benefits outweigh the health disadvantages associated with performing multiple social roles. This oversimplification fails to take into account the interaction effects of the specific roles and combination of roles that we each play, which may lead to role conflict—the psychosocial distress experienced when an individual is forced to play one or more incompatible roles. For example, the beneficial health effects of being married and employed (e.g., social support and increased income) may be offset when they are combined with the parental role in their impact on women's health. Modifications to the role accumulation hypothesis now "recognize that the health effects of a role may vary depending on the other roles a woman holds" (Waldron, Weiss, and Hughes 1998, 217). Maclean, Glynn, and Ansara (2003, 1) add that "more recent research indicates that involvement in each role has both harmful and beneficial effects, and the balance between these varies depending on characteristics of the role, the specific combination of roles, and the socio-economic context of women's lives." As illustration, in a Canadian longitudinal study of employed women and men, Janzen and Muhajarine (2003, 1492) explain that "men and women occupying the same types of roles may experience them in profoundly different ways." These researchers found that women who occupied the "triple roles" of mother, wife, and worker had more positive health outcomes than women who occupied one or two of these roles. The study revealed the same pattern for men at a later life stage. Interestingly, the researchers found that these patterns of role occupancy and health were independent of social class effects. That is, more roles were healthier for women at all levels of income adequacy. However, the researchers note that their study sample was not sufficiently representative of low-income or unemployed people. On balance, the majority of published studies find support for the role accumulation hypothesis, and yet more research is required to understand how roles combine with other aspects of social location to influence health (Klumb and Lampert 2004).

The Role Strain Hypothesis

In contrast to the first hypothesis regarding gender differences in health, the **role strain hypothesis** emphasizes the harmful effects of women's roles. This hypothesis proposes that multiple roles (such as parenting and being employed) result in role overload and role conflict for women. The increased stress and excessive demands on time and energy associated with performing multiple roles (i.e., the well-known double day) contribute to higher levels of psychological distress

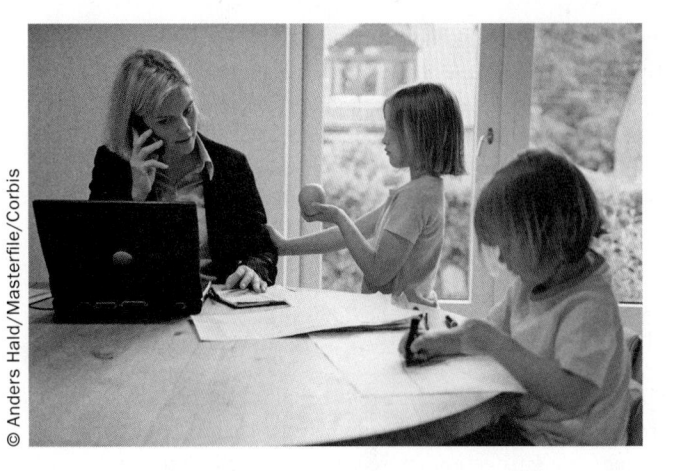

The role strain hypothesis suggests that multiple roles can result in higher levels of stress and poorer health. Women's health can be negatively affected by the stress caused by playing a role as primary caregiver for their children, spouses, and aging parents while also working outside the home.

and poorer health for women. "Thus, the combination of employment and motherhood may have particularly harmful health effects for women who combine full-time employment with parental responsibility for young children and/or many children" (Waldron, Weiss, and Hughes 1998, 218). In their gendered role as primary caregiver for their children, spouses, and aging parents, women experience considerable stress and time constraints and may neglect their own health needs. In other words, trying to live up to the social expectations associated with performing caring and nurturing roles may have adverse effects on women's health. In evaluating the role strain hypothesis, Janzen and Muhajarine (2003, 1492) note that "Interestingly, although experience and common sense strongly suggests that role overload is experienced by many employed parents, empirical research indicates that, on average, adults who occupy more roles experience better physical and psychological well-being than those who have fewer roles." However, research has also found that Canadian women identify stress as their major health concern (Walters 1992). This stress is typically associated with women's family and employment responsibilities and their worries about other matters such as marital conflict and domestic violence. Additionally, social role research consistently shows that single-parent mothers are the most vulnerable to the adverse health effects of role strain (Maclean, Glynn, and Ansara 2003). Other hypotheses regarding gender differences in health can also be found in the literature, such as the social acceptability hypothesis and the risk-taking hypothesis.

The Social Acceptability Hypothesis

The **social acceptability hypothesis** (e.g., Hibbard and Pope 1986) suggests that due to socialization into patriarchal gender roles, women are more willing to adopt the sick role (i.e., they are more willing to admit to being sick and to accept help in dealing with their health problems). As illustration, Turcotte (2011, 19) reports that "in 2009, of females aged 12 and over who described their mental health as fair or poor, 17% had seen a psychologist in the previous year, compared with 11% of males." This leads her to conclude that "Since women have a greater tendency to ask for help, it is also more likely that they will be diagnosed with a mental health problem." According to this hypothesis, women are more likely to report experiencing symptoms because it is more socially acceptable for them to do so. However, other research casts doubt on this hypothesis, concluding that there is little evidence to support it (Macintyre, Ford, and Hunt 1999). One of the obstacles in fully testing the social acceptability hypothesis is the difficulty of comparing the reporting of symptoms with actual morbidity as revealed by objective biophysical measurement. Despite this challenge, we do know that there are gender differences in the use of social support networks in relation to health concerns. Kandrack, Grant, and Segall (1991, 583) explain how "assessment of the use of informal social networks for discussions of health problems suggests that women talk to, or use a greater number of persons in their networks." In fact, significant differences were found between women and men in the use of specific members of their social networks as health consultants. While men rely on their spouses for social support related to their health concerns, women are more likely to turn to friends and their children as health resources. Women not only discuss their health more freely, but they also engage in a wide variety of other health-protective actions, including seeking early medical care. Qualitative research focusing on the embodied aspects of health (Saltonstall 1993) reveals that while both genders ground their understanding of health in the body, women and men have different conceptualizations of health and how best to pursue it. As Saltonstall (1993, 12) explains, "the doing of health is a form of doing of gender." Feminist health sociologists point out that gendered health behaviours are enacted according to the sexist norms of patriarchal culture.

Within patriarchal culture, men have been socialized traditionally to deny that they are experiencing symptoms of illness and disease and are reluctant to adopt the sick role (with its associated behavioural expectations such as dependency). To illustrate, in a study of health and the gendered dimensions of African Canadians' cancer experiences, Evans and a team of community researchers (2005) explored the intersections of gender and ethnicity with breast and prostate cancer in Nova Scotia. Consistent with previous research (Cameron and Bernardes 1998), they found that men do not like to discuss prostate cancer, viewing it as a threat to stereotypical depictions of masculinity and, in particular, Black masculinity. Men are not likely to seek professional help until their symptoms have become impossible to ignore any longer (or, in the case of married men, until their wives have finally persuaded them to go to the doctor). Cameron and Bernardes (1998, 683) report that "although there was variation among the men in the study, for many men the onset of symptoms did not lead immediately to help-seeking. For some it did not come until a health crisis occurred or a particular incident which acted as a trigger to consult." Evans and her team of researchers found that African-Canadian men expressed an extreme reluctance to submit to digital rectal exams (DREs), viewing such medical screening as emasculating. Evans and colleagues explain that "As the managers of health in their families and communities, women were more likely to know about health resources, including the time and location of an annual men's health clinic. They also expressed sympathy for men wanting to avoid DREs because of the association between the penetration of men's bodies, homosexuality, and compromised masculinity" (2005, 266). These findings reflect common gender role assumptions about sexuality and women's responsibility for family health matters.

This type of research shows that men's gender performance affects their health and illness behaviour. An extreme example of this behaviour is provided by Long (1993), whose research describes a farmer who severed his finger while harvesting, wrapping his finger in a handkerchief, and waiting until the end of the workday before seeking medical care. The social acceptability hypothesis suggests that there may be a complex link between acknowledging illness, seeking care promptly, getting early intervention, receiving frequent treatment, one's eventual health status (and perhaps life expectancy), and the performance of gender. In other words, women admit to experiencing more ill health but ultimately may live longer than men because they are willing to take prompt health action and to seek early treatment.

The Risk-Taking Hypothesis

In a discussion of changing gender roles, Waldron (1997) proposed another hypothesis related to patriarchal culture as a possible explanation for gender differences in health and illness behaviour. The **risk-taking hypothesis** shifts the emphasis somewhat and suggests that men are socialized to take risks, while women are socialized to be more cautious and more concerned about taking care of their health. "Consequently, males engage in more risky behavior, while females engage in more preventive and protective behavior, as well as more treatment seeking and self-care for illness" (Waldron 1997, 303). Criticizing the absence of gender-sensitive men's health research from a feminist perspective, Courtenay (2000b, 1387) observes that "The consistent, underlying presumption in medical literature is that what it means to be a man in America has no bearing on how men work, drink, drive, fight, or take risks." Despite these sexist, taken-for-granted beliefs, an extensive review of large-scale studies, national data, and meta-analyses (i.e., studies combining the results of other studies in one large analysis) by Courtenay (2000a) systematically demonstrates that males of all ages are more likely than females to engage in more than 30 behaviours that increase the risk of disease, injury, and death! Box 6.3 provides an illustration of one such risky behaviour that has recently taken off in popularity, often with devastating consequences for the men involved.

As previously explained, researchers guided by the feminist paradigm understand gender as a set of socially constructed relationships, which both women and men perform in varying degrees, based on differing social locations. In other words, gender is something we "do" or, as Courtenay (2000b, 1387) puts it, "is better understood as a verb than a noun." Social scientific study of gender and men's health makes frequent reference to the term "hegemonic masculinity" (coined by Connell [1995], a leading figure in the sociology of masculinity) to understand the relationship between the performance of gender and men's behaviour. **Hegemonic masculinity** refers to the culturally dominant ideal of what it means to be male and how masculine men are supposed to behave within patriarchal society. In North America today, the hegemonic form of masculinity (i.e., the one that is most prominent, idealized, and unquestioned in our culture) is that of the individualistic, independent, domineering, rational, tough, aggressive, and exploitative heterosexual male. Hegemonic masculinity is a cultural ideal embodied in heterosexual, highly educated, and successful men of European ancestry with high socioeconomic status. Health beliefs and behaviours are one of the main means by which boys and men in our health-conscious society "do gender" and attempt to display hegemonic masculinity. In the context of hegemonic masculinity, as Courtenay (2000b, 1388) explains,

> The social practices required for demonstrating femininity and masculinity are associated with very different health advantages and risks. Unlike the presumably innocent effects of wearing lipstick or wearing a tie, the use of health-related beliefs and behaviours to define oneself as a woman or a man has a profound impact on one's health and longevity.

Developing a theoretical framework for understanding men's health based on the influence of masculinity across the life course, Evans and colleagues (2011, 13) explain that "Given that social constructions of masculinity shape men's perceptions of health and illness and their subsequent health care practices, hegemonic masculinity and traditional beliefs about manhood are the strongest predictors of individual risk behaviour over the lifecourse." In other words, patriarchal

Box 6.3 Gendered Risk-Taking and Health

"Car surfing" is a term introduced in the mid-1980s to describe a thrill-seeking activity that involves riding on the exterior of a moving motor vehicle while it is being driven by another person. While data on the prevalence of health risks are not yet available in Canada, the United States Centers for Disease Control and Prevention identified 58 reports of car-surfing deaths and 41 reports of non-fatal injury from 1990 through August 2008. Most of the injuries were among males (70 per cent) and persons aged 15 to 19 years (69 per cent) (CDC 2008). In Canada, police have laid criminal charges against youth who were driving when their friends were killed while car surfing. Why do young men engage in such obviously risky behaviour?

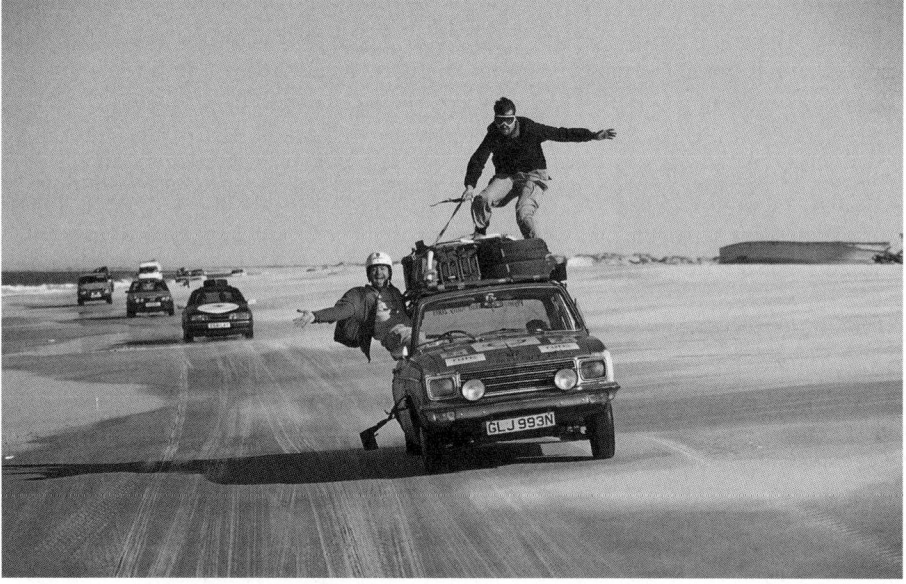

© james cheadle/Alamy Stock Photo

ideologies of masculinity can be dangerous for both women's and men's health! A few examples from the research illustrate the relationship between hegemonic masculinity and health.

Violence against women in Canada represents a major threat to population health. Data from a Canadian study (Cohen and Maclean 2003) show that totalling the various modes of intimate partner abuse (physical, sexual, emotional, and financial), the reported rate of "any" abuse was 21.2 per cent among Canadian women. In other words, one in five Canadian women is a victim of some form of abuse! The health effects of violence against women are lengthy and include, but are not limited to, physical injury and disability; mental and emotional distress, including low self-esteem, anxiety, depression, suicidal thoughts, and post-traumatic stress disorder; substance abuse; higher risk of sexually transmitted infections and diseases; and increased vulnerability to a range of chronic diseases such as diabetes, heart disease, and fibromyalgia. Despite these adverse effects, efforts to address this major social disparity in health have emphasized the response of the criminal justice system to the neglect of the health-care system (Fisher et al. 2007). Increasingly, Canadian health researchers (e.g., Crooks et al. 2007) are calling for recognition that in addition to being a criminal justice issue, violence against women is a population health issue that requires an understanding of the role played by men, boys, and masculinity in violence against women. Applying a social determinants of health approach to intimate partner violence, a team of Canadian health researchers estimate the economic health costs attributable to violence for women who have left violent relationships (a subset of all victims of intimate partner abuse) to conservatively be in the order of $6.9 billion per year (Varcoe et al. 2011). These findings led the researchers to conclude that "consequences and costs attributable or partially attributable to experiences of violence endure long after women have 'left'" (2011, 376).

While hegemonic masculinity is centrally connected to the subordination of women, it also harms men's health. As Courtenay (2000b, 1389) explains,

> By dismissing their health care needs, men are constructing gender. When a man brags, "I haven't been to a doctor in years," he is simultaneously describing a health practice and situating himself in a masculine arena. Similarly, men are demonstrating dominant norms of masculinity when they refuse to take sick leave from work, when they insist that they need little sleep, and when they boast that drinking does not impair their driving. Men also construct masculinities by embracing risk. A man may define the degree of his masculinity, for example, by driving dangerously or performing risky sports—and displaying these behaviours like badges of honor. In these ways, masculinities are defined against positive health behaviours and beliefs.

Reframing gendered health disparities in terms of hegemonic masculinity allows Courtenay to suggest that the real issues may have to do with men's under-reporting of health concerns and their underutilization of health care. It is not just stereotypically masculine or "macho" heterosexual men whose health suffers as a result of hegemonic masculinity. Evans and co-researchers (2011, 9) explain that "Men who belong to subcultures categorized by marginalized masculinities based on race, ethnicity or sexual orientation experience poorer health outcomes than other groups of men." As illustration, in a patriarchal context of hegemonic masculinity, gay and bisexual men may use their bodies as dangerous mediums for protesting against such cultural norms. In explaining the connection of hegemonic masculinity to risk-taking behaviours of gay men that may put them at increased risk of sexually transmitted infection, Connell (1995, 153) cites the coming-out narrative of one young gay man: "Rage, rage, rage! Let's do everything you've denied yourself for 25 years. Let's get into it and have a good time sexually." However, in conceiving of gay oppression as a largely psychological and individualistic determinant of gay men's health, traditional health promotion activities show a medico-centric bias in that "like mainstream health research and practice, gay men's health focuses attention on the mental and physical functioning of the individual, ignores the social and structural determinants of health, and directs health intervention squarely on the individual" (Aguinaldo 2008, 87). The relationship between risk-taking, sexuality, and gender is complex. Clearly, as evidenced by higher rates of smoking among young females, women are not risk-aversive. Given this complexity, future health research that considers these intersections of diversity is needed.

Toward an Intersectional Theory of Health and Gender across the Life Course

There are still many unanswered questions about the link between gender and health. For example, we still do not know the extent to which changes in socialization have had an effect on gender differences in health behaviour or whether social trends, such as increasing numbers of female-headed households, will translate into an eventual change in gender patterns of health and illness behaviour. This has important implications for the role played by women as health-care providers in both the family and the formal health-care system. Armstrong (2010) draws attention to the fact that the current emphasis in health-care reform on fiscal constraint, cost-effectiveness, and efficiency avoids issues such as equity and the increased burdens faced by women as caregivers and health-care workers. As she (2010, 331) explains, "Health care is profoundly gendered. Women and men use the health care system differently once they enter it. Women also provide the overwhelming majority of care, although they are a minority of those in positions of power within health care services and policy organizations." These issues are neglected because historically a woman's major role has been uncompensated care for dependants and family members (Armstrong et al. 2002). Women's caring work begins early and continues throughout their lives, usually starting with motherhood (if not marriage), then in middle age caring for older relatives (typically parents), and then caring in old age for disabled husbands. Caregiving has been largely invisible and unpaid.

Feminist researchers such as Oakley (1994) highlight the difference between valued societal work in terms of output and wages and the devalued labour of nurturance and health maintenance. This distinction reflects the sexist discrepancy between the public sphere of men as instrumental, competitive, and rational and the domestic sphere of women as expressive, nurturing, and emotional. One consequence of differential socialization into these types of sexist roles is that women may have difficulty setting limits on expectations of themselves and others about how much care to provide. Typically, women believe that they should be able to provide all of the care that is needed (Segall and Chappell 2000). This situation is further compounded by the fact that health-care administrators (e.g., hospital discharge planners) often assume that women are able and willing to provide care for those being discharged from health-care facilities. In contrast, it is assumed that men will need formal assistance. Women who work in the paid labour force and provide extensive informal care for family members have two jobs. "As a result, it is their leisure and discretionary time that decrease, and their personal health that may be adversely affected" (Segall and Chappell 2000, 35).

Commenting on the well-established relationship between gender and health, Macintyre, Hunt, and Sweeting (1996) ask: are things really as simple as they seem? As you might anticipate from the information presented in this chapter, the answer to this question is no—gender differences in health are more complicated than conventional wisdom suggests. Without denying that there are gender differences in a number of health outcomes, these researchers (1996, 621) argue that the picture "presented in much recent sociological and epidemiological literature has become oversimplified, and that over-generalization has become the norm, with inconsistencies and complexities in patterns of gender differences in health being overlooked." Their findings reveal that gender differences in morbidity and mortality vary according to the condition in question (e.g., psychological versus physical symptoms) and according to stage of the life course.

Sociological explanations for gender differences in health focus on structural inequalities (such as gender differences in socioeconomic status) and the link between social roles and the gendered experience of health and illness. As we have seen, while there are a number of competing hypotheses that explain gender differences in health to a certain extent, none has yet emerged as the single best explanation for these differences. What is clear is that gender interacts with other factors, such as social class, ethnicity, and stage of the life course, to produce specific patterns in health outcomes (Benoit et al. 2009). For example, Turcotte (2011) reports that older women and those who have lower levels of education are less likely to positively self-evaluate their health. Studies have made an effort to address gender differences in health in later life (Arber and Cooper 1999) and to include life stage in analyzing the relationship between social role occupancy and health for women and men (Janzen and Muhajarine 2003). Outlining the need to adopt an intersectional perspective on men's health across the life course, Evans and colleagues explain that "In addition to multiple masculinities across the category 'men,' what it means to be a man and practices of masculinity change in response to locale, life events and aging across the lifespan. For men, age has a significant impact on health in light of age related constructions of masculinity" (2011, 10). Arber and Cooper (1999, 61) make the point that "older people have tended to be neglected in research on gender differences in health compared with at other stages of the life course. Similarly, there has been a lack of research on how class intersects with gender and age in later life." According to these researchers, such omissions are surprising for a number of reasons, including the fact that women outnumber men in later life. Since women generally outlive men, older age groups are predominantly female. The purpose of their research was to examine different age groups (with an emphasis on women and men over the age of 60) rather than to assume that the relationship between gender and health remains constant throughout the life course. Arber and Cooper (1999, 75) characterize their research results as a "new paradox," since they found "that older women have a more positive self-assessment of their health status than men, once age, class, income and their greater level of functional disability are taken into account." While this finding may initially seem somewhat inconsistent with the preceding discussion of gender differences in health and illness (i.e., women experience more illness episodes than men and are apparently sicker), it underscores the need for an intersectional analysis of health incorporating the combined effects of social determinants such as class, gender, and ethnicity across the life course.

In struggling to interpret the findings of research that examined the influence of social structural factors and psychosocial resources on gender differences in health, Walters, McDonough, and Strohschein (2002, 687) conclude that "the embeddedness of gender in all social relationships may make it impossible to separate gender from the very life circumstances that we examine in order to understand gender patterns in health." They assert that the complexity of the relationship between gender and health means that further mixed-method research is required in order to produce more satisfactory explanations of why being a woman or a man has such important effects on life chances and health. Likewise, Griffith (2012, 107) contends that "An intersectional approach is consistent with the focus and goals of men's health disparities research because it helps researchers consider how masculinities and social determinants of health combine and why they affect men's health and differences in health outcomes among men." Armstrong (2010, 331–2) reaches a similar conclusion, explaining that a fully developed understanding of the intersectionality of health needs to move toward a more comprehensive sex- and gender-based analysis:

> All populations are gendered. Of course, other social locations linked to age, culture, income, disability, and racialization—to name only some—also matter. But these,

too, are divided by gender, intersecting with other social and physical locations. Being gender-sensitive means much more than analyzing data by sex; it means recognizing how gender shapes and is shaped by conditions, practices, and relations, including relations of markets, of power, and of inequality. It means understanding how gender intersects with other locations.

Like so much of the research reviewed in this chapter, these studies demonstrate that gender differences, while important determinants of disparities in health between women and men, are not solely responsible for health outcomes. Each of us has many identities, some of which are more significant in certain social locations than in others. Furthermore, our social locations vary throughout the life course as we age. The challenge for advancing health research is to understand how diverse social locations overlap to shape population health over time.

A systematic sex- and gender-based analysis of disparities in health between women and men is an important step toward understanding the relationship between gender and health. However, as Hankivsky and Christoffersen (2008, 273) conclude, "Persistent and increasing inequities within the group 'women' are challenging Canadian researchers to move beyond gender based analysis and to engage in broader frameworks of analysis that move beyond the assumed norm of the 'white, middle-class heterosexual woman.'" This means that if meaningful progress is to be made in addressing health disparities between women and men, research must advance beyond merely describing existing health differences between the genders to testing theories that explain the complex interactions that occur across the life course among all dimensions of social location and health outcomes. Research must move toward exploring what Hankivsky and Christoffersen (2008, 273) term the "intersecting axes of oppression that affect health." As Hankivsky (2012a, 1713) explains, this is the potential of intersectional analyses of gender and health: "In the fields of women's health, men's health, and gender and health, the promise of an intersectionality analysis is that it advances a new order of complexity for understanding how sex and gender intersect with other dimensions of inequality . . . to create unique experiences of health." Benoit and Shumka (2009, 27) warn that "Failing to examine gender and sex within the context of other fundamental determinants homogenizes the experiences of women (and men), reifying existing inequalities while at the same time overlooking important sources of within-group inequity." What is needed to address disparities in health is an intersectional understanding of health as it develops across the life course.

Chapter Summary

In this chapter, we have seen that gender has profound effects on the pursuit of health and wellness. Whether a person is born a girl or a boy and how she or he is socialized to perform the various social roles associated with femininity and masculinity shape health and wellness. Though culturally variable, there are gender differences in life expectancy and in the major causes of death. We know that women are diagnosed as suffering from more ill health than men and that there are gender differences in the use of formal health care. We also know that gender differences in health behaviour have to do with elements of the culture such as the medicalization of women's lives and differences in gender role socialization. Finally, we know that there are pronounced social inequalities in the living and working conditions of women that have harmful health effects. It should be clear that the relationship between gender and health is far too complex to be described by the simple adage "women are sicker, but men die quicker." While patterns of gender differences in health are variable, the defining feature of sociological perspectives on these disparities is that gender differences are best accounted for by socio-cultural factors interacting with biologically based sex differences. Finally, we also know that in order to develop a satisfactory understanding of the relationship between gender and health, we need to move toward an intersectional approach, which understands gender as one of many potential sources of health inequity that unfold across the life course. Ethnicity is an important dimension of social location that intersects with gender and social class as a determinant of health. In the next chapter, we expand our consideration of the structural factors that shape health to examine the relationship between health and ethnicity.

Study Questions

1. The adage "women are sicker, but men die quicker" is sometimes used to summarize gender disparities in health. Provide research examples that show how this adage is an oversimplification of how women and men differentially experience health and wellness.
2. Summarize what is known about gender differences in mental health and emotional well-being.
3. How do the different health and health-care experiences of women and men reflect the historical fact that women's bodies and lives have long been the target of medical consumerism and medicalization?
4. Summarize the different hypotheses that explain gender differences in health in relation to the performance of gender roles.
5. Use examples to illustrate how patriarchal ideologies harm both women's and men's health.
6. What would intersectional analysis that adopted a life course perspective add to our understanding of gender and health?

Recommended Readings

Annandale, E. 2009. *Women's Health and Social Change*. London: Routledge.

Benoit, C., and L. Shumka. 2009. *Gendering the Health Determinants Framework: Why Girls' and Women's Health Matters*. Vancouver: Women's Health Research Network.

Bird, C., and P. Rieker. 2008. *Gender and Health: The Effects of Constrained Choices and Social Policies*. New York: Cambridge University Press.

Courtenay, W. 2011. *Dying to Be Men: Psychosocial, Environmental, and Biobehavioral Directions in Promoting the Health of Men and Boys*. London: Routledge.

DesMeules, M., D. Stewart, A. Kazanjian, H. Maclean, J. Payne, and B. Vissandjée, eds. 2003. *Women's Health Surveillance Report: A Multidimensional Look at the Health of Canadian Women*. Ottawa: Canadian Institute for Health Information.

Spitzer, D. "Engendering health disparities." 2005. *Canadian Journal of Public Health* 96: S78–96.

Recommended Websites

Canadian Institutes of Health Research—Institute of Gender and Health:
www.cihr-irsc.gc.ca/e/8673.html

Canadian Women's Health Network:
www.cwhn.ca

Gender and Health—Collaborative Curriculum Project:
www.genderandhealth.ca

The Source for Women's Health:
www.womenshealthdata.ca

Addressing Sources of Inequality and Health Disparities: Ethnicity

Learning Objectives

This chapter expands our examination of sources of inequality and disparities in health beyond socioeconomic status and gender by considering

- the relationship between social exclusion, racism, and the health of Aboriginal peoples;
- the healthy immigrant effect;
- ethnic group differences in perception and understanding of symptoms, health-care behaviour, and the social determinants of health;
- explanations of ethnic differences in health and illness; and
- the link between ethnicity, religion, and health.

Health and Ethnicity

In addition to socioeconomic status and gender, there is another socially constructed division by which people are systematically sorted and which affects the pursuit of health and wellness. Like gender, ethnicity is a group identity that is performed by people. As Smaje (2000, 115) explains, "Race or ethnicity denotes relations between people and not substantial qualities possessed by them." Smaje means that ethnicity, like gender, is a dynamic and changing socially constructed way of categorizing people. While there is a growing body of research looking at the relationship between health and ethnicity in Canada, particularly Aboriginal health status, which has been extensively studied, the relationship between health and ethnicity has received less research attention than the link between health disparities and other sources of inequality such as socioeconomic status and gender. Canada's long history of immigration and increasing cultural diversity highlights the importance of understanding ethnicity as a key aspect of the pursuit of health and wellness.

According to Statistics Canada, "Canada is a nation with an ethnocultural mosaic as indicated by its immigrant population, the ethnocultural backgrounds of its people, the visible minority population, linguistic characteristics and religious diversity" (2013c, 6). The 2011 *National Household Survey* (which replaced the more detailed long-form census in 2010) shows that one in five of Canada's population, or 20.6 per cent, are immigrants (Statistics Canada 2013c). This means that Canada has the highest proportion of foreign-born among G8 countries. Since 2000, more than 2 million immigrants arrived in Canada. One in four children in Canada is either an immigrant or the child of immigrant parents (Statistics Canada 2008b). The survey shows that Canada's 6-million-plus visible minorities represent 19 per cent of the non-Aboriginal population. The *Ethnic Diversity Survey* reveals that one-half of the Canadian population feels a strong sense of belonging to ethnic or cultural groups. Additionally, six-and-a-half million Canadians report that maintaining ethnic customs and traditions is important. One-third of Canadians with family living abroad report having transnational (i.e., back and forth) contact with their countries of origin. Nearly one-quarter of Canada's visible minority population report that "they felt uncomfortable or out of place because of their ethnocultural characteristics all, most or some of the time" (Statistics Canada 2003, 16). The 2011 census shows that more than 200 languages were reported as either home language or mother tongue (Statistics Canada 2012c). Wang (2014, 90) notes that "20.6% of Canadians (6.8 million people) reported a mother tonque other than English or French." Nearly three-quarters of Canadians reported a religious affiliation, with two-thirds of Canadians, or more than 22 million people, saying they are Christian (Statistics Canada 2013c). In such a multicultural context, ethnic and religious diversity is an important social determinant of health and wellness.

Before discussing what is known by health researchers about the relationship between health and ethnicity, it is necessary to say a few words about interrelated terms that are used by social scientists to conceptualize ethnicity. **Ethnicity** is a complex and multi-dimensional phenomenon that includes culture, ethnoculture, ethnic ancestry/origin, ethnic identity, language, religion, and race or some mixture of all these elements (Aspinall 2001; Isajiw 1993). **Culture** is a very general term that denotes "a complex collection of values, beliefs, behaviours, and material objects shared by a group and passed on from one generation to the next" (Ravelli and Webber 2016, 121). This understanding of culture allows us to view **ethnic groups** as socially based groupings that exist within a particular cultural framework. In other words, ethnicity is a shared (whether perceived or actual) group identity that is rooted in some element of culture, such as custom, language, religion, history, or a mixture of these factors. As such, it is possible to define **ethnoculture** as cultural features associated with ethnic groups that support patterns and processes of ethnic identification.

Despite the centrality of culture to social life, Li (1999, 9–10) explains that there is a problem with what he refers to as "the unrefined use of the all-embracing concept of 'culture' to account for all aspects of behaviours that seemingly relate to race and ethnicity." He goes on to detail three specific problems associated with cultural explanations of human behaviour. First, Li (1999, 11) notes that "Since culture is largely people's responses to external conditions, it is not static." Culture continually changes and adapts to changing social circumstances. Li adds that "Second, people of the same ethnicity do not necessarily share a common culture. . . . It is therefore incorrect to assume that people with the same ethnic label would necessarily have a common culture." Thus, ethnicity shapes behaviour in diverse ways. The final objection Li (1999, 12) raises with respect to cultural explanations of behaviour is that "conceptually, almost every aspect of human life can be included under the rubric of culture: hence it can explain no aspect of human life." This means that culture is such a general concept that it has little explanatory power. For these reasons, health researchers need to clarify which aspect of ethnoculture they are studying. The point of this discussion is that, like health, ethnicity is a multi-dimensional concept that can be measured in several different ways.

Two commonly used measures of ethnicity in population health research are ethnic ancestry/origin and ethnic identity. **Ethnic ancestry/origin** refers to the place where an individual or her ancestors were born. In surveys, this is typically indicated by the country of birth of either the respondent or her distant relatives. Research has compared the health status of "native-born" Canadians (those whose country of birth is Canada) with "foreign-born" (those who live in Canada but were born in another country). Aspinall (2001, 832) elaborates: "The two types of questions are quite different conceptually. Country of birth questions collect data for geographically defined countries of birth, while ethnic origin/ancestry questions collect data for ethnic groups which may be located within one or many countries, with some countries being home to more than one distinct ethnic or cultural group." More than 200 ethnic origins were reported in the 2011 *National Household Survey*, with 13 of these origins reported by at least 1 million people (Statistics Canada 2013c). **Ethnic identity** is even more complex to define and measure because ethnicity is only one of many possible dimensions by which a person may locate and understand herself within the world. As Frideres (1999, 89) puts it, "All of us have many different identities and we easily shift their priority and nature as we move from one milieu to the next." Measures of ethnic identity found in population health surveys typically list a variety of ethnic groups and ask respondents to indicate to which group they consider they belong (Aspinall 2001). From a salutogenic perspective, it is interesting to note that there is evidence that a strong sense of ethnic identification can alleviate the adverse effects of discrimination on mental health for minority group members (Mossakowski 2003). It appears that pride and participation in ethnocultural practices are beneficial for the pursuit of health and wellness!

Understanding the link between ethnicity and health is further complicated by the fact that ethnicity is a dimension of social location that intersects with other dimensions, such as socioeconomic status and gender, across the life course. This means that teasing out the effects that ethnicity has on health and health behaviour from other aspects of social location poses a challenge for health research. You should be aware of this as we review ethnic differences in health. In the following section, examples from research will be cited to summarize the available information on ethnic differences in health. Then the discussion will consider explanations that have been offered by researchers to explain ethnic differences in health.

Ethnic Differences in Health

Vissandjée and colleagues (2003, 1) summarize ethnic differences in health by stating, "The body of research on the relation between ethnic background and health suggests that immigrant subgroups may be vulnerable in terms of health status, health service use and determinants of health." Additionally, Canadian researchers have systematically documented the fact that Aboriginal peoples have numerous negative health outcomes associated with a long history of social exclusion. We now know that factors such as a person's skin colour, immigration and refugee status, timing and length of migration, ethnic origin and identification, and social exclusion are powerful aspects of social location that influence the pursuit of health and wellness. Box 7.1 outlines major research findings concerning ethnic differences in health.

Box 7.1 Ethnic Differences in Health

- Aboriginal peoples have poorer health outcomes because of social exclusion and racism.
- There is a "healthy immigrant effect" that deteriorates over time.
- There are ethnic differences in perception and understanding of symptoms.
- There are ethnic differences in health-care behaviour.
- There are ethnic differences in the social determinants of health.

Aboriginal Peoples Have Poorer Health Outcomes Because of Social Exclusion and Racism

There is no clearer evidence of the social determinants of health than the health status of Canada's Aboriginal peoples. Canada's long history of socially excluding Aboriginals has had tremendous negative consequences for the health and well-being of its First Nations, Métis, and Inuit people. You will recall from Chapter 5 that "social exclusion" is a term used by researchers and policy activists to describe the systematic exclusion of a group of people from the wider society's economic, political, and social resources (Galabuzi 2012). Racism is a key dimension of social exclusion in Canada, which has harmed the health of Aboriginals (Reading 2013). As Galabuzi (2012, 107) explains, "in relation to oppressions arising from colonization, Aboriginal people experience persistent income and health inequities, which are exacerbated by colonial relations and structural racism in Canada." In a report by the Senate of Canada on population health, Reading points out that the social exclusion of Aboriginal peoples has historically been and continues to be a feature of Canadian society:

> The process of dislocation as a result of colonization rendered many Aboriginal people and communities as socially excluded from the rest of Canada. The social exclusion led to marginalization in education, employment, housing, health care and many other services which effectively created a two-tiered society in Canada; one standard for Canadians and the other for Aboriginal peoples (2009, A-1).

Aboriginal peoples in Canada are classified into four general categories: North American (First Nations) Indians registered under the Indian Act, North American Indians not registered under the Indian Act, Métis, and Inuit. The 2011 *National Household Survey* reports that 1,400,685 people, or 4.3 per cent of the total Canadian population, have an Aboriginal identity (Statistics Canada 2013a). Statistics Canada cautions that because of non-reporting by members of First Nations on-reserve communities, this number underestimates the actual Aboriginal population. Children and youth make up just under half of Canada's recorded Aboriginal population, and approximately one-third of them live with a lone parent (Statistics Canada 2013d). Several government and research reports document the social exclusion and health of Aboriginal peoples, dramatically illustrating the interrelationship between the two (e.g., Adelson 2005; Allan and Smylie 2015; Curtis 2007; Health Canada 2009; National Collaborating Centre for Aboriginal Health 2012; Reading 2009; Smylie 2009; Statistics Canada 2008a). As Anaya (2014, 4) makes clear, Canada's Indigenous population is very diverse: "There are currently 617 First Nations or Indian bands in Canada representing more than 50 cultural groups and living in about 1,000 communities and elsewhere across the country." Given this diversity, it is important to recognize that just as the negative health effects associated with patriarchy do not accrue to all women, health disparities associated with colonialism are not experienced by all Aboriginals in the same way.

Social exclusion associated with living in poverty has been profound for many Aboriginal peoples. For example, in 2005 the median income for Aboriginal women was $16,079 and $22,386 for Aboriginal men, compared to $21,765 for non-Aboriginal women and $33,214 for non-Aboriginal men in Canada (Aboriginal Affairs and Northern Development 2012). Just over one-quarter of First Nations people between the ages of 25 and 64 who live on reserves have a total annual income of less than $5000 (Health Canada 2014a). In fact, according to the Association of Faculties of Medicine of Canada (2015), Aboriginal identity along with socioeconomic status are the "two most prominent sources of health inequity in Canada." Additionally, unemployment rates, incidence of low educational attainment, and welfare dependency are higher among Aboriginals (Health Canada 2014a). As depicted in Box 7.2, the desperate housing conditions in many First Nations and Inuit communities rival those of developing nations.

In addition to poor housing conditions, environmental threats such as pollution and food insecurity represent persistent threats to the health of Aboriginal peoples. Shah (2004, 271) offers the following explanation of the linkages between food insecurity, environmental degradation, and poor Aboriginal health outcomes:

Box 7.2 The Housing Crisis of First Nations People in Canada

It is not uncommon for multiple families with many different generations to be crowded into a single rundown house. Health Canada (2014a) reports that Aboriginal peoples living on reserves are six times more likely than non-Aboriginals to live in a crowded dwelling (defined as one or more people per room) and 14 times more likely to live in a home requiring major repair. Housing on reserves frequently lacks central heating, proper ventilation systems, and adequate water and sanitation facilities and exposes people to fire hazards from wood stoves and overcrowding (Health Canada 2009). Half of First Nations people living on reserve report mould or mildew (i.e., known health threats) growing in their homes (Health Canada 2014a). Thirty-nine per cent of First Nations communities' water systems inspected were categorized as high-risk (Health Canada 2014a). How might such poor housing affect the pursuit of health and wellness of Aboriginal people?

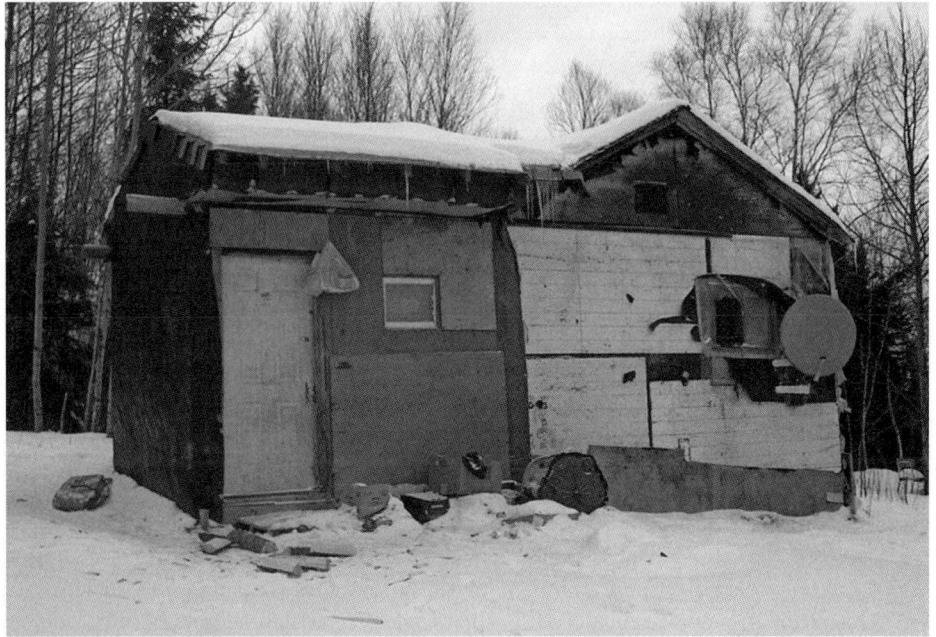

A photo taken on 2 December 2011 of a house on the Wasagamack First Nation in northern Manitoba.

Many Aboriginal people in Canada, particularly in remote communities, experience all or most aspects of food insecurity due to low incomes, safety risks due to pollutants in the traditional food supply, quality problems associated with inappropriate shipping, handling, and home preparation of commercial foods, and disruptions in shipping or changes in animal migratory patterns.

The *First Nations Regional Health Survey* (RHS) shows that "[m]ore than half (54.2 per cent) of First Nations households were categorized as being 'moderate' to 'severely' food insecure" (First Nations Information Governance Centre 2012, 81). The survey also provides information on the types of community challenges identified by Aboriginal peoples. For instance, alcohol and drug abuse was identified by 82.6 per cent of First Nations adults surveyed, housing by 70.7 per cent, and employment or the number of jobs by 65.9 per cent. Other community challenges identified included education and training opportunities, funding, health and control over decisions. While the number of identified community challenges varied by the age of respondents, no gender differences were observed. Two-thirds of the First Nations adults, who identified community challenges, perceived no improvement or worsening of these aspects of community life during the year prior to the survey. With such extreme examples of social exclusion, it is little wonder that Aboriginal peoples suffer from poorer health outcomes than the general Canadian population.

The life expectancy of First Nations people registered under the Indian Act (amounting to about half of the Aboriginal population) and Inuit is five to fourteen years shorter than for non-Aboriginal Canadians (Statistics Canada 2008a). The Senate reports that "past and present studies have proven that Aboriginal peoples in Canada bear disproportionately higher burden of some chronic illnesses than do non-Aboriginal Canadians" (Reading 2009, A-4). Aboriginal people are increasingly affected by conditions such as cancer and heart disease. Many Aboriginal communities have higher rates of infectious diseases, such as tuberculosis and AIDS, than non-Aboriginal Canadians. Monette and colleagues (2011) report that although Aboriginals accounted for only about 4 per cent of the Canadian population in 2006, they accounted for 8 per cent of AIDS cases in Canada and 12.5 per cent of new infections. As highlighted by the H1N1 flu pandemic in 2009, death rates among Aboriginal adults from infectious and parasitic diseases are consistently above national levels, reflecting differences in living conditions and lifestyle. Frideres (2011, 129–30) notes that "about 20 percent of all new STDs yearly (chlamydia, gonorrhea, syphilis) originate from individuals claiming to be members of First Nations." Elias (2014) points out that official vital statistics that estimate the infant mortality rate for First Nations to be twice that of the general Canadian population actually underestimate the full extent of infant mortality among Aboriginals! The leading causes of death among Aboriginal infants—respiratory ailments, infectious and parasitic diseases, and accidents—are indicators of inadequate housing, unsanitary conditions, and poor access to medical facilities. Children in Aboriginal communities also have higher rates of accidental death and injury, as well as poisoning, than other Canadian children.

Owing in large part to intergenerational trauma caused by the terrible legacy of physical, emotional, and sexual abuse in residential schools, the incidence of violence, physical and sexual abuse, substance dependence, and suicide is higher in Aboriginal communities (Frideres 2011). **Intergenerational trauma** refers to negative emotional effects stemming from an initial terrible experience felt throughout the life course and reproduced through subsequent generations as a legacy of suffering. In the case of the government-funded and church-operated **residential schools**, which removed First Nations children from their families and communities with the goal of assimilating them into mainstream Canadian culture, just over half of the 70 to 80 thousand Aboriginal people who attended these schools report that it had a negative impact on their health and well-being (Health Canada 2014b). Many Indigenous people who were emotionally harmed in the residential schools passed this harm onto their children and grandchildren (Frideres 2011). The life course concept of "linked lives" wherein "events that affect one person also affect other persons in their network" helps us to understand the lasting harm of intergenerational trauma (Gee, Walsemann, and Brondolo 2012, 969). In this way, the social structures of intergenerational trauma stemming from colonialism spread and continue to harm Aboriginals. Evidence of this is that the suicide rate among First Nations people is three times higher than the national average (Health Canada 2014b). Particularly saddening is the high number of Aboriginal youth who take their lives. Health Canada (2014b, 12) reports that "suicide accounted for 28.9% of deaths among 10–14 year olds, 30.1% of deaths among 15–19 year olds, and 23.6% of deaths among 20–24 year olds." Research by Elias and colleagues (2012) links intergenerational trauma associated with residential schools to increased risk of suicide thoughts and behaviour among Aboriginals.

Figure 7.1 shows that First Nations people are much more likely to die because of accidents or poisoning than are non-Aboriginal Canadians. Waldram, Herring, and Young (2006, 103) explain that "Among the most serious health problems affecting Aboriginal people in the decades since the end of the Second World War, particularly the younger age groups, are injuries sustained as a result of accidents and violence." Substance abuse was a factor in almost a third of injuries reported in the *First Nations Regional Health Survey* and in 70 per cent of injuries related to assault (First Nations Information Governance Centre 2012).

After providing an excellent review of the links between the social determinants of health, the health status of Aboriginal peoples, and both historical policy developments that produced health disparities and current efforts to address these inequities, Smylie (2009, 294) offers this summary:

> Although rates of infectious disease and mortality, including infant mortality rates, improved over the course of the 20th century, persistent disparities continue and improvement appears to have levelled off over the past decade. . . . Health status disparities persist and chronic disease rates continue to rise despite federal/provincial/territorial governments' increased investment in health services and programs for on-reserve First Nations and northern Inuit communities.

Linking Aboriginal disparities in health to colonization, Shah (2004, 267) explains that "Four centuries of colonization—being subjugated and stripped of their land, religion, culture, language, and autonomy—have taken their toll on the physical, mental, emotional, spiritual, and cultural health of Aboriginal communities." In fact, in keeping with a social determinants of health perspective, it is possible to view colonization as what we referred to in Chapter 4 as an upstream determinant of Aboriginal health (Loppie, Reading, and Wein 2014). Colonization set the stage for further downstream Aboriginal health disadvantage. Research has revealed that Canadian Aboriginal experience of health disparities matches a global pattern of adverse health effects originating with colonization (Locust 1999). First, as Indigenous populations are colonized,

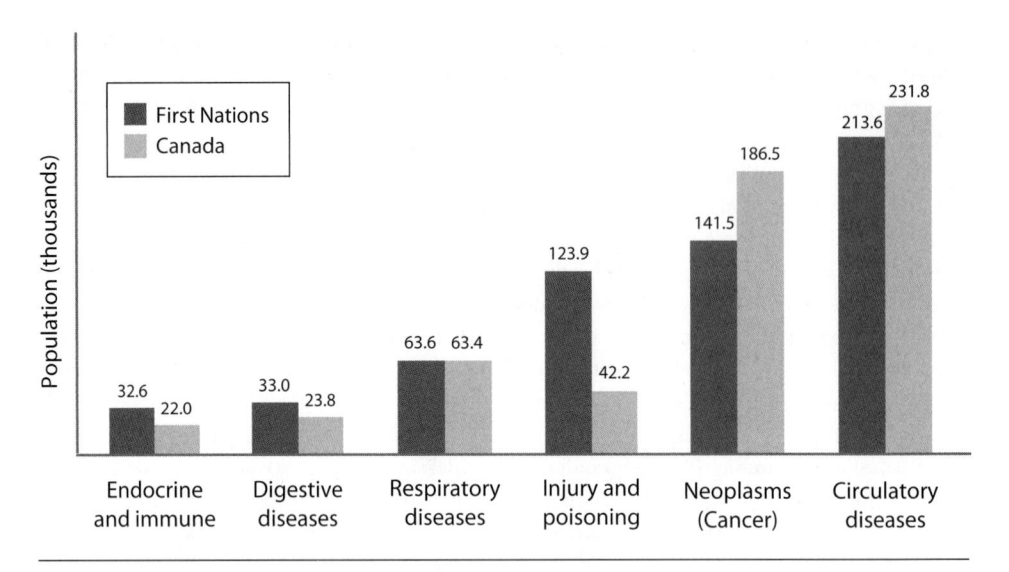

Figure 7.1 Age-standardized Leading Causes of Death in First Nations, 1999, and in Canada, 1998

First Nations have much higher rates of death caused by injury and poisoning than the general Canadian population. In which ways might this be attributable to the social exclusion facing Aboriginals in Canada?

Note: Ranking based on mortality (deaths per 100,000 population) for First Nations in 1999.

Source: Health Canada 2003. © All rights reserved. Adapted and reproduced with permission from the Minister of Health, 2016.

they are subject to famine, high rates of infectious disease, and high mortality (especially among infants and children). As time unfolds and the social exclusionary effects of colonization become institutionalized, infectious disease gives way to chronic and degenerative health problems. For example, type 2 diabetes is now a major chronic health problem among Aboriginals, while it was unheard of before 1940! The World Health Organization (2008, 36) points out that because of the legacy of colonization that has taken their land and imposed social, economic, and political structures upon them, "Indigenous Peoples' unique status must therefore be considered separately from generalized or more universal social exclusion discussions." Following on this, we can see that Aboriginality is a unique aspect of social location that intersects with other factors, such as socioeconomic status and gender, to jeopardize the health of Aboriginal peoples. The World Health Organization (2008, 157) concludes that "The persistent inequity in the health conditions of Indigenous populations goes to the heart of the relationship between health and power, social participation, and empowerment."

Despite recent efforts by Aboriginal communities to empower themselves and regain control over health-care services, access to effective and culturally safe health care remains a significant obstacle to Aboriginal health (Benoit, Carroll, and Chaudhry 2003). Adelson (2005, S46–7) describes how "mainstream biomedical health care, as it has evolved in relation to Aboriginal communities, has been shaped by a century of internal colonial politics that have effectively marginalized Aboriginal peoples from the dominant system of care." As a result, many Aboriginals encounter racism as part of their experience with mainstream health care. Racism jeopardizes the quality of care received by Aboriginals and often further threatens their health and well-being. As discussed in the opinion editorial presented in Box 7.3, a highly publicized and widely known example of this is the extreme case of "fatal racism" (Allan and Smylie 2015, 27) experienced by Brian Sinclair, a 45-year-old Winnipeg man who died from a treatable bladder infection after spending 34 hours in the emergency waiting room of the Health Sciences Centre and being repeatedly overlooked by the doctors, nurses, and medical aids at the emergency triage desk.

Frideres (2011, 117) explains how "The negative attitudes of professional medical practitioners are expressed more or less openly, making encounters with health-care providers unpleasant for many First Nations people." In response to racism encountered by Aboriginals and other minority groups within the Canadian health-care system, many hospitals are adopting models of intercultural care in an attempt to address the needs of people from minority backgrounds, such

Box 7.3 Brian Sinclair: Victim of Racialization, Medicalization, or Both?

On 21 September 2008 an Aboriginal man named Brain Sinclair was found dead. Though he was mentally and physically disabled, an addict, and socially excluded, Brian Sinclair's body was not found, as you might suspect, in some anonymous Winnipeg back alley. Rather, a horrified member of the public discovered Brian's body in the waiting room of the Emergency Department at Winnipeg's Health Sciences Centre.

According to a chief medical examiner's inquest, Brian Sinclair died from a treatable bladder infection after spending 34 hours in the hospital's waiting room and being repeatedly overlooked by the doctors, nurses, and medical aides at the emergency triage desk. Indeed, though Brian Sinclair went to the hospital for medical help, he was never triaged despite being seen by 17 different hospital staff and attempts by several bystanders in the emergency room to get him help. Brian Sinclair's tragedy prompted a provincial inquiry led by Provincial Court Judge Tim Preston. The inquiry, which lasted 10 months and heard from 80 witnesses, refused to consider what role racism and stereotyping played in Mr Sinclair's death. Instead, the inquiry's 63 recommendations focus on less contentious issues such as the design of the emergency department and patient flow systems. For their part, Brian Sinclair's family and Aboriginal groups refused to continue participating in the inquiry into his death when Judge Preston ruled that social determinants, such as the role played by race, poverty, and disability, were outside the scope of the inquiry.

Others have, however, pointed to racism and racialization as factors in Brian Sinclair's death. Several experts have pointed to the racism faced by Aboriginals in the Canadian health-care system, which can lead to both stereotyping and poor health outcomes experienced by Aboriginals. Sociologists use the term racialization to describe the processes by which people are systematically categorized and socially excluded according to perceived racial differences. In Brian Sinclair's case, he became stereotyped as "just another mentally ill and addicted, homeless Indian," and the Health Sciences Centre was often where he went or was taken for help. With nowhere else to turn, the hospital came to be seen as the institution to deal with his socially excluded "master status" of "drunken, disabled Indian." Racialization is a means by which individuals, such as Brian Sinclair, are

Continued

stereotyped into particular kinds of people, such as "drug addicted Indian" and then socially excluded. In our culturally diverse society, racialization is commonplace. Easy to perceive physical differences are used to profile others. This is the essence of racialization.

As Dr Alika Lafontaine, vice-president of the Indigenous Physicians Association of Canada, points out, physicians and other health-care professionals are not immune to stereotyping (*Winnipeg Free Press*, 4 March 2014). Indeed, Dr Lafontaine argues that being able to quickly sort patients out into patterns is fundamental to the effective practice of modern medicine. This type of profiling is the first step in making medical diagnoses needed to treat patients.

The tragedy is that, as Dr Lafontaine points out, Brian Sinclair appears to have been profiled not on the basis of his medical status so much as his social status. Dr Catherine Cook, the Winnipeg Regional Health Authority's vice-president of population and Aboriginal health, agrees with Dr Lafontaine, telling the inquiry that "you start wondering if [the] stereotype of aboriginal people comes to mind instead of the actual situation" (*Winnipeg Free Press*, 26 February 2014). Because of racialization, health-care professionals may see racial differences instead of medical issues.

Racialization is so embedded in the Canadian health-care system that hospitals such as the Health Sciences Centre are trying to address it through special Aboriginal health programs, such as cultural sensitivity training for staff and hiring Aboriginal staff to treat Aboriginal patients. Dr Cook told the inquiry, "aboriginal patients are more comfortable receiving care from aboriginal health-care workers." Like many, Brian Sinclair himself categorized people according to race. The inquiry heard that Sinclair refused to accept placement with a foster family because they were white. Racism entails a corrosive distrust and fear of others. Recognizing the racially divided character of Canadian society, health-care policies are being implemented to try and ensure that people aren't discriminated against on the basis of racial categorizations. Some polices are based on a racialized belief that certain types of people should be involved in caring for "their own kind." But these policies themselves are racialized and miss a fundamental point when it comes to formal health care. As Dr Alika Lafontaine points out, racism makes the power imbalance that is basic to biomedical health care even worse for Aboriginals in Canada (*Winnipeg Free Press*, 17 December 2014 A9).

It wasn't racialization alone that led to Brian Sinclair's death. His life of extreme poverty and substance abuse became medicalized at the same time it was racialized. As we will learn in Chapter 10, medicalization is the term used by sociologists to describe the process by which aspects of life come to be understood as medical issues requiring intervention and control on the part of medicine. We expect medicine to solve life's problems and, in return, have given health-care professions more power over our lives. Addiction is but one of many troubling aspects of everyday life that are increasingly being defined as medical issues requiring formal medical care. Poverty, addiction, disability, and social exclusion are all forms of social suffering that have been given medical meanings.

Only in a society that has so totally come to understand the human condition in terms of the ideas, images, language, and practices offered by biomedicine can this sort of medicalization of social suffering be possible. Brian Sinclair's experience vividly illustrates that it was a combination of racialization and medicalization that ultimately lead to his dehumanization and death. Brian Sinclair was the victim of both racialization and medicalization.

This is a revised version of an earlier opinion editorial by Christopher J. Fries, which appeared in the *Winnipeg Free Press*, 22 May 2010.

as Aboriginals and immigrants (Douglas 2013). Douglas (2013, 40) offers the following description of the challenges a culturally diverse population presents to formal health care in Canada:

> The problem is that the old, authoritarian models of health care delivery assumed that the population was homogenous, that everyone could be treated in the same way, and that everyone would do as they were told. This no longer holds true of even the European-descended segments of the population, much less for those who do not recognize the cultural authority of biomedicine.

The growing diversity of the Canadian population is challenging the authority of health-care professionals and reshaping the medical encounter. Douglas (2013) explains that models of intercultural care in Canada range from cultural sensitivity through cultural competency to cultural safety. The basic rationale underlying all these models of **intercultural care** is that a one-size-fits-all approach to health care harms the safety and effectiveness of medical care offered to individuals from diverse ethnic backgrounds. Rather, health-care professionals must provide care that recognizes the cultural uniqueness of individual patients from different ethnic backgrounds (Hole et al. 2015). It should be obvious that intercultural care is closely related to Canada's official policies of multiculturalism and, as such, is hotly debated (Kirmayer 2011; Rosenberg et al. 2007). **Cultural sensitivity** emphasizes an awareness on the part of doctors and nurses that patients may come from different cultural backgrounds. According to **cultural competency**, doctors and nurses are expected to understand how ethnocultural diversity affects the behaviour of specific patient subpopulations such as ethnic groups and to tailor care accordingly.

Cultural safety is the most demanding and promising of the approaches to dealing with ethnocultural diversity in health care. It originated in response to the racism encountered by the Maori, New Zealand's Indigenous population. **Cultural safety** is an approach to intercultural care that relies on the mutual accommodation of both patients and medical personnel within the medical encounter. While both parties are expected to be aware and respectful of cultural differences, cultural safety gives the patient the power to judge whether a particular health-care professional or treatment is, in fact, culturally safe. Cultural safety then amounts to a fundamental challenge to the medical dominance traditionally associated with biomedical health care. Despite this, cultural safety has been endorsed by the Canadian Nurses Association, the Canadian Association of Schools of Nursing, and the Canadian Medical Association (Douglas 2013). There is, however, a lack of consensus among health researchers as to whether cultural safety constitutes a meaningful and workable response to the challenges posed by Canadian ethnocultural diversity and the racism encountered by Aboriginals in the Canadian health-care system (Josewski 2012). As Douglas (2013, 45) concludes, "Canadian health care professionals are unlikely to implement cultural safety if it means compromising their own values or those of mainstream Canadian society. In essence, the professionals need to feel as culturally safe as much as the patients do."

In terms of future research and policy, Adelson (2005, S59) tells us that "the path towards a reduction in disparities in First Nations, Métis and Inuit health status is ultimately linked to a larger political will and attendant policy framework that will effectively acknowledge the relationship between inequality and ill-health." She warns us that traditional epidemiological research on Aboriginal health disparities fails to understand the "diversity among and between Aboriginal populations" (2005, S47). Based on a review of existing research, Bombak and Bruce

(2012, 2) highlight the importance of moving toward an intersectional understanding of Aboriginal health: "Given the diversity of living conditions experienced by indigenous peoples globally, intersectionality theory is an important consideration in understanding indigenous health and health inequities." Allan and Smylie (2015) offer the additional caution that because most government surveys do not include people living on reserves and under-represent the population of Aboriginals living in urban areas under conditions of homelessness and poverty, there is a serious lack of data regarding the full extent of health disparities faced by First Nations peoples in Canada. More research is needed that involves Aboriginal peoples in the process of investigating the social inequalities that lead to disparities in health and developing policies that recognize Aboriginals as active participants in addressing these disparities. An example of this type of research is provided by Allan and Smylie's (2015) comprehensive review of the role of racism in the health and well-being of Indigenous peoples in Canada, which employed a mixed-method research design under the direction of Indigenous elders, whose narratives guided the research process. These researchers emphasize that future research is needed to address "the complex relationship between racism, trauma, Indigenous identity and Indigenous health," utilizing concepts such as "historic trauma, historic loss trauma, soul wound, residential school syndrome, and intergenerational trauma" (Allan and Smylie 2015, 19). Allan and Smylie's review (2015, 1) convincingly demonstrates that

> Policies and practices emerging from imperialistic and colonial ideologies have been extremely destructive to the health and well-being of Indigenous peoples, cutting across the broad spectrum of social determinants of health, impacting access to education, housing, food security, employment and health care, and permeating societal systems and institutions that have profoundly impacted the lives and well-being of Indigenous peoples.

Perhaps most notable of all, Indigenous people have a holistic understanding of health and wellness from which we could all learn and benefit (Adelson 2000). As Shah (2004, 267) explains, "Aboriginal people define health and illness in terms of balance, harmony, holism, and spirituality rather than in terms of the Western concepts of physical dysfunction and disease within the individual." He points out that this holistic and integrative understanding of health is embodied in the "medicine wheel" concept of some First Nations. Box 7.4 depicts the medicine wheel.

While the exact origins of the medicine wheel are debated (Kehoe 1990; Nicholas 2008), one thing that does seem clear is that Indigenous knowledge, such as a holistic vision of health and wellness, provides a theoretical basis for future research on health disparities guided by an intersectional paradigm and employing mixed methods to understand how ethnicity influences health across the life course. Lemchuk-Favel and Jock (2004) point out that Aboriginal understandings of holism and wellness embedded with the medicine wheel are similar to the social determinants of health perspective advocated by the World Health Organization. Additionally, as Estey, Kmetic, and Reading (2007, 444–5) point out, the holistic perspective First Nations have of health and wellness is complementary to a life course perspective: "The importance of intergenerational relationships, community well-being, and holistic understandings of health in Aboriginal communities is complemented by a life course perspective that examines the influence of a combination of biological, social, and environmental processes across all life stages—from prenatal life to infancy to the elder years." Emphasizing the resiliency of

Box 7.4 Indigenous Understanding of Health and Wellness: The Medicine Wheel

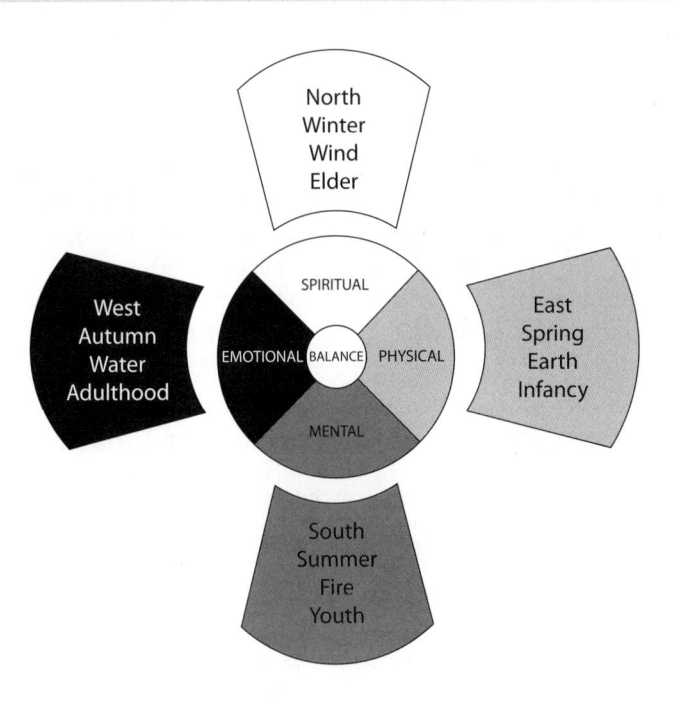

Figure 7.2 The Medicine Wheel

The National Collaborating Centre for Aboriginal Health (2013, 5) explains that "Aboriginal approaches to health are often rooted in a holistic conception of well-being involving a healthy balance of four elements or aspects of wellness: physical, emotional, mental and spiritual. These four elements are sometimes represented in the image of the medicine wheel." Irvine (2009, 28) explains that while there are many different forms of the medicine wheel, they all share the belief that "the circle symbolizes the foundational cultural understandings of wholeness, interconnectedness, and balance." There are a number of complex meanings represented in the medicine wheel. The four quadrants simultaneously represent: the four peoples of humanity (Yellow, Red, Black, White); the four directions (east, south, west, north); the four seasons; the four elements; the four stages of the life course (infancy, youth, adult, elder); and the four aspects of a life well lived (physical, mental, emotional, and spiritual). In this extremely sophisticated model, the pursuit of health and wellness is the ongoing process of balancing each of these elements in holistic fashion.

Source: Based on http://connectability.ca/Garage/wp-content/uploads/workshops/medicine_wheel/medicine_wheel.html. This is an excellent and highly informative online tutorial on the medicine wheel by Peggy Pitawanakwat. Used by permission of Peggy Pitawanakwat.

Aboriginal peoples in the face of health disparities wrought by colonialism, the First Nations Information Governance Centre (2012) explains that aspects of the medicine wheel, such as a focus on community wellness, are central in Aboriginal understandings of health and wellness. The Centre's "Power of Data" stories provide many important examples of First Nations communities that illustrate the resiliency and innovation of Aboriginal peoples in their pursuit of health and wellness. They cite survey research by Graham and Leeseberg Stamler (2010) that shows that First Nations "respondents identified such elements as a clean environment, a society free from racism, the presence of political autonomy, control over local issues by a majority of the residents, and employment on the reserve, as components of health" (First Nations Information Governance Centre 2012, 190). Finally, as Frideres (2011, 115) observes, "For First Nations people well-being results when a balance or harmony among these elements is established by the individual and/or community." All things considered, it seems clear that Aboriginal conceptions of health and illness are at present an underutilized but potentially very productive theoretical basis for future intersectional health research incorporating a life course perspective on health and wellness.

The Healthy Immigrant Effect Deteriorates over Time

The preceding section clearly demonstrates that the social determinants of health have extremely negative consequences for the health status of Aboriginal peoples. What is the impact of living in Canada on the health status of immigrants? The answer may surprise you. Many studies have shown the existence of a **healthy immigrant effect** whereby immigrants to Canada typically arrive in better health than those born in Canada. This should not surprise us, given that individual health status is one of the most important criteria used by the Government of Canada to screen those who attempt to immigrate to this country. Further, only those who are healthy enough to withstand the stresses of migration are likely to decide to uproot and move from one country to another. In effect, immigrants to Canada often self-select on the basis of their individual health status. It is believed that this initial health advantage is due, at least partly, to health selectivity and other factors such as occupational and lifestyle differences between immigrants and the Canadian-born. That is, Canadian immigration policy favours people who do not have major health problems and people who are skilled or are professionals. These are the same individuals most likely to have healthy lifestyles and to report positive health status (Perez 2002). More surprising, however, is what happens to the health of immigrants over time as they live in Canada and adopt a Canadian lifestyle.

Several studies using population health survey data to explore immigrant health have found that immigrants have better self-rated health status, less chronic disease, less disability, and lower all-cause and avoidable mortality than native-born Canadians. However, after approximately four to ten years, as immigrants become acculturated, their health appears to converge with or even overshoot (i.e., become worse than) the patterns found among the general non-Aboriginal population. Ng, Pottie, and Spitzer (2011, 1) point out that "The transition to poorer health has been found in general self-reported health, mental health status, the prevalence of chronic diseases, and birth and death outcomes." However, as Beiser (2005) and, more recently, De Maio (2010b) point out, many of the earlier studies that supported the existence of a healthy immigrant effect that deteriorates over time were cross-sectional in nature (e.g., Dunn and Dyck 2000; Gee, Kobayashi, and Prus 2004; Newbold and Danforth 2003; McDonald and Kennedy 2004; Perez 2002).

Such cross-sectional studies rely on comparing the health of more recent immigrants to that of those who arrived during earlier waves of immigration. This is problematic, because the patterns of immigration to Canada have changed markedly over the years, with people coming from different parts of the world and experiencing very different social determinants of health depending on the historical period in which they immigrated. In effect, cross-sectional studies of the healthy immigrant effect face the challenge of comparing very different types of immigrants. For example, a study by McDonald and Kennedy (2004) used data from multiple cross-sections of the *National Population Health Survey* (NPHS) and the *Canadian Community Health Survey* (CCHS) to attempt to account for differences in region of origin and period of arrival. They found that while immigrant health outcomes appear to converge with those of native-born Canadians for all groups of immigrants, those arriving from countries that are predominantly English-speaking and culturally similar to Canada have patterns of chronic disease that are more similar to those of the Canadian-born. These researchers also found that year of arrival is an important determinant of immigrant health status. Such research highlights the importance of remembering that just as women do not represent a homogeneous group, nor do immigrants or members of ethnic groups. Rather, immigrants have unique life histories shaped by a diversity of factors, such as country of birth, year of arrival, and the experience of social exclusion. These factors intersect to shape immigrant health. For this reason, it is better to study the same group of immigrants over time (i.e., longitudinal research) to gain a greater understanding of the many factors influencing their health across their life course (as they live and age in Canada).

Several more recent Canadian studies have adopted longitudinal research designs more in keeping with life course perspectives on health in an attempt to learn how the health status of immigrants changes over time and what factors are responsible for these changes. Set within the social determinants of health framework, Newbold (2005) used data from four waves of the NPHS to look at the factors associated with changes in immigrant self-rated health status. He identified immigrants who reported a change in their health status from healthy to unhealthy and analyzed the extent to which this transition could be explained by socioeconomic status, demographic variables, lifestyle factors, and health-care utilization. The findings indicate that native-born Canadians were at significantly less risk than the foreign-born to experience a decline in self-rated health. Based on his analysis, Newbold (2005, 1367–8) concludes that "Given that the decline in self-assessed health occurs over a very short period, it is unlikely to reflect the uptake of unhealthy lifestyles after arrival." Instead, Newbold believes that differences in the social determinants of health, such as working and living conditions, explain transitions of immigrants to poorer self-rated health.

The *Longitudinal Survey of Immigrants to Canada* (LSIC) has been a data source for several studies analyzing the health trajectories of immigrants to Canada (e.g., De Maio and Kemp 2010; Fuller-Thomson, Noack, and George 2011; Kim et al. 2013; Newbold 2009; Ng, Pottie, and Spitzer 2011; Setia et al. 2011a, 2011b). The LSIC is a three-wave study that followed a panel of immigrants who arrived in Canada between October 2000 and September 2001 for four years. The purpose of the survey was to "study how newly arrived immigrants adjust over time to living in Canada" (Statistics Canada 2003, 5). De Maio and Kemp (2010) used data gathered from the LSIC to assess transitions in self-rated health status and self-rated emotional health of immigrants to Canada measured in three waves: six months after arrival in Canada, two years after arrival, and four years after arrival. As depicted in Table 7.1, these researchers found that both health indicators worsened over time for immigrants. They also found that visible minorities and immigrants who

Table 7.1 Health Transitions of Immigrants to Canada (Weighted Percentages)

"In general, would you say your health is . . ."

	Wave 1	Wave 2	Wave 3
Excellent	43.0	30.2	23.0
Very Good	35.4	40.1	37.2
Good	18.6	24.3	31.8
Poor	0.6	0.9	1.4

"Have you experienced any emotional problems?"

	Wave 1	Wave 2	Wave 3
Yes	5.1	30.0	28.6
No	94.9	70.0	71.4

Source: De Maio and Kemp 2010.

experienced discrimination were most likely to experience decline in self-rated health status. Explaining that the deterioration of the healthy immigrant effect over time demonstrates the importance of the social determinants of health, De Maio and Kemp (2010, 662–3) state that "Indeed, the health transition of immigrants may be a key signal of the importance of the social determinants of health, or factors outside of the formal health care system that influence patterns of morbidity and mortality throughout the lifecourse." The results of this study have been confirmed by subsequent research (Fuller-Thomson, Noack, and George 2011; Kim et al. 2013; Setia et al. 2011a).

As listed in Box 7.5, explanations for the deterioration of the healthy immigrant effect emphasize converging lifestyles, the effects of stress associated with resettlement (Beiser 2005), and differential access to culturally competent and appropriate health care (McDonald and Kennedy 2004).

Convergence explanations contend that as immigrants acculturate to life in Canada, over time they adopt unhealthy behaviours (e.g., smoking, alcohol abuse, and high-fat diets) while surrendering health-protective behaviours that were part of their culture of origin. As McDonald

Box 7.5 Explanations for the Deterioration of the Healthy Immigrant Effect

- Converging lifestyles
- Resettlement stress
- Differential access to health care

(2006, 3) explains, "if health behaviours converge to native-born levels with additional years in Canada, it seems reasonable to think that it is changing personal behaviours that are contributing to changes in health outcomes." Unfortunately, the LSIC does not contain variables that measure lifestyle behaviours such as patterns of diet and exercise or smoking and alcohol consumption. This means that researchers interested in the convergence explanation have had to rely on other data sources to investigate the relationship between immigrant health status and lifestyle behaviours. McDonald (2006) used data from the NPHS and CCHS to investigate the degree to which weekly alcohol consumption, binge drinking, smoking, participation in vigorous physical activity, and daily intake of five or more servings of fruits and vegetables converged with native-born Canadians' habits for three groups of immigrants. He found no evidence that the measured health lifestyle behaviours of immigrant women converged with those of native-born women. However, McDonald did find that for most immigrant men, both alcohol consumption and smoking increase with time spent in Canada. He also found differences in participation in physical activity and the consumption of fruits and vegetables. These results led McDonald (2006, 19–20) to conclude that while his findings "provide some evidence that health behaviours converge over time to comparable native-born levels . . . the persistent differences in the health behaviours among some immigrants and visible minority groups suggests that maintenance of ethnic or home-country attitudes and beliefs persists in some dimensions even if the individual has been in Canada for many years."

A second explanation focuses on the stressful effects of resettlement (e.g., unemployment, poverty, social exclusion) as sources of cumulative negative health effects. As illustration, Kim and his co-researchers found that immigrants males from West Asia and China showed increased rates of poor health, leading them to conclude that "ethnic disparities in immigrant health were determined by postimmigration experiences such as acculturative stress and discrimination" (2013, 101). Kim and colleagues found evidence of even greater health deterioration among women immigrants, who also experienced poorer employment opportunities than male immigrants. Ng, Pottie, and Spitzer found that immigrants who had poor proficiency in either official language were more likely to experience a deterioration in self-reported health, leading these researchers to conclude that "This suggests that the benefits of acquiring official language skills may not only be social and economic, but may also be associated with the maintenance of health" (2011, 7). Finally, Setia and colleagues (2011a) found that both male and female immigrants who did not experience discrimination in Canada were less likely to report poor self-rated health.

McDonald and Kennedy (2004) note that another possible explanation for the apparent worsening over time of immigrant health in Canada may have to do with newly arriving immigrants having less access to the health-care system because of language and cultural barriers to utilization. As these barriers diminish with length of time in Canada, immigrants may be increasingly diagnosed with health problems that previously went unrecognized. However, these researchers found that immigrant use of formal health-care services, such as visits to family physicians and access to such preventive screening services as blood pressure checks, converges rapidly with that of native-born Canadians. These results are supported by Fuller-Thomson and colleagues (2011), who found that among the immigrants who reported a two-step decline in self-rated health status, 27.2 per cent also reported problems in accessing health care compared with 18.5 per cent of those with no decline in self-rated health. In addition, those who reported fair or poor health were significantly more likely to receive medical attention in the previous 12 months than immigrants who reported excellent or very good health. A study by Setia and colleagues (2011b) reaches a similar conclusion: "In general, there is little evidence that immigrants have worse access to health-care than the Canadian-born population." Overall, research has provided evidence supporting the converging lifestyle and resettlement stress explanations, which appear to interact to produce immigrant differences in health (Beiser 2005).

The decline in the health of immigrants who have moved to a country such as Canada, with a well-developed health-care system founded on the principles of universality and comprehensiveness, clearly shows the importance of social inequalities in the production of health disparities. De Maio (2010b) concludes his extremely thorough review of Canadian health research on the healthy immigrant effect by arguing that by learning more about the health transitions of immigrants, we can develop better theories and methods for understanding the social determinants of health. Noting that "Understanding the health transitions of immigrants is a way of examining how the social determinants of health and the formal health care system overlap to produce and sustain population health," De Maio (2012b, 959) concludes by calling for the use of intersectional models and longitudinal research to better understand immigrant health.

As with other aspects of social location, intersectional research is required to tease apart the ways in which intersecting inequalities, such as socioeconomic status, gender, ethnicity, immigration, and age, collectively produce disparities in population health. There has been little qualitative research on the healthy immigrant effect. One notable exception is Dean and Wilson's study, which used interviews with 23 immigrants to Canada "to gain insight into immigrants' perspectives of health change over time" (2010, 1220). The majority of Dean and Wilson's participants reported either improved health or no change over the period of their lives in Canada. In contrast, a minority reported a decline in health status, attributing their worsening health to stress associated with lack of employment or natural life course changes, such as aging and child bearing, rather than acculturation to an unhealthy lifestyle or lack of access to health care. These researchers conclude by suggesting that "more research is needed to understand the pathways through which stress among recent and mid-term immigrants and aging among longer-term immigrants are linked to a decline in health status" (2010, 1226). Summarizing the nature of the intersectional puzzle that confronts health researchers trying to understand the healthy immigrant effect, Spitzer (2012, 113) writes that "The question remains as to why certain groups of new comers, particularly racialized and female populations, are more apt to report a decline in their health status over time than others." This is a reason for the use of mixed-methods research designs to better understand the health transitions of migrants from an intersectional perspective. In any event, the decline of the healthy immigrant effect over time challenges our lay belief that living in Canada is good for our health!

Ethnic Differences in the Perception and Understanding of Symptoms

In a discussion of cultural determinants of health-related behaviour, Segall (1988, 249) states that "cultural context shapes prevailing beliefs regarding the cause of illness and appropriate forms of treatment. Whether a person is sensitive to feelings of discomfort, how symptoms are perceived and evaluated, and whether or not the individual decides to seek medical care are largely matters of cultural prescription. Even the individual's view of the physician as a relevant helper depends in part upon cultural background." More recently, Bombak and Bruce (2012, 1) note that "Evidence suggests that ethnic groups differ in their self-perceptions of health, their conceptualization of what constitutes health, and the determinants that factor into their self-assessments of health." In other words, the meaning of health, as well as the extent to which emotional expressions of symptoms such as pain are expected (or permitted) during sickness and the type of treatments selected, are all culturally patterned. Our perception and understanding of bodily symptoms is mediated through culture. Thus, conceptions of health and illness and beliefs about the meaning and management of the illness experience are, to an extent, ethnocultural products.

The impact of ethnicity on the perception and understanding of symptoms has been investigated by social scientists for quite some time (Rollman 2004). Studies of the influence of broad social and ethnocultural factors on health- and illness-related behaviour typically focus on subcultural groups, such as ethnic and religious groups. For instance, Kopec and colleagues (2001) found that cultural factors such as ethnocultural identification have an effect on the reporting of chronic pain and mental health problems. The study, which used data collected in the *NPHS*, found that "factors commonly associated with health status in individuals, such as socioeconomic status and chronic conditions, do not explain the variation in the Health Utilities Index across different cultural/ethnic groups in Canada. Although the healthy immigrant effect is likely responsible for some of this variation, considerable differences exist within the immigrant and Canadian-born populations" (2001, 47). A qualitative study by Barkwell (2005) of 18 Ojibway cancer patients, caregivers, and healers in a Manitoba reserve and 13 health-care professionals from a nearby hospital found a marked contrast in how the two groups understood pain. The Ojibway had a holistic understanding of their pain that contrasted with the doctors' and nurses' unidimensional understanding of pain as a biophysical sensation. An experiment that compared undergraduate university students of Chinese ancestry with students from European backgrounds by placing their lower arms in ice water found that the Chinese had lower tolerance for pain and more negative cognitive and emotional reactions to pain stimuli (Hsieh et al. 2010).

There is a long history of studies that investigated cultural differences in the expression of symptoms associated with illness and disease. These studies report that the number of symptoms presented and the willingness of the individual to present pain as a symptom varies among the members of different ethnic groups (e.g., Lipton and Marbach 1984; Zola 1964; Zborowski 1969). In one such early study, Zborowski analyzed styles of pain expression and found that there are ethnic differences in both the meaning attached to pain and in behavioural responses to pain. Rollman (2004) offers a critical appraisal of such research, noting that early studies often lacked scientific rigour and sometimes perpetuated cultural stereotypes. Rollman (2005) is equally critical of more recent studies of the relationship between ethnocultural factors and the experience of pain, noting that this area of research has become dominated by experimental psychological studies that lack both ecological validity and clinical relevance.

In summary, while the evidence indicates that within any given society there are important ethnocultural differences in lay beliefs about the nature of ill health, there remain unanswered questions concerning the relationship between ethnicity and the perception and understanding of symptoms. For instance, researchers are trying to disentangle how much of the variance between ethnic groups is the result of biophysical differences between population groups as opposed to socio-cultural factors (Campbell and Edwards 2012). Highlighting the fact that there is more to the experience of pain than its biological aspects, Shavers, Bakos, and Sheppard (2010, 193) write that "The pain response is not restricted to a physiological reaction to the exposure to noxious stimuli or tissue injury but encompasses emotional and behavioral responses as well. These responses have as their foundation variations in cultural perceptions, expectations, and past experiences which are known to differ among race/ethnic groups." Failure to understand ethnocultural variation in responses to symptoms such as pain acts as a barrier between socially excluded minorities and effective health care (Shavers, Bakos, and Sheppard 2010). As with most aspects of health, the experience of pain is multi-dimensional and affected by numerous aspects of social location. Campbell and Edwards (2012, 228) conclude their review by noting that "In the future, it would be helpful for more studies to report on and describe the ethnic characteristics of their samples and delve into differences or similarities that exist between groups in order to elucidate the mechanisms underlying these differences." This underscores the need for further research on the perception and understanding of pain that is cognizant of intersections of diversity. While sociologists such as Zola (1964) initiated social and behavioural studies of the relationship of ethnicity to the perception and understanding of symptoms such as pain, this field of research is now dominated by experimental psychology. Few contemporary sociologists focus on ethnicity and the experience of pain. This is regrettable, given the discipline's established record of rigorous conceptualization and measurement of ethnocultural factors. Future research needs to explore how, in a transnational context characterized by increasing globalization and migration of both people and culture, individual responses to the embodied experiences of illness and pain are influenced by intersecting socio-cultural factors to which we are all exposed in contemporary social life. Health sociology has much to offer this undertaking.

Ethnic Differences in Health-Care Behaviour

Researchers have known for some time that ethnicity also informs people's beliefs about adopting the sick role (e.g., Segall 1976b) and their willingness to consult a physician and make use of formal health-care services (e.g., Harwood 1981; Mechanic 1963; Suchman 1964). Leduc and Proulx (2004, 15) offer the following summary of research that has looked at the connection between ethnicity and health-care behaviour:

> Several studies have highlighted the role of ethnocultural affiliation in determining the utilization of health services. In fact, affiliation, regardless of the way it is measured, has been reported to influence not only the decision to utilize formal health services, but also the choice of primary healthcare services, the quantity and quality of services provided by professionals, and compliance with recommended treatment regimens. Ethnocultural affiliation remains an important determinant of the health services utilization even after factors such as income, education, severity of illness, age, and sex are taken into account.

Canadian studies have provided evidence that demonstrates the importance of ethnoculture for the health-care behaviour of both laypersons and health-care professionals such as physicians and nurses. For instance, in their study of the narratives of health-care utilization by young immigrant families in Quebec, Leduc and Proulx (2004) found that use of formal health-care services by newly arrived immigrants followed a three-phase trajectory—of making contact, selection, and consolidation of health-care services—which was shaped by the migration experience rather than by ethnic affiliation. In other words, they found that factors associated with being an immigrant, such as living and working conditions and length of stay, were more critical determinants of health-care behaviour than membership in specific ethnic groups. As these researchers conclude (2004, 23), "For this reason, it is impossible to state that there is a typical Lebanese, Algerian, Sri Lankan, or Vietnamese way of utilizing health services."

Another Quebec study, by Blais and Maiga (1999), posed the question, "Do ethnic groups use health services like the majority of the population?" Controlling for factors such as socioeconomic status, gender, age, access to health-care facilities, and self-rated health, these researchers found that while immigrants were no more likely to be hospitalized, attend an outpatient clinic, or go to an emergency department than native-born Québécois, they were more likely to seek specialist care. The researchers speculate that among the possible reasons for this pattern is that ethnic minorities may be more likely to be shunted by family physicians over to other specialists for care. A study by Gee, Kobayashi, and Prus (2007) using the CCHS found that Asian-born female immigrants have a significantly decreased likelihood of having had a mammogram in the past year compared to Canadian-born women. These researchers note that their findings are supportive of the results from Hislop and colleagues' (2000) research, which showed that Chinese-Canadian women in British Columbia received less screening for breast and cervical cancer. These findings led Gee, Kobayashi, and Prus (2007, 22) to speculate that "there may be ethnocultural differences in a fear of clinics, labs, and hospitals due to negative attitudes and behaviours of family physicians in some communities." Xiong and co-researchers (2010) confirm that Asian immigrant women make much less use of preventative screening for cervical cancer even after controlling for factors such as length of residency, demographic differences such as age, health status, lifestyle factors, and socioeconomic status. More generally, Omariba (2015, 5) notes that "relative to the native born, Canadian immigrants' use of preventive health services is low." For these reasons, in an effort to provide culturally appropriate health care to members of ethnic groups, government agencies in Canada have undertaken health promotion campaigns such as that depicted in Box 7.6, which target members of specific ethnic groups.

From these studies we can conclude that ethnicity is an important basis of identity that informs health-care behaviour. It works in concert with other aspects of social location, such as socioeconomic status, gender, and age, to influence how one uses formal care to pursue health and wellness. Noting that "Health behaviors are important pathways that link racism and other basic causes to health outcomes," Williams and Mohammed (2013b, 1215) argue that structural interventions that reduce barriers to health-promoting behaviours faced by socially excluded groups are effective means of addressing ethnic disparities in health. As with ethnic differences in perception and understanding of symptoms, future research needs to be directed at understanding how ethnicity and other aspects of social location intersect to produce variations in the utilization of health-care services among differing ethnocultural affiliations. It is equally important to apply a life course perspective that accounts for how patterns of health-care utilization change as we age. Fostering cross-cultural understanding between physicians and their patients can inform the development of Canadian health-care policy and practice that is sensitive to variations among a multicultural population, enhancing the health care provided to all Canadians.

Ethnic Differences in the Social Determinants of Health

Since John Porter's 1965 description of Canada as a "vertical mosaic," there has been widespread recognition among social scientists that Canadian society is stratified along ethnic lines. In an important early study of **ethnic stratification**, or the unequal distribution of wealth, power, and privilege on the basis of ethnic group membership, Porter documented the existence of a social hierarchy of occupations, income, and prestige in terms of ethnic group membership, with those of British origins coming out on top, followed by French Canadians, persons of other European origins, and, finally, blacks and Aboriginals at the bottom. More recent studies have found continued support for the finding that visible minorities remain economically disadvantaged within Canadian society (Pendakur and Pendakur 2010). Gee, Kobayashi, and Prus (2007, 13) summarize this body of research by noting that "Recent studies on the ethnic dimensions of income

Box 7.6 Ethnoculturally Targeted Health Promotion Campaigns

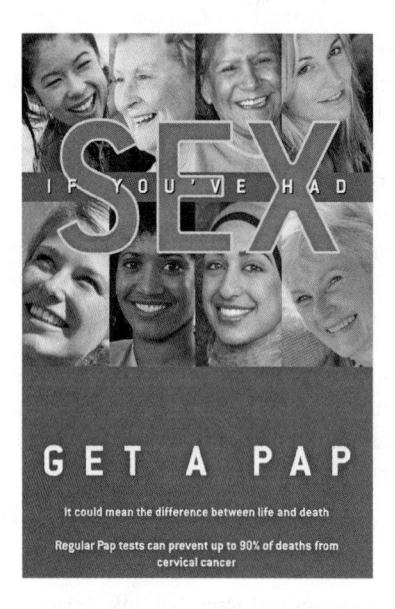

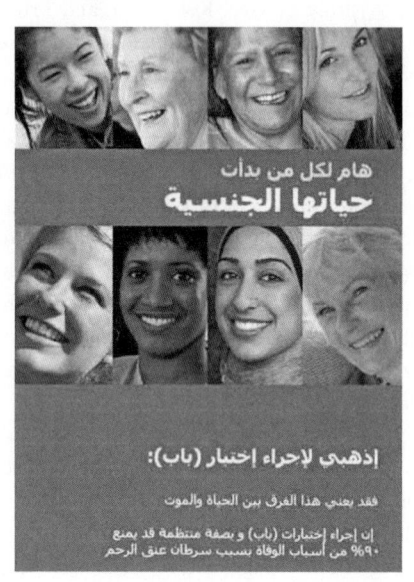

(Included with permission from Cancer Care Nova Scotia's Cervical Cancer Prevention Program. Cancer Care Nova Scotia is a provincial program of the Nova Scotia Department of Health and Wellness.)

Recognizing the importance of ethnocultural affiliation for health-care behaviour, Cancer Care Nova Scotia launched a culturally sensitive health promotion campaign encouraging women to attend medical screenings for cervical cancer, featuring advertisements presented in the languages of different ethnic groups.

inequalities, using different data and employing somewhat differing ethnicity categorizations and sets of control variables, converge on one main finding—that visible minorities and Aboriginals earn less income than European-origin Canadians." Systemic discrimination and prejudice means that members of certain ethnic groups occupy social locations that make them vulnerable to a variety of forms of social inequality. This, in turn, has direct consequences for the pursuit of health and wellness. For example, because of the ethnic stratification of Canadian society, ethnic group differences exist in life expectancy, infant mortality, and virtually all of the indicators of population health.

However, as with gender, there are important between- and within-group differences in the health status of ethnic group members. This means that ethnic differences in health defy easy summary. Most Canadian population health studies looking at the issue of health and ethnicity compare aggregate ethnic groups, such as Aboriginals and visible minorities versus whites, foreign-born versus Canadian-born, and anglophone and francophone versus allophone. In an effort to answer the question "what is the extent of ethnocultural-based health inequalities in the

Canadian context?" Prus and Lin (2005), using the CCHS, document differences in the physical health of 21 ethnocultural groups. Consistent with existing literature, these researchers report that visible minorities generally have better physical health than white Canadians. This finding is surprising, given that, in general, visible minorities are economically disadvantaged in Canada. However, the socioeconomic status of ethnocultural groups in Canada is variable, and not all members of ethnic groups share this health advantage. Some ethnic groups are wealthier and healthier (e.g., Japanese) than others (e.g., Aboriginals). Prus and Lin (2005, 18) summarize their findings by saying that health differences between ethnic groups are, in large part, attributable to differences in social determinants of health, such as socioeconomic status, and conclude that "Social structural factors are generally more important than behavioural ones in explaining ethnocultural-based differences in health."

Wu and colleagues (2003) used data from the NPHS to explore ethnic differences in mental health and emotional well-being. Similar to patterns in physical health, they found that East and Southeast Asians, Chinese, South Asians, and blacks experience the lowest rates of depression in Canada. Aboriginals report the highest rates of depression. These researchers (2003, 438) note that other aspects of social location, such as socioeconomic status, gender, marital status, and social support, mediate these effects and conclude that "in any case, we cannot assume that visible minority status automatically translates into comparatively poor mental health." These results reflect the variable patterns between the social determinants of health and ethnic differences in health.

In several studies, Veenstra (2009; 2011a; 2011b; 2012; 2013) has investigated the effects of racialization on health. As discussed earlier, **racialization** refers to the processes by which people are systematically categorized and sorted into inferior social statuses according to perceived racial differences. As such, racialization is a precursor to **racism**—the prejudicial treatment of groups and individuals according to subjective understandings of race. Explaining that "racialization is not simply reducible to race," Teelucksingh (2007, 647) argues that "Racialization is not an isolated process, but rather is an interrelated component of numerous other political, economic and gender discourses." In Canada, Aboriginals, visible minorities, and recent immigrants are among racialized groups; they suffer numerous and overlapping forms of oppression. In introducing his analysis, Veenstra (2009, 539) explains that "Because processes of racialization are fundamentally processes of power and inequality, they likely have repercussions for health and well-being and, therefore, deserve attention from population health researchers." Veenstra's research bears this out. Based on an analysis of data from the CCHS, he found that while no racial/cultural identification had significantly better self-rated health scores than whites, respondents with Aboriginal or Aboriginal/white and visible minority identifications had some of the highest risks for diabetes, hypertension, and fair/poor self-rated health. Using data gathered from a telephone survey of respondents living in Toronto and Vancouver, Veenstra (2011b; 2012) further documented the negative health effects of racialization for black Canadians.

To further understand the complex relationship between racialization and poor health outcomes, Veenstra (2011a; 2013) has turned to intersectionality theory. While intersectionality will be more fully considered in the next chapter, for now it is helpful to note that Veenstra (2013, 16) explains that "Intersectionality theory presents a sophisticated framework for conceptualizing the nature of relations of power pertaining to racism, sexism, classism and heterosexism in modern societies and possesses enormous potential for providing insight into the nature of inequalities." Applying intersectionality to the determinants of self-rated health, Veenstra (2011a) found that socioeconomically disadvantaged homosexuals and South Asian women were the groups most at multiple jeopardy for poor or fair self-rated health. He concludes that racial identities are themselves multi-dimensional, adding to the complexity of ethnic differences in health and illness (Veenstra 2011b).

Research on health and ethnicity increasingly makes clear that like other aspects of social location, ethnocultural identification is uneven and the health of ethnic group members is shaped by a number of intersecting factors, such as socioeconomic status, gender, and stage of the life course. While the experience of systemic racism, prejudice, and racialization is pathogenic, these factors interact with additional aspects of social location to produce individual variations in health. The challenge for researchers remains to tease apart the overlapping contributions of social determinants of health in order to understand how individual health outcomes are influenced by ethnicity interacting with other social and cultural factors.

Explanations of Ethnic Differences in Health and Illness

Explanations of ethnic differences in health and illness generally fall under three broad categories (Wu and Schimmele 2005). Because of the biologically deterministic heritage described in the introductory chapter, biomedical researchers have sought to explain health and illness disparities among ethnic groups in terms of biophysical attributes such as genetic influences. In contrast, social scientists point to cultural differences in health and illness behaviours of different ethnic groups to account for disparities in health (i.e., the cultural behavioural perspective). Finally, informed by the political economy approach of the conflict paradigm, ethnic differences in health and illness have also been attributed to socioeconomic differences. In reality, all three explanations (listed in Box 7.7) intersect in complex biosocial ways to produce ethnic disparities in health. This is to say that health disparities among ethnic groups are the result of biological, cultural behavioural, and socioeconomic factors interacting with one another. Let's briefly examine each of these explanations.

Box 7.7 Explanations of Ethnic Differences in Health and Illness

- Biological determinist explanations
- Cultural behavioural explanations
- Socioeconomic explanations

Biological Determinist Explanations

Reflecting a medico-centric bias, population health policies have sought to address ethnic disparities in health by focusing on presumed biological differences between ethnic groups. Unfortunately, this has often been to the exclusion of addressing the socio-cultural differences and socioeconomic inequalities that give rise to health disparities. As illustration, Poudrier (2007, 238) points out how the biologically determinist hypothesis of the so-called "thrifty gene" as an explanation for the high rates of diabetes among Aboriginals puts the focus on biological factors while minimizing "environmental and lifestyle factors such as age, stress, poor nutrition, sedentary lifestyles, as well as low socio-economic status, and social marginalization." The "thrifty gene" (Neel 1962) is an unproven hypothesis that attempts to explain the high incidence of diabetes among particular populations, such as American Aboriginals, in terms of an alleged genetic propensity of groups with a hunter-gatherer ancestry to accumulate and store body fat purportedly necessary to survive periods of famine. The idea is that under the supposed living conditions of early hunter-gatherers, such a genetic adaptation would confer a survival advantage. However, under the "obesogenic" (James 2008) conditions of our fast-food culture, those with the so-called thrifty gene are now alleged to be at greater risk of obesity-related disease such as diabetes. Though the "thrifty gene" hypothesis has little current scientific support (Genné-Bacon 2014; Speakman 2013), it is an excellent illustration of the popular appeal of biological determinist explanations for ethnic differences in health. As Poudrier (2007, 256) explains, "the focus on gene sequencing diverts attention from other basic health requirements like food security, employment and safe environments." Williams and Sternthal (2010, S17) argue that "Views of race that focus on biology can divert attention from the social origins of disease, reinforce social norms of racial inferiority, and promote the maintenance of the status quo. If racial differences in health are caused by inherent genetic differences, then social policies and structures that initiate and sustain the production of disease are absolved from responsibility." The problem is, as Krieger (2003, 195) critically points out, "Myriad epidemiological studies continue to treat 'race' as a purely biological (i.e., genetic) variable or seek to explain racial/ethnic disparities in health absent consideration of the effects of racism on health." Though biology is a major determinant of health, explanations that attempt to explain ethnic disparities in health solely in terms of biological differences between so-called racial groups have proven fruitless.

Despite its popularity in everyday talk, the term "**race**" is a scientifically discredited concept. Biological science has demonstrated that besides differences in the average proportions of genetic material based on ancestral geographic origin (i.e., "geographical race"), there are no racially based biological differences among human beings (Collins 2004). These ancestral geographic differences do influence the probability of genetically influenced diseases within certain population subgroups. (The best known examples are Tay-Sachs disease among Ashkenazi Jews and sickle-cell anemia among African Americans.) However, "genetic variation is often greater within racial/ethnic groups than between them" (Wu and Schimmele 2005, 710). This means that the "recipe to bake the human cake" contains the same "ingredients" for every human being. While there are some differences in the amount of the ingredients between particular population groups—some might have more "sugar" while others might have more "spice"—these differences are less important for health than the differences between individuals! For these reasons, in describing a 1995 United Nations Educational, Scientific and Cultural Organization (UNESCO) statement on race issued by a group of the world's leading scientists, Katz (1995, 4–5) writes that "The same scientific groups that developed the biological concept [of race] over the last century have now concluded that its use for characterizing human populations is so flawed that it is no longer a scientifically valid concept. In fact, the statement makes clear that the biological concept of race as applied to humans has no legitimate place in biological science."

Social scientists point out that while race is recognized as a scientifically discredited concept, as a social construction it still has important consequences for people's lives, bodies, and health. Duster (2003, 264) explains this by paraphrasing a well-known sociological adage from the symbolic interactionist paradigm in terms of embodiment: "If humans define situations as real, they can and often do have real biological and social consequences." This means that to say that race is a social construction is not to deny that racialization has profound and objective consequences for behaviour and health. Distinguishing individuals according to observable biophysical differences (i.e., racialization) is basic human social behaviour (Dovidio and Gaertner 2004). What must be remembered is that these racialized distinctions are not supported by a scientific understanding of human biology. However, processes of racialization are "capable of affecting biochemical, neurophysical, and cellular aspects of our bodies that, in turn, can be studied scientifically" (Duster 2003, 263). As the sociology of the body paradigm points out, society shapes the human body, which also shapes society! While there is no such thing as "race," there are important ethnocultural differences among groups, and there certainly is racialization, racism, and ethnic stratification. All of these factors have very real consequences for the pursuit of health and wellness.

Because of the legacy of race relations between whites and blacks in the United States, race is still used by influential American social scientists (e.g., Duster 2003; 2015), although in international social and behavioural research "race" has been rejected as a useful concept in favour of "ethnicity." Unfortunately, this change in terminology has not worked itself fully into population health research or health promotion literature, much less popular thought. Additionally, despite prominent calls for a limited use of the concept of race in biomedical research (e.g., Schwartz 2001), racialized terminology is often employed to the neglect of examining the consequences of cultural behavioural and socioeconomic differences for ethnic group health disparities. This reality prompted Wu and Schimmele (2005, 710) to write that "The association between race/ethnicity and health disparities needs to be placed in the social context of racial/ethnic hierarchies rather than simply described in terms of biological or genetic differences." This means that ethnic disparities in health are best understood with reference to social inequality among ethnic groups and processes of social exclusion.

Cultural Behavioural Explanations

As Chapter 4 discussed, lifestyle behaviours are a major determinant of health. Segall (1988, 249) explains that "It is evident that culture plays a broad part in shaping people's ideas about health and illness and their subsequent treatment activities." This, in turn, influences differences in health outcomes associated with membership in various cultural groupings. Evidence of this is the negative consequences of unhealthy lifestyles for Aboriginal peoples in Canada. Another example is that the healthy immigrant effect is, in part, attributable to differences in health practices and health-protective actions that are part of recently arriving immigrants' ethnocultural lifestyles, which are, in many regards, healthier than those of native-born Canadians (Beiser 2005). Further, researchers have shown that ethnocultural identification is an important determinant of health-care behaviour even after factors such as socioeconomic status, gender, age, and health status are taken into consideration (Leduc and Proulx 2004). Cultural behavioural explanations for ethnic differences in health and illness examine the contribution of lifestyle differences among ethnic groups to health disparities.

Describing the relationship between cultural racism, stereotyping, and poor health outcomes, Williams and Mohammed (2013a,1161) explain how those subjected to racism may internalize "the dominant society's beliefs about their biological and/or cultural inferiority": "By fostering the endorsement of beliefs about the innate deficiencies of one's self and one's group, internalized racism can lead to lower self-esteem and psychological well-being, which in turn could adversely affect health and health behavior in multiple ways." These researchers note that psychological distress, overweight and obesity, alcohol consumption, and high blood pressure are all associated with internalized racism, which they describe as the "stereotype threat." As Berger (1963, 102 [sic]) remarked, one of the most harmful aspects of racism is how it affects one's self-concept: "The most terrible thing that prejudice can do to a human being is to make him tend to become what the prejudiced image of him says that he is." In this manner cultural stereotypes get under the skin of socially excluded individuals and negatively affect the pursuit of health and wellness. Culture provides a conceptual framework whereby individuals understand and act in society. Thus, behaviour, including health behaviour, is bound up with the norms and values that are a part of the individual's cultural life. As Williams and Mohammed (2013a, 1158) describe, "Communication factors that shape health knowledge, attitudes, and behavior, such as access to and the use of various media sources, attention to health information, trust in the sources of information, and the processing of information, all vary by race-ethnicity and SES." Working in concert with biological and socioeconomic factors, cultural behavioural factors have marked consequences for the pursuit of health and wellness. However, more research is required to better understand issues such as which groups are most vulnerable to the negative health effects associated with racism, the causal pathways between racism and health, and how racism intersects with other dimensions of social inequality to jeopardize health (Williams and Mohammed 2013a). Once again, the challenge for future health research is to tease apart the relative contributions each of these factors makes to an overall explanation of ethnic disparities in health.

Socioeconomic Explanations

Explaining the socioeconomic perspective on ethnic differences in health, Prus and Lin (2005, 4) write that "Socioeconomic status is important since it mediates the relationship between race/ethnicity and health. Socioeconomic status, in turn, is important because it influences well-known determinants of mental health such as access/utilization of healthcare services, physical environment (e.g., housing), and chronic stress." As Wu and Schimmele (2005) point out, health researchers believe that socioeconomic factors affect health primarily through two intersecting mechanisms: First, individuals with lower socioeconomic status have less access to effective health care. Second, owing to their social exclusion, people with lower socioeconomic status are exposed to poorer living and working conditions, the material prerequisites for good health. By definition, socially excluded minority group members have lower socioeconomic status. Thus, researchers believe that much of the difference in population health outcomes among ethnic groups can be explained by the socioeconomic disadvantage associated with social exclusion of minorities. Writing in the American context, Williams and Sternthal (2010, S19) assert that "Recent research continues to find that SES differences among the races account for a substantial component of the racial-ethnic differences in health." Yet they caution that SES intersects with ethnicity in an extremely complex fashion. While socioeconomic status has been shown to shape health outcomes, there is evidence that socioeconomic inequality alone does not fully account for ethnic disparities in health (Kobayashi and Prus 2005; Wu and Schimmele 2005).

Wilkinson and Pickett (2010, 168) note that "research shows that the health of ethnic minority groups who live in areas with more people like themselves is sometimes better than that of their more affluent counterparts who live in areas with more of the dominant ethnic group." Restated, less well-off minority group members who live in areas with higher concentrations of people from their minority group have better health than better-off minority group members who live in areas in which they are a visible minority. This "ethnic density effect" points to the importance of factors other than SES in ethnic disparities in health (Das-Munshi et al. 2010; Jurcik et al. 2013; Pickett and Wilkinson 2008). The **ethnic density effect** refers to health benefits associated with living in a neighbourhood with a high concentration of others from one's own ethnic group. Additional evidence for an ethnic density effect comes from a Canadian study of immigrant mental health that found that incidence of depression decreased among immigrants and visible minorities living in areas with higher concentrations of immigrants whereas it increased among whites living in these areas (Stafford, Newbold, and Ross 2010). Hence, despite the commitment of many Western nations to ethnic diversity in the form of official polices that promote multiculturalism, research suggests that it is social cohesion rather than ethnocultural diversity that is beneficial to the pursuit of health and wellness. There is evidence that communities have better population health if high levels of social cohesion exist. Ethnically connected communities tend to be communities with high levels of social cohesion (Breton 1991; 2005). Socially cohesive societies are characterized by high levels of membership and participation in community group activities, particularly those structured around religion (Breton 2012). It is noteworthy that research has found that religious involvement can act as a health-promoting buffer against the negative mental health consequences of discrimination faced by minority group members (Bierman 2006; Ellison et al. 2008). For these reasons, an analysis of ethnicity and health is incomplete without consideration of the well-established relationship between religion and health.

Ethnicity, Religion, and Health

The complex relationship among ethnicity, religion, and health is highlighted by an Italian-American town named Roseto (in Pennsylvania). The "Roseto effect," first documented in the 1960s, is often cited to illustrate the population health effects of socially cohesive community relationships. Researchers found that in Roseto, the incidence of heart attack was half that in four nearby communities (Stout et al. 1964). What could account for such a startling difference? The "usual suspects" of lifestyle behavioural factors were ruled out because the lifestyles in the surrounding communities were similar to Roseto's in terms of smoking, fat intake, diet, and exercise levels (Bruhn et al. 1966; Lynn et al. 1967). So the "Roseto effect" had to somehow be related to the characteristics of the community of Roseto itself rather than to the individuals living there. Roseto was described by early researchers as an "ethnic enclave" (Bruhn and Wolf 1979, vii). By this they meant that Roseto was populated almost exclusively by Italian immigrants who maintained ethnic traditions of Catholic Church participation, strong family and social ties, and a high rate of intra-ethnic marriage (i.e., marrying within the same ethnic group); characteristics of a culturally homogenous ethnic enclave. In other words, Roseto had a high level of social cohesion based on shared religion and ethnicity among its residents. A 50-year comparison of mortality rates in Roseto and adjacent communities suggests that when risk factors such as smoking and being sedentary are taken into account, it appears that changes in the health status of residents of this town reflect differences in level of family ties, ethnic and social homogeneity, and cohesive community relationships (Egolf et al. 1992).

For many years, the Italian immigrants who settled in Roseto retained the low levels of coronary heart disease enjoyed by their ancestors who remained in Italy. However, as Roseto became more diverse and people assimilated into mainstream American culture, traditional family-centred social life centred around religious ritual declined, the community became less socially cohesive, and the incidence of heart disease increased (e.g., death rates went up for heart attack). Egolf and her co-authors provide the following account of what changed (1992, 1090): "Roseto was shifting from its initially highly homogeneous social order made up of three-generation households with strong commitments to religion and to traditional values and practices to a less cohesive, materialistic, more 'Americanized' community in which three-generation households were uncommon and inter-ethnic marriages became the norm." The explanation offered for the "Roseto effect" is that a stable family structure and supportive social relationships associated with Italian ethnic group membership in a socially cohesive and ethnically homogenous community provided protection against heart attacks and contributed to health and longevity. Thus, ethnocultural homogeneity and shared religion were found to be related to positive health outcomes.

While religion and ethnicity are two different concepts, they are conceptually interrelated (Breton 2012). **Religiosity** refers to the degree of adherence to and participation in religious belief and practice. Numerous studies have considered the relationship between religiosity and health and have concluded that religious group membership is associated with positive mental and physical health outcomes (George, Ellison, and Larson 2002). George and colleagues (2002, 190) note that "people who attend religious services once a week or more typically have fewer illnesses, recover more quickly from illness, and live longer than individuals who attend less frequently." However, there is not yet agreement as to what it is precisely about religiosity that plays a role in the successful pursuit of health and wellness. Part of the challenge in understanding just what it is about religion that is good for health is that religiosity, like health, is a multi-dimensional phenomenon. As Aukst-Margetić and Margetić (2005, 370) point out, "Religious involvement could be associated with, or mediated by, a variety of demographic, psychosocial, and physiological variables, such as age, gender, race/ethnicity, social support, psychological well-being, health practices such as exercise, diet and smoking."

Such factors, which are associated with religiosity, have well-known health effects. For example, as will be considered in Chapter 9, researchers have established that social support is a key determinant of health. Religious groups often provide their members with social support in its varied forms. Another possible mechanism whereby religiosity might benefit health is through the encouragement of health-protective behaviours (i.e., prohibitions against smoking, drinking, and promiscuous sex) and health-promoting practices (i.e., guidelines concerning diet and rest) (George, Ellison, and Larson 2002). For example, members of the Mormon Church are well known for their healthy lifestyles. George and colleagues (2002, 193) point out that "most, if not all, religions teach their members to respect and take care of their bodies." A final mediating factor through which religiosity may shape health is via psychosocial resources such as Antonovsky's sense of coherence (discussed in Chapter 4). There is a limited but intriguing body of research that suggests religiosity/spirituality can be understood as an engine that powers sense of coherence (Idler 1987; Kark, Carmel, et al. 1996; Kark, Shermi, et al. 1996). George, Ellison and Larson (2002, 195) remind us that "Antonovsky also pointed out that individuals are likely to develop a SOC (or lack of it) based on the belief systems of their cultures and the social institutions in which they participate." Faith in a higher power may allow people to believe that life is meaningful, predictable, and manageable.

With reference to future research in the area of religiosity and health, George and colleagues (2002, 190) argue in their comprehensive review that "Given the accumulating evidence that religious involvement is or can be beneficial to health, a critical next step is to identify the processes and mechanisms by which religion exerts its salubrious effects." As they point out, however, we need to realize that it is also possible for religiosity to harm health, such as in cases in which religious convictions are at odds with medically necessary treatment. Hotly debated contemporary examples are people who, owing to their religious beliefs, refuse medical treatment for themselves or their children (such as blood transfusions). Lastly, in thinking about the relationship between religiosity and health, we also need to be aware that as social and behavioural scientists, health researchers are limited by our secular commitments in fully understanding the complex nature of spiritual faith and health.

Toward an Intersectional Theory of Health and Ethnicity across the Life Course

Canadian research on health and ethnicity has produced a mixed yield. Researchers have established the harmful health consequences of social exclusion of Aboriginal peoples in Canada and have also systematically documented deterioration of the healthy immigrant effect over time. There is some descriptive information on the relationship between ethnicity and perception and understanding of symptoms, but more sociological research is needed to understand the mechanisms underlying observed differences. While we know that there are profound differences in social determinants of health among ethnic groups, we still have a lot to learn about how structural and behavioural factors intersect with and are mediated by ethnocultural factors to produce ethnic differences in both health-care behaviour and resulting health disparities throughout the life course. De Maio (2010b, 16) explains that "this area of research could benefit from a closer integration with the rapidly growing literature on intersectionality." We need to be aware that structures of inequality (such as class, gender, and ethnicity) intersect with each other and that their combined impact on health may change across the life course. As illustration, Castañeda and her co-authors (2015) point out that immigrant health status is shaped by the social determinants of health that migrants faced prior to migration and by the changing conditions they encounter in their destination countries. De Maio (2010b, 10) agrees, stating that "the factors driving the health transitions of immigrants may be life-stage dependent." In a detailed and important contribution to the life course literature on immigrant health, Vang and colleagues (2015, 7) note that because "immigrants' health advantage varies across the life-course and within each stage of the life-course, by different health outcomes . . . the healthy immigrant effect is not a universal phenomenon." In their systematic review of the literature guided by a life course perspective, these researchers found that "The healthy immigrant effect appears to be strongest during adulthood but less so during childhood/adolescence and late life." Williams and Mohammed (2013a,1165) echo calls for further research from a life course perspective, noting that "At the present time, we do not clearly understand how the age of onset of experiences of discrimination and the accumulation of such experiences over the life course affect the onset and course of illness." Gee, Walsemann, and Brondolo (2012, 972) summarize existing research in the area of life course studies of racism as follows:

> Many studies have investigated the relationship between discrimination and health. For the most part, these studies suggest that discrimination is related to illness. Yet, major questions remain as to how experiences of discrimination may vary across the life course, whether discrimination at specific developmental periods may be more harmful than at other ages, and how these experiences may accumulate over time. A life course perspective provides a key way to integrate a large body of research on discrimination and health.

To gain a better understanding of the complex relationship among ethnicity, age, and health, an increasing number of researchers are adopting a life course approach in their studies of social inequalities and health disparities. However, it is clear that though the life course perspective has been around for decades, it has not yet realized its full potential to contribute to social and behavioural studies of how sources of inequality and health disparities affect the lifelong pursuit of health and wellness.

Similar to calls for sex- and gender-based analysis, health researchers such as Hankivsky (2012b) have strongly encouraged others working in this field to deepen their engagement with cultural diversity in its varied forms. While population health surveys are a rich source of data on ethnic disparities in health, Aspinall (2001, 837) cautions that "The danger of the routine use of such Census categories in studies of disadvantage, mediated by discrimination and other processes, is the reification of group labels and the support their usage lends to the view that groups like 'Indian' or 'Black African' are homogeneous wholes." This means that quantitative data analysis tends to oversimplify the lived experience of ethnoculture and its health consequences. Aspinall also warns that individualistic ethnic identifications of the sort readily identifiable in qualitative research run the risk of missing broad, societal level disparities in the health status of racialized groups. For these reasons, future research intended to expand our understanding of the effects of the intersections of diversity on population health must systematically employ the type of mixed-methods research described in Chapter 3. Quantitative research is well suited to mapping social structural inequalities and resulting disparities in health, while qualitative research may dig deeper into the relationships among the variables thus identified. The challenge for health researchers in the future will be to use the sociological imagination to combine both streams of data in developing a comprehensive understanding of the ongoing intersections of diversity and health across the life course.

Chapter Summary

The purpose of the discussion was to highlight the importance of ethnic diversity as a vital component of social inequality and a major determinant of health. In view of Canada's immigration patterns and the increasingly ethnocultural character of the country, it was argued that we need to learn more about the part played by ethnicity, in conjunction with social and economic factors, in shaping health beliefs and behaviour and, ultimately, the health status of Canadians. The many poor health outcomes experienced by Canada's Aboriginal peoples were emphasized. These outcomes include higher morbidity rates (for both acute infectious diseases and chronic conditions), higher rates of suicide and accidental deaths, and shorter life expectancy than non-Aboriginal Canadians. To illustrate the fact that ethnic group membership and ethnic identity are important determinants of health and wellness, ethnic differences in perception and understanding of symptoms and health-care behaviour were reviewed.

From a sociological perspective, critical importance is typically attached to processes of social exclusion in accounting for these types of ethnic disparities in health. A number of alternative explanations for ethnic differences in health and illness were considered, including biological determinist, cultural behavioural, and socioeconomic. Although they each focus on different explanatory factors (i.e., biophysical properties, cultural norms and values that shape our beliefs and practices, and ethnic stratification based on the unequal distribution of wealth), all three explanations intersect in complex biosocial ways to produce ethnic disparities in health. Furthermore, the discussion demonstrated that ethnicity is a dimension of social location that intersects with socioeconomic status, gender, and age to collectively influence population health. In addition, the contribution of these types of structural factors to the creation of disparities in health varies at different stages in the lifecycle. As we have learned, people experience social structures, such as class, gender, and ethnicity, differently depending on their age.

The chapter also raised the question, "is living in Canada good for your health?" and examined apparent changes in the "healthy immigrant effect" to try to find an answer. According to convergence explanations, as immigrants acculturate to life in Canada, they adopt unhealthy lifestyle practices while surrendering some of the health-protective behaviours that were part of their original cultural context. Other accounts focus on the stressful effects of resettlement (such as poverty and social exclusion) as sources of negative health outcomes. Overall, research evidence supports both of these explanations and suggests that they interact to produce differences in the health status of immigrants. As pointed out, however, clarification of the healthy immigrant effect requires more longitudinal studies of immigrant groups over time to document what happens to their health across the life course. The chapter concludes with a call for a clearly formulated intersectional approach that incorporates a life course perspective on how structures of inequality change over time and the ways in which this is reflected in health disparities. The life course perspective makes it clear that the foundations of health are established early in life and that the pursuit of health and wellness is an ongoing, lifelong process. It is time to take a closer look at the conceptual components of an intersectional model of health across the life course.

Study Questions

1. Why do health researchers need to clarify which aspect of ethnoculture they are studying?
2. How is the health status of Canada's Aboriginal peoples clear evidence of the social determinants of health?
3. Provide explanations of the healthy immigrant effect and why it appears to decline over time.
4. Summarize what is known about the relationship between ethnicity and the perception of symptoms and health-care behaviour.
5. What is the relationship between the social determinants of health and ethnic differences in health?
6. Summarize the explanations of ethnic differences in health and illness.
7. Outline the advantages of using a life course perspective for studying ethnic differences in health and wellness.

Recommended Readings

Adelson, N. 2005. "The embodiment of inequity health disparities in Aboriginal Canada." *Canadian Journal of Public Health* 96: S45–61.

Beiser, M. 2005. "The health of immigrants and refugees in Canada." *Canadian Journal of Public Health* 96: S30–44.

Frideres, J.S. 2011. *First Nations in the Twenty-first Century.* Don Mills, ON: Oxford University Press.

Kobayashi, K. 2003. "Do intersections of diversity matter? An exploration of the relationship between identity markers and health for mid- to later-life Canadians." *Canadian Ethnic Studies* 35: 85–98.

Reading J. 2009. *A Life Course Approach to the Social Determinants of Health for Aboriginal Peoples.* Ottawa: Senate Subcommittee on Population Health.

Smylie, J. 2009. "The health of Aboriginal peoples." In D. Raphael, ed., *Social Determinants of Health: Canadian Perspectives*, 280–304. Toronto: Canadian Scholars Press.

Waldram, J.B., D.A. Herring, and T.K. Young. 2006. *Aboriginal Health in Canada: Historical, Cultural, and Epidemiological Perspectives.* 2nd edn. Toronto: University of Toronto Press, 2006.

Vang, Z., J. Sigouin, A. Flenon, and A. Gagnon. 2015. "The healthy immigrant effect in Canada: A systematic review." *Population Change and Lifecourse Strategic Knowledge Cluster Discussion Paper Series* 3(1): Article 4.

Recommended Websites

National Aboriginal Health Organization (NAHO):
www.naho.ca

Report of the Royal Commission on Aboriginal Peoples:
www.ainc-inac.gc.ca

Teachings of the Medicine Wheel:
http://connectability.ca/Garage/wpcontent/uploads/workshops/medicine_wheel/medicine_wheel.html

Recommended Audiovisual Sources

Race: The Power of an Illusion. Three-part educational documentary series produced by California Newsreel and originally broadcast by PBS, 2003.

"When the bough breaks." From *Unnatural Causes: Is Inequality Making Us Sick?* Seven-part documentary series exploring racial and socioeconomic inequalities in health produced by Vital Pictures, Inc., and California Newsreel and originally broadcast by PBS, 2008.

"Becoming American." From *Unnatural Causes: Is Inequality Making Us Sick?* Seven-part documentary series exploring racial and socioeconomic inequalities in health produced by Vital Pictures, Inc., and California Newsreel and originally broadcast by PBS, 2008.

8 Unravelling the Mystery of Health: An Intersectional Model of Health across the Life Course

Learning Objectives

This chapter concludes our exploration of general determinants of health by outlining an intersectional model that uses sociological theory to conceptualize intersecting effects of structural and behavioural factors on health across the life course. The chapter examines

- the intersectionality of health disparities;
- how lifestyle factors relate to health disparities;
- the limits of individualized health promotion responses to health disparities; and
- an intersectional model of health, which uses sociological theory to highlight that health disparities result from the lifelong interplay of life chances and life choices.

The chapters in this part of the text should have made one point clear: society can make you healthy, or it can make you sick! We learned that healthy biological development requires a healthy environmental context; problems in the natural and built environments can lead to health problems; lack of access to health care can harm health; and social inequality, whether based on socioeconomic status, gender, ethnicity, or age, leads to health disparities. Further, as a life course perspective makes clear, the effects of these intersecting structures of inequality change over time as one ages. One could easily reach the conclusion that it truly is a mystery how anyone manages to stay healthy! In this chapter, we will unravel the mystery of health by explaining how society, through the mechanisms of health lifestyles, shapes the pursuit of health and wellness across the life course.

Let's begin by considering the intersectionality of health disparities based on socioeconomic status, gender, ethnicity, and age. Then we will summarize how lifestyle factors relate to disparities in health. This will set the stage for a critical look at individualized health promotion responses to health disparities. The chapter concludes by presenting an intersectional model of health, which uses sociological theory to highlight the fact that health disparities result from the ongoing interplay of life chances and life choices across the life course.

Intersectionality and Health Disparities

In terms of health disparities, who are the most vulnerable members of Canadian society? The existence of the social gradient in health provides clear evidence that one's position in the social hierarchy affects life chances, including chances of being healthy or becoming sick. But do all people in the same social class position experience similar health disparities? Restated, do other structures of inequality, such as gender, ethnicity, and age, compound socioeconomic inequality, making some people more vulnerable to disparities in health?

If you are poor, is it better or worse for your health if you are a woman? Research shows that the effects of income inequality are particularly negative for women, meaning that it is worse for your health to be an impoverished woman than to be an impoverished man. If you are an impoverished woman, is it better or worse for your health to be white? Evidence suggests that the effects of poverty on health are especially negative for racialized groups who experience social exclusion. If you are a poor, non-white woman, is it better or worse for your health to be an older adult? Again, research has shown that older, non-white women who live in poverty are among the most vulnerable members of society in terms of disparities in health. In fact, when the combined effects of socioeconomic status, gender, ethnicity, and age are considered, older Aboriginal women are among the most vulnerable members of Canadian society in terms of their health status. This illustrates that in addition to the social gradient in health, there are a range of social and cultural hierarchies based on factors such as gender, ethnicity, and age that intersect to affect the pursuit of health and wellness. In other words, just as health is multi-dimensional, so too are health inequalities!

What have we learned about intersecting sources of inequality that can harm health? O'Campo and Dunn (2012, 4) sum up existing research by stating that "What holds this large body of mostly problem-focused research together is the repeated finding that health status is not distributed equally in society and that persistent differences exist between groups along a number of axes of social differentiation, including gender, income, education, race, ethnicity, immigration status and housing status, to name a few." How then can we make sense of the multi-dimensional nature of health inequality? As each of the chapters in this part of the text has shown, while much has been learned, researchers need to develop a better understanding of the intersectional forces affecting health over time if we are to be successful at unravelling the mystery of health and addressing health disparities that accumulate throughout the life course. As Veenstra (2011a, 2) points out, it is here that the intersectionality of health comes in: "Intersectionality theory presents a new way of understanding social inequalities that possesses potential to uncover and explicate previously unknown health inequalities."

General determinants of health intersect to compound the root causes of health inequalities (Veenstra 2013). A key issue for researchers trying to address health disparities is to understand whether some determinants are more important than others. If so, which ones, in what contexts, and at what points during the life course? In what ways do determinants of health interact with one another? The conventional approach to understanding determinants of health has been to conceptualize them as separate, temporally bounded categories. Connell (2012, 1667) terms this "a categorical approach" and argues that "Regrettably, much of the 'intersectionality' literature simply combines a categorical approach to one dimension of difference with a categorical approach to another. This adds little to an understanding of social dynamics." Admittedly, this is how general determinants of health were presented to you in Chapter 4. First, we briefly considered biology and then moved to lifestyle behavioural factors, followed by environmental factors, and, finally, the use of formal health-care services. While such a presentation makes sense for teaching and learning purposes, as Connell and other intersectional theorists point out, the determinants of health are not, in reality, reducible to separate categories. Rather, it is possible to understand the determinants of health as "complex social locations that shape the experience of health in important ways" (Hedwig 2007, 1). Furthermore, the timing of the experience of structures of inequality, such as socioeconomic status, gender, and ethnicity, also matters. Hankivsky (2014, 10) explains that "Intersectionality emphasizes the importance of time and space . . . privileges and disadvantages, including intersecting identities and the processes that determine their value, change over time and place." This is why it is necessary to develop an intersectional model if we are to unravel the mystery of health as it unfolds across the life course.

Hankivsky and Christoffersen (2008, 276) maintain that "intersectionality challenges dominant analyses of health determinants by revealing how to better conceptualize the cumulative, interlocking dynamics that affect human experiences, including human health." In this way, characteristic of feminist methodology, intersectional health research crosses the broad societal level of patriarchal domination and the individual level of the lived experiences of women. This means that, according to the perspective offered by intersectional analysis, health outcomes are produced by combined and overlapping structures of inequality. As Oxman-Martinez and Hanley (2005, 4) elaborate, "Health disparities must be understood within a context of intersecting domains of inclusion, exclusion and inequality." Sources of inequalities such as position on the social gradient and those based on gender, ethnicity, or age can overlap, placing disadvantaged individuals at multiple jeopardy for poor health outcomes.

Intersectional analysis is an approach that employs mixed-methods research to study factors interacting across the macro and micro levels of social analysis based on the realization that each of us occupies different social locations and has varying life chances throughout the course of our lives. Returning to the example of an older Aboriginal woman living in poverty, an intersectional analysis of health would realize that her gender is one factor alongside other factors such as Aboriginality and socioeconomic status, all of which contribute to her lived experience of health as she ages. Bauer (2014, 11) points out that "the intersectional approach assumes that an individual's experience, and their health, are not simply the sum of their parts, and that, for example, what it means to be a woman and what the health implications are, may be different for Aboriginal women versus non-Aboriginal women." This means that the entirety of an older Aboriginal woman's social location must be taken into account to understand the health disparities that affect her. Hankivsky and Cormier (2009, 5) explain that "At the core of an intersectional model is the understanding that individuals occupy complex and dynamic social locations, where specific identities can be more or less salient depending on the historical or situational context." In the case of the older Aboriginal woman, factors such as gender, Aboriginality, socioeconomic status, and age all affect her pursuit of health and wellness. Further, from a life course perspective, the timing of exposure to sources of inequality matters, with certain points in the life course (e.g., childhood) being particularly vulnerable to sources of inequality. Intersectional researchers believe that in order to understand how differing social locations affect aspects of lived experience, such as disparities in health, a theoretical understanding of these intersections needs to be developed. As we learned in Chapter 6, intersectional analysis has been especially important in feminist analyses of inequality.

It is possible to trace the conceptual origins of intersectional analysis to the wave of thought that characterized the feminist paradigm beginning in the 1960s, which argued that women could not be reduced to a single homogeneous category united in difference from men. Instead, feminist researchers argued that women are a very diverse social group characterized by a multitude of socioeconomic, ethnic, and other differences in social location. At the same time, the newly emerging women's health movement "aimed to take bodies back from the institutions of medicine and reframe knowledge and experience in ways not configured by sexism and androcentrism" (Tuana 2006, 2). Following on these feminist ideas, intersectional researchers argue that "because gender differences and inequities in any particular time and place combine with the effects of other forms of social division such as class and ethnicity, not all women or all men experience gender or gender-related health problems or issues in the same way" (Hankivsky and Christoffersen 2008, 277).

The feminist realization that women with diverse social locations face inequality in different ways and have different lived experiences prompted social scientists to adopt a new way of thinking about inequality and disparities in health. Intersectional analysis sees socially constructed categories of class, gender, ethnicity, and age as interacting over time in dynamic fashion across the macro and micro levels. Describing the research methods employed by intersectional analysis, Hankivsky and Cormier (2009, 21) contend that "this approach prioritizes the use of a mix of methods to realize the demands of a multi-dimensional research analysis." Mixed-method research designs, employing both qualitative and quantitative methods, are necessary in order to understand the many intersecting dimensions of social location and health (Fries 2009).

Intersectional analysis argues that in order to understand how society affects health, we need to move from describing inequalities based on socioeconomic status, gender, ethnicity, and age separately to developing theories that allow us to understand their lifelong, complex intersections. Referring to the familiar epidemiological triad of agent, host, and environment, Cockerham (2007, 10) explains the central role played by health lifestyles in an intersectional understanding of health disparities by noting that "Health-related lifestyles are of particular relevance as a social mechanism producing positive or negative health outcomes. Such lifestyles have multiple roles in that they function as a collective pattern of behavior (agent) that is normative (environment) for the individual (host)." In order to understand the intersectionality of health disparities, researchers need to understand the central role played by lifestyle behaviours in such inequalities. This is because health lifestyles act as a bridge connecting the macro level of social structures with the micro level of individual experience and behaviour. In the next section, we will look at the relationship between lifestyle behaviours and health.

Lifestyle Behaviours and Health

Chapter 4 identified lifestyle behaviours as one of the four major determinants of health. Doubtless, behaviours such as smoking, alcohol and drug abuse, lack of exercise, eating high-fat and sugary foods, and having unprotected sex can make you sick. According to the World Health Organization (2014c), diseases linked to unhealthy lifestyles, such as heart and lung diseases, stroke, cancer, and diabetes, are responsible for 16 million premature deaths worldwide. In Canada, there is an abundance of evidence concerning the relationship between lifestyle behaviours and population health status. Population health surveys, such as the *Canadian Community Health Survey* (CCHS), collect a great deal of information about lifestyle behaviours that are recognized to be determinants of health. Reviewing this data supports the conclusion that approximately half of all Canadian deaths are related to unhealthy behaviours, including smoking, alcohol abuse, infrequent exercise, obesity, and unsafe sex!

Smoking

Despite declining smoking rates, this unhealthy behaviour remains one of the most important causes of illness and premature death in Canada. In 2013, 19.3 per cent of Canadians were smokers, compared to 22 per cent in 2005 and 26 per cent in 2001 (Statistics Canada 2014b). While the prevalence of smoking continues to decline, Reid and colleagues (2015) report that this decline appears to be slowing. The decrease in the rate of smoking was observed for both men and women and across all age groups, though smoking has been declining more among men than among women. While smoking has been declining in the Canadian population as a whole, one disturbing finding is that the highest prevalence rates are found among young adults (between the ages of 20 and 35). In 2013, 17.9 per cent of 20- to 24-four-year-olds and 18.5 per cent of those between the ages of 24 and 35 were current smokers despite the known health risks (Reid et al. 2015). While among adult smokers more men than women smoke (16.0 per cent of men and 13.3 per cent of women), this gender difference narrows among those under the age of 25. Smoking among young women in particular has important implications for population health. It not only directly affects the health of the women themselves, but smoking (as well as alcohol use) during pregnancy has been linked to lower birth weights and other negative birth outcomes. In other words, children born under these circumstances begin life at a disadvantage. As the life course perspective makes clear, the negative effects of early life events are sometimes not evident until much later in life. As with many lifestyle behaviours, serious and wide-reaching health outcomes result from smoking. Baliunas and colleagues (2007) found that smoking accounted for 16.6 per cent of all deaths in Canada in 2002 and that 515,608 years of life were lost prematurely in that year because of smoking!

Alcohol Use

While there are health benefits associated with the consumption of moderate amounts of alcohol, "for most people, more than two drinks a day does more harm than good" (Rehm, Geisbretch, et al. 2006, 79). The World Health Organization (2014c) notes that 5.1 per cent of the global burden of disease and 5.9 per cent of all deaths globally were attributed to alcohol. This prompted the Sixty-Third World Health Assembly of the WHO held in May 2010 to pass a resolution calling for governments around the world to control the negative health consequences of alcohol. Canadian researchers have documented the relationship between alcohol and negative health effects. For example, Rehm and colleagues (2006, 3) note that "Alcohol has the highest prevalence of consumption in the Canadian population among psychoactive substances. The vast majority of adult Canadians (almost 80 percent of the population aged 15 and above) consumed alcohol within the last year.... About 21 percent of Canadians reported drinking above the low risk guidelines." The health benefits associated with moderate consumption of alcohol have mainly to do with the beneficial effects on cardiovascular health. However, as Rehm and colleagues (2006) note, age is highly correlated with the amount of alcohol consumed, with light to moderate drinking occurring mostly among those in older age groups. Additionally, the health benefits of alcohol apply mainly to people over the age of 45 (Rehm, Patra, and Popova 2006). While the social and health benefits associated with alcohol consumption are modest, what cannot be denied is the clear evidence that alcohol is also related to numerous social and health costs, such as accidents, violence, criminality, disease, death, and disability. As illustration, Rehm, Patra, and Popova (2006) note that more than 60 causes of death have been attributed to alcohol consumption. Shield and colleagues (2012) find that alcohol accounted for 7.7 per cent of deaths in Canada among those under 65 years of age in 2005 and that 134,555 years of life were lost prematurely in that year because of alcohol. These findings prompted the researchers to declare that "alcohol is clearly a major contributor to mortality and potential years of life lost, and has a significant public health impact in Canada" (2012, 9).

Physical Activity

Another lifestyle behaviour that has been consistently linked to health is participation in leisure-time physical activity. Research has established that the single best lifestyle behaviour contributing to good health is regular physical activity (e.g., Frankish, Milligan, and Reid 1998).

Activities such as walking, jogging, exercising, and participating in sports have numerous benefits for physical and mental well-being. Regular physical activity is the single best thing you can do for your health! Despite the well-known health benefits of active living, 3.2 million deaths per year worldwide are attributable to insufficient physical activity (World Health Organization 2014c). "Globally, in 2010, 20% of adult men and 27% of adult women did not meet WHO recommendations on physical activity for health. Amongst adolescents, aged 11–17 years, 78% of boys and 84% of girls did not meet these recommendations." Unfortunately, at least half of Canadians are inactive, and 85 per cent of adults do not meet the latest physical activity guidelines of 150 minutes per week of moderate-to-vigorous physical activity accumulated in at least 10-minute bouts (Colley et al. 2011). The rules of thumb provided by health researchers are clear: Your total weekly physical activity should amount to two and a half hours of moderate-to-vigorous physical activity spread throughout the week. Regardless, Janssen (2012) estimates that physical inactivity cost $6.8 billion, or 3.8 per cent of total health-care costs, in Canada in 2009! This leads him to conclude that "physical inactivity has surpassed epidemic proportions in Canada and accounts for a significant portion of health care spending" (2012, 806). More encouraging news is that there has been an increase over the past decade in the level of physical activity reported by Canadians.

To illustrate, many people who were classified as inactive (based on average daily physical activity) in the 1994 *National Population Health Survey* (NPHS) were classified as moderately active (an increase of 15 per cent) or active (an increase of 10 per cent) by 2006 (Gilmour 2007). Hurst (2009) finds that between 1992 and 2005, overall Canadian participation in active leisure increased from 20.9 per cent to 24.3 per cent. These are positive changes, since "even moderate levels of activity confer health benefits, and for most people, additional health benefits may be derived by becoming more active" (Frankish, Milligan, and Reid 1998, 287). Unfortunately, while most Canadians are engaging in more leisure-time physical activity, 8 per cent of Canadians still report no or very little physical activity, meaning that they have inactive leisure time, are sedentary during the workday, and walk or bicycle as a means of transportation less than two hours per week (Gilmour 2007). Perhaps not surprisingly, health researchers (e.g., James 2008; Sarma et al. 2014) have established a link between sedentary lifestyles and the obesity epidemic that plagues countries such as Canada.

Obesity

Canadians are getting fatter. Twells and colleagues (2014) report that "Between 1985 and 2011, the prevalence of adults in the overweight category increased by 21% from 27.8% to 33.6%, and the prevalence of obesity (BMI ≥ 30.0) increased 200% from 6.1% to 18.3%." These researchers point out that even more worrisome from a population health standpoint is that while all three classes of obesity increased over this period, the highest proportionate increases were seen in the higher obese classes. Based on their analysis of these trends, Twells and her co-researchers predict that by 2019, most (55.4 per cent) of the Canadian adult population will be categorized as overweight (34.2 per cent) or obese (21.2 per cent), the prevalence of obesity in classes I, II, and III will increase to 14.8 per cent, 4.4 per cent, and 2.0 per cent, respectively, and that half of the Canadian provinces will have more overweight or obese adults than normal-weight adults.

The Canadian increase in BMI mirrors an international trend of increasing body weight, the health consequences of which are now becoming apparent on a global scale. The World Health Organization (2014a, xiv) cautions that "Worldwide, the prevalence of obesity has nearly doubled since 1980. In 2014, 11% of men and 15% of women aged 18 years and older were obese. More than 42 million children under the age of 5 years were overweight in 2013." The BMI is a measure for

Box 8.1 Slurpee Capital of the World . . .

To commemorate Manitoba's sixteenth consecutive year of being named the Slurpee Capital of the World, staff of the 7-Eleven convenience store chain create the world's largest Slurpee drink at 711 litres in the parking lot of the 7-Eleven store at 119 Salter Street, Winnipeg.

Once again, Manitoba has had the dubious distinction of being named "the Slurpee Capital of the World" for consuming the most of the sugary frozen drink per capita. 7-Eleven Canada will not disclose how many Slurpees were consumed to win the title, citing confidentiality. What is not confidential is that in 2008–9, approximately 2.4 million Canadians, or 6.8 percent of the nation's population, had diabetes (Public Health Agency of Canada 2011). According to the Public Health Agency of Canada (2011, 96), "a diet high in sugar, fat, or processed foods has contributed to increased overweight, obesity and risk of diabetes." The agency notes that obese adults are two to four times more likely to have type 2 diabetes. The World Health Organization (2014a) notes that policies and interventions that have proved effective in various countries around the globe for reducing the prevalence of obesity and diabetes include: agricultural subsidies to encourage the production and consumption of fruits and vegetables; "junk food taxes" on foods high in sugar, salt, and caffeine; and regulating the marketing of foods and non-alcoholic beverages to children. What additional measures can you think of to reduce the prevalence of obesity and diabetes?

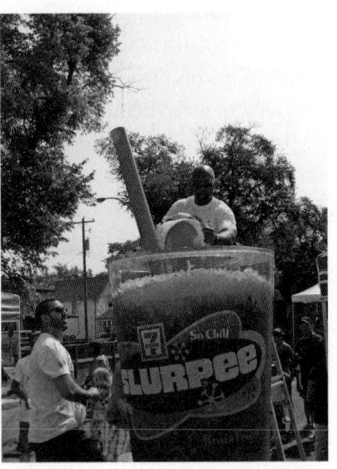

---

classifying human weight and assessing health risks. While it is known that obesity is linked to a host of negative health outcomes, including high blood pressure, diabetes, joint problems, cardiovascular disease, and cancer, it is also apparent that from a sociological perspective, diagnostic cut-off points for "normal" BMI are socially constructed. The BMI is a measure of human weight that is subject to controversy. Describing the complex social and political history of the BMI, James (2008, 338) notes that "one also has to recognize that all the choices of cutoffs—whether for designating hypertension, glucose tolerance or hyperlipidaemia (i.e., obesity)—are very arbitrary."

While diagnostic criteria may be culturally arbitrary, there is widespread consensus among health researchers that we are facing a global epidemic of obesity: "Although the epidemic of obesity really started to increase markedly in the 1980s it is only since 1997 that WHO and many national governments have recognized the importance of obesity as a major public health problem affecting both the developed and the developing world" (James 2008, 341). In Canada, despite a widespread cultural desire to be thin, the age-adjusted obesity rate increased from 13.8 per cent measured in the 1978–9 *Canada Health Survey* to 23.1 per cent of Canadians by the time of the 2004 CCHS. Tjepkema (2005, 3) notes that "the obesity rate of every age group except 65 to 74 rose during this period. The most striking increases were among people younger than 35 and 75 or older. For instance, the percentage of 25 to 34 year olds who were obese more than doubled, rising from 8.5 percent in 1978–1979 to 20.5 percent in 2004. The extent of the increase among people aged 75 or older was about the same: from 10.6 percent to 23.6 percent." Le Petit and Berthelot (2006) found that nearly a third of NPHS respondents who were classified as having normal weight in the 1994–5 survey had become overweight by the 2002–3 wave of the survey and approximately a quarter of those who were overweight in 1994–5 had become obese by the time of the follow-up survey. The study also showed that only about 10 per cent of those who were overweight in 1994–5 had managed to return to a normal BMI after eight years. Particularly worrisome is that the prevalence of childhood obesity is increasing, with data from the *Canadian National Longitudinal Survey of Children and Youth* showing that 19 per cent of children aged 2 to 11 were overweight and 18 per cent were obese (Hejazi et al. 2009). In his overview of the public health burden of obesity in Canada, Janssen (2013, 96) sums up these statistics by noting that "At present, approximately 8 million Canadians are obese, which represents 26% of adults and 12% of school-aged children" and that "Obesity places a large economic burden on the country, accounting for $3.9 billion in direct health care costs and $3.2 billion in indirect costs in 2006." Clearly, obesity is another lifestyle behaviour that has far-reaching health consequences across the life course.

Explanations for the obesity epidemic include physical inactivity, shifts toward high-fat and sugary processed foods (as illustrated by Box 8.1), the design of the built environment, and perpetuation of medical consumerism and consumer culture (Oliver 2005). These factors combine with human biology to produce an "obesogenic environment" (James 2008, 347) in which all but a few are guaranteed to gain weight. Starky (2005, 7) explains that "the problem of overweight and obesity should be framed in the context of a population health approach which considers and acts upon the broad range of factors and conditions that have a strong influence on body weight." James (2008, 347) concludes by explaining the intersectional nature of the policy and practice response that is required to address the obesity epidemic: "The problem is so severe that an overwhelming medical crisis is inevitable unless the problem is seen as a huge multidimensional issue which requires everybody to change their policies and practice. This means that it is no longer reasonable to simply specify the individual changes needed but now every branch of society has to be involved if we are to avoid an overwhelming financial and societal burden." Obesity provides a clear example of the intersectional nature of health disparities that cannot be addressed through a focus on the lifestyle behaviours of individuals.

Unsafe Sex

Human sexuality is a key aspect of the pursuit of health and wellness. However, unsafe sexual practices such as unprotected sex, early age at time of first intercourse, and promiscuity can harm health, increasing the risk of sexually transmitted infections and unwanted pregnancies. The Public Health Agency of Canada (2015) reports that since the late 1990s, sexually transmitted infections of chlamydia, gonorrhea, and syphilis continue to rise despite extensive public health campaigns. Between 2003 and 2012, rates of reported cases of chlamydia increased by 57.6 per cent, gonorrhea by 38.9 per cent, and syphilis by 101 per cent. While rates of HIV/AIDS have gradually declined since 2008, 2090 new cases were reported in 2013, representing a slight decrease from the 2099 cases reported in 2012 and the lowest number of annual infections since reporting began in 1985 (Public Health Agency of Canada 2014). Intersecting forms of social exclusion based on socioeconomic inequality, gender, ethnicity, and sexual orientation overlap to shape individual risks of sexually transmitted infection. McKay (2004) cautions that Canadian youth and young adults are the group most at risk of sexually transmitted infection. Using data from the CCHS, Rotterman (2012) found that 9 per cent of 15- to 24-year-olds reported first-time sexual intercourse at an age younger than 15, 35 per cent of those aged 15 to 17 years reported having had sexual intercourse with more than one partner in the previous 12 months, and 20 per cent in this age group did not use condoms during their most recent sexual intercourse. A study of teenagers and mothers of teenagers found that 69 per cent of teens could not find the sexual health information they were looking for and 62 per cent reported obstacles in obtaining information on healthy sexual practices (Frappier et al. 2008).

Given the abundance of evidence regarding the link between lifestyle behaviours and health, you might wonder what the big mystery is when it comes to the pursuit of health and wellness. People just need to be responsible and avoid these unhealthy behaviours or change their behaviour so that they live healthy lifestyles in order to be healthy, right? This apparently straightforward solution forms the basis of the individualized health promotion response to disparities in health. The next section will show that there are problems with this line of reasoning, which means that individualized health promotion is not the solution to the mystery of health or an effective means to address health disparities.

Individualized Health Promotion

Since the 1970s, the promotion of healthy lifestyles has become official and highly visible public policy in societies such as Canada. In an early article, Kickbusch (1986, 118) noted that "there is almost no agreement either in theory or practice as to what constitutes a 'lifestyle.'" Despite this fact, lifestyle is a concept that remains popular in health research and in health promotion campaigns. Simply stated, **lifestyle** refers to a way of life or a style of living that reflects the beliefs, attitudes, and values of the individual and the groups to which she belongs, as well as patterns of behaviour that are shaped by life circumstances and socio-cultural context. Lifestyles, thus, consist of a number of different components but essentially focus our attention on socially and culturally determined health-related behavioural patterns. Sociological analysis suggests that a process of change is occurring and that healthy lifestyles are an increasingly important component in both everyday life and official government strategies for population health promotion (Baum and Fisher 2014). This focus on individualized health promotion has aptly been described as an instance of "lifestyle drift": "the tendency for policy initiatives on tackling health inequalities to start off with a broad recognition of the need to take action on the wider social determinants of health (upstream), but which, in the course of implementation, drift downstream to focus largely on individual lifestyle factors" (Hunter et al. 2009, 3). A deceptively simple and, as it turns out, inaccurate idea has guided the increasing tendency of government efforts to promote population health by raising health consciousness: this idea takes evidence concerning the relationship between lifestyle behaviours and health as its starting point and concludes that the best way to improve population health is by promoting healthy lifestyles.

Based on a belief in the connection between individual health consciousness and preventive health behaviour, governments use health promotion campaigns to increase both our personal level of health consciousness and general public awareness of the importance of engaging in health-protective behaviours. The idea is that this will encourage individuals to engage in healthy

Box 8.2 An Example of Health Promotion

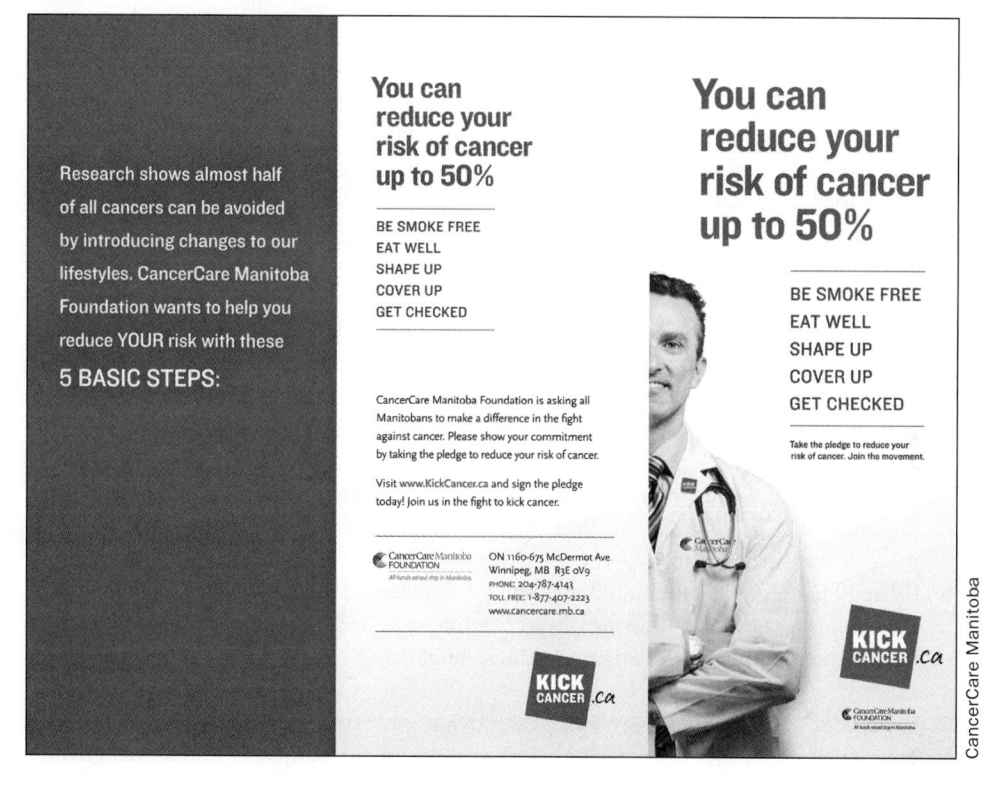

Research shows almost half of all cancers can be avoided by introducing changes to our lifestyles. CancerCare Manitoba Foundation wants to help you reduce YOUR risk with these **5 BASIC STEPS:**

You can reduce your risk of cancer up to 50%

BE SMOKE FREE
EAT WELL
SHAPE UP
COVER UP
GET CHECKED

CancerCare Manitoba Foundation is asking all Manitobans to make a difference in the fight against cancer. Please show your commitment by taking the pledge to reduce your risk of cancer.

Visit www.KickCancer.ca and sign the pledge today! Join us in the fight to kick cancer.

CancerCare Manitoba FOUNDATION
ON 1160-675 McDermot Ave.
Winnipeg, MB R3E 0V9
PHONE: 204-787-4143
TOLL FREE: 1-877-407-2223
www.cancercare.mb.ca

KICK CANCER.ca

You can reduce your risk of cancer up to 50%

BE SMOKE FREE
EAT WELL
SHAPE UP
COVER UP
GET CHECKED

Take the pledge to reduce your risk of cancer. Join the movement.

KICK CANCER.ca

CancerCare Manitoba

The Kick Cancer campaign emphasizes that by engaging in these five behavioural lifestyle practices Manitobans can reduce their risk of cancer up to 50%.

A review demonstrated that such mass media campaigns to encourage physical activity do not work; people remember the advertisements but don't change their behaviour (Marcus et al. 1998). Sociologically, we are forced to ask what other reasons might government-funded agencies such as CancerCare Manitoba have for undertaking such health promotion campaigns?

behaviours, which together are supposed to form healthy lifestyles. In turn, it is hoped that this will lead to improved population health. Thus, **health promotion** is a state-sponsored process aimed at getting people to take control over and improve their health by providing health-related education and information. Box 8.2 provides an example of a recent health promotion campaign. In evaluating lifestyle-focused health promotion, we need to ask two interrelated questions: First, are healthy lifestyles really a matter of individual choice? Second, is there such a thing as a healthy lifestyle? The answers provided by health research conducted from a sociological perspective might surprise you.

The Individualization of Health Lifestyles

Providing citizens with information and advice to help them look after their health and wellness seems like a sensible thing for governments to do. However, the sociological imagination enables health sociologists to challenge this common-sense assumption, pointing out that the current political focus on individual responsibility for health, described as "the new public health" (Petersen and Lupton 1996), differs from older public health measures enacted by governments to promote the health of their citizens. By focusing on upstream determinants of health such as affordable housing, safe workplaces, unpolluted water and air, and affordable, nutritious food, early public health initiatives tried to provide citizens with the material conditions conducive to good health. With the neo-liberal attack on the welfare state, these old strategies of public health have given way to a newly individualized public health promotion that creates an "imperative of health" (Lupton 1995) through which individuals are encouraged to become health-conscious medical consumers, paying attention to health risks in their individual behaviour. Individuals are held personally accountable for adoption of so-called healthy lifestyles or blamed for the failure to do so should their health suffer.

Rose (1999, 86–7) offers the following description of the pursuit of health under the new public health:

> In the new modes of regulating health, individuals are addressed on the assumption that they *want to be healthy*, and enjoined to freely seek out the ways of living most likely to promote their own health. Experts instruct us as to how to be healthy, advertisers picture the appropriate actions and fulfilments and entrepreneurs develop this market for health. Individuals are now offered an identity as consumers—offered an image and a set of practical relations to the self and others [original emphasis].

Rather than as "citizens," the new public health treats us as "consumers"; we are supposed to be vigilant of risks to our health and actively seek out information, products, and services that we are to use in the individualized pursuit of health and wellness. Healthy living has become synonymous with buying the "right" products and services to look after the body. Box 8.3 provides an illustration of the new public health message.

Cockerham (2000, 160) explains that the theoretical perspectives that inform the new public health originate within psychology (e.g., the health belief model and the stages of change model) and, as a consequence, lead to the individualization of health lifestyles: "The standard public health approach treats health behavior and lifestyles as matters of individual choice and targets the individual to change his or her harmful health practices largely through education." This approach to population health promotion meshes well with other beliefs that characterize neo-liberalism, such as ideas concerning the importance of personal autonomy and individual responsibility. Within our culture, it is taken for granted that health is a personal matter. Working from a political economy perspective, however, health sociologists point out how this individualization of health lifestyles leads to blaming the victim for her health problems. In turn, this serves to let governments off the hook when it comes to ensuring that they provide citizens with material conditions necessary for good health: "If you become sick, it isn't because of society, it's because of your own bad choices." As illustration, consider the excerpt from a *Maclean's* article presented in Box 8.4.

When it comes to lifestyle behaviours, arguments such as those illustrated in Köhler and Righton's *Maclean's* article are examples of commonplace misconceptions. You often hear that

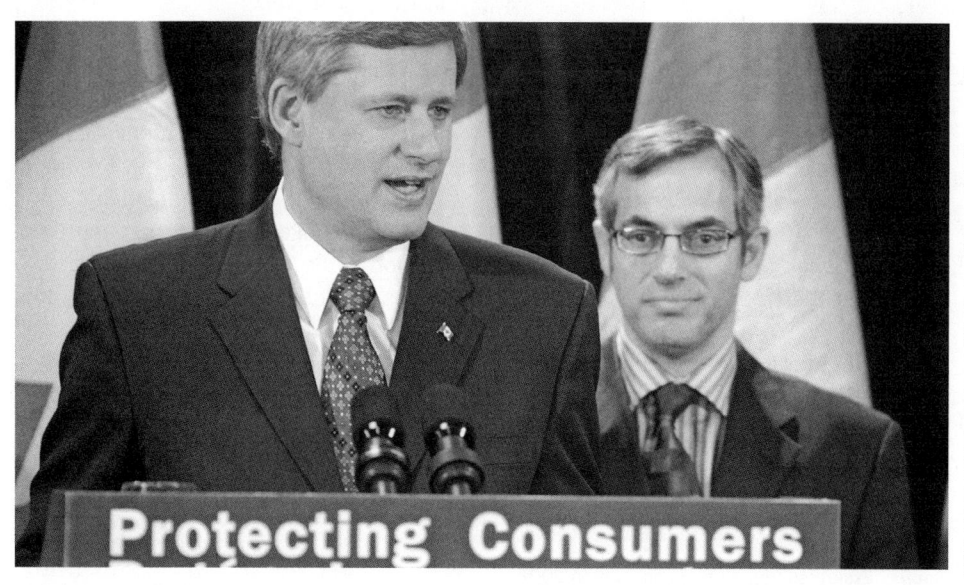

Box 8.3 "The New Public Health"

Former prime minister Stephen Harper announces changes to Canada's food and product safety laws, 8 April 2008. The press release from the Prime Minister's Office reads, in part, "Public access to information about product safety would also be improved, giving Canadians more control over their own health protection." Notice that the podium sign does not read "Protecting Canadians" or "Protecting Citizens." Under the new public health, citizens are transformed into consumers who are individually responsible for their health.

individuals can freely choose pathogenic or salutogenic behaviours. However, such politically loaded beliefs ignore the sociological insight that lifestyle choices are influenced by our social location. Whether people smoke, abuse alcohol, are sedentary, eat poorly, or practise unsafe sex reflects, to a great extent, broad social determinants such as how much money you have to spend on food, your exposure to mass media and popular culture, how your educational background equips you to understand mixed messages and conflicting information about health, the type of environment in which you live and work, and what stage of the life course you are in. Researchers have known for some time that health risk behaviours follow the social gradient! This is true for smoking (Poland et al. 2006), alcoholism (Rehm, Geisbrecht, et al. 2006), physical inactivity and sedentary behaviour (Gilmour 2007; Hurst 2009; Nandi, Glymour, and Subramanian 2014), diets lacking in nutrition (Ricciuto and Tarasuk 2007), obesity (Janssen 2013), and pretty much any unhealthy behaviour:

> Overall, the lifestyles of the upper and upper-middle classes are the healthiest. Virtually every study confirms this. These classes have the highest participation in leisure-time

Box 8.4 Overeaters, Smokers, and Drinkers: The Doctor Won't See You Now

At issue: health care for patients with self-destructive vices—overeating, smoking, drinking or drugs. More and more doctors are turning them away or knocking them down their waiting lists—whether patients know that's the reason or not. Frightening stories abound. GPs who won't take smokers as patients. Surgeons who demand obese patients lose weight before they'll operate, or tell them to find another doctor. Transplant teams who turn drinkers down flat. Doctors say their decisions make sense: why spend thousands of dollars on futile procedures? Or the decision is the product of frustration: why not make patients accountable for their vices? Others call it simple discrimination. But in a health system with more patients than doctors can treat, where doctors have discretion over whom they'll take on, some say it's inevitable that problem patients will get shunted aside in favour of healthier, less labour-intensive cases.

So here's the question: if people won't stop hurting themselves, can they really expect the same medical treatment as everyone else? Health care in Canada is supposed to be about equal treatment for all comers. For some doctors, however, there are patients who are less equal than others.

Source: Excerpted from Köhler and Righton 2006.

---

sports and exercise, healthier diets, moderate drinking, little smoking, more physical checkups by physicians, and greater opportunities for rest, relaxation, and coping with stress. The upper and upper-middle classes are also the first to have knowledge of new health risks and, because of greater resources, are most able to adopt new health strategies and practices (Cockerham 2007, 62).

To answer the question concerning whether lifestyles are a matter of individual choice, research clearly shows that lifestyle behaviours are linked to structures of inequality and are formed by locations in the social structure, such as socioeconomic status, gender, ethnicity, and age. The social gradient is not explained by differences in lifestyle behaviours or individual lifestyle choices. Since the Whitehall Studies (discussed in Chapter 5), researchers have known that what is typically considered "lifestyle" accounts for only one-third of the difference in disease rates between those at the top of society and those at the bottom. Restated, when lifestyle choices such as smoking, drinking, physical activity, and diet are controlled for in studies of the social patterning of illness and disease, they account for less than one-third of the difference in rates of disease! This means that health disparities cannot be addressed through an individualized lifestyle focus. Frohlich, Corin, and Potvin (2001, 784) offer the following critique of the conceptualization of lifestyle underlying individualized health promotion: "The individual is seen to be ultimately responsible for her/his behaviour as if there were no systemic influences, sociocultural context, or social meaning ascribed to the behaviour. This has led to an understanding of lifestyle that views the individual in a sort of behavioural vacuum; outside sociocultural influences, struggling to master her/his vices."

Despite such sociologically informed criticism, victim-blaming is still prevalent in the media and popular culture (see Box 8.4). This perspective continues to assert that lifestyle factors are the major cause of illness and disease, especially among the lower social classes. This individualization of the causes of illness takes the focus off the ways in which structures of inequality contribute to poor health.

Evidence from studies of social class and health lifestyles (e.g., Blaxter 1990; Dumas, Robitaille, and Jette 2014) suggests that the experience of social exclusion thwarts the adoption of healthy lifestyles. Bearing the weight of structural inequalities such as unsafe living and working conditions undermines sense of coherence while engendering powerlessness and lack of control. The result is that those who are socially excluded have much less success in adopting healthy lifestyle practices, and their health suffers as a result. This is exactly what studies of the social gradient in health show. Cockerham (2000, 169) summarizes this by noting that "Overall, it would appear that . . . disadvantaged life chances reduce the opportunities for positive health behaviours or reduce their effectiveness." Additionally, the research of Macintyre and colleagues (Macintyre, McKay, and Ellaway 2005, 313) has shown that "those at risk of ill health may be less likely to acknowledge the social gradient of health." Those who suffer poor health outcomes attributable to social exclusion are the most likely to internalize public health discourses of individual responsibility for health and accept personal blame for their illnesses. This somewhat counterintuitive finding is made easier to understand in light of the insights of Bourdieu's sociological theory. In his analysis of the perpetuation of class-based inequalities through consumption, Bourdieu (1984, 177) points out that the experience of social exclusion transforms structures of inequality into a fatalistic self-fulfilling prophecy because of the way lower social classes come to understand structures of inequality in a manner that embodies "a virtue made of necessity," making their oppression seem inevitable. Research by Dumas, Robitaille, and Jette (2014, 15) used Bourdieu's theory to explore the issue of habit versus choice in the health behaviours of young underprivileged women. They conclude that "The concepts of habitus, practical sense and 'choice of the necessary' show the complexity of understanding lifestyles by calling attention to the limitations of knowledge-based or strictly individual approaches to behaviour modifications." Such research (see also Lindbladh and Lyttkens 2002) has clearly established the futility of individualized health promotion in the face of structures of inequality.

Research shows that health promotion directed at the modification of individual lifestyle behaviours is unsuccessful at producing either lifestyle changes or improvements in population health. Simply stated, the notion that population health can be improved through the promotion of healthy lifestyles is, at best, misguided. At worst, it amounts to blaming the victim. Social epidemiologists have shown that interventions directed toward encouraging individuals to modify unhealthy behaviours by providing health information have consistently failed. Describing the results of "the largest, most ambitious, and most expensive experiment ever designed to see if by getting people to change high risk behaviours, the coronary heart disease death rate could be reduced"—the Multiple Risk Factor Intervention Trial (MRFIT)—renowned social epidemiologist Leonard Syme (see Box 8.5) states that "The message from this extreme example is very clear and well-known: it is very difficult for people to change high risk behaviours even when they really want to and even when every effort is made to help them" (1994, 80).

Hansen and Easthope (2007) explain that despite the success of social epidemiology in demonstrating that lifestyle behaviours and their health effects are socially patterned by structures of inequality, population health promotion approaches focused on individual risk factors are a mainstay of the new public health. Abel (2007, 44) calls our attention to the fact that not

> **Box 8.5** Leonard Syme (1932–)
>
> - Considered the "father of social epidemiology" because of his landmark studies of social determinants of health and health inequity, such as the Multiple Risk Factor Intervention Trial (MRFIT) study
> - Researches psychosocial risk factors such as job stress, social support, poverty, and social inequalities in health
>
> "As individuals, we are ultimately responsible for our own health and our own behaviour. But it is naïve to think that we are free agents in this. All of us are influenced by forces in the community that shape our choices and preferences" (1994, 82).

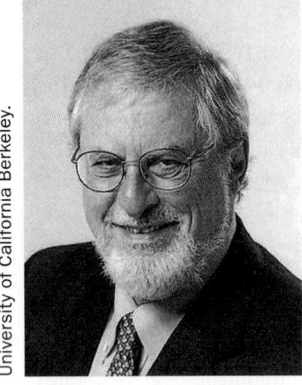

only are health disparities socially produced, leading to the perpetuation of social inequality, but also that the conditions that make people healthy are socially produced:

> In the social epidemiological tradition, it is the social inequality in the "distribution of illness" rather than social inequality in the "production of health" on which public health research and policy seems to be concentrated. It is therefore time to push further with a new focus on the distribution of health rather than disease and to include in our theories explanations of social inequalities in the means for producing health at the societal and the individual level.

Abel points out that the societal contributions to producing health are overlooked in most research. In keeping with the transformation of the field from medical sociology to health sociology, it is necessary to direct research toward understanding how people with advantaged social locations produce health through healthy lifestyle behaviours. The sociological imagination allows us to understand that rather than saying some individuals have unhealthy lifestyles, it is more accurate to say that our society is itself unhealthy. Because of social exclusion, some members of society are more vulnerable to this unhealthy culture than others are.

Extensive studies have shown that it is almost impossible for people to change their lifestyles in the absence of changes to their social environment. Research shows that people change their health behaviour not when encouraged to do so through education or mass media campaigns but, rather, when made to do so through aspects of the social context such as legal and structural measures. The clearest illustration of this comes from efforts to decrease smoking. Cockerham (2007, 2) notes that "smoking is associated with more diseases than any other health-related lifestyle practice." But you already know that: research shows that more than 85 per cent of Canadians, smokers and non-smokers alike, know that smoking causes disease (Siahpush et al. 2006). Awareness of the negative health consequences of smoking is not, however, what has produced the most dramatic decreases in smoking rates among Canadians. Health promotion campaigns that focus on informing people of the already widely known health risks associated with smoking don't get people to quit smoking. Rather, it was when smoking became a highly stigmatized, inconvenient, and expensive activity that smoking rates began marked decline. These social changes were brought about by changes in public policy, such as bans against smoking in public and in workplaces and tax increases on tobacco products (Kreindler 2008). What the smoking example shows us is that the most effective to change unhealthy lifestyle behaviours is to change the social environments that produce them in the first place. Money spent by health promotion campaigns aimed at raising individual health consciousness would be better spent on addressing the upstream social determinants of health. Public policy can encourage healthy behaviour by making that behaviour easier, cheaper, and more convenient than less healthy choices (Kreindler 2008).

In summary, those with disadvantaged social locations are more likely to adopt health risk behaviours as a means of coping with their difficult social circumstances. As Walters (2003, 3) explains, "Such 'unhealthy' lifestyles are culturally appropriate responses to the social context that prompts depression and despair." Furthermore, lifestyle practices such as smoking or eating habits that are established at an early age are resistant to change. The health consequences of lifestyle behaviours such as smoking or overeating may not become fully apparent until later. In other words, we need to adopt an intersectional perspective to fully appreciate the complex ways in which lifestyle behaviours function as health determinants across the life course. We will return to this topic later in the chapter when we present an intersectional model of health and health lifestyles across the life course, but before doing this, we need to take a critical look at the research concerning health behaviours and health lifestyles.

Remennick (1998, 27) explains the belief about individual responsibility for health that underlies the new public health: "The premise behind this type of thinking is that people get sick or injured and die prematurely not because of their lacking access to resources such as good housing, education and health care but due to self inflicted hazards like substance abuse, poor eating habits and violence." Explaining health outcomes by pointing to individual behaviour has a long history. As Hansen and Easthope (2007, 8) explain, "Relationships between the ways people live and the illnesses they develop have always been a focus for healers, western and non-western." What is novel about the new public health is the moral imperative that personal responsibility for health has taken on in our culture. Research informed by the sociology of the body paradigm has shown how, in our culture, we judge people by the appearance of their bodies and how they treat their bodies (e.g., Giddens 1991). Everybody is encouraged to reflect upon the conditions of bodily existence, especially health lifestyles. This accounts for the popularity of television shows such as "The Biggest Loser." The imperative of health has become a spectator sport, with those who manage to discipline their bodies through bodily regimens of diet and exercise among our culture's biggest winners! However, the sociological imagination forces us to step outside of this ethnocentrism, allowing us to see that "health lifestyles are not just matters of individual psychology, but a form of behavior grounded in social structure and societal influences" (Cockerham 2000, 160). Consider as illustration the unhealthy behaviour discussed in Box 8.6.

Based on neo-liberal ideas about individual responsibility for health, new public health promotion initiatives provide information to consumers intended to facilitate the development of healthy lifestyles. The rationale behind such health promotion strategies is simple: health is highly valued in our individualistic culture, and by providing individuals with information on how to stay healthy, governments promote healthy lifestyle behaviours among the population because once people know what behaviours are considered healthy, they should engage in these behaviours and good health will result. Unfortunately, while this line of reasoning might seem straightforward enough, a review of the latest statistics concerning the relationship between lifestyle behaviours

Box 8.6 Tanning Beds: A "Healthy" Glow?

According to the World Health Organization (Leading Edge 2009) tanning beds are a "category one carcinogen"—the highest cancer-causing risk (cigarettes are also in this category). In 2015, the Canadian Cancer Society estimated that 6800 Canadians would be diagnosed with melanoma (the most dangerous type of skin cancer) that year, with about 1150 resulting in death (Canadian Cancer Society Advisory Committee on Cancer Statistics 2015). The World Health Organization warns that in those under age 30, the use of tanning beds raises the risk of melanoma by 75 per cent. Do you engage in this unhealthy behaviour despite known health risks? If so, can you rightly be described as having a healthy lifestyle? If you tan and develop skin cancer, should you be blamed and denied medical care?

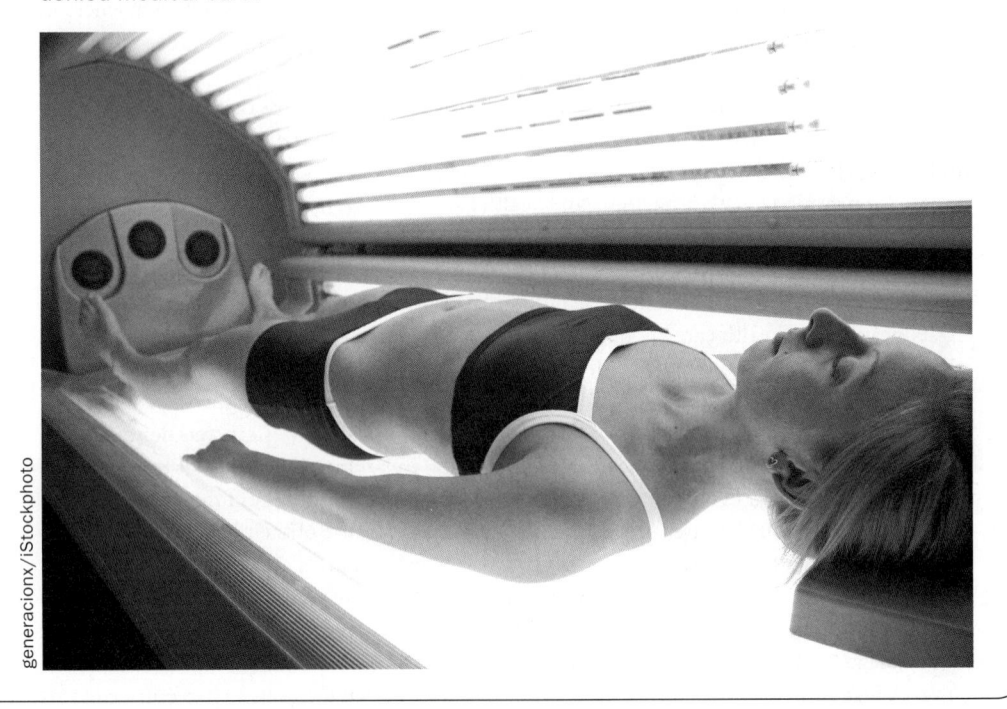

and population health shows that it is not. The practice of indoor tanning, discussed in Box 8.6, provides an example. It is well known that tanning increases the risk of skin cancer. Despite this, cultural standards of beauty make this unhealthy behaviour highly seductive in our society, especially among youth (Vannini and McCright 2004). Governments have endorsed an individualized approach to health promotion for the past four decades, yet the latest evidence indicates that approximately half of all Canadian deaths are related to unhealthy behaviours. Research on individualized health promotion shows that it doesn't work for the majority of the population and that it is especially ineffective among those who experience social exclusion. As Baum and Fisher (2014, 215) conclude, strategies of individualized health promotion "tend to assume that people are blank sheets ready to be receptive to health promotion messages. The reality is that people's lives reflect a range of factors, including their current social and economic resources, and risk factors are accumulated over the lifespan, with negative conditions in early life being particularly damaging." Further, research leads us to question whether there is such a thing as a "health lifestyle"!

Health Lifestyles or Health Behaviours?

Over several decades, health researchers (e.g., Calnan 1989; Harris and Guten 1979; Krick and Sobal 1990; Kronenfeld et al. 1988; Newsom et al. 2005) have tried to determine whether a set of personal health practices forms what could be understood as a "health lifestyle." The results of this research have important consequences for the new public health promotion, because if it is possible to demonstrate that there is such a thing as a coherent health lifestyle causally related to positive health outcomes, then it should theoretically be possible to improve population health by getting individuals to adopt healthy lifestyles. The general research strategy in this field of inquiry is to begin by measuring the frequency with which respondents engage in a variety of health behaviours similar to those in Box 8.7. The specific health behaviours vary from study to study but typically include personal health practices such as alcohol consumption, smoking, stress management, seat belt use, diet and nutritional intake, maintenance of proper weight, getting sufficient sleep, engaging in regular exercise, leisure activities, self-examination, and preventive medical and dental checkups. The number of specific health behaviours investigated ranges from four health behaviours (e.g., Newsom et al. 2005) to 18 health behaviours (Krick and Sobal 1990) to as many as 30 thirty health behaviours (Harris and Guten 1979).

After the number and type of personal health practices have been documented, the next step is generally a correlation analysis to test the strength (and significance) of the association between each of the individual health behaviours measured. A number of studies have taken the analysis one step further by subjecting the data collected on health behaviours to factor analysis. This is a statistical technique that helps to determine the degree to which these individual practices form clusters of related behaviours. In other words, the intent is to try to reduce the range of individual health practices measured to a limited number of interpretable dimensions or major types of health behaviour. Without getting lost in the statistical details of this research, the purpose of the following discussion is to highlight the key findings of studies that have investigated the degree to which health behaviours are part of an overall health lifestyle.

Steele and McBroom (1972), in an early study, examined the degree of association among a number of indicators of health behaviour (i.e., preventive actions such as physical checkups and dental visits) and found that consistent forms of behaviour were limited to a very small proportion of the respondents in their study. For the majority of respondents, analysis revealed that health behaviours are not mutually reinforcing. That is, just because individuals engaged in some health behaviours did not necessarily mean that they engaged in others. In their study, Mechanic and Cleary (1980, 808) report that health behaviours "were either independent of one another or only modestly correlated." Other studies report essentially the same findings. For example, Lau, Hartman, and Ware (1986, 37) examined the usual types of health behaviours and found that, consistent with prior research, "these preventive behaviors do not correlate very highly with each other" and, therefore, do not form a good summary scale. Kronenfeld et al. (1988, 322) report that results of correlation analysis revealed "only about a third of the interrelationships between the six habits were strong enough to reach statistical significance, and even then with only modest levels of correlation." They conclude that personal health practices do not represent a single

Box 8.7 A Healthy Lifestyle Self-Test

Respond to each of the following statements with a YES or NO based on the extent to which they apply to your health-related behaviour. Place a check mark next to each statement with a YES answer.

- ❏ I have never smoked cigarettes.
- ❏ I am careful not to drink alcohol when taking certain types of medication (e.g., medicine for colds and allergies).
- ❏ I always read and follow the label directions when using prescribed and over-the-counter drugs.
- ❏ I eat a variety of foods each day, such as fruits, vegetables, whole-grain breads, and lean meats.
- ❏ I limit the amount of fat and cholesterol I eat.
- ❏ I limit the amount of salt I eat by not adding salt to my food at the table.
- ❏ I do vigorous exercises for 15–30 minutes at least three times a week (e.g., running or swimming).
- ❏ I use part of my leisure time to participate regularly in activities that increase my level of fitness (e.g., gardening, bowling, or golf).
- ❏ I find it easy to relax and express my feelings freely.
- ❏ I have close friends and relatives whom I can talk to about personal matters and call on for help when needed.

Count your number of check marks: How many health behaviours do you engage in? The items included in the list cover a variety of aspects of our daily lives that affect our health. If you are able to check most or all of these 10 items, then your personal health practices might enable you to claim that you have a healthy lifestyle. If you are able to check only some of these items, then you might want to reconsider your personal health practices and the steps that might enable you to develop healthier lifestyle behaviours. Finally, if you are unable to check any of these items (or very few), then your personal practices may be hazardous to your health!

---

dimension of health behaviour. Krick and Sobal (1990, 20) also examined the relationship between health behaviours in an effort to learn "whether there is an overall positive health orientation that results in the adoption of health behaviors as a set, or whether health behaviors are more independently determined." Despite their use of more rigorous measures than previous studies, Krick and Sobal's findings support the view that health behaviours are multi-dimensional in nature.

A few studies (e.g., Newsom et al. 2005; Norman 1985; Stephens 1986) used Canadian data and basically came to the same conclusion—that health behaviours are essentially unrelated. For example, Norman (1985) studied the interrelationships among health behaviours in an undergraduate university student population. Overall, Norman (1985, 410) found that there is a low degree of interrelationship between health behaviours and concludes that "individuals reporting health promoting actions in one behavioural domain were usually no more or less likely than others to engage in the other health behaviours." Stephens (1986) found weak or non-existent correlations between the health practices studied among a large sample drawn from the general Canadian population. Most recently, in a correlation study that used data from four population health surveys, Newsom and colleagues (2005) found that smoking, exercise, diet, and alcohol consumption had a shared variance of only about 1 per cent. This finding prompted the researchers to describe the notion that individual health consciousness underlies health lifestyles as a "myth."

In summary, different investigators have assessed the relationship between specific health behaviours. The most consistent finding is that diverse individual health behaviours are not closely correlated with each other. For the most part, these health practices are independent of one another, although in some cases they are actually negatively correlated with each other. In other words, rather than forming an overall health lifestyle, health behaviour is multi-dimensional. Is it possible to identify the specific health practices that make up each of these behavioural dimensions? Calnan (1989, 131) concludes that the "evidence from empirical research has shown that the strength of statistical relationships between types of health-related behaviours are at best modest." According to existing research, there is no such thing as a coherent health lifestyle! Rather, there is a continuum of behaviours running from salutogenic to pathogenic, with most people demonstrating a mix of behaviours, some good for health, others bad (Blaxter 1990). It is important, therefore, to critically examine health promotion efforts that simply encourage the adoption of healthy lifestyles.

Despite the fact that the individualized lifestyle approach used in the new public health lacks a sociological imagination, fails to recognize the existence of a social gradient in health behaviours, and is not based on a clear understanding of what combination of health practices actually constitutes the behavioural pattern associated with a healthy lifestyle, individualized health promotion continues to be emphasized by neo-liberal governments (Baum and Fisher 2014). Lifestyle health behaviour remains a central feature of the new public health despite the fact that we have little clear evidence as to which behaviours actually constitute a healthy lifestyle. There are a variety of reasons why this may be the case.

One factor is that as a result of population aging, prevalent health-care needs have changed. Chronic degenerative diseases and an emphasis on long-term care, rather than cure, have largely replaced acute infectious diseases. The management of chronic conditions in an aging population poses new challenges for the organization and delivery of appropriate health-care services. In turn, this has translated into a greater emphasis on lifestyle behaviours that might delay the onset of some chronic conditions and as a means of managing the daily demands of living with chronic illness. As Baum and Fisher (2014, 217) put it, "The dominant public discourse that has since developed has portrayed chronic diseases as an outcome of poor individual 'lifestyle' choices, from which it is an easy step to see them as preventable through lifestyle changes encouraged by behavioural messages."

In addition, the emphasis on lifestyle behaviour is likely to persist because of the widespread belief that healthful living is a desirable alternative to relying on expensive, sophisticated medical technology and institutionally based health-care services. Baum and Fisher (2014, 217) contend that "The dominant biomedical model of disease and treatment that drives most health policy also reinforces individualism and directs the bulk of resources to medical services and research." Obviously, lifestyle changes in level of physical activity and in dietary practices that might result in maintaining heart health are preferable to relying on costly medical procedures such as bypass or transplant surgery to deal with cardiovascular disease. This perspective is reinforced by ongoing efforts of governments to control rising health-care costs. Promoting healthy living and preventive medical behaviour (e.g., screening programs and early detection) are seen as cost-effective alternatives to the present emphasis of the formal health-care system on disease intervention and treatment. Shifting responsibility for health to individuals allows neo-liberal governments to attempt reductions in health-care spending.

Finally, the pursuit of a wellness-oriented lifestyle is a deeply ingrained cultural component in societies such as Canada. Baum and Fisher (2014, 217) explain that "The individualism of neoliberal theory offers little space to support a view that health is primarily created by the structures which powerfully shape people's lives, including the dominant economic structure." The new public health approach is likely to persist, because lifestyle behaviours (e.g., diet and exercise) are believed to be within the control of the individual and because of the prevailing belief that compared to other major determinants of health, lifestyle has "the largest and most unambiguously measurable effect on health" (Evans and Stoddart 1990, 1355). Within consumer culture, health has become a valued commodity and a moral obligation. The widespread belief in the moral correctness of a healthy lifestyle promises to make this concept even more difficult to abandon.

We are left, then, with the unsolved mystery of health. On the one hand, we are committed to promoting the adoption of healthy lifestyle behaviour. On the other hand, current research indicates that personal health practices are essentially separate behavioural dimensions that follow the social gradient. In other words, it is not safe to assume that promoting one type of health behaviour will translate into the adoption of other health-protective behaviours, especially among those who are socially excluded. Stated another way, research has been unable to demonstrate that these health activities are actually part of a lifestyle behavioural pattern. At the same time, we know that lifestyle behaviours are related to one's social location and that social exclusion acts as a barrier to their adoption. Consequently, we must question whether it is possible to effectively promote healthy lifestyles in contrast to discrete health behaviours targeted to specific subpopulations. Does all of this mean that health lifestyles are unimportant for understanding the pursuit of health and wellness and addressing health disparities? The answer is a resounding no. However, the concept of a healthy lifestyle requires sociological clarification before it is possible to promote the adoption of wellness-oriented lifestyle behaviour that will result in improvements in the health of all Canadians.

The social determinants of health that we have explored in this part of the text have direct and indirect effects on health disparities. For example, Chapter 5 explored the direct effects of social structure on health in terms of socioeconomic status and in terms of the social class gradient. A direct effect on health is apparent when a social structural factor (such as socioeconomic status) is related to health while controlling for other factors such as gender, ethnicity, and age. This allows researchers to say that socioeconomic status has a direct effect on health. However, the intersectional perspective, explained at the beginning of this chapter, argues that the whole picture of health is more complicated than direct effects alone. In other words, social structural factors can also have an indirect effect on health, one that is mediated by other factors. Indirect effects of social determinants of health are those that are culturally mediated through lifestyles. This discussion of direct and indirect effects reflects a dichotomy that has characterized population health research (Abel 2007). However, in reality, health outcomes are shaped by both direct and indirect effects. Unfortunately, this reality is often lost in health research, which dichotomizes social determinants of health into either material or cultural factors. Rather than studying these effects separately, intersectional analysis argues that we need to understand how the two act together to influence each other and affect health outcomes. This means that health researchers wishing to address disparities in health must ask how structures of inequality (i.e., material factors) are channelled through lifestyles (i.e., cultural and behavioural factors) to produce health disparities across the life course. This question, which will be discussed shortly, represents one of the most important issues in sociological theory, the structure–agency question.

Theorizing the Intersectionality of Health

There is widespread agreement among researchers that health disparities can only be understood with reference to the social context of health and disease. For instance, Adelson (2005, S46) states that "in any analysis of health disparities . . . it is as crucial to navigate the interstices between the person and the wider social and historical contexts as it is to pay attention to the individual effects of inequity." In other words, in order to understand health disparities so that we can do something about them, we need to realize that individual differences in health are socially produced by wider social and cultural inequality within society. As Spitzer (2005, 2) explains, "A review of the literature suggests that health inequities emerge from the dynamic intersections of the demands of multiple gender roles, environmental exposures, the threat and consequences of gender violence, workplace hazards, economic disparities, the costs of poverty, social marginalization and racism, aging, health conditions and interactions with health services and health behaviours." In other words, instead of a single source of health disparities, inequalities in health arise out of a dynamic intersection of many different structures of inequality. In terms of C. Wright Mills' sociological imagination, we need to understand "intersections of history and biography" if we are to unravel the mystery of health and address disparities in health.

Unfortunately, as Bauer (2014, 11) points out, "Population health research has been increasingly critiqued for its failure to explicitly acknowledge the theory (or lack of theory) underlying analyses, and for the failure of research teams to deliberately consider theoretical frameworks on which their research may then be built." This means that, for the most part, the sociological imagination has been lacking as health researchers have tried to understand disparities in a way that moves beyond simply describing group differences in population health (Dunn 2006). Walters (2003, 4) describes the intersectional puzzle facing health researchers: "The challenge we face is to develop frameworks of understanding that allow us to see pathways of influence from the societal level to individuals and their experience of illness, and to document how the influence flows in both directions, the ways in which the biological experience of disease has social costs." What is needed to unravel the mystery of health is a theoretical perspective that uses an intersectional framework to put together factors such as socioeconomic status, gender, ethnicity, age, and social exclusion to form an integrative and systematic account of how a diversity of social locations affects the individual pursuit of health and wellness across the life course. Because of its emphasis on the relationship between the individual and society, our best hope of understanding these dynamic intersections rests with the sociological imagination that lies at the heart of sociological theory.

Health Lifestyles and the Structure–Agency Issue

The challenge for health sociologists is to understand how social structural factors, such as socioeconomic status, gender, ethnicity, and age, intersect with individual behavioural factors (e.g., health behaviours) to affect health outcomes. Cockerham (2005, 51) explains the connection between health disparities and health lifestyles in this way: "When applied to health lifestyles, the question is whether the decisions people make with respect to diet, exercise, smoking, and the like are largely a matter of individual choice or are principally shaped by structural variables such as social class position and gender?" Our culture places high value on health, and it is generally assumed that good health is valued by everyone. However, "the lack of healthful behavior on the part of many people leads us to question this assumption" (Bruhn et al. 1977, 209). The research reviewed in this chapter demonstrates that there is no clear relationship between most personal health practices. In fact, many of our everyday health-related behaviours are inconsistent or, in some cases, even detrimental to health. For example, an individual might be fully aware that smoking is bad for health but continue to smoke because it is a pleasurable activity and one that she feels is helpful in managing stress. Another individual might fully agree that exercise is beneficial for health but find that engaging in regular physical activity is difficult and unenjoyable and, as a consequence, be sedentary. Common sense tells us that there should be a concrete relationship between health beliefs and health behaviours, but in reality, human behaviour is seldom this straightforward. As a result, we must question the meaning of a healthy lifestyle.

In an insightful early article concerning the role of structure and agency in health lifestyles, Williams (1995, 580) explains that "Whilst there appears to be a logical connection between concepts of health, beliefs about health maintenance, and health-related forms of behaviour, empirical evidence suggests that their importance may in fact have been overestimated, and that the relationship between knowledge and action is a problematic one." He (1995, 581) goes on to point out that this question is part of a much larger issue in sociological theory: "A key question in this respect concerns how, exactly, we are to theorise the structure–agency problem in relation to health-related behaviour?" Cockerham (2000) and Williams (1995) are among the first of an increasing number of health sociologists who are realizing that understanding the relationship between health disparities and health lifestyles necessitates consideration of the structure–agency issue (e.g., Abel 2007; Frohlich, Corin, and Potvin 2001; Abel and Frohlich 2012; Frohlich and Potvin 2010; Korp 2008, 2010; Maller 2015; Pescosolido, McLeod, and Alegría 2000; Rütten and Gelius 2011; Veenstra and Burnett 2014; Williams 2003). Abel and Froehlich (2012, 237) conclude that "Today there is a near unanimous recognition that concern with the production and reproduction of health inequalities must take into account both the social structure and individual agency to be given credence."

The structure–agency issue lies at the heart of the sociological enterprise and has been the subject of extensive theoretical inquiry within sociology (e.g., Archer 2003; Cockerham 2005). In keeping with the idea that the task of sociology is to understand intersections of history and biography (Mills 1959), sociological theory conceptualizes how and why individuals produce social phenomena (groups, institutions, social structures, society, etc.) and how and why social phenomena, in turn, act to produce individuals, individual behaviour, and individual personality. The task of sociology is to explain how the macro affects the micro and vice versa, or how "history and biography intersect" to produce social phenomena and behaviour, or how structure and agency interact to shape our lives. The structure–agency issue is foundational for sociology! You should be forewarned against the temptation to view this issue as "merely" theoretical or philosophical in nature: the question of the nature of the relationship between individual and society has direct bearing on how we understand the pursuit of health and wellness and has implications for such real-world issues as the extent to which individuals can and should be held personally responsible for unhealthy behaviours. Arriving at a sociological understanding of the relationship between knowledge and behaviour is crucial to unravelling the mystery of health.

Social structure refers to relatively stable patterns of behaviour that we learn from our society's culture, are observable, and have a material quality. For example, a person's socio-economic status can be inferred by observing such things as the neighbourhood in which she lives, what kind of car she drives, how much money she has, and what she does to earn a living. In a similar manner, studies of the social gradient show that knowing an individual's health behaviours and status can help us infer her social class membership. Consider, as illustration, who is more likely to smoke, a rich person or someone who is poor? Research demonstrates that smoking prevalence is highest among those with lower socioeconomic status (Hiscock et al. 2012). In this way, social class and other observable patterns of behaviour, such as gender, ethnicity, and age, are considered by sociologists to be social structures. Social structures provide the societal patterns our lives follow. Cockerham (2007, 53) notes that "sociological concepts reflecting literally all theories of social life attest to the fact that *something* (namely structure) exists beyond the individual to give rise to customary patterns of behavior" [original emphasis]. While such patterns are important for understanding social life, they are not all there is to human behaviour; there is also agency. **Agency** refers to the ability of individuals to act as self-conscious, wilful social agents and to make free choices about behaviour, including health behaviour.

The **structure–agency issue** raises the very complex sociological and, indeed, philosophical question: Is there such a thing as human free will (i.e., agency) in the face of society's systems of social control (i.e., social structure)? In terms of the mystery of health, the critical question to ask is: Are health behaviours really an expression of an individual's agency, or is there a social structural context to our health lifestyles that influences health behaviour? Frohlich, Corin, and Potvin (2001, 781) comment on the importance of addressing the structure–agency issue in population health research:

> What is missing is a discussion of the relationship between agency (the ability for people to deploy a range of causal powers), practices (the activities that make and transform the world we live in) and social structure (the rules and resources in society). Without such an understanding, factors associated with people's disease experiences within a context tend to be denuded of social meaning.

Despite the centrality of this issue for sociology, no definitive answers exist. Instead, numerous perspectives concerning structure–agency have been advanced by social theorists. How this question is answered and whether agency or structure is seen as the most important factor in explaining behaviour depends on the theoretical paradigm that guides the social researcher. For instance, the structural functionalist and conflict paradigms give more weight to structural explanations of behaviour, while the symbolic interactionist paradigm focuses on the agency of individuals in shaping interaction. Both the feminist and sociology of the body paradigms view behaviour as a consequence of the interaction of structure and agency.

As Cockerham, Rütten, and Abel (1997) note, one of the first sociological theorists to conceptualize behaviour in terms of structure–agency was the German sociologist Max Weber (1922). According to Weber, lifestyles are produced by the dialectical interplay of what he called "life choices" with "life chances." Building on the work of Weber, these researchers suggest that **life choices** refer to the decisions that people make in their selection of lifestyle behaviours, while life chances are the probabilities of translating these choices into action. In other words, life choices involving decisions about smoking, alcohol use, diet, and exercise are expressions of agency. However, and this is where the sociological imagination is demonstrated in understanding health lifestyles, such life choices are made in the context of life chances. In other words, the choices we make in life are constrained by structural conditions such as our socioeconomic status, gender, ethnicity, and age. Hence, **life chances** are aspects of the social structure that provide a social context for behaviour that shapes our individual life choices. Consequently, lifestyle behaviour and health are related to social location and result from the interplay of choice and chance (e.g., which foods you choose to eat is related to the amount of money that you have available for groceries). Based on this conceptual approach, Cockerham (2007, 56) proposes that **health lifestyles** be defined as "collective patterns of health-related behavior based on choices (i.e., agency) from options available to people according to their life chances (i.e., structure)." Sociologically, this is a very useful definition in that it points out that health lifestyles arise from the intersectionality of structure and agency and serve as a central mechanism for disparities in the production of health. The question for health researchers and promoters remains: How do health behaviours that are built into our culture become ingrained in our daily embodied practices of living as a routine part of family life, recreation, and work, forming an overall pattern of a wellness-oriented lifestyle? As the next section describes, health researchers are increasingly turning to the sociological theory developed by Pierre Bourdieu to answer this question.

Pierre Bourdieu and a Relational Theory of Health Lifestyles

A theoretical perspective that researchers are increasingly finding useful as a guide for understanding intersecting health disparities is the relational sociology developed by Pierre Bourdieu (e.g., Bourdieu 1990; Bourdieu and Wacquant 1992; see Box 8.8). As Poland and colleagues (2006, 60) explain, Bourdieu's theory allows us to understand how lifestyle behaviours "are generated at the intersection of social structure (norms, resources, policy, institutional practices that organise society), and agency (individual action, volition and sense of identity), and manifest concretely in specific places (for example, neighbourhoods)." Working within the sociology of the body paradigm, Bourdieu argues that it is necessary to understand the embodied basis of what he calls

Box 8.8   Pierre Bourdieu (1930–2002)

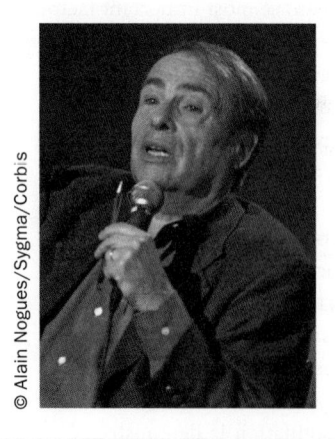

- The foremost sociologist of the late twentieth century
- Developed reflexive sociology, which highlights the role played by various types of "capital" in perpetuating social inequalities
- A leading theorist in the sociology of the body paradigm who developed the concept of "habitus" as an explanation of society and behaviour

"Health-oriented practices such as walking and jogging are also linked to the dispositions of the culturally richest fractions of the middle classes and the dominant class" (1984, 214).

"the logic of practice" (1990). Williams (1995, 582) offers the following explanation of Bourdieu's perspective on "the logic of practice" in social life:

> That is to say, most of us, most of the time, take ourselves and the social world around us for granted; we do not think about what we do because, quite simply, we do not have to. Indeed, the business of social life would be impossible if it were not taken for granted most of the time: imagine the absurdity of having to keep an active file in our heads of each and every social rule and regulation!

For Bourdieu, the logic of practice explains how social structures become embodied within individuals, leading to the reproduction of structures of inequality unthinkingly in social behaviour. As Williams (1995, 598) and many other health sociologists contend, "Much of Bourdieu's argument concerning the logic of practice and its determinants can profitably be used in order to understand and explain health and lifestyles." Bourdieu's relational sociological theory is gaining in popularity among researchers as a way of understanding health disparities (e.g., Buzzelli 2007; Carpiano 2008; Gatrell, Popay, and Thomas 2004; Dumas, Robitaille, and Jette 2013; Lynam and Cowley 2007; Pinxten and Lievens 2014; Singh-Manoux and Marmot 2005; Veenstra 2007; Veenstra and Burnett 2014).

Bourdieu's approach is described as "relational" because he understands society as a multi-dimensional "social space" made up of overlapping and interconnected cultural fields (Fries 2009). These fields shape the human body and influence behaviour according to each individual's lifelong journey through social space. His goal is to offer an account of how individuals and society relate to produce behaviour. Bourdieu argues that the cultural fields in which we are socialized and in which our identities form and our bodies develop shape our habitus as the embodiment of our movement through various cultural environments across our life course.

The habitus rests upon socialization experiences through which social structures of our surrounding environments form our beliefs, values, and attitudes about the nature of social reality. Thus, the habitus reflects the social structures among which it develops. These structures become embodied within the habitus as culture literally shapes our bodies. This happens throughout the life course through the biophysical effects of behavioural patterns such as diet or exercise. For Bourdieu, habitus is key to understanding the structure–agency issue in that it provides a mechanism linking social structure (i.e., life chances) and agency (i.e., life choices). Habitus, in turn, influences our position in social space as structures of inequality become internalized by individuals, are embodied, and are thereby reproduced in behaviour according to this unthinking logic of practice. As Bourdieu (1992, 113) explains the logic of practice, "The social world doesn't work in terms of consciousness; it works in terms of practices, mechanisms and so forth." Bourdieu's relational sociological theory allows us to understand how biosocial outcomes, such as health, are the unique and dynamic product of social history and individual biography.

For Bourdieu, the task of social science is to understand how social structures influence individual expressions of agency and, in turn, how social behaviour serves to reproduce the reality that is society (Fries 2009). In this way, Bourdieu's goal was to fulfill what C. Wright Mills (1959) famously described as "the promise" of "the sociological imagination." Bourdieu, like Mills before him, viewed understanding the relationship between structure and agency as central to sociology. Society affects individual behaviour, which, in turn, in its totality reproduces society. This insight is perhaps the ultimate sociological realization.

In keeping with Bourdieu's emphasis on the logic of practice in understanding behaviour, if most behaviour is habitual, as embodied in the habitus (rather than consciously learned), then it follows that this is the case for health behaviour. We incorporate health beliefs into our habitus based on structures of inequality that are dominant within the cultural fields surrounding us as we age. Following Bourdieu, the reason researchers have been unable to identify a single behavioural pattern that constitutes a health lifestyle is that there is no such thing as a "lifestyle" in the conventional, individualized sense! With the logic of practice, Bourdieu argues that people don't consciously choose how to behave; we just behave, and how we "just behave" is embodied within our habitus. As Williams (1995, 583) argues,

> Much of what we commonly and unthinkingly refer to as "health-related behaviour"—itself an analytical or second-order construct—is in fact, when viewed in the context of actors' daily lives, part and parcel of a practical rather than an abstract logic. In other words, "health-related behaviour" is itself a routinised feature of everyday life; something which is woven into its very fabric.

We perform many health behaviours by habit as part of the logic of practice that becomes embodied within us over the course of our lives. Think, for example, about how much of your health-related behaviour you just do, without stopping to think about it! We don't think of daily habits of living that affect health, such as eating breakfast or trying to get enough rest, necessarily as health behaviour. Rather, such practices either are or aren't part of our habitus, and we do them unreflectively. Sure, you can consciously decide whether you're going to go to the gym after class today or instead go home and eat a big piece of chocolate cake, but in the totality of your behaviour, such choices are ingrained within your habitus as part of your location in the structures of social space that form our health lifestyles. The consequences of these behaviours, in turn, collectively shape your health status. In reviewing theoretical problems associated with the health lifestyle discourse as found in individualized health promotion, Korp (2010, 806) concludes that "Bourdieu's understanding of lifestyles is thus fundamentally different from the sort of analyses that stress conscious and intentional choices as a fundamental principle of the construction of lifestyles."

As Williams (1995) points out, understanding health behaviour in terms of the logic of practice has serious implications for health research. He notes that when researchers ask people to tell them how a person should try to stay in good health, most will be able to say all the right things. This doesn't mean, however, that they are practising any of these health behaviours. Despite this, individualized approaches to understanding the relationship between health-related knowledge and health behaviour often adopt this approach. This likely accounts for the mixed findings on the relationship between health knowledge and health behaviour that were described earlier in the chapter. Stated differently, Bourdieu's approach helps to make sense of the seeming paradox that when sociologists ask people about their health beliefs, they are able to say all the right things and explain what counts as health behaviour and yet they may not behave this way in their own lives. The implication is that if researchers want to understand the relationship between health knowledge and health behaviour, they need to focus on actual health behaviours as a way of revealing the logic of practice underlying health lifestyles. This is one of the advantages of health diaries—they allow researchers to focus on actual health behaviours in order to determine how these behaviours relate to structures of inequality.

Applying Bourdieu's theory to the mystery of health in terms of the structure–agency issue suggests a reframing of the health lifestyle research question in a way that can address some of the methodological limitations plaguing this area of study. Rather than asking whether there is a pattern of correlated behaviours that together constitute a health lifestyle, researchers guided by an intersectional perspective should ask: How is social location related to collective patterns of lifestyle behaviours? In other words, the intersectional model suggests that instead of looking for associations between health behaviours with statistical techniques such as correlation and factor analysis (typical strategies in health lifestyle research), it makes more sense to assess the common social structural factors (such as socioeconomic status, gender, ethnicity, and age) associated with engaging in healthy and unhealthy behaviours, using statistical techniques such as correspondence analysis to map the social space of health lifestyles.

Hankivsky and Christoffersen (2008) point out that Bourdieu's theory of social relations and his insights into the role power plays in these relations have a lot in common with the intersectional perspective. While Bourdieu (e.g., 1984) saw social class as a major source of oppression in society, his relational model also describes how other structures of inequality, such as gender (e.g., Bourdieu 2001), shape the habitus. His theory does this by focusing on how, in addition to material conditions, cultural factors contribute to social inequality. Bourdieu saw the cultural fields that make up society as being characterized by a variety of categories of power, which he called "species of capital" (Bourdieu and Wacquant 1992, 114). For Bourdieu, the economic relations of social class, while an important type of capital, are not the only type of power that affects people's lives, bodies, and health. Other types of power, such as those stemming from cultural difference (i.e., "cultural capital") or linked to a person's social relations and group membership (i.e., "social capital") or even a person's unique embodiment (i.e., "physical capital"), intersect in complex ways to shape the habitus across the life course.

As discussed in Chapter 5, cultural capital includes non-material resources, such as forms of knowledge, skill, or expertise that are accorded value within a field, and their material representations, such as certifications, qualifications, and diplomas. Just what constitutes cultural capital is the object of social struggle within particular cultural fields. Next, with his treatment of **social capital**, Bourdieu demonstrates how people construct social relations to accumulate social power through interpersonal relations. Third, for Bourdieu the human body is yet another bearer of social value, what he describes as bodily or **physical capital**. All of these types of capital interact to influence behaviour and shape health outcomes through their lifelong effects on the habitus.

As illustration, Bourdieu's conception of cultural capital informs us that a person's social location influences access to cultural resources such as medical knowledge and, therefore, health behaviour. In other words, our health beliefs are a form of cultural capital related to our positions in social space. For example, in North America most people know smoking is harmful. Indeed, most of us received this cultural capital early in the life course as we learn in elementary school that smoking is bad for your health. However, because of social exclusion, some might not receive this knowledge. Perhaps they were raised in a social environment in which family members and peers smoked, thereby delivering the implicit message to them as children that smoking is an acceptable part of life. As teens they adopt this unhealthy behaviour and later in life experience health consequences such as lung cancer. This example shows that the structures of inequality that normalize smoking and other unhealthy behaviours are embedded in the habitus of the socially excluded. Canadian research has shown that the social exclusion of Aboriginal peoples is related to the increased consumption of tobacco in places such as bingo halls, where communities gather and which serve as a refuge from marginalization (Bottorff et al. 2009). In this way, health behaviour and health lifestyles are unconsciously influenced by what Bourdieu calls cultural capital.

In this perspective, social inequality, including health disparities, is produced not only through observable differences in material conditions related to structures of inequality (i.e., living and working conditions) but also through hidden cultural differences (i.e., lifestyles) mediated through the habitus. According to Abel (2007, 43), this is what is so useful about Bourdieu's approach to understanding inequality for health researchers: "Most often missing in public health research however, are cultural factors that link material and social resources, social structure and health."

Following Bourdieu's relational sociology, we come to understand four fundamental points about health lifestyles and the production of health as summarized in Box 8.9. In developing his "health lifestyle theory" over the course of several publications Cockerham (2000; 2005; 2007; 2013; Cockerham, Rütten, and Abel 1997) highlights three points concerning health lifestyles in a sociological perspective, to which we can add a fourth point in keeping with the life course paradigm.

Box 8.9 Health Lifestyles according to Bourdieu's Relational Sociology:

- are a collective phenomenon; shared by groups within society
- represent patterns of consumption, not production
- are shaped by the dialectical interplay between life choices (i.e., agency) and life chances (i.e., structure)
- are accumulated across the life course as part of socialization and have enduring health consequences

First, health lifestyles "are associated with status groups, therefore they are principally a collective, rather than individual phenomenon" (Cockerham 2000, 162). Bourdieu shows how lifestyle choices depend on ideas about the body (reflected through the habitus) held by different groups within society. A well-known example provided by Bourdieu (1984) relates to differing attitudes and beliefs members of different social classes have about the effects of food and exercise on the body in terms of health, strength, and beauty. Bourdieu's survey research showed that the upper classes prefer food that is light and tasty (i.e., "a delight for the taste buds"), while the lower classes favour food that is hearty and filling (i.e., "sticks to your ribs"). The upper classes prefer tennis, while the lower classes prefer rugby. Varying social locations mean that not everyone accumulates the same cultural capital in the same manner; hence, different groups in society have differing logics of practice and differing health lifestyles. In other words, different habitus associated with different locations in social space support different health lifestyles. Bourdieu shows how "having used their bodies all day in what often amounts to physically demanding work, the working classes may have little time or inclination for the 'pretensions' of exercise such as jogging or 'keep fit'" (Williams 1995, 595). Similarly, sociology professors who write health textbooks likely have both the time and the money to exercise in expensive CrossFit® gyms, while students working extra jobs to pay for university tuition have neither. Thus, some social locations support health behaviours while others may discourage healthy lifestyles. Think, for example, of people who live in violent neighbourhoods and can't safely exercise outdoors. Unhealthy lifestyles become embodied within the habitus of the socially excluded, and structures of inequality are reproduced through apparently individualistic health behaviours that are actually rooted in society.

The second point about health lifestyles that arises from Bourdieu's theory is that they "represent patterns of consumption, not production" (Cockerham 2000, 162). Although positive health lifestyles are intended to produce good health, the ultimate aim of such lifestyles is to be healthy in order to be able to work, feel and look good, participate in sports and leisure activities, and enjoy life. Investing in health builds a health reserve (Herzlich 1973) of physical capital that can be exchanged for other forms of capital. Considering the link between health lifestyles, consumption, and medical consumerism, Cockerham (2005, 55) explains that "health lifestyles are supported by an extensive health products industry of goods and services (e.g., running shoes, sports clothing, diet plans, health foods, club and spa memberships) promoting consumption as an inherent component of participation." Realizing the intimate connection of our bodies to our self-identity, companies market health-care goods and services not so much on the basis of the actual products they sell but, rather, on the statements that the consumption of these products make about our lifestyle. However, not all people have social locations that allow them to be able to afford to participate in consumption-driven health lifestyles. There are inequalities in the social production of health, since not everyone can afford gym memberships, yoga classes, and expensive running shoes. Box 8.10 provides an illustration of the lifestyle marketing of health and wellness.

Third, health lifestyles "are shaped by the dialectical interplay between life choices (i.e., agency) and life chances (i.e., structure)" (Cockerham 2000, 162). This means that both

Box 8.10 The Lifestyle Marketing of Health and Wellness

Health and wellness retailers such as Lululemon understand that in today's health-conscious society, health and wellness are linked to lifestyle expressions of identity. Their goal is to sell health lifestyles through the consumption of their products and services. How do your health lifestyle purchases make statements about how you like to think about yourself?

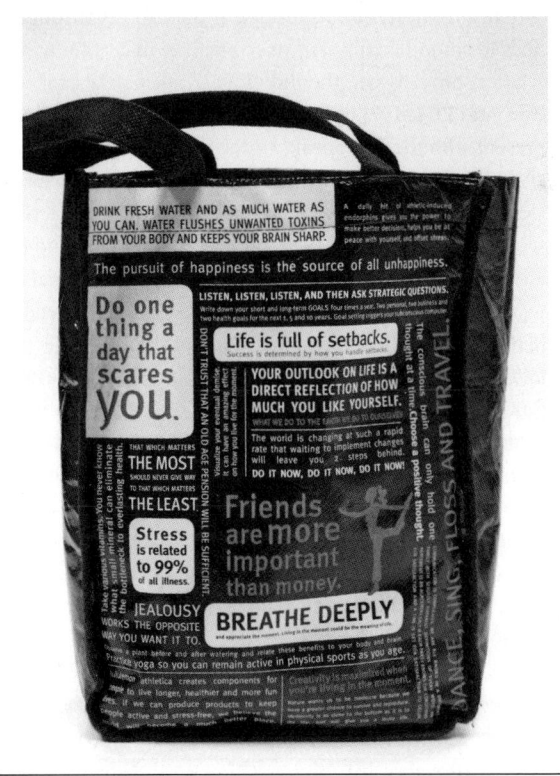

The Canadian Press

agency and structure play a role in the formation of health lifestyles. Health lifestyles are not solely the product of an individual's choices: agency is always constrained by structural conditions, and so too are health behaviours! We can understand lifestyles not merely as markers of social difference but, rather, as the central means through which disparities in health are produced and reproduced throughout the life course. Habitus provides the linking mechanism between social structure and individual health behaviours, beliefs, and outcomes. As such, Bourdieu's conception of lifestyles provides us with a theoretical explanation of the existence of the social gradient in health risk behaviours. Consider the following from Cockerham (2000, 168):

> A person's class position provides structural boundaries to the options that he or she can successfully execute in life. Thus, the health lifestyles of the upper and upper-middle classes—featuring more healthy diets, greater opportunities for relaxation and coping with stress, higher levels of participation in sports and leisure-time exercise, more physical checkups by physicians, and other preventative-care activities—assist the affluent in living a healthier and longer life. The lower class, in turn, has choices and opportunities for health lifestyles that are much more limited and confronts lessened life expectancy than the classes above.

In other words, past and present life chances affect our life choices, which further reproduce life chances and shape future health outcomes.

Finally, applying Bourdieu's theory to health lifestyles reminds us that our health reserve is affected not only by personal health behaviour but also by broader societal conditions that structure health lifestyles as a feature of the habitus throughout the life course. Habitus, referring as it does to embodied dispositions to behave in certain ways, is a valuable tool for conceptualizing the relationship between the individual and society as it unfolds across the life course. Veenstra and Burnett (2014, 192) point out that habitus is "A phenomenon that mediates past experiences and present stimuli . . . It speaks to the ways in which past experiences in social settings and presently available chances and opportunities manifest themselves in relatively durable dispositions that inform the future choices that people make and the actions they may take." This means that social structures, such as socioeconomic status, gender, and ethnicity, are embedded within the habitus and shape health lifestyles throughout our lives. Social structures and the behaviours that go along with them are reproduced in the embodied experiences and behaviours of individuals. As such, habitus is a developmental concept in that one's trajectory through social space, with its attendant forms of capital, continually shapes and reshapes the habitus and the behavioural dispositions that flow from it. This embodied learning of health lifestyles operates at multiple levels "ranging from structured pathways through social institutions and organizations to the social trajectories of individuals and their developmental pathway" (Elder 1994, 5).

It is through these health lifestyles that society and culture literally get under your skin! This helps us to understand why health lifestyle behaviours, such as smoking, are socially graded. Individuals from low SES backgrounds internalize behaviours that are regarded as acceptable in those social contexts. Baum and Fisher (2014, 216) elaborate the significance of Bourdieu's relational theory for understanding health lifestyles across the life course:

> Bourdieu (1984) bridges the agency–structure divide with his theory that explains how individuals accumulate durable and transposable values and dispositions through

socialisation and then adapt their ambitions and actions to the social circumstances and context of their lives. He maintains that values, beliefs and worldviews are created through the habitus, which reflects and helps to maintain class, gender or cultural position, and can be more or less supportive of health promotion practices in everyday life. Bourdieu sees that economic capital is maintained and reproduced through cultural, social and symbolic capital and these capitals are crucial in determining opportunities to adopt healthy lifestyles over the life course.

Furthermore, individuals who share similar social locations share a group habitus, which is consistent with the life course principle of linked lives. Cockerham (2013, 148) describes the habitus by explaining that "One of its principal functions is that of providing a unity of style linking the practices of a single agent to a class of agents that brings together agents or individuals who are very similar to each other and different from members of other classes." Similarly, Bourdieu (1977, 85) states that "Though it is impossible for all members of the same class (or even two of them) to have the same experiences, in the same order, it is certain that each member of the same class is more likely than any member of another class to have been confronted with the situations most frequent for members of that class." This similarity of social conditioning gives rise to collective patterns of behaviour that are recognized as health lifestyles. It should be obvious that habitus is a concept that captures the essence of the life course perspective's linked lives.

Health lifestyles are accumulated across the life course as part of socialization and have enduring health consequences. As Blaxter (2003, 81) explains,

> There are period effects of living through epidemics, economic depression, or traumatic eras of history, and long-term consequences of general changes in social conditions and lifestyles which do not have causes specific to the individual though they affect individual bodies. Thus the determinants of health capital are cohort-specific and not entirely individual: the concept links the individual lifetime with the temporal movement of social history.

Such a model represents an intersectional life course perspective on health disparities. Developments in epigenetics show that social conditions have intergenerational biophysical consequences for health. This means that in much the same way that economic capital can accumulate over generations and be inherited by individuals, so too can health capital. This leads to different groups having unequal reserves of health capital across the life course based on differences in social location and health lifestyles.

Abel (2007, 45) argues that Bourdieu's theory of social relations is well suited to addressing health disparities: "As Bourdieu's approach integrates different levels of analysis, his work becomes a particularly useful venue into health promotion issues, that typically link individual behaviour to different levels of collectivity including families, peer groups, communities etc." Thus, health research guided by Bourdieu's relational sociology is, by definition, intersectional in that the habitus develops throughout the life course in relation to a variety of interacting material and cultural factors. The next section closes this chapter by presenting an intersectional model of health and health lifestyles across the life course based on Bourdieu's insights into lifestyles and social inequality.

An Intersectional Model of Health and Health Lifestyles across the Life Course

A model for understanding health guided by Bourdieu's theoretical perspective conceptualizes health as a complex biosocial phenomenon that changes over time. That is, health emerges irreducibly from intersecting biological and social contexts. As depicted in Figure 8.1, the centrepiece of an intersectional model for understanding health as a biosocial reality is the realization that the categories of analysis typically employed in the health determinants framework are dynamic (rather than static) overlapping constructions. Biological factors are frequently understood as though they were distinct from social factors in health research. However, in light of insights provided by Bourdieu's conceptualization of habitus, an intersectional approach recognizes that biological bodies are shaped by, and themselves shape, society and culture. Tarlov (1996, 84) provides an excellent description of this when he writes that "Human bodies in different social locations become crystallized reflections of the social experiences within which they have developed." As the sociology of the body paradigm makes clear, biological factors, such as biophysical endowment, genetic traits and predispositions, sex, and racial characteristics, are important bases of embodiment. However, social factors, such as the socio-cultural environment in which one's habitus develops, are also key in explaining health outcomes. This means that biological development occurs within a socio-cultural context that is itself a complex biosocial reality. Thus, as indicated by the overlapping circles in Figure 8.1, health is a biosocial reality: arising from biological and social factors that must be conceptualized as intersecting (i.e., together they shape the biosocial reality that is health).

The model presented in Figure 8.1 is intended to summarize the information discussed in this chapter and illustrate an intersectional model of health across the life course inspired by the sociological imagination. In keeping with Bourdieu's relational sociology, the figure shows habitus as a mechanism that mediates between social structure and agency. The habitus is a developmental concept in that it changes throughout the life course, shaping what Wadsworth (1997) terms the health trajectory. The large arrows running clockwise around the conceptual model are intended to symbolize this developmental process as the habitus is shaped by changing social structures from infancy, through youth and adulthood, to the elder stage of life. Wadsworth (1997) contends that the advantage of a life course approach to the study of health inequalities is its ability to provide evidence of the ways in which time-associated biological and social vulnerability contribute to the lifelong development of the individual's health trajectory. The concept of a **health trajectory** focuses attention on changes in the patterns of health experienced over time. According to Henly, Wyman, and Findorff (2011, S7), "health trajectory research is the longitudinal investigation of the health and illness of individual persons, families, groups or populations over time." The important point is that health trajectories develop over a lifetime and are the product of cumulative risk and health protective factors (Halfon and Hochstein 2002). Consequently, "applying a life course perspective challenges researchers to consider the dynamic process and multidimensional nature of health and well-being in adulthood" (Liu, Jones, and Glymour 2010, 490).

The arrow pointing from the social structural side of the upper overlapping circles to "health as a biosocial reality" represents the direct effects that life chances associated with structures of inequality have on health as they shape the habitus in an ongoing developmental process. But as discussed, health lifestyles reflect particular habitus and also mediate the effects of social structure on health. The interaction effect on health shared by the habitus and health lifestyles is

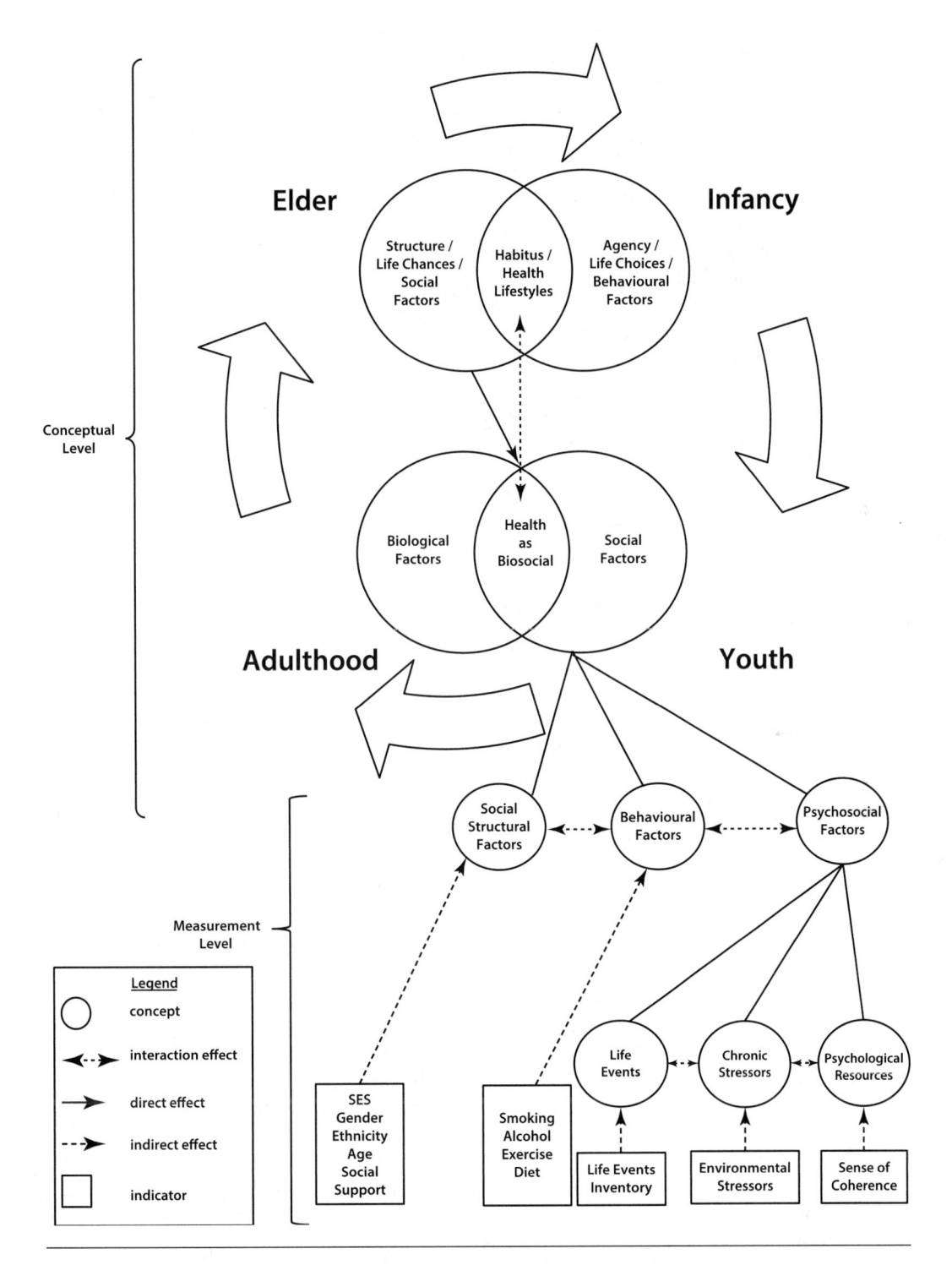

Figure 8.1 An Intersectional Model of Health As a Biosocial Reality Unfolding Across the Life Course

indicated by the dashed, double-headed arrow connecting these elements. Note that these three elements constitute a self-repeating relationship in that the habitus continuously structures particular health lifestyles, which are associated with particular health outcomes, which reciprocally both influence health lifestyles and shape the habitus throughout the life course.

Moving down a conceptual level and following Denton, Prus, and Walters (2004), the social determinants of health (i.e., "social factors") can be grouped into three broad categories: social structural factors, behavioural factors, and psychosocial factors. Social structural factors include patterned elements of social life, such as socioeconomic status, gender, ethnicity, and age. In addition, networks of social support, which will be discussed in Chapter 9, are key structural determinants of health. At the measurement level, these macro-level structural determinants tend to be measured by researchers using quantitative methods, such as statistical analysis of population health survey data, to derive indicators such as socioeconomic status (explained in Chapter 5).

Behavioural factors refer to lifestyle behaviours, such as tobacco and alcohol consumption, regular exercise, and diet. Many studies have documented the fact that routine personal practices aimed at protecting health and preventing illness contribute to good health while other personal practices contribute to ill health. It is important to recognize that behavioural factors share an interaction effect with both social structural factors and psychosocial factors. That is, as symbolized by the dashed, double-headed arrows, behavioural factors are influenced by and influence both social structural factors and psychosocial factors, which have separate and combined effects on health. It is equally noteworthy that studies have demonstrated that behavioural factors earlier in the life course, such as obesity and level of physical activity, have health effects later in life (Pluijm et al. 2007; van Oostrom et al. 2012). Health lifestyle behaviours themselves also tend to develop across the life course. For example, Cockerham (2013, 141) describes how "Age affects health lifestyles because people tend to take better care of their health as they grow older by being more careful about the food they eat, resting and relaxing more, and either reducing or abstaining from alcohol use and smoking."

Psychosocial factors are those that "in contrast to social structural factors . . . operate at the individual, subjective level" (Denton, Prus, and Walters 2004, 2586). However, from a sociological perspective, although factors such as "life events," "chronic stressors," and "psychological resources" may be expressed individually, these too are patterned by social location and follow a social gradient across the life course. Stressful life events experienced throughout life, such as the death of a spouse or friend, financial difficulties, marital breakdown, or change in residence, have important long-term effects on health and wellness. Research has shown that exposure to such stressful life events places individuals at greater risk for a host of negative health impacts, such as psychological distress and mental disorders, poor physical health, and substance abuse. In addition, research has looked at the relationship between chronic stressors—"ongoing and difficult conditions of daily life" (Denton, Prus, and Walters 2004, 2586)—and illness. For example, McDonough and Walters (2001) found that exposure to chronic stressors associated with social life problems, financial troubles, relationship difficulties, children (i.e., parenting-related), environmental issues, family health, and job strain were all positively associated with distress and, to a lesser extent, chronic health conditions. The effects of such stressors may not be readily apparent, instead having consequences for health much later in life, as with the case of Cohen's (2004) study of childhood socioeconomic status and immuno-vulnerability to infection by the cold virus (described in Chapter 2).

Research oriented by Antonovsky's goal of unravelling the mystery of health has also looked at the way in which psychological resources, such as "sense of coherence," "mastery," and "self-esteem," can act as salutogenic factors, enhancing health. The connection between psychological resources and health is a challenging one to study because of problems involved in operationalizing these resources, as well as the complicated task of measurement. Nevertheless, specific aspects of these resources have received study. For example, sense of control and high self-esteem have been found to be consistently correlated with health, measured in terms of functional ability, self-rated health, and depressive symptoms (Baltes, Wahl, and Schmid-Furstoss 1990; Krause, Herzog, and Baker 1992; Turner and Noh 1988).

Psychosocial factors and behavioural factors also interact with social structural factors, such as socioeconomic status, mediating their effects on health. In Denton, Prus, and Walters' (2004, 2587) words, "Lifestyle behaviours, exposure to stressful life events, the experience of chronic stress and the level of psychological resources are rooted in the social structural context of people's lives." One's control over one's own actions and feelings of contributing to the larger society are of particular importance for health (Syme 1994). The Determinants of Health Working Group of the National Forum on Health notes that individual agency in dealing with life's challenges might be explained through concepts such as self-esteem, sense of control over one's life, and resiliency (Renaud et al. 1996). The idea is that individual psychological resources embodied within habitus mediate the relationship between social structural factors and health. Such interpretations argue that the habitus intervenes between position within society and health; the psychosocial realm is of critical importance. For example, Krause (1987) reports that individuals who perceive they have more control in their lives are less likely to become depressed in the face of stress. In other words, individuals have a degree of agency in that we are active participants in, not passive recipients of, social forces.

More and more research is establishing the intersectionality of biological, social, and psychological factors in health as they intersect across the life course. Consider the case of immune system functioning as an example of the biosocial complexity of health. The immune system is the body's primary defence against bacteria, viruses, and cancer. Stress alters the immune system. The nervous and immune systems communicate with each other so that the social environment can influence biological responses through its input to the nervous system (Evans and Stoddart 1990). Biological responses, however, include more than the immune system. Our hormonal systems also respond to stress. Research aimed at understanding the linkages between the social environment, our emotional and biological responses, and our biology is an area of much attention at present.

A number of researchers have investigated the biological pathways through which social factors affect our health (e.g., Cohen, Tyrrell, and Smith 1991; Cohen 2004; Glaser et al. 1992). Research such as this is becoming more prominent in contributing to our understanding of the intersectionality of health. Writing from a sociology of the body perspective, Williams (2003) locates both feelings and emotions within our biological makeup, and yet, he notes, they are relational in nature. That is, they are elaborated through cultural meaning. He argues that individuals on different steps of the social hierarchy have differential empowerment. Those who are more disempowered experience greater feelings of stress, hopelessness, depression, insecurity, and lack of coherence. What is clear is that there are intersectional bases of health that are only beginning to be acknowledged within the health sciences. While data are now available establishing a linkage between social factors and health, an intersectional understanding of mechanisms through which biological changes interact with and result from these social factors has not yet been fully demonstrated through empirical research. The next frontier as we move to unravel the mystery of health is to undertake studies guided by an intersectional model that recognizes health as a complex biosocial reality that unfolds across the life course with the passage of time.

The challenge that awaits health researchers is understanding the intersection of biosocial risk factors that have lifelong, but sometimes not readily apparent, health effects. Commenting on the intersections of different social locations, the life course, and health outcomes, Spitzer (2005, 90) explains that "individuals occupy various locations on our social landscape that can change throughout the life cycle; each position offers a range of potential opportunities and experiences, oppressions and insights. The pathways by which persons can be constituted as vulnerable—or conversely, placed on the road to good health—depends in part on where one is located in this social tableau." An increasing number of studies explicitly focus on the ways in which social determinants, such as socioeconomic status, gender, and ethnicity, intersect over the life course to shape health. Furthermore, this appears to be an international trend. For example, Mishra and colleagues (2004) studied Australian women, at mid-life and later life, to explore whether socioeconomic gradients in health vary over time and with age. The purpose of this research was to attempt to determine at what point in the life course SES gradients in health get wider (or narrower) and what causes change to occur. Similarly, building on past British studies, Graham (2002) adopts a life course approach for outlining a conceptual model to guide social research on the dynamic relationship between socioeconomic status and health. She argues that the ultimate objective is to build an interdisciplinary strategy for explaining health consequences of social inequality and to provide evidence necessary for government initiatives intended to pursue "inter-sectoral policies to tackle the social determinants of health inequalities" (2002, 2013).

Chapter Summary

This chapter began by demonstrating that there are series of overlapping structures of inequality that together produce disparities in health. The case for using an intersectional perspective to understand the multi-dimensional nature of health disparities was made by arguing that in order to appreciate how society affects health, we need to move from describing inequalities based on socioeconomic status, gender, ethnicity, and age separately to developing theories that allow us to recognize their complex intersections. It was suggested that health lifestyles act as a key mechanism in the social production of health. We saw that there is conclusive evidence that establishes the direct causal relationship between particular lifestyle behaviours and health outcomes. The best example of this is the well-known relationship between tobacco use and cancer.

Awareness of such causal connections has led public health promoters to engage in individualized health promotion campaigns aimed at raising health consciousness through education. The line of reasoning behind encouraging health and wellness behaviours is that, when taken together, this will produce a population with the type of healthy lifestyles recommended by the new public health. This reasoning has led to widespread victim-blaming, which individualizes "the imperative of health" as each person's moral responsibility. The idea that we should deny medical treatment to those who smoke or have other unhealthy lifestyle behaviours is a remarkable example of this.

There is little evidence that health behaviours cluster together to form what could be called a healthy lifestyle. That is, most people's behavioural repertoires include healthful and harmful practices. For example, a person may exercise regularly and yet consume large amounts of caffeine. In addition, evidence suggests that individualized health promotion campaigns aimed at raising health consciousness are not very successful at modifying health risk behaviours. This is especially the case for those at the lower levels of the social gradient. A clear illustration of this is the failure of the Multiple Risk Factor Intervention Trial (MRFIT project) to demonstrate that lifestyle interventions change people's behaviours. What such studies do show us is how hard it is to change lifestyle behaviours.

The only public policy measures that have been shown to be unambiguously successful at getting people to change their behaviours are government regulatory measures such as enforced laws (e.g., those requiring seat belt use or prohibitions on smoking) or higher taxation on health-harming products and services (e.g., the well-known "sin taxes" on alcohol and tobacco). The political irony is that these are the types of public policy measures most opposed by neo-liberals, while the "govern through individual freedom" type of public policy favoured by the right wing doesn't work in the case of health promotion. The complexity of these issues clearly demonstrates the need for a sophisticated theoretical approach to understanding the relationship between health knowledge and health behaviours.

This relationship represents a specific instance of what sociologists refer to as the structure–agency question. The relational perspective on social life developed by Pierre Bourdieu was applied to unravelling the mystery of health across the life course. Using Bourdieu's perspective to theorize the relationship of health knowledge and health behaviours in terms of the structure–agency question led us to understand four fundamental points about health lifestyles. First, health lifestyles are a collective rather than individual phenomenon. This is because different habitus associated with different locations in social space support different health lifestyles. Second, health lifestyles represent patterns of consumption, not production. This means that we pursue particular health lifestyles (with associated health behaviours) not because we want to produce health as an end product but, rather, because of what we hope this investment in our physical capital will allow us to achieve—that is, consumption. Although positive health lifestyles are intended to produce good health, the ultimate aim of such lifestyles is to be healthy in order to use health for some other purpose, such as the ability to work, feel and look good, participate in sports and leisure activities, and enjoy life. Third, health lifestyles are formed through the dialectical interplay of agency (choices) and structure (chances). This means that health lifestyles are not simply a product of an individual's choices (agency): agency is always constrained by structural conditions, and so too are our health behaviours! This is why individualized health promotion campaigns directed at improving population health through raising individual health consciousness are misguided, and denying medical care to people with unhealthy lifestyles is uninformed! The final point that arises from conceptualizing health lifestyles in this way is that they accumulate across the life course as part of socialization and have enduring health consequences.

While in our individualistic culture we usually consider lifestyles an individual choice, health sociologists point out that aspects of our position in the social structure, such as social class, gender, ethnicity, and age, act to socially pattern lifestyles among groups of people within society. Those who suffer social exclusion also suffer poorer life chances, which produce poorer lifestyle choices, which lead to poorer health. Linking health disparities and the unequal patterning of the life chances that produce both health lifestyles and health outcomes highlights the complex connections between the major determinants of health. According to Moss (2002, 651), "Recognizing how inequality and disparities among gender and income (as well as ethnic) groups create a burden of psychosocial, functional, and health risks, brings us to the threads of human life that create and support well-being. These threads, woven into a cloth that we call social capital, include kin and community ties and social networks." The next chapter will explore the hidden depths of health care by discussing the relationship between lay beliefs, social support, informal care, and the pursuit of health and wellness.

Study Questions

1. Outline the problems associated with an individualized health promotion response to disparities in health that focuses on lifestyle factors.
2. Explain the difference between health promotion and medical consumerism.
3. Explain the relevance of the structure–agency issue for understanding the connection of health beliefs to health behaviour and addressing health disparities.
4. Sociologically, why is it useful to define health lifestyles as "collective patterns of health related behavior based on choices (i.e., agency) from options available to people according to their life chances (i.e., structure)" (Cockerham 2007, 56)?
5. Explain the connection of the habitus and the forms of capital to health lifestyles.
6. Explain the four fundamental points about health lifestyles that arise from Bourdieu's relational sociology.
7. How does an intersectional model of health and health lifestyles make it clear that health is a biosocial reality that is shaped across the life course?

Recommended Readings

Blaxter, M. 1990. *Health and Lifestyles*. London: Routledge.

Bourdieu, P., and L. Wacquant. 1992. *An Invitation to Reflexive Sociology*. Chicago: University of Chicago Press.

Cockerham, W.C. 2013. *Social Causes of Health and Disease*. 2nd edn. London: Polity.

Hankivsky, O. 2014. *Intersectionality 101*. Vancouver: Institute for Intersectionality Research and Policy.

Hansen, E., and G. Easthope. 2007. *Lifestyle in Medicine*. New York: Routledge.

Oliver, J.E. 2005. *Fat Politics: The Real Story behind America's Obesity Epidemic*. New York: Oxford University Press.

Recommended Website

The Institute for Intersectionality Research and Policy (IRPP) at Simon Fraser University: www.sfu.ca/iirp

Recommended Audiovisual Sources

Ghost in Your Genes. Documentary film broadcast on PBS, 2007.

Pierre Bourdieu: Sociology Is a Martial Art (La Sociologie est un sport de combat). Documentary film directed by Pierre Carles, 2002.

Super Size Me. Documentary film directed by Morgan Spurlock, 2004.

Part Three

Pursuing Health and Wellness

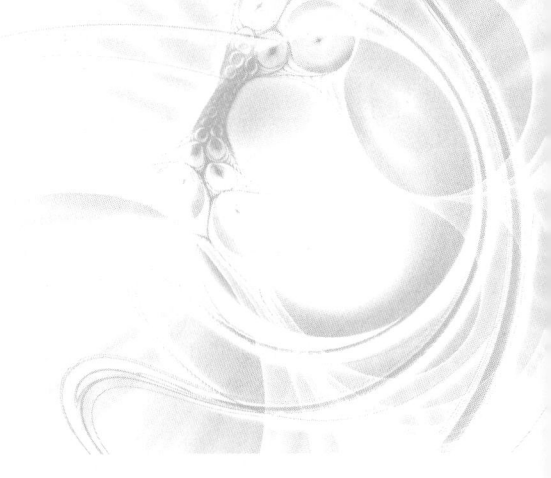

Part Three, Pursuing Health and Wellness, contains four chapters. The first three chapters explore the ways in which the informal and formal components of the health-care system contribute to population health. The final chapter summarizes the key issues discussed throughout the book and concludes by raising some unanswered questions about the prospects for achieving a healthy future.

Chapter 9 examines the nature and extent of self-health management and the relationship between lay explanatory beliefs, everyday self-care behaviour, supportive social networks, and population health. The evidence presented in this chapter clearly illustrates the fact that people play a critical role as primary providers of informal health care and are not simply consumers of formally provided medical goods and services. The chapter highlights the contributions made by the hidden components of the health-care system to the production of health.

The next two chapters shift the focus to the formal health-care system. Chapter 10 examines the development of the biomedical model of disease and the social construction of biomedical knowledge. The discussion summarizes the process by which biomedicine attained and maintains its position of dominance in health care. The chapter critically assesses the link between biomedical care and population health by exploring the increasing tendency in contemporary society to understand aspects of human experience as medical issues requiring biomedical intervention and the resulting medicalization of beings and bodies.

Chapter 11 expands the discussion of formal health care to include complementary and alternative health-care providers. The chapter explores medical pluralism by examining the use of alternatives to biomedicine in the pursuit of health and wellness. The cultural origins of medical pluralism are summarized, along with sociological explanations for the increasing popularity of complementary and alternative medicine. The chapter concludes with a discussion of the compatibility of biomedical, complementary, and alternative forms of health care and the prospects for developing an integrative medicine as part of a future formal health-care system.

Chapter 12 begins with a summary of the critical components of a sociological analysis of healthy societies and healthy people, including a theoretically based perspective, an intersectional life course model of health, and a mixed-methods approach to measuring the dimensions of health. The discussion highlights the importance of structural determinants of population health and the complex relationships between sources of inequality, such as socioeconomic status, gender, and ethnicity and health disparities.

The chapter then comments critically on the shared personal, professional, and public responsibility for health and briefly considers examples of policy initiatives with the explicit goal of reducing social inequalities in health and achieving a healthier future. The chapter ends by raising several unanswered questions about central issues that continue to be the focus of ongoing debates in the field of population health promotion. For example, is it possible to implement healthy public policies that would include structural interventions and effectively redress social inequalities in health? These types of issues must be resolved if we are to become more successful at facilitating the pursuit of health and wellness and achieving healthy societies and healthy people.

Discovering the Hidden Depths of Health Care: Lay Beliefs, Social Support, and Informal Care

Learning Objectives

This chapter explores self-health management and the relationship between informal care and population health by examining

- lay explanatory beliefs about health maintenance and illness management;
- the distinction between popular and professional conceptions of health and illness;
- self-care health beliefs and behaviour;
- social support and helping networks and their influence on health;
- the process of making sense of sickness and maintaining a healthy self-identity; and
- the contribution of informal care to the pursuit of health and wellness across the life course.

The Iceberg of Health Care

When you hear the term "health care," what comes to mind? Perhaps you think about hospitals, doctors with stethoscopes, and nurses busily rushing around wards. Maybe you think about medical technology, such as x-ray machines and CT and MRI scans, or taking prescribed medications. While these are important components of what health sociologists describe as formal care, there is a great deal more to health care than formal medical and hospital services. After reading this chapter, when you hear the term "health care" you'll think about an iceberg. That's right, "the iceberg of health care"!

The iceberg metaphor has been used a number of different ways by health researchers. For example, the types of action people undertake on their own to deal with everyday illness episodes and common symptoms have been described in terms of "the iceberg of morbidity" (Verbrugge 1986; Verbrugge and Ascione 1987; Kooiker 1995; Idler and Benyamini 1997). Verbrugge (1986, 1195) suggests that the image of an iceberg reflects the way we experience health problems in our daily lives. In describing the iceberg of morbidity, she states that

> above water is visible, or measured morbidity. This is diseases and injuries that propel permanent limitations, medical services, and death. Below water is the larger expanse of unmeasured morbidity. This is day-to-day problems that prompt self-care or no care. Moving from bottom to top, one encounters more serious health problems and more intensive professional care.

Research indicates that people engage in a variety of self-care practices to take care of routine health problems. They typically discuss symptoms with family and friends to gain support and advice, restrict daily activities, and take non-prescription drugs before making a decision to seek professional health care. In fact, "for most symptoms of daily life, people opt to do something on their own without medical help" (Verbrugge and Ascione 1987, 549). The health problems for which people seek formal medical care actually represent a small percentage of the total illness experienced.

The iceberg metaphor has been used in other ways. For example, researchers have commented on the "injury iceberg" (Sahai et al. 2005; Hanson et al. 2005). Sahai and colleagues point out that in Canada, injury is the leading cause of preventable morbidity and potential years of life lost, and they use the iceberg image to illustrate the fact that "minor" injuries are often under-reported. Detected and treated injuries are just the tip of the iceberg. The largest part of the injury iceberg remains unseen (or submerged) because injury statistics are generally poorly documented. Verbrugge (1990) contends that there is another type of iceberg—that is, the "iceberg of disability," which is used to demonstrate that we do not fully understand the impact of physical, mental, and social disabilities on people's daily lives because much of it is hidden. We know a good deal about ways in which essential activities of daily living are affected by disability because they are visible (e.g., work loss days) but less about changes that occur in optional activities, such as social interaction and leisure participation.

It should be noted that physicians have also recognized that symptoms presented by patients to formal health-care providers are only a small fraction of the wide range of health problems people routinely experience. For example, Frankel (1991) makes reference to the "iceberg of morbidity" when discussing the extent of untreated illness. More recently, McAteer, Elliott, and Hannaford (2011) conducted a community-based survey in an attempt to learn more about the size of the "symptom iceberg." Studies of interaction between patients and physicians provide "clear evidence for the existence of a submerged part of the iceberg" (Biderman and Antonovsky 1988, 176) and highlight the implications for clinical practice of not seeking medical care for prevalent, treatable conditions such as urinary infections (Last and Adelaide 2013; Minassian et al. 2012). In an editorial in the *British Medical Journal*, Jones (2000, 596) asserts that the "iceberg of illness" is an important concept in understanding the relationship between self-care and medical care and "one that healthcare systems ignore, Titanic-like, at their peril."

Finally, the iceberg analogy has even been applied to national and international health policies. According to Baum (2009, 957), one of the main messages repeatedly offered by the Commission on the Social Determinants of Health is that governments need to "avoid tip of the iceberg solutions." All of the available evidence supports the argument that it is time for health policies to go beyond the tip of the iceberg and look below the surface to find more effective ways to achieve greater health equity and to improve population health. As illustrated by Box 9.1, the iceberg metaphor is used in this chapter to inform our analysis of the informal and formal components of the health-care system and to highlight the hidden depths of health care.

Hidden Components of the Health-Care System

According to Verbrugge (1986, 1210), the iceberg of morbidity consists of distinct layers with permeable boundaries. "Each layer is a different accounting of health events. Daily symptoms are at the bottom, symptoms treated by oneself next, then problems which cause short term restricted activity, conditions which cause long term limitation next, visits to health professionals, hospital episodes and then death at the top." The layers above the water involve contact with health

Box 9.1 The Iceberg of Health Care

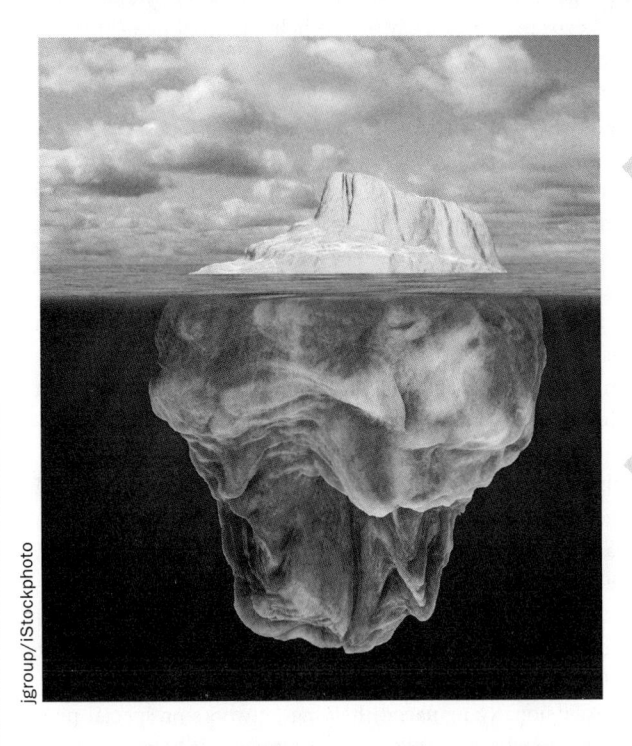

← Formal care *

← Informal care **

* Formal care—the visible part of the iceberg (above the waterline)—includes physicians and professional health-care providers, hospitals and health-care institutions, the pharmaceutical industry, and medical technology.

** Informal care—the invisible part of the iceberg (below the waterline)—includes lay health beliefs, self-care practices, mutual aid and social support networks, and self-help groups. Because of the depth of the iceberg, we have to probe deeper to discover the hidden parts of the health-care system.

professionals and the formal part of the health-care system and are routinely measured (e.g., we have extensive data documenting health-care utilization patterns). Layers below the water represent hidden and, consequently, informal components of health care that are more challenging to study. We need to make greater use of both quantitative and qualitative methods (such as health diaries) to gain a greater understanding of ways in which informal care contributes to the pursuit of health and wellness across the life course. For example, Verbrugge and Ascione (1987, 561) state that "diary data help reveal the iceberg of morbidity—the whole array of symptoms people experience and health actions taken for them."

We can visualize an iceberg of health care composed of a number of layers. In exploring the hidden parts of health care, we are going to start at the bottom of the iceberg and work our way up to the surface. The base of the iceberg consists of lay beliefs about health and illness. Calnan (1987, 8) contends that we possess a "complex system of ideas about health and its maintenance and illness and its management." We have personal beliefs about the meaning of good health and ideas about what keeps us healthy. Lay beliefs help us to define health and to select wellness-oriented behavioural practices that we think will protect our health. We also have personal ideas about what makes us sick. Lay beliefs help us to interpret the causes of ill health and to decide who are relevant helpers and the most effective ways to handle illness experiences. In other words, we all have a complicated body of knowledge and beliefs about health and illness. Lay explanatory beliefs are of vital importance because they guide our pursuit of health and wellness and provide an interpretive framework for making sense of prevalent conditions such as sickness. At the same time, beliefs cannot be directly observed and are difficult to measure. As such, they are the bottom layer of the iceberg. Lay beliefs about health and illness give meaning to the ways in which we experience changes in our health status and may guide health actions. Calnan (1987) asserts that these complex beliefs about health maintenance and illness management enable laypersons to attend to their own health requirements and to make critical judgments about the use of appropriate health-care practices, including self-care.

Moving up to the next layer of the iceberg, we find a wide variety of self-care behavioural practices that people routinely engage in to try to maintain good health and to manage illness episodes. We have learned a good deal about self-care behaviours, although there is still a lot left to learn about this component of the hidden health-care system. The next layers of the iceberg consist of supportive social networks. Researchers now recognize that social support is crucial for health, and informal caregivers, such as family and friends, play a critical part in the pursuit of health and wellness. Finally, just below the waterline, the iceberg of health care includes a layer of organized (and sometimes professionally managed) helping networks or special purpose self-help groups. Alcoholics Anonymous is probably the best known self-help group. As illustrated in reality television shows such as "Celebrity Rehab," these helping networks bring together people who are facing a common health problem to support them in their efforts to deal with issues such as addiction, abuse, bereavement, and body image and weight management, as well as a variety of mental and physical illnesses (e.g., depression, breast and prostate cancer, diabetes, and heart disease). This component of the health-care system bridges an important gap between informal self-care and formal medical care and is more visible than other types of social support.

Lay Beliefs about Health Maintenance and Illness Management

We all deal with health-related concerns on a daily basis. Everyone accounts for health and illness using socially patterned beliefs or shared ideas about the nature of the world to give meaning to these everyday experiences. **Lay beliefs** are understood by health sociologists as comprising ideas and perspectives employed by ordinary people to make sense of and find meaning in their everyday life experiences, such as health and illness. Lay conceptions of health and health-protective behaviours (i.e., routine self-care practices that we believe to be part of a healthy lifestyle) are important personal determinants of population health. In addition, the effects of structural determinants, such as SES, on our health status are mediated through the beliefs we hold about sources of good health and ill health, the personal meaning attached to being healthy, and ideas about the best ways to maintain health and manage illness.

A number of years ago, Blaxter (1997) pointed out that the way people think about causes of health and illness and their beliefs about sources of health inequalities have seldom been studied. Popay and colleagues (1998) argue that this is an oversight, since lay beliefs about the nature and causes of inequalities in health play a critical part in shaping personal health-care practices. In their opinion, the meanings that people attach to life experiences such as health and illness "in narrative form could provide invaluable insights into the dynamic relationships between human agency and wider social structures that underpin inequalities in health" (Popay et al. 1998, 636). This highlights the importance of gaining a greater understanding of the processes by which lay beliefs help people connect their life experiences with health inequalities to structural factors (such as social location) and guide actions they undertake to maintain good health and manage illness. In other words, we can learn a lot about how social location shapes health and health behaviour by studying people's lay beliefs.

While lay health beliefs are extremely important, they are also very difficult to study. Consequently, researchers have focused on health-related behaviours that can be directly observed and measured and operate on the assumption that behavioural practices reflect underlying beliefs about the world. Radley and Billig (1996) maintain that if you listen carefully when people talk about their "state of health," you can learn a great deal about their conceptions of health and illness. Litva and Eyles (1994) provide an example that illustrates this point. While participants in their study acknowledged that smoking is bad for health, some of them were able to justify continuing this practice. "While smoking is seen as affecting health in general, it is also sometimes seen as a reasonable risk to undertake in order to deal with a far more serious threat to healthiness—stress" (Litva and Eyles 1994, 1086). The personal meaning of health held by these individuals enables them to accept the fact that smoking is hazardous to health in general, but, at the same time, they continue to believe that smoking may be beneficial to their sense of healthiness since it helps them to manage stress (or to keep their weight under control). This research suggests that people make distinctions between the ways in which major determinants affect the health of the general population and the impact these factors have on their personal sense of healthiness.

Health researchers (Levesque and Li 2014, 633) argue that "the way health is defined and conceptualized represents a guide for actions; health behaviors and practices are thus informed by the conceptions of health held by individuals." Despite this widely accepted theoretical assumption, they contend that past efforts to measure conceptions of health and illness have been limited and that the link between everyday lay explanatory beliefs and personal health practices has still not been fully investigated. Qualitative approaches are typically recommended as the best way to uncover lay health and illness beliefs. In order to move beyond the recurrent descriptive themes identified in past research (and discussed in the following sections), Downey and Chang (2013) employ a mixed-method approach to develop a Lay Concepts of Health Inventory. Their objective is to transform qualitative data (such as open-ended descriptions of what health is) into a valid quantitative measure of lay health and illness beliefs. In their opinion, "while the complex relations between health concepts and behaviours are of central interest to researchers and practitioners, they can only be speculated about in the absence of reliable measurement tools of lay concepts of health" (2013, 819). Although this inventory shows promise, Downey and Chang acknowledge that it needs further validation to ensure that it is conceptually sound and captures the multi-dimensional nature of lay health beliefs. Consequently, researchers have more work to do if we are to gain a better understanding of lay conceptions of health and illness, as well as the relationship between beliefs, behaviour, and health status.

Lay Beliefs about Good Health: The Meaning of Wellness

What do people mean when they say they are in good health? Do members of the public think about good health and wellness in terms other than the absence of disease? Do lay beliefs include positive aspects of health and well-being? What are the most prevalent lay beliefs about maintaining good health? There are still more questions than answers when it comes to lay conceptions of good health. Because of the emphasis of past research on illness behaviour and formal medical care, we have learned a great deal about people's ideas regarding the causes and consequences of sickness, but we know less about lay beliefs regarding sources of good health and the meaning of wellness. This is unfortunate, given the earlier discussion of the importance of adopting a salutogenic perspective to unravel the mystery of health.

Although only a limited number of researchers have investigated lay beliefs about good health, there have been some exceptions (e.g., Levesque, Li, and Bohemier 2013; Downey and Chang 2013; Asbring 2012; d'Houtaud and Field 1984; Herzlich 1973). With the transformation of medical sociology into health sociology and the shift in research focus from patient illness behaviour to population health behaviour, lay conceptions of good health are receiving more attention. Unfortunately, research continues to concentrate primarily on lay beliefs about illness management and pathways to formal care. Lay beliefs apparently reflect the general view that health is a multi-dimensional concept that incorporates physical, psychological, and social components. The results of an early study by Baumann (1961) suggest that we make judgments about health based on an appraisal of all of these components. This study identified three general orientations or lay conceptions of good health: a **symptom orientation** based on the belief that good health means an absence of symptoms of illness (i.e., a physical component), a **feeling-state orientation** based on the belief that good health means a sense of well-being (i.e., a psychological component), and a **performance orientation** based on the belief that good health means being able to carry out one's usual daily activities (i.e., a social component). These findings indicate that health is not a unitary concept but a multi-dimensional one, even in the layperson's mind!

While people may think about health in terms of physical, psychological, and social dimensions, it is the individual's interpretation of the personal meaning of good health that determines which component is highlighted. Lay conceptions may reflect a negative view, such as health as the absence of disease, illness, and disability, or more positive aspects of health, such as psychosocial well-being, fitness, and the ability to function in one's daily life (Levesque, Li, and Bohemier 2013). As Williams (1983, 189) explains, "Although health can be used to mean simply the absence of disease, it is also used in a far more complex and positive sense." There is growing awareness on the part of the public that the absence of illness and disease is not the same as being well, and, according to Hughner and Kleine (2004), "lay health worldviews" include a range of ideas about health and wellness. Let's briefly review the major thematic conceptions of the differing meanings of health and wellness. As we do this, consider your own beliefs, comparing how you think about good health to the major themes that have been identified in the research literature (see Box 9.2).

The negative conception of **health as the absence of illness and disease** has been identified in several studies (e.g., Levesque and Li 2014; van Dalen, Williams, and Gudex 1994; d'Houtaud and Field 1984; Williams 1983; Herzlich 1973). Researchers suggest that most members of the public have conceptions of good health that are formed in relation to beliefs about illness. It has been argued that the meaning of health must be understood in relation to the individual's experiences with illness and disease. Herzlich (1973, 55) referred to this negative conception as

> **Box 9.2 Differing Meanings of Health and Wellness**
>
> - Health as absence of illness and disease ("health-in-a-vacuum")
> - Health as fitness
> - Health as sense of well-being
> - Health as functional ability
> - Health as a resource for living (health reserve)

"health-in-a-vacuum" and stressed that this lay definition hinges on what is absent or missing from the individual's life (i.e., illness).

The belief that good health simply means not being ill can be expressed in a number of different ways. Generally, it means freedom from symptoms of ill health, such as having no aches or pains. Alternatively, it may mean not having anything more serious to deal with than a cold. In other words, it is possible to experience a common health problem and still believe that you are a healthy person. This negative conception of health may also mean not having any serious diseases such as cancer. It is interesting to note that this lay conception of good health is related to a sense of wholeness. In fact, the terms "healthy" and "whole" are both derived from the same Old English root word—*hoelth*, and this connection seems to be evident in contemporary lay beliefs. Thus, the layperson may have a symptom orientation to health and believe that the absence of illness means she is a hale (whole) and hearty (healthy) person.

Blaxter (1990) has described a variation on this theme as "health despite disease." She points out that it is important to recognize that the presence of disease is not incompatible with a conception of good health. According to Levesque, Li, and Bohemier (2013, 220), many people believe that they can still be healthy "despite an illness, as long as their disease is under control and does not interfere with their daily functioning." Research indicates that older adults living with multiple chronic conditions typically report that they are in good health for their age (Segall and Chappell 1991). Such findings suggest that this conception of good health is tied to the belief that the individual is managing her conditions effectively. Thus, it is possible to reconcile chronic illness with the personal meaning of good health.

In this conception, health is defined in negative terms by what is absent or has not occurred and is tied to lay beliefs about illness. In contrast, studies have identified lay beliefs that focus on the presence of indicators of good health rather than the absence of indicators of ill health. These conceptions emphasize positive aspects of health and wellness, such as fitness, healthiness, and functional ability. Each of these conceptions will be briefly examined, as well as a final lay conception that characterizes health as a resource for living.

Health as fitness has been identified by researchers such as van Dalen, Williams, and Gudex (1994). Ideas about fitness generally include both physical and psychological dimensions of health. This notion of health is reflected by the individual who believes that to be healthy, "one has to be both physically and mentally fit." Thus, lay beliefs about health as fitness combine being physically active and having a healthy body with psychological energy and vitality. The term "vitality" refers to being able to meet demands, being lively, or being "full of life." According to van Dalen, Williams, and Gudex (1994, 252), "positive health, it seems, is about being fit, energetic, and feeling on top of the world." Similarly, Levesque and Li (2014) report that some health definitions emphasize factors such as level of energy, feeling well emotionally, and having good cognitive functions. This conception of health is clearly tied to a sense of healthiness or well-being and the social capacity to perform well roles.

The lay conception of **health as a sense of well-being** emphasizes positive aspects of health similar to Baumann's (1961) feeling-state orientation discussed earlier. A sense of well-being is based on psychological and social components of health, reflecting feelings of happiness and healthiness along with rewarding relationships. For example, Litva and Eyles (1994, 1085) define healthiness as "an individualistic sense of well-being which is linked to a psychological (as opposed to the physical) state." At the psychological level, van Dalen, Williams, and Gudex (1994) suggest that this conception of health reflects feelings such as being relaxed, contented, and confident. In addition, health as a sense of well-being has a social dimension that is based on having close ties to family members and friends and meaningful interpersonal relationships with others in the community (Levesque and Li 2014). Herzlich (1973) characterized these beliefs about good health as a sense of balance in everyday life (i.e., mind, body, and spirit are in harmony). For example, an individual might believe that she is a healthy person because she feels that everything is going well or all parts of her life are working right. Thus, this conception of good health as a positive feeling-state may be expressed in terms of her level of satisfaction with quality of life.

A conception of **health as functional ability** is reflected by lay beliefs about individual ability to carry out daily tasks and cope with demands of everyday life and social roles. For example, Calnan (1987, 18) points out that an important meaning of health for the typical layperson is the "capacity to achieve preferred goals or perform certain functions." This conception of health, which Levesque and Li (2014) label as "functionality" or the ability to function in one's daily life, emphasizes being able to do things or, in Baumann's terms, a performance orientation. A Canadian study (Mansour 1994) reported that health was frequently defined as the ability to perform functions of daily living (i.e., health is being able to do things by yourself). This conception of good health as social capacity is based on lay beliefs about the importance of being able to perform usual well roles and tasks without restrictions. In other words, good health means being able to do what you want to do, when you want to do it. In addition, this lay conception of health includes the capacity to function as expected by others at home and at work. Health as functional ability is tied to beliefs about physical and psychological fitness (e.g., being fit for activities such as child care, housework, or paid labour) and a sense of well-being (e.g., having the energy and enthusiasm necessary to carry out normal well roles).

Finally, the lay conception of good **health as a resource for living** combines the social, psychological, and physical dimensions. Herzlich (1973, 56) used the term "reserve of health" to describe this resource for living. According to Herzlich, our **health reserve** has a physical basis and is associated with factors such as a person's constitution and temperament (e.g., being energetic and having personal strength and vitality). Herzlich characterizes health reserve as a capital asset to be managed. A good analogy might be an inheritance (for example, money we received from a grandparent when we were born). We can place this money in a bank account or another type of investment and withdraw funds as necessary to cover expenses. We may have limited expenses and spend the money slowly, or we may have major expenses and go through it quickly (e.g., university tuition). We may also have unexpected expenses. In any case, if we simply withdraw funds, this asset will eventually be depleted. In contrast, by carefully investing the money and making occasional contributions, our savings reserve can increase and offer us future financial security.

Similarly, health can be viewed as an asset to be managed. Although this reserve of health is shaped to a certain extent by heredity (i.e., genetic makeup) and early childhood experiences, there is evidence that it is affected over the life course by personal health practices. On the one hand, self-neglect (e.g., lack of physical activity) and harmful personal practices (e.g., smoking) can deplete this reserve. As a result, we may increase our susceptibility to serious illness and, in some cases, premature death. On the other hand, healthy lifestyle practices help to strengthen this reserve and potentially increase health expectancy. In other words, if you take care of yourself (avoid known health hazards and engage in health-protective behaviour), you may add years of good health to your lifespan (i.e., build up your assets).

It is important, however, to recognize that our health reserve is affected not only by personal health behaviour but also by broader societal conditions. Today, health is increasingly seen as a resource that is shaped not only by lifestyle activities and behaviours but also by structural factors explained in the chapters in the preceding part of the book. It is important to note that health as a resource for living consists of a combination of physical fitness, a sense of psychological healthiness or well-being, and the social capacity to perform expected well roles and that all three are necessary for the pursuit of health and wellness. Sociologically, this conception makes a lot of sense, because it reflects the multi-dimensional biopsychosocial reality of health. Furthermore, it is consistent with the salutogenic understanding of the continuum of health as described by Antonovsky. The pursuit of health and wellness involves an ongoing process of adapting to changing social conditions, and an individual's ability to adapt effectively is, in turn, a product of their health reserve.

Lay Illness Belief Dimensions: The Meaning of Sickness

We all become ill at times throughout life and develop explanatory beliefs that help us to interpret the meaning of what we are going through and decide on a course of action. Zola (1972a) argued that we are all confronted at some point with an inevitable search for the meaning of misfortune and suffering. For example, when we experience sickness (particularly in the case of serious health problems), a series of questions arise. We struggle to find answers to questions about the onset and treatment of each condition, such as: What caused the problem? How should it be handled? At the same time, we struggle to find answers to questions we have about the meaning of health problems for our present and future, such as: Why is this happening to me? What will the outcome be? The biomedical model and health-care professionals may be able to provide reasonably complete answers to the first set of questions. Scientific explanations of disease, however, typically do not provide adequate answers to questions such as: Why me? Murray (1990, 84) explains that "the response to these questions goes beyond the search for causes and becomes a quest for meaning." Lay explanatory beliefs and common sense understandings of the way in which the world works give meaning to our illness experiences.

Lay illness explanatory beliefs develop over time as people struggle to make sense of sicknesses they experience. Lay explanations of chronic illnesses such as arthritis or high blood pressure, which become an enduring part of life, are likely to be more developed than lay beliefs about acute illness episodes (except recurring ones such as the "common" cold). People who have lived with chronic illness for a number of years have had ample opportunity to formulate beliefs about the causes and consequences of their health problems and the best course of action for dealing with the symptoms. What types of lay beliefs regarding the meaning and management of sickness have health researchers identified? The following discussion highlights the major illness belief dimensions that have received the most research attention. Many studies in this area focus on illness beliefs held by older adults who live with multiple chronic health problems. The illness

Box 9.3 Illness Belief Dimensions

- Causality
- Controllability
- Susceptibility
- Seriousness

belief dimensions examined most frequently are listed in Box 9.3. It is important to recognize that these dimensions are not mutually exclusive.

The process of making sense of sickness generally begins with the individual's ideas about the causes of the health problems that she is experiencing. Internationally renowned British sociologist Mildred Blaxter (see Box 9.4) (1983) contends that the search for causal explanation is a common aspect of lay illness experience. In her words, "It is a common finding that one of the things which most concerns patients, when they are given a diagnosis, is to know not simply the name of their disease but also its cause" (1983, 59). According to Blaxter, the importance attached to understanding **causality**, or the origins of disease, reflects the influence of the biomedical model on lay illness beliefs. Apparently, most members of the lay community (like health-care professionals) operate on the assumption that every identified disease has a specific underlying cause or combination of causal factors.

The middle-aged, working-class women interviewed by Blaxter typically rejected "natural degenerative processes" associated with aging as the cause of their conditions. The most prevalent categories of cause cited by respondents were infection, heredity, family susceptibility, and environmental factors. Environmental explanations were the most popular and included working in unpleasant and stressful conditions, poor housing, and, in some cases, a harsh climate.

Box 9.4 Mildred Blaxter (1925–2010)

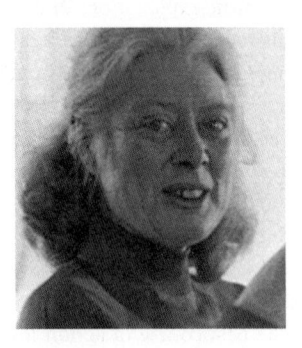

- Internationally renowned UK sociologist
- Played a leading role in the first UK Health and Lifestyle Survey (1990)
- Published extensively in the areas of social inequalities and health and cycles of disadvantage
- Served as editor of major journals, such as *Sociology of Health and Illness* and *Social Science and Medicine*

"[I]t is necessary to distinguish, not only between public and private accounts, but also between the cause of illness and the cause of health, . . . and between what is held to affect the health of society in general and what is perceived as influential in one's own life" (1997, 755).

Blaxter (1983, 63) concluded that "to find a cause in the environment was more acceptable than to locate responsibility in one's own body." According to her study, illness is primarily attributable to external causes. These women's beliefs about the causes of their conditions helped them to make sense of their diagnoses and had direct effects on their help-seeking behaviour.

Pill and Stott (1982; 1985), following Blaxter, argue that beliefs about illness causation are related to the acceptance of personal responsibility for health (i.e., for both staying healthy and becoming ill). These researchers distinguish between causes that are within versus those that are outside of the individual's control. The majority of working-class women who participated in these studies expressed the belief that causes are external to the individual and were characterized as having fatalistic views regarding sources of illness. For example, they attributed the onset of illness to factors such as the environment, heredity, and family susceptibility. A smaller proportion accepted some responsibility for health maintenance and acknowledged that day-to-day lifestyle choices regarding diet, exercise, and other personal practices have important implications for future health and the onset of illness. Once again, virtually none of the women in these studies mentioned "the wearing out of bodily systems or ageing as explanations for illness causation" (Pill and Stott 1982, 45).

Lau and Hartman (1983) also differentiated between external (not my fault) versus internal (my fault) reasons for becoming ill. Many respondents gave several different reasons for getting sick (including, in some cases, both external and internal factors). Despite these multiple responses, it should be noted that most external causes were believed to be sufficient by themselves to be *the* primary cause of illness (e.g., contagious disease or the weather). In contrast, internal causes (e.g., not taking care of oneself or not getting enough sleep) were only believed to contribute to the onset of ill health in combination with other factors. From these studies we can conclude that lay beliefs about causes of illness minimize the importance of personal responsibility for health (i.e., internal causes) and attach greater significance to social and physical environmental factors (i.e., external causes). These findings raise questions about the wisdom of continuing to pursue the type of individualized health promotion approach described in the previous chapter.

Research also suggests that there are age differences in causal attributions for illness. While studies of middle-aged respondents (e.g., Blaxter 1983; Pill and Stott 1982, 1985) report that illness was seldom attributed to the aging process, studies of older adults found that they seem ready to make attributions to internal physical processes (such as biological aging) rather than to the environment. For example, Stoller (1993) used a health diary method to explore causal attributions for symptoms experienced by older adults and categorized responses as either medical or non-medical interpretations. These older adults attributed symptoms to three medical (professional) interpretations (i.e., a flare-up of a chronic disease or condition, other medical conditions, or something they caught from someone else). Four non-medical (popular) interpretations were also evident in their health diaries (i.e., normal aging, lifestyle, stress, and weather or season of the year).

Stoller's findings demonstrate that older adults generally make attributions that combine internal and external causal factors when interpreting the meaning of health problems. It is significant to note that more than half of the older adults attributed at least one symptom to normal aging. In other words, they normalized symptoms such as fatigue and joint or muscle pain by characterizing them as "something that happens to most people as they get older" (Stoller 1993, 67). Since older adults expect to have to deal with illness in later life, it may be viewed as a normal part of aging (Gibson and Boiko 2012). This research suggests that as people move through the life course, they tend to use normal aging as an explanation for common symptomatic conditions and declining functioning, although these changes in health are not universal consequences of the aging process.

It seems that when people of all ages experience misfortune in their lives, such as sickness, they search for a causal explanation to help make sense of what is happening to them. Lundell, Niederdeppe, and Clarke (2013, 1126) suggest that lay beliefs about causality and responsibility provide "the natural starting point for talking about health." For example, Prior, Evans, and Prout (2011, 927) explored the ways in which older adults talk about the symptoms and causes of the common cold and influenza (flu) and report that their respondents identified "a wide range of causative agents." Causes of the flu included viruses, bugs and germs, the environment in general, being wet and wearing damp clothes, and the coughs and sneezes of other people. However, they caution that an understanding of the part played by these factors must take into account lay beliefs about a person's resilience, immunity, and overall healthiness.

In summary, causality is typically attributed to either internal or external factors. In lay illness explanations, causation is attributed to factors that are considered either non-modifiable (e.g., heredity) or modifiable (e.g., unhealthy lifestyle practices). As the research demonstrates, beliefs about causality are quite comprehensive and include complex combinations of natural factors (e.g., germs, climate), the aging process, social factors (e.g., stress, occupational and environmental conditions), and, occasionally, supernatural factors (e.g., God's will). Further research is required to clarify the relationship between social location (e.g., gender and ethnicity), beliefs about causality, and interpretations of the meaning of specific symptoms and illness conditions.

Controllability has been identified as another key lay illness belief dimension. This explanatory belief refers to the extent to which individuals believe that illness is controllable and can be managed by either the sick person or another person, such as a health-care professional. "Controllability reflects whether anyone or anything can influence the course of the disease" (Turk, Rudy, and Salovey 1986, 470). Studies frequently differentiate between internal and external health control beliefs. Personal (or internal) self-control beliefs refer to sense of mastery of health and illness. External beliefs refer to provider-control beliefs (i.e., faith in health-care professionals) and chance health outcome beliefs (i.e., the idea that factors affecting health are beyond everyone's control) (Lau and Hartman 1983; Seeman and Seeman 1983).

The focus in this case is primarily on lay ideas about the course of the illness rather than the cause of the illness. This dimension includes beliefs about whether the individual is responsible for health and the extent to which she believes that personal actions are important in avoiding illness and taking care of health problems. Many studies have explored the issue of control in the context of both health and illness behaviour. For example, Lee and colleagues (2014) found that public discourse on health risk in Canada is associated with people's beliefs concerning individual control, personal agency, and responsibility. They conclude that "the findings of the present study point to the high value that Canadians place on health, as well as the strong sense of control and personal agency that they place over health risks" (2014, 132). Past research has shown that a sense of control is associated with self-rated health and self-initiated preventive care, as well as behaviour during illness episodes such as the use of physician services and compliance with medical treatment.

For example, Calnan (1989) examined the link between lay beliefs about control and specific preventive health behaviours such as exercise and smoking cessation, while Peterson and Stunkard (1989) took a more general approach and explored the potential value of the concept of personal control for the field of health promotion. According to Peterson and Stunkard, personal control reflects people's sense of mastery of the environment and their beliefs about how effective they are at bringing about positive events in their lives (such as health and well-being). They assert that there is a well-established connection between internal personal control beliefs and health that is supported by a growing body of research demonstrating "that belief in one's competence is closely tied to physical well-being, while a belief that one is helpless is associated with mortality and morbidity" (1989, 822). These researchers argue that the explanation for this relationship stems from the fact that people who strongly believe in personal control are more likely to adopt healthy behavioural practices. Such findings make sense in light of Antonovsky's "sense of coherence" described in Chapter 3.

Causality and controllability are clearly interrelated. Many discussions of these first two lay belief dimensions concentrate on the notion of personal responsibility. For example, Turk, Rudy, and Salovey (1986, 469) acknowledge that controllability "bears some resemblance to the personal responsibility dimension." Similarly, Lee and colleagues (2014) contend that public views about the controllability of health risks emphasize individual responsibility for health. In neo-liberal culture, there is a widespread belief that one means of asserting control over illness experiences is to assume responsibility for the factors that caused the health problem. In other words, attributing illness to internal causes (such as behavioural practices) may enhance the individual's sense of control over the course of the condition. Calnan (1987, 54–5) states that "the extent to which people feel in control of their health appears to depend on a number of different but interrelated elements. The first one involves their theories about disease causation and the extent to which their actions or the actions of others are imputed as a significant influence in causation." It may be possible to distinguish between personal responsibility for the onset of ill health (i.e., the cause) and a sense of personal control over the course of the condition and its management. However, responsibility for illness outcomes combines beliefs about both the causality and controllability of specific illness conditions, and, consequently, it is very difficult to separate these two lay illness belief dimensions.

Another illness belief dimension "claimed to be important in explaining health actions is perceived vulnerability to illness in general or to a specific disease" (Calnan 1987, 41). **Perceived susceptibility** is defined as the degree to which a person believes that she is vulnerable to or might experience health problems. Discussions about illness susceptibility beliefs generally include notions of illness danger or threat, as well as risk versus resistance and weakness versus strength. Studies have examined both disease-specific and general vulnerability to illness. For example, Evans and colleagues (2007) investigated lay beliefs about influenza and found that feeling vulnerable was linked to respondents' views about the need for immunization. According to Williams (1983), beliefs about illness vulnerability may be expressed in terms of "centres of weakness" that have a bodily focus. In other words, perceived susceptibility is related not only to our ideas about the nature of illness but also to our beliefs about how our bodies function. In Williams' words, "The usual way in which my respondents defined such a centre of weakness was in terms of an organ, limb or part of the body which has tended to collect varying diseases or symptoms at different times" (1983, 191). The chest was identified as the most vulnerable part of the body, although the heart, back, stomach, legs, eyes, and nerves are common sites of susceptibility. Based on such beliefs, an individual might be convinced that she is at particular risk of developing chest colds or pneumonia. Apparently, these areas of vulnerability are related to people's beliefs about their susceptibility to illness and the types of health problems they expect to experience. Although the link between perceived health risks and the process of aging has received limited research attention, there is evidence that an individual's sense of vulnerability increases with age (Lee et al. 2014). Consequently, these researchers conclude that "further research on the health risk representations, perceptions of control and health risk decisions of older adults would be fruitful to determine how these evolve over the life course" (2014, 131).

Finally, lay ideas about the seriousness of illness have been identified as an important belief dimension. Turk, Rudy, and Salovey (1986) suggest that **seriousness** consists of individual beliefs about whether the condition is long-lasting and difficult to cure and requires medical attention. Conditions that are difficult to manage and require professional health care are generally interpreted as serious. The relationship between time and seriousness is more problematic. Initially, symptomatic conditions that persist and do not respond promptly to intervention may be interpreted as serious. However, if conditions become chronic in nature and last for a long time, they may become normalized and, eventually, perceived as less serious. In addition, seriousness has also been related to other factors, such as whether the illness is familiar or recognizable versus unknown. Conditions that are familiar to us (e.g., colds), that we have had past experience handling, and that typically do not result in long-term problems are less likely to be perceived as a serious threat to our health.

Health researchers have learned a good deal about some belief dimensions, such as causality and controllability, and much less about beliefs regarding susceptibility and seriousness. In addition to these four belief dimensions, analysis of the content of lay illness explanations also needs to be broadened. There are other lay illness beliefs that warrant research attention, such as beliefs about stability versus changeability. This dimension refers to beliefs about whether symptoms and illnesses are stable or change over time. Although Turk, Rudy, and Salovey (1986) report that stability was the weakest of the dimensions investigated, it appears to be an important aspect of lay illness beliefs. Further research is needed to address the fact that this dimension includes beliefs about whether symptoms and illness are temporary or permanent (i.e., stable over time), as well as beliefs about whether symptoms and illness are predictable versus random in both occurrence and outcome (i.e., stable across situations). We also need to learn more about the ways in which these types of beliefs shape our personal health practices.

Both conceptual clarification and improvements in methodology are necessary if we are to gain insight into the extent to which our health-related behaviours reflect underlying lay beliefs about health and illness. At the conceptual level, future research needs to specify precisely the nature of lay belief dimensions and clarify relationships between these explanatory beliefs. In other words, we need to pay more attention to the linkages between lay beliefs. Future research might also assess more carefully the precise manner in which these belief dimensions are related to social location and function as coherent explanatory styles (i.e., patterned ways of conceptualizing good health and explaining sickness when it occurs throughout our lives). Research methods must also be improved if we are to gain a better understanding of lay health and illness beliefs. What is the best way to measure implicit lay conceptions of good health or unstated common sense ideas about sickness? This is not an easy question to answer because of the depth of the hidden parts of the health-care system. Longitudinal studies, prospective research designs, and the use of qualitative methods, such as illness narratives, would enable investigators to assess the impact of personal health history (i.e., age of onset and years lived with specific illness conditions) and life course transitions on lay beliefs about health maintenance and illness management. Future studies must concentrate on developing measures of underlying beliefs and recognize that ability to verbalize lay explanatory beliefs may vary widely. In summary, then, a variety of conceptual and methodological issues must be addressed. These are important issues that speak to real world debates such as the current controversy over vaccinations. Greater conceptual clarity and improved measurement are essential if future research is to be successful at improving our knowledge about the complex processes by which lay explanatory beliefs shape our understanding of the meaning of good health, help us to interpret changes in health status and make sense of sickness, and influence the type of actions we undertake to maintain health and manage illness.

There is also a need to address the origin of lay beliefs about health and illness. How do people acquire the types of explanatory beliefs just reviewed? To what extent are lay beliefs separate and distinct from expert medical knowledge? A number of researchers have debated this issue (e.g., Kangas 2002; Prior 2003; Shaw 2002). Shaw (2002, 289) argues that the term "lay beliefs" is somewhat misleading, since our ideas and knowledge about health and illness primarily come from "internalizing medical or professional constructions of the world." As a result, he contends, the way people view health and illness is ultimately shaped by medical rationality and the biomedical model. In contrast, Hughner and Kleine (2004, 416) assert that lay beliefs about health and illness "do not directly correspond to those of professionals, nor are they watered-down versions of what is taught in medical schools." They conclude that the perspective (or health world view) of lay people draws upon a wide variety of information sources and is not limited to the professional health-care sector. In a discussion of diversity in lay health understandings, Hughner and Kleine (2008) provide evidence that prevailing lay ideas vary considerably in terms of the meaning of health, perceived self-efficacy and self-care practices, and the extent to which they align with conventional biomedical or alternative health belief systems. In addition, Gibson and Boiko (2012, 158) argue that we need to find a way of "disentangling the complex relationships that emerge in accounts of illness" and focus greater research attention on the structural aspects of illness accounts. At present, we don't have a precise understanding of the processes by which people acquire health-related beliefs or the relationship between lay and expert knowledge about health and illness. Ideas about what it means to be healthy, how we become sick, and the best ways to handle illness are products of subtle, but complex, processes of informal socialization in the socio-cultural context of family and friends and exposure to mass media, along with formal learning in educational settings and, of course, contacts with professional health care.

Popular and Professional Health Belief Systems

Beliefs about health, illness, and healing vary widely. As depicted in Figure 9.1, researchers over the years have used a variety of terms to categorize health belief systems as being either: folk and primitive or scientific (King 1962); lay or professional (Freidson 1970a; 1970b); non-Western or Western (Pfifferling 1975); traditional or modern (New 1977); and popular or expert (Blumhagen 1980). Despite diversity in classification, all health belief systems shape our conception of good health and wellness and provide us with an interpretive framework for making sense of sickness. O'Conner (1995, 22) offers the following description of health belief systems:

> Health belief systems weave together attitudes toward health and illness, and theories of disease etiology and remediation. In addition they articulate these within a larger cultural framework of other important beliefs and values—for example, those dealing with religious, moral, and ethical concerns; with family and community relations and the requirements of reciprocal responsibility; with the nature of the universe, the world, or Nature, and the rightful place of humanity in them; with human nature and the capacities and limitations of the human body, mind, and spirit, and so on.

Drawing upon this, it is possible to define a **health belief system** as a systematic set of ideas with regard to health, healing, and self-care that are shaped by aspects of culture and social location. Both popular (i.e., non-scientific, traditional, lay) and professional (i.e., scientific, modern, expert) health beliefs offer ways of understanding the nature of everyday health concerns and attributing meaning to illness experiences.

Popular and professional conceptions of health and illness are based on systems of meaning that attempt to explain the onset, course, progression, and resolution of sickness (Pfifferling 1975). Health belief systems frame the way we think about illness experiences and the language we use to describe changes in health status. They guide the course of action we select to manage our health-care needs and to try to overcome illness (i.e., self-care). Thus, each health belief system helps to resolve the uncertainty and anxiety that often accompany the onset of illness. Health beliefs also serve to rationalize treatment choices and to pattern expectations about the course and outcome of illness experiences. Therefore, in a sociological perspective, formal biomedical knowledge, like informal lay health knowledge, "may be seen as just another set of ideas validated by social consensus" (Dingwall et al. 1977, 11). We will return to this point in Chapter 11 when we examine medical pluralism and alternatives to biomedical knowledge and practice.

For now, as depicted in Figure 9.1, it is essential to recognize that a reciprocal relationship exists between popular and professional systems of belief and practice (Press, 1980). Although this relationship is rather uneven in nature because of the dominance of biomedicine, laypersons and health-care experts continuously exchange ideas about health and illness. There are many elements that are common to both, and since these two systems of thought are not mutually exclusive, an understanding (or, for that matter, even an acceptance) of biomedicine does not necessarily mean rejection of traditional lay health beliefs. For example, Segall and Chappell (1991) studied older adults' ideas about the meaning and management of chronic illness and found that most respondents believed that medical care is necessary for conditions such as high blood pressure, while at the same time many also believed that some home remedies are better than

Popular Sector
"folk/primitive"
"lay"
"non–Western"
"traditional"

Everyday Health Beliefs and Practices

Professional Sector
"scientific"
"expert"
"Western"
"modern"

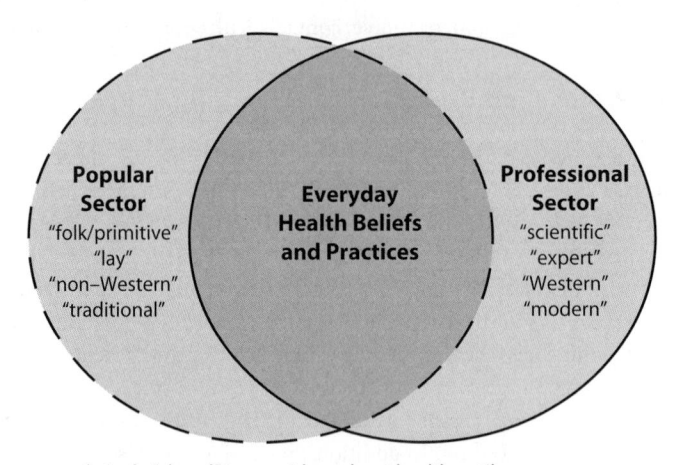

— relatively "closed" to new ideas about health until scientifically verified.
-- relatively "open" two-way exchange of ideas about health.

Figure 9.1 Pluralistic Health Belief System

prescribed drugs for treating sickness. Segall and Chappell (1991, 130) conclude that "although scientific, medical understandings of the causes and consequences of sickness may be prevalent in the lay community, they appear to operate selectively in conjunction with enduring popular health beliefs in giving meaning to the experience of chronic illness."

Apparently, in societies in which both popular and professional health belief systems coexist, people take a practical approach to managing illness and may use what each system has to offer as long as it results in favourable health outcomes. For example, prescribed medications, such as antibiotics, may be combined with traditional home remedies, such as the ever-popular chicken soup. Individuals may selectively engage in health actions based on a combination of popular and professional beliefs, relying on some form of self-treatment for familiar conditions (such as a sore throat) and, at the same time, consulting a range of health-care professionals (such as physicians and chiropractors) for other conditions. As illustrated by Figure 9.1, everyday health beliefs and practices incorporate many basic tenets of biomedicine along with traditional lay understandings of health maintenance and illness management derived from prevalent popular ideas about health and wellness, such as those in the mainstream media.

Popular and professional health beliefs can and do exist in the same social settings. It could be argued that while these belief systems offer competing frameworks for understanding health and illness, their fundamental relationship may also be characterized as complementary rather than contradictory in nature. It seems that "popular belief systems are different from, yet linked to, expert belief systems" (Blumhagen 1980, 197). Figure 9.1 illustrates that there is a constant ongoing interchange of ideas about health and illness between the popular and professional components of the pluralistic health belief system existing in societies such as Canada. Elements of both belief systems blend together in everyday ideas about health and illness and our health-care practices. Lay beliefs about health and illness often include a diverse mixture of both scientific and other forms of knowledge. In our complex culture, a wide array of sources of information is readily available. While universities and laboratories are important sources of knowledge, they are not the only ones available to the layperson (Gabe, Bury, and Elston 2004). For example, as we saw in Chapter 7, ethnic and Indigenous cultural traditions also offer people information and knowledge with which to understand their bodies and health. Health advice offered by celebrities, such as Jenny McCarthy, Angelina Jolie, or Gwyneth Paltrow, is for some, another source of health-related information. In fact, in a book provocatively entitled *Is Gwyneth Paltrow Wrong about Everything?* Caulfield (2015) points out that celebrity culture is an important source of unscientific health information often adopted uncritically by a willing public. Caulfield (2015, 304) warns that "The bulk of health and beauty products and recommendations peddled by or through celebrities are either useless or harmful or both." The significance of particular forms of knowledge in shaping health beliefs and behaviours varies depending on aspects of social location such as socioeconomic status, gender, ethnic background, and stage in the life course.

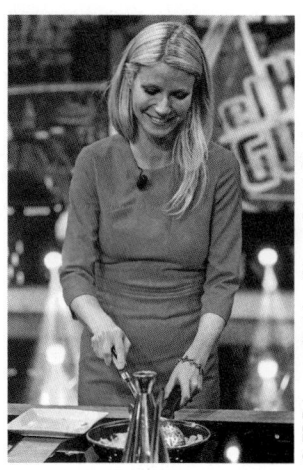

Lay beliefs about health can be influenced by many sources, including celebrities. For example, Gwyneth Paltrow, pictured here during a television appearance, provides health and nutritional advice on her lifestyle website called Goop. Paltrow and other celebrities have been criticized for offering health and wellness advice and accused of holding health-related beliefs that may not be scientifically substantiated.

It is important to recognize that the lay sector of the health belief system is relatively "open" to new ideas and techniques in contrast to the essentially "closed" expert sector. (The dashed line around the popular sector in Figure 9.1 is intended to symbolize this difference in permeability.) Biomedicine has obviously had a major impact on lay beliefs and practices. At the same time, popular health practices have at times influenced the professional health-care system. However, these practices must pass tests of scientific validation to be transformed into officially recognized therapies (Fries 2005). Malacrida (2015) points out that a good example of this mutual influence can be found in changing practices for handling childbirth and maternity care. Within the past century, we witnessed the virtual elimination of the lay midwife in this country (i.e., an experienced female member of the family or community who handled delivery of newborn children in the home) and the emergence of obstetrics as a medical speciality. Because of the dominance of the professional health-care sector, a medically trained specialist became the legitimate birth attendant, and the modern hospital became the legitimate birthplace for the majority of babies. Currently, there is growing evidence that traditional beliefs and practices related to midwifery have resurfaced and that midwifery has moved from lay practice to a regulated health-care profession. For example, in several Canadian provinces trained midwives now have legal status and are therefore legitimate birth attendants, and home births have become more frequent (Bourgeault et al. 2012; Burton and Ariss 2014). Benoit and colleagues (2005, 732) point out that although Canada has been slow to reorganize the maternity-care system and to include a role for the midwife, "in recent years, much to the chagrin of the medical profession, some provincial governments have enacted policies integrating certified trained midwives and a homebirth option into the formal healthcare system."

The key point is that health belief systems are not static. They are dynamic cultural constructions that are constantly adapting to broad societal changes. At the same time, traditional lay health beliefs and practices are highly resilient, shifting and adjusting to the pressures of biomedicine. We all negotiate the cultural value we attribute to ways of knowing, whether it is primarily scientific or traditional, based on our social location and experiences in the world. In a complex, pluralistic society such as Canada, with such a diversity of ways of knowing, many people pick and choose the elements with which they construct their lay beliefs about health and illness—a little science here, a little traditional knowledge there, as well as a dash of celebrity advice. In fact, it seems that traditional beliefs about health and illness are given up very slowly, and many persist along with the latest in medical knowledge. To test this assertion, review the popular beliefs about health listed in Box 9.5, and count the number of statements that you believe are correct. This list of health beliefs was derived from a dictionary of medical folklore (Rinzler 1981). They are characterized as popular because they are part of the collective wisdom of the lay community. You are probably familiar with many of these health beliefs. Which beliefs do you share?

Some of these popular health beliefs blend lay wisdom passed on informally from generation to generation along with formal knowledge supported by scientific medical evidence. For example, eating carrots may be good for your eyesight—but do you know the full explanation for this relationship? Carrots, like squash and corn, contain vitamin A, which helps to protect you from night blindness. Eating carrots once in a while is good for your health, but the popular health belief could have been that eating squash is good for your eyes! Similarly, eating onions may be good for your heart, not just because an older relative recommended it but because the essential oils in onions (and garlic) help to reduce cholesterol. Finally, based on traditional lay beliefs, the root of the licorice plant has been used as part of folk medicine practice as a laxative and a digestive aid for many years. There is evidence that one of the substances in licorice root (carbenoxolone)

> **Box 9.5 Popular Health Beliefs Self-Test**
>
> Do you believe the following?
>
> ❏ Eating carrots improves your vision.
> ❏ If your feet get wet, you will get a cold.
> ❏ Sleeping with the window open will cause head colds.
> ❏ Bowels should move every day.
> ❏ Eating garlic protects you from germs.
> ❏ Eating onions is good for your heart.
> ❏ Eating licorice is good for digestion.
> ❏ Your muscles turn to fat as you age.
> ❏ You should tilt your head back to stop a nosebleed.
> ❏ Getting chilled means you are more likely to catch a cold.
> ❏ You should put butter on a burn.
> ❏ You should feed a cold and starve a fever.

protects the lining of the stomach against erosion by stomach acid. Thus, these types of beliefs may persist because they are supported by both past practice and contemporary scientific proof.

In contrast, some of the other beliefs listed in Box 9.5 persist despite the fact that they are inconsistent with scientific explanations of the causes of disease and recommendations of medical professionals. For example, according to biomedicine, you are not more likely to get a cold if you sleep with the window open or get your feet wet (despite what your mother may have told you when you were younger). Getting chilled isn't a cause of a cold, but it may be one of the first noticeable symptoms of a cold. "Only viruses cause true colds, which are viral infections" (Rinzler 1981, 5). Other health beliefs on this list contradict current medical advice. For example, cold water is a much better first-aid treatment for a burn than putting butter on it. Cold water is more effective at soothing pain and preventing scarring, while butter increases the chances of infection. Finally, rather than tilting your head back to stop a nosebleed, it is actually recommended that you tilt your head slightly forward and pinch the bridge of your nose so that a clot will form and stop the bleeding.

In summary, laypersons draw upon both popular and professional systems of belief and practice in dealing with everyday health concerns. In our daily lives, we are continuously involved in negotiating the personal meaning of health and illness and making decisions about specific health actions. This self-care process is guided by our health beliefs. The content of contemporary health beliefs shapes our health maintenance behaviour and illness management practices and reflects a combination of elements derived from both the biomedical model and traditional lay ideas about health and wellness.

Self-Care Beliefs and Behaviour

A symbolic interactionist approach to understanding the interpersonal meanings of health and illness emphasizes the subjective processes by which beliefs help us to give personal meaning to health and to the social experience of illness. The individual's definition of the situation helps her to make sense of sickness and decide on the best course of action to maintain good health and manage illness. For example, an individual may think that it is very important to get an annual physical examination for preventive purposes and to bring potential symptoms of illness to the attention of a physician immediately. In contrast, a friend or co-worker of this individual might believe that annual examinations are a waste of time and that these types of health concerns can be handled by self-care (e.g., by getting more rest or by becoming more active). In the latter case, the person might be skeptical about the effectiveness of professional medical care and believe strongly in personal responsibility for health. Self-care beliefs, like other ideas about health and illness, are shaped by factors such as personal health history (e.g., childhood diseases) as well as the health experiences of others (e.g., a family member's experience with cancer).

Self-Health Management

The way people think about health and illness today reflects a complex, holistic health model that is not solely reliant on the expertise of biomedicine (Iedemaa and Veljanova 2013). For example, O'Sullivan and Stakelum's (2004, 41) study of lay health understandings suggests that there has been a shift "away from the biomedical paradigm and a move toward the more holistic paradigm, which stresses the role of the self and lifestyle in the production and maintenance of one's health." Green (1985) introduced the term **self-health management** to reflect the fact that members of the public routinely engage in personal health practices, including health-protective and illness treatment activities. Self-health management consists of a wide range of health-related behaviours that are an expression of personal autonomy and active involvement in a complex decision-making process. Although self-health management is a vital part of the hidden health-care system, we may not be fully aware of the implications of everyday activities or decisions we make about what to eat each day, whether to exercise, and how to spend leisure time. These life choices affect health status and have significant consequences for the pursuit of health and wellness.

In addition to these positive health actions, we routinely engage in a variety of self-care practices to manage illness experiences. We monitor our health status on a regular basis, evaluating the meaning of symptoms and changes in bodily conditions, and decide on an appropriate course of action. "Most people experience symptoms of ill health most of the time, and most of these niggling

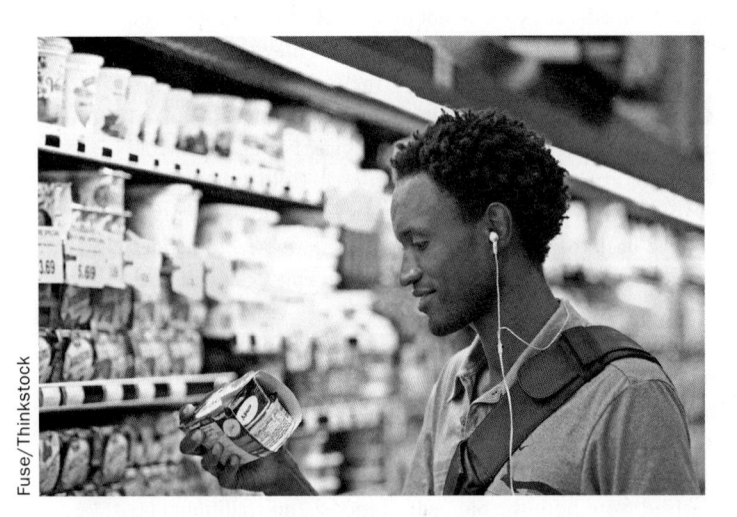

Self-care can involve a variety of activities—including regulatory behaviours, such as choosing healthy foods that allow you to eat a balanced diet. What are your personal self-care health practices? To what extent do you take personal responsibility for the decision-making process involved in maintaining your health?

complaints are never dealt with by the formal health-care system. While professionals only see the tip of the illness iceberg, the vast majority of health issues are dealt with by people acting for themselves, drawing on advice and using products provided by an ever-increasing array of corporations, governments and interest groups" (Ziguras 2004, 2). Responses to illness may involve self-treatment using non-prescription medications, natural remedies, or lifestyle changes. For example, Statistics Canada (2001) reports that the majority of Canadians who have colds or the flu take care of themselves rather than seeking formal care. Approximately two-thirds (63 per cent) of those who experienced cold or flu symptoms initially engaged in some type of self-treatment (such as taking over-the-counter medication, vitamins, or herbal supplements or getting more rest and using home remedies). In addition, self-health management may include talking to family members and friends to gain information and support or eventually consulting a wide range of formal health-care practitioners (including traditional and alternative healers). In each case, the critical factor is that these self-care behaviours all involve lay-initiated health action.

Self-health management is related to the notion that we each possess a reserve of health that needs to be managed. Healthy lifestyle practices and effective self-care behaviour help to strengthen this reserve and increase our health expectancy. According to Green (1985), self-health management is a multi-faceted concept. While the terms "self-health management" and "self-care behaviour" are often used interchangeably, Green argues that they do not have the same meaning and that self-health management is a broader concept that includes self-care. This argument could be extended to suggest that self-health management incorporates different (but interrelated) types of informal health-care behaviour: self-care practices, mutual aid, and membership in self-help groups.

It is important to understand that self-care does not simply mean taking care of oneself! **Self-care** encompasses the many everyday health-care activities that lay people informally undertake to manage personal and family health concerns. Think about the range of health-care practices that typically take place in the context of family life. Researchers informed by the feminist paradigm point out that it is generally women, in their roles as wives and mothers, who are responsible for the nutritional needs of the family and deciding whether children (or other family members) take vitamins or other supplements and get enough rest. In addition to these self-care health-protective behaviours, the wife/mother family role often includes responsibility for responses to illness. This type of self-care behaviour ranges from evaluating symptoms experienced by family members (e.g., taking a child's temperature) to deciding when to consult a health professional to making doctors' appointments. As the primary manager of family health care, the wife/mother role includes self-care activities such as ensuring that physicians' recommendations are followed (e.g., changes in dietary practice), prescribed medications are taken as directed, and follow-up appointments are arranged. While these types of health practices are referred to as self-care, they are generally part of the management of ongoing family health (including the health of children, spouses, and, quite often today, elderly parents). Thus, self-care is a fundamental part of self-health management and more accurately refers to everyday informal health care (e.g., Kickbusch 1989).

Mutual Aid

Self-health management also includes mutual aid. This term refers to ways people informally come together to offer each other mutually beneficial forms of support or reciprocal assistance.

In other words, **mutual aid** takes the form of collective activities, such as the types of social support exchanged by members of informal social networks typically made up of family and friends. In some cases, mutual aid might mean having a close friend or family member serve as a confidant or sympathetic listener who provides emotional support and encouragement. In other instances, it might mean practical assistance with daily activities, such as help with shopping, banking, or transportation. This type of informal care plays an important part in helping to meet health and social needs. We will return to the topic of mutual aid and helping networks when we examine the relationship between social support and health in the next section.

Self-Help Groups

Finally, self-health management may include joining a self-help group. This type of health behaviour involves participating in more formally organized group activities. **Self-help groups** are generally small, voluntary special-purpose organizations that are intended to help people deal with specific common health-related problems (e.g., Alcoholics Anonymous). Self-help groups bring together people who have a shared health concern to enable them to help themselves and often fill a gap that may exist between informal caregiving networks and formal professional health care.

Toward an Alternative Model of Health Care

Although self-care and mutual aid refer to personal and family practices that influence health and self-help refers to more visible, organized health-related group activities, they are all examples of the "hidden health care system" (Levin and Idler 1981). In other words, personal self-care behaviours and mutual aid or participation in self-help groups are part of lay self-health management. To acknowledge the meaning and impact of self-health management, we have to modify our approach to the study of health care. This conceptual shift means that we will have "to lay to rest the assumption that 'health care' in this society is synonymous with professional medical care" (Levin and Idler 1981, 2). The point is that professionally provided medical care does not equate with the totality of health care! We have to change the way we think about the formal part of the health-care system and discover the hidden depths of the iceberg of health care, including the informal contributions made by members of the lay community as producers of health. Based on their exploration of the border between self-care and professional care, Kielmann and colleagues (2010, 55) argue that this paradigm shift not only "repositions patients from being passive recipients of expert care to active partners who share responsibility for their medical care" but also means that there must be changes in the fundamental organization of the health-care system. To understand the way in which we each contribute to the production of health, we are now going to take a closer look at self-care as the foundational component of the health-care system and then turn our attention to the link between social support, helping networks, and health.

The Canadian health-care system is organized on the basis of formal medical care (i.e., the visible part of the iceberg), not informal self-care. If we are to shift the focus away from consuming health care to producing health, our understanding of the health-care system must expand to include not only the dominant biomedical model but also the hidden parts of the iceberg, including the self- (lay) care model! Based on the biomedical model, members of the public have been viewed essentially as consumers of medical goods and services (e.g., prescribed medication and physician and hospital services). Health professionals, particularly physicians, have, in turn, been viewed as the legitimate providers of these medical goods and services and have dominated the health-care system and our pursuit of health and wellness. The role of governments in this country (based on this model) has been to regulate formal medical care, including the provision of physician services and the consumption of prescribed medications through programs such as medicare. Part A in Figure 9.2 illustrates the formal medical-care model and the typical relationships between participants in the visible part of the health-care system.

Looking below the surface of the water at the whole iceberg of health care and substituting the informal self-care model (for medical care) changes the nature of relationships between all of the participants in the health-care system. Recognizing that self-care is the basic component of health care changes the way in which members of the lay community are viewed. This model acknowledges that ordinary people are, in fact, primary *providers* of health care (as well as consumers of formal medical-care services). Furthermore, this model acknowledges the fact that members of the public are actively involved in managing their health as a part of everyday life. The self-care model of health also recognizes that utilizing professional medical care is only one of the available options for members of the lay community. You may decide to handle your health concerns by using some form of self-treatment, by consulting members of your informal supportive networks, by using the services of a range of alternative health practitioners, or by going to see the doctor. In other words, once we can see the whole iceberg, including the hidden depths of health care, and once self-care replaces medical care as the central component of the health-care system, health professionals are viewed as one of many formal and informal community resources available to the layperson for the purpose of self-health management.

The role played by government in the health care system also changes in the self-care model. Instead of simply continuing to try to regulate public access to medical and hospital services, governments are under increasing pressure to try to find ways of facilitating self-health management and decreasing the consumption of professional medical-care services. A number of years ago, the Canadian government identified informal self-care (along with mutual aid) as a critical health promotion mechanism (Epp 1986). Governments, at different levels, have been working for some time on strategies for facilitating self-care behaviour and fostering healthy environments in the hope of creating healthy communities and, ultimately, reducing disparities and improving the health of the Canadian population. Part B in Figure 9.2 illustrates the informal self-care model and changes in relationships within the health-care system (e.g., the directions of the arrows connecting the basic parts of the health-care system change).

Self-care has been consistently described as the basic level of health care practised by members of the public (e.g., Dean 1981; Fries 2013, 2014; Levin and Idler 1983; Levin, Katz, and Holst 1976; Williamson and Danaher 1978). In fact, informal lay self-care that takes place on a daily basis constitutes the dominant form of health care. According to Pickard and Rogers (2012, 102), "self-care is above all an embodied practice, grounded in the context of everyday life." The everyday practices by which we look after our bodies reflect how we think about our bodies and ourselves. In an early discussion of lay initiatives in health, Levin, Katz, and Holst (1976) defined self-care as a process by which the layperson functions on her own behalf to promote health, to prevent illness, and to detect and treat disease when it occurs. According to this definition, the layperson is the primary provider of health care and, therefore, producer of health. Dean (1981) contends that self-care includes not only health-protective behaviours, utilization of preventive medical services, symptom evaluation, and various self-treatment practices but also interaction with the formal medical-care sector. It is important to note that "this conceptualization does not present self-care and professional care as mutually exclusive, but rather as integral and inter-related

**Part A
Formal Medical Care Model**

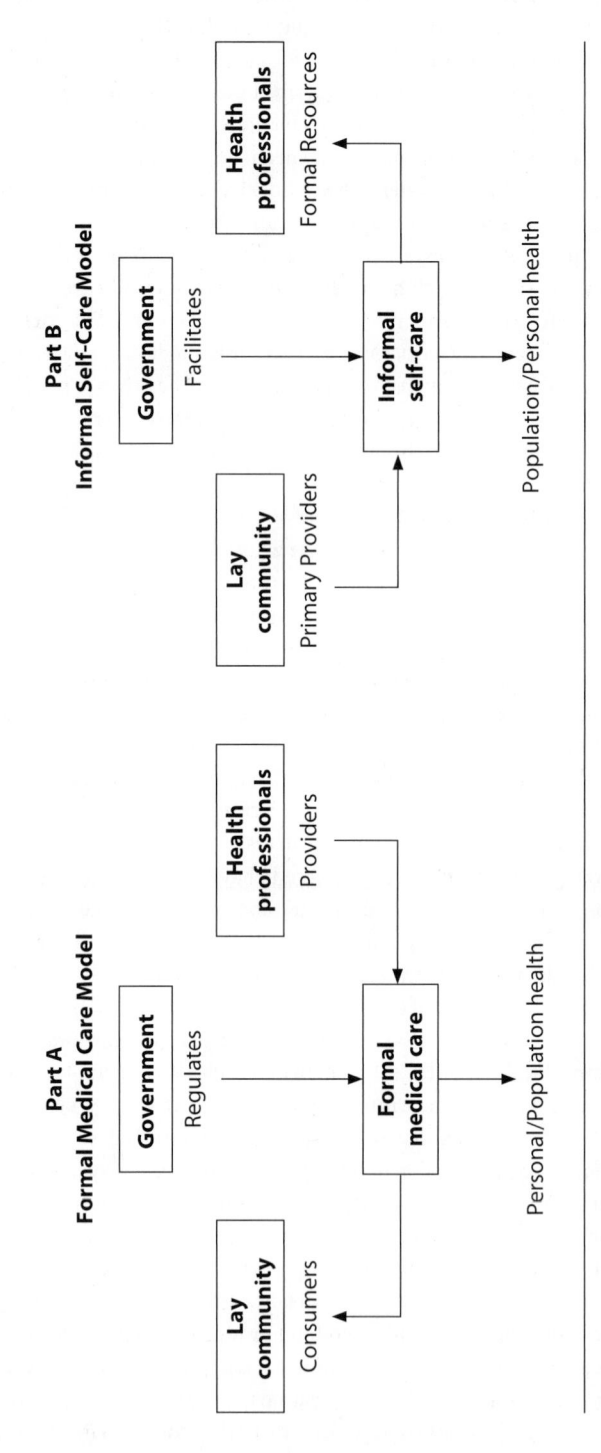

Government — Regulates
Health professionals — Providers
Lay community — Consumers
Formal medical care
Personal/Population health

**Part B
Informal Self-Care Model**

Government — Facilitates
Health professionals — Formal Resources
Lay community — Primary Providers
Informal self-care
Population/Personal health

Figure 9.2 Alternative Models of Health Care

components of the health care system" (Segall and Goldstein 1989, 154). While self-care practices appear to be expanding in scope and importance, Ziguras (2004, 10) argues that it is the visibility of self-care that has increased dramatically "because health researchers have 'uncovered' the previously 'hidden' realm of self-care practices of lay people, and because of the development of the more visible forms of self-care advice such as self-help groups and self-help books."

Members of the lay community are active providers of health care in addition to being consumers of professionally provided health-care services, and this has to be taken into account if we are to gain a greater understanding of the factors that shape health status. Self-care includes a broad range of potential behaviours, such as

- health maintenance activities;
- illness prevention, symptom evaluation, and self-diagnosis;
- self-treatment (both self-medication and non-medication practices);
- self-referral and the use of informal social networks as a health resource;
- consultation with a variety of non-medical, complementary, and alternative health-care providers; and
- the use of professional medical services.

In each case, the critical factor is that these self-care behaviours are lay-initiated and are undertaken as a result of a self-determined decision-making process. Self-care (as an aspect of self-health management) involves the exercise of lay control over the health-care decision-making process and management of health-care resources. Self-care behaviour incorporates notions of autonomy, influence, and responsibility for health decisions and care.

Dimensions of Self-Care Behaviour

Within the range of self-care behaviours, it is possible to distinguish between specific types of self-care. It is important to note that self-care "is both reactive (concerned with the management of symptoms associated with existing acute and chronic health conditions) and proactive (focused on the prevention of illness through healthy lifestyles)" (Clarke and Bennett 2012, 212). The following discussion builds on Barofsky's (1978) typology of self-care behaviour, which differentiates between regulatory, preventive, reactive, and restorative self-care. The distinguishing features of these four types of self-care are summarized in Figure 9.3. The first two types of self-care can be characterized as health behaviour, since they refer to health maintenance and illness-avoidance activities. **Health behaviour** refers to routine health-protective activities, including personal self-care regulatory and preventive practices (e.g., exercise, nutrition), risk reduction, and disease prevention (e.g., smoking cessation). **Regulatory self-care** consists of daily habits of living that affect health (e.g., health maintenance activities such as eating a balanced diet, getting enough sleep, and being physically active). This type of self-care takes place within the context of everyday life and may not be viewed as actions that are explicitly intended to improve health and well-being. For example, eating breakfast may be a part of your daily routine (i.e., a familiar, long-term habit) and, therefore, not likely to be thought of within a self-health management frame of reference, although this practice does affect health.

Preventive self-care consists of deliberate health actions undertaken to reduce the risk of illness. Many of these practices are also a part of everyday life but have an explicit illness-avoidance focus and are intended to prevent the onset of diseases (e.g., regularly brushing and flossing

```
Health behaviour
    ├──► Regulatory self-care
    │     Health maintenance and health protective activities
    └──► Preventive self-care
          Illness avoidance and risk reduction practices

Illness behaviour
    └──► Reactive self-care
          Evaluation and response to symptoms

Sick role behaviour
    └──► Restorative self-care
          Management of chronic conditions
```

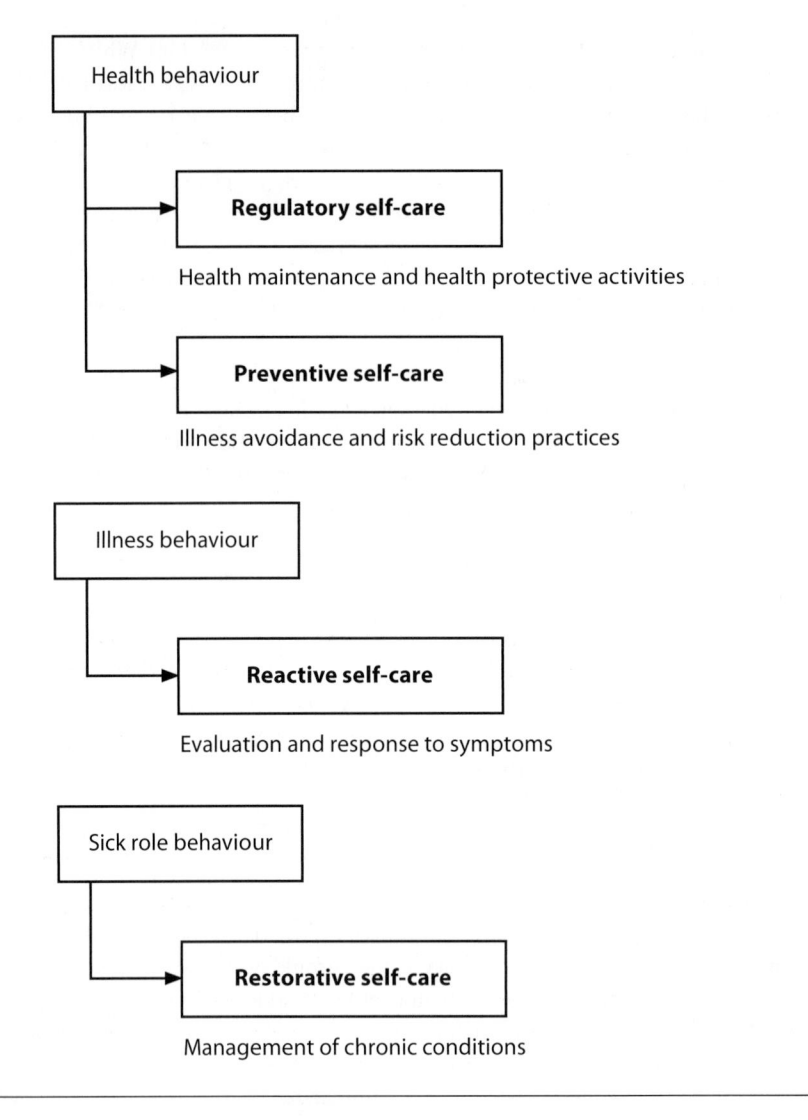

Figure 9.3 Dimensions of Self-Care Behaviour

your teeth to avoid dental cavities and gum disease). Other preventive self-care practices include weight loss (dieting) or restricted daily intake of salt or sugar to try to avoid certain health conditions (e.g., hypertension, diabetes). Self-examination is another example of a preventive self-care behaviour that might be routinely practised (for the early detection of growths that might be indicative of cancer or other health problems). Finally, this dimension of self-care includes periodic self-selected illness-avoidance activities, such as the use of professional preventive services for blood pressure measurement, breast examination, or a general physical check-up. Together, regulatory and preventive self-care practices reflect a range of health behaviours undertaken by people who believe that they are healthy for the purpose of protecting their health.

The third type of self-care can be characterized as illness behaviour, since it comprises activities undertaken by people who feel ill to interpret the meaning of symptoms and determine an appropriate course of action for managing health problems. **Illness behaviour** refers to the perception and evaluation of the meaning of daily symptoms (e.g., perceived seriousness, causal attributions) and reactive self-care practices, including self-medication and illness-related activity restrictions (e.g., sick days). **Reactive self-care** is based on recognition and evaluation of symptoms and includes self-initiated responses to symptoms that have not been diagnosed by a physician. When we feel ill we go through a process of interpreting the meaning of symptoms we are experiencing in an effort to decide whether they are familiar, whether we have dealt with them before, and whether we can handle them on our own (Twaddle 1974). According to Barofsky (1978), the primary form of treatment for this type of symptom-induced self-care behaviour is self-medication (using the vast array of over-the-counter drugs that are available to us, along with the growing number of natural health products now on the market). This dimension of self-care also involves use of many non-medication self-treatment practices, such as getting more rest or cutting down on usual daily activities. According to Dean (1986, 275), "lay care provided in the community constitutes the dominant proportion of care in illness." Hughner and Kleine (2004, 395) agree that lay people "make most decisions regarding whether and when to seek care, whom to consult and whether to comply. Estimates indicate that between 70 and 90 percent of sickness is managed solely within the lay domain in western societies." If the symptoms do not respond to self-treatment, however, a decision may be made to consult a formal health-care practitioner.

The final type of self-care can be described as sick role behaviour because it comprises the activities of people who believe they are sick for the purpose of getting well. **Sick role behaviour** refers to both informal and formal help-seeking behaviour, such as lay consultation and the use of formal health-care services. Sick role behaviour generally involves some degree of neglect of one's usual duties (e.g., sick leave), becoming dependent on others for care, and receiving treatment. In the case of an acute infectious disease (e.g., the flu), the goal is recovery and a return to good health and the performance of one's usual well roles as soon as possible. In contrast, if the individual is experiencing chronic degenerative disease (e.g., arthritis), the goal becomes adaptation or learning to live with the condition. **Restorative self-care** may mean overcoming the health problem in the case of acute disease or adjusting one's daily life to achieve an optimum level of functioning in the case of chronic disease.

Barofsky (1978) originally defined restorative self-care as compliance with a professionally prescribed treatment regimen of medication and behavioural changes. It was limited to self-care behaviours such as taking medication as prescribed and following doctors' orders. In current research, restorative self-care still refers to the routine activities of those living with medically managed chronic illnesses. To illustrate, managing a chronic condition such as diabetes may involve self-care practices on the part of the individual, such as monitoring blood glucose levels at home and following a modified diet based on the recommendation of health-care professionals. This type of self-care behaviour, however, reflects both medical advice and the exercise of personal autonomy, since it is ultimately based on lay decision-making in the selection of health-care practices. It recognizes the fact that adopting the sick role does not mean that we lose our ability to make health-related choices. For example, you may decide not to have a prescription filled or make the follow-up appointment that the doctor recommended. Consequently, restorative self-care may reflect voluntary adherence to recommended health-care practices rather than mandatory compliance. Members of the lay community (even when they are sick) continue to be active participants in the health-care process instead of simply becoming passive recipients of professional medical care.

Because of the limitations of the original sick role concept formulated by Parsons (as discussed in Chapter 2) and the prevalence of self-care behaviour, Segall (1997) argues that a redefined, non-medicalized concept is required for the study of health-related behaviour that takes these self-care dimensions into account. It is important to clearly distinguish between the informal sick role and the formal patient role and to recognize that it is possible to enter and exit the sick role without seeking the assistance of health-care professionals. Research evidence demonstrates that the majority of everyday health problems are self-managed and may never be brought to the attention of the formal health-care system. By situating the modified sick role in the context of lay health beliefs and behaviour and acknowledging the importance of informal care, "this nonprofessional reconceptualization of the rights and duties associated with the sick role should more accurately reflect the everyday health and illness experiences of the individual and more fully recognize the pervasive nature of self-care" (Segall 1997, 297).

While behavioural dimensions of the modified sick role were influenced to some extent by Parsons and the structural functionalist paradigm, the reformulated rights and duties differ in a number of significant ways. The revised set of reciprocal role relationships reflects the fact that we are all active participants in the health-care process, that informal care and supportive social networks play a crucial role, and that routine self-health management involves both health-protective behaviour and responses to illness. The modified sick role concept includes rights and duties that encompass both health behaviour and illness behaviour. It recognizes the right of the individual to make decisions about health-related matters and to make use of informal care and the types of support offered by members of one's social networks (e.g., family and friends). At the same time, the occupant of the modified sick role has an obligation to engage in health maintenance and illness-avoidance activities as well as trying to overcome illness. While health and illness are still portrayed as social roles, the modified sick role concept acknowledges the significant part played by self-health management in the pursuit of health and wellness.

In summary, the defining characteristic of self-care, as a component of self-health management, is the individual's capacity to exercise autonomy in the decision-making process involved in maintaining health, achieving symptomatic relief, and managing chronic illness. Self-care embodies self-health management skills such as self-diagnosis and health status assessment, self-treatment of common illness symptoms, and self-monitoring and management of chronic illness. Self-care behaviour serves a number of important functions by contributing to the maintenance of good health and by shaping responses to everyday illness episodes as well as the daily challenges involved in managing long-term chronic conditions. "Research on self-care indicates that gender, age, health status, and socio-economic status are important factors shaping and constraining the individual's engagement in various health practices" (Clarke and Bennett 2012, 212) Unfortunately, there are gaps in this area of research and an incomplete understanding of the full range of behaviours that constitute self-health management, the factors that shape different dimensions of self-care behaviour, and the efficacy of self-care practices in health maintenance and illness management. Consequently, there is more to learn about the effectiveness or the limits of self-care behaviour.

Lupton (2013) contends that new forms of self-care are starting to emerge as a result of advances in digital health technologies. In her words, we are witnessing "an imminent revolution in healthcare, preventive medicine and public health driven by the use of new digital medical and health-related technologies, variously termed 'digital health,' 'eHealth,' 'Medicine 2.0' or 'Health

2.0'" (2013, 256). So-called "digitally engaged patients" will be better equipped to perform health maintenance and illness management self-care tasks in their daily lives as a result of their ready access to digitalized health information systems and their ability to conduct medical consultations via digital media and to use wireless mobile digital devices to self-monitor various components of their health and well-being (such as HealthKit and Fitbit technology and smartphone apps to track the number of steps walked and stairs climbed as well as nutritional information about the type of food items consumed).

Lupton (2014) explains that ongoing developments in digital technologies have had a major impact on the health-care activities of both professional practitioners and lay people. The constantly expanding range of technologies related to health available to the general public supports critical self-care routines (such as self-monitoring of health status). According to Lupton (2014, 1346), laypeople are now able

> to access an array of social networking platforms such as PatientsLikeMe . . . , where they can exchange their experiences with other members of the site, contribute to aggregated data that are used by site members and medical researchers and sign up to drug trials. They can upload photographs and videos showing the bodily signs and symptoms of their condition, using services such as Instagram and YouTube and create Facebook pages on their condition to share information and comments.

These developments in digital health technologies may signal not just new forms of self-care but also the potential for significant expansion of our capacity to function effectively as informal care providers and producers of health.

Social Support, Helping Networks, and Health

Self-health management also typically involves discussions with family members and friends who make up our social networks. Ongoing interaction with members of our social networks is a vital part of health and illness behaviour (Smith and Christakis 2008; Ashida and Heaney 2008; Sinding 2004). Based on a review of the literature on social support, caregiving, and aging, Chappell and Funk (2011, 363) conclude that "social support is now recognized as an important (non-medical) determinant of health and well-being." Informal helping networks have an extensive capacity to aid us in dealing with health maintenance and illness management. For example, our first response to health concerns is generally to turn to family members, friends, or co-workers to gain practical assistance, a sympathetic ear, or advice. Social support takes many different forms, including: **instrumental support** (functional assistance offered by social network members, such as help with housework, transportation, and banking, as well as other activities of daily living); **emotional support** (having companions or confidants with whom we feel comfortable discussing personal matters and sharing feelings and who offer concern, encouragement, and acceptance that makes us feel we are cared for and valued—also referred to as appraisal support); and **informational support** (advice, suggestions, and other information offered by social network members that helps us to make critical decisions about appropriate health care activities). Lay social networks are involved in making diagnoses, medicating and treating health problems, and making referrals to health-care professionals, as well as providing assistance with activities of daily living (such as shopping and meal preparation). According to Wilkinson and Marmot (2003), good social relations and strong supportive networks have a powerful protective effect on health. Research indicates that meaningful social relationships contribute as much to the maintenance of good health as "established risk factors such as smoking, obesity, and high blood pressure" contribute to the onset of ill health (Richmond, Ross, and Egeland 2007, 1828)! There is, however, still a good deal more to learn about the salutary effects of social support and the ways in which this hidden component of informal health care affects our health and well-being.

In 2012, more than 2 million Canadians received care in their own homes for long-term chronic illnesses or age-related needs (Sinha and Bleakney 2014). Based on an analysis of data from the 2012 *General Social Survey*, these researchers report that the vast majority of participants (88 per cent) in this national study rely on help from family members, friends, and neighbours (either in combination with or instead of using professional services). These social networks typically include a number of different people, such as a spouse or common-law partner, grown children, and siblings as well as other extended family members, friends, and neighbours. The most common type of informal care received is transportation (e.g., assistance with attending medical appointments or participating in social events), followed by domestic help (e.g., meal preparation, laundry, and cleaning), home maintenance, and outdoor tasks. In addition to these types of instrumental support, three-quarters of the care recipients also state that they receive important emotional support from family and friends. For example, they indicated that family members and friends "spent time with them, engaged in conversation, cheered them up or provided other forms of emotional support" (Sinha and Bleakney 2014, 13). Using the same data source, Turcotte (2013) asserts that most people, at some time in their lives, will provide informal care to a family member or friend to help them deal with long-term health conditions or problems related to aging. In fact, some Canadians who are primary caregivers for family members provide support that is "equivalent to a full-time job" (2013, 3).

As discussed in Chapter 4, being a part of a social network and having close ties to family and friends provide us with **social support** that enhances our sense of self-worth and the resources that we have available for dealing with life's challenges, and it results in health benefits. When it comes to social support and heath, perception may be as important as reality. It may be equally important to perceive that social support is available if you need it (i.e., that there are people in your social networks whom you can confide in and count on for help) as it is to actually receive social support. Stephens and colleagues (2011) describe perceived support as the person's belief that the members of their social networks are actually supportive in a variety of ways. "These two dimensions do not appear to be interchangeable as beneficial effects of perceived support may be obtained in the absence of any actual support being provided" (Uchino 2009, 54). Uchino recommends a life course approach for clarifying the ways in which perceived and received support interact with each other over time and collectively influence our health. While we may not yet fully understand the different ways in which these dimensions of social support are related to health outcomes, perceived support may be as significant a determinant of health as received support!

Does social support have an ongoing effect on our health, or does it become a significant factor only during times of stress? This question has received a good deal of research attention. Numerous studies have examined the association between stressful life events (social stressors) and health outcomes (such as psychological distress) and the ways in which this relationship is affected by individual coping skills (such as sense of mastery) and supportive social networks (e.g., Gadalla 2009). There is evidence that social support has both direct and indirect effects on health and well-being (Clarke 2008; Stansfeld 2006). For example, social support is an important part of everyday life, and membership in supportive social networks directly enhances health, regardless of how stressful life circumstances happen to be (direct effect). In other words, there are direct physical and mental health benefits associated with being a part of a supportive social network. In addition, social support buffers the negative effects of stressful life events on our health (indirect effect). In this case, it is argued that the effects of social support are most evident during times of stress, when supportive social relationships help "to moderate the impact of acute and chronic stressors on health" (Stansfeld 2006, 151). According to this view, social support protects our health and well-being by intervening between the stressful life events and health outcomes (such as psychological distress and physical illness).

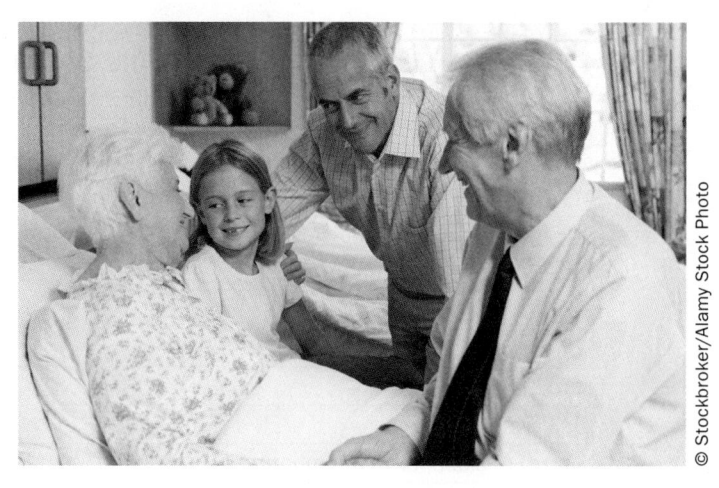

Supportive social networks such as families are an invaluable health resource.

Despite the fact that there is now a substantial body of evidence showing that social support generally contributes to positive health outcomes, we still "do not know how social ties or social support actually work to sustain or improve health and well-being" (Thoits 2011, 145). While the results of their research highlight the indirect association of social support with better health, Segrin and Domschke (2011, 228) state that "there are undoubtedly various mechanisms by which social support benefits health." Consequently, there have been repeated calls for researchers to focus their attention on identifying the intervening mechanisms or psychosocial pathways through which social support is linked to physical and mental health (e.g., Thoits 2011; Uchino et al. 2012). One of the potential pathways that has been investigated is the link between social support, health-protective behaviours (e.g., being physically active and avoiding smoking), and positive health outcomes (Harvey and Alexander 2012; Fiori and Jager 2011; Umberson, Crosnoe, and Reczek 2010). This approach is based on the assumption that "health behavior occupies a pivotal position in theoretical models that seek to explain when and how social ties affect health" (Umberson, Crosnoe, and Reczek 2010, 140). What is particularly noteworthy about these studies is that they adopt a life course perspective and argue that we need longitudinal data to be able to examine the ways in which various social relationships influence health behaviours at different life stages and ultimately over time affect our pursuit of health and wellness.

The Holmes-Rahe Life Event Inventory in Table 9.1 measures the extent to which stressful life events contribute to health problems. The life-change units that apply to each of the events experienced in the previous two years of an individual's life are added, and the total score provides an estimate of level of stress, which has been shown to be a predictor of illness. When you think about each of the events that has occurred in your life, try to recall how it affected your health, how you dealt with the stress, and the extent to which the types of support provided by members of your social networks played a part in your response.

Table 9.1 Life Event Inventory: The Social Readjustment Scale

In the past 24 months, which of these life events have happened to you? Check the box next to any event that has occurred in your life in the past two years. There are no right or wrong answers. The aim is to identify which of these events you have experienced.

Life Events	Life Changes Units	
Death of spouse	100	
Divorce	73	
Marital separation	65	
Jail term	63	
Death of close family member	63	
Personal injury or illness	53	
Marriage	50	
Fired at work	47	
Marital reconciliation	45	
Retirement	45	
Change in health of a family member	44	
Pregnancy	40	
Sex difficulties	39	
Gain of new family member	39	
Business readjustment	39	
Change in financial state	38	
Death of close friend	37	
Change to different line of work	36	
Change in number of arguments with spouse	35	
Mortgage over $100,000	31	
Foreclosure of mortgage or loan	30	
Change in responsibilities at work	29	
Son or daughter leaving home	29	
Trouble with in-laws	29	
Outstanding personal achievement	28	
Spouse begins or stops work	26	
Begin or end school	26	
Change in living conditions	25	
Revision in personal habits	24	
Trouble with boss	23	
Change in work hours or conditions	20	

Change in residence	20	
Change in schools	20	
Change in recreation	19	
Change in church activities	19	
Change in social activities	18	
Mortgage or loan less than $30,000	17	
Change in sleeping habits	16	
Change in number of family get-togethers	15	
Change in eating habits	15	
Vacation	13	
Christmas alone	12	
Minor violations of the law	11	
Your score is:		

Score of 300 or more: susceptible to stress-induced health problems and at risk of illness
Score between 150 and 299: moderate risk of illness in the next two years
Score of 150 or less: relatively low risk of illness

It is possible to complete this inventory online. Your total score will be automatically calculated by clicking on the "Calculate Results" button. You may also click "Reset" to take the inventory again. (See Recommended Websites at the end of this chapter.)

Source: Adapted from Holmes and Rahe 1967.

As previously described, mutual aid refers to the collective activities in which people informally engage to exchange mutually beneficial or reciprocal forms of social support. In other words, mutual aid is characterized by reciprocity or balanced, equitable exchanges in people's interactions with members of their social networks. We generally find relationships that are reciprocal to be rewarding. These types of interpersonal relationships are more meaningful and enjoyable because we receive as much as we give to others. Evidence suggests that reciprocal relationships are health-protective, while relationships that do not involve this type of give-and-take have either no effect or a negative effect on health. Belonging to supportive social networks may contribute to positive health outcomes for all participants. Clarke (2008, 181) reinforces this point by stating that it is "worth emphasizing that the health benefits associated with social support are not limited to those who receive it; those who provide support can benefit as well."

Stansfeld (2006, 148) contends that "social support has a positive effect on many different aspects of both physical and mental health." A growing body of research has documented the salutary effects of supportive social networks on a variety of health outcomes, such as morbidity and mortality rates (Segrin and Domschke 2011; Cheng and Chan 2006; Poortinga 2006), depression (Ostberg and Lennartsson 2007), and self-rated health (Gadalla 2009). In contrast, there is evidence that social isolation leads to ill health. For example, Shields (2008, 1) reports that "people who are socially isolated and have few ties to other individuals are more likely to suffer from poor physical and mental health and to die prematurely." Fortunately, factors such as the level of social support received have been found to reduce loneliness and improve well-being in later life (Chen and Feeley 2014).

For many years, research emphasized the beneficial effects of social support on health and well-being. There is now growing recognition that informal social networks are also potential sources of stress and that there are many opportunities for problematic social exchanges within families (Funk 2010). "It should be noted that not all social relationships are beneficial and pleasant and that frequent social contact may actually increase the chances of conflicts, disputes, or strained relations (i.e., negative social interactions)" (Chen and Feeley 2014,143). Gallant (2003, 172) points out that "because of misconceptions or a lack of understanding, friends and family members may behave in unsupportive or inappropriate ways, offer well-intentioned advice that conflicts with self-management recommendations, or directly or indirectly promote unhealthy behaviors." According to Turcotte (2013), there can also be negative consequences for caregivers' physical and mental health, their ability to participate in the paid labour force, and the time they have for other social activities. Available evidence on the negative aspects of social support "challenges the idea that social support is universally beneficial for well-being" (Chappell and Funk 2011, 363). In other words, the relationship between social support and health outcomes is complex, and not all social networks are good for your health!

In concluding our look at the link between social support and health, as illustrated by Box 9.6, it is important to note that "social support operates at both an individual and a societal level" (Stansfeld 2006, 162). Evidence of the health benefits derived from belonging to supportive social networks can be found in an analysis of data from the *Canadian Community Health Survey* (*CCHS*). The findings of this survey demonstrate that at the individual level, approximately two-thirds of those who felt a strong or somewhat strong sense of connection to their community reported that they are in excellent or very good general health (Shields 2008). In other words, people with a strong sense of community belonging are more likely to state that they are in good physical and mental health. While the proportion of women and

Box 9.6 Major Findings concerning Social Support and Health

- At the individual level, social integration is positively linked to mental and physical health and lower mortality rates.
- Perceived emotional support leads to better physical and mental health and helps to buffer the impact of major life events.
- The most powerful form of support is an intimate and confiding reciprocal relationship.
- At the societal level, socially cohesive societies have better population health.

Source: Thoits 1995; White 2002.

men who reported a strong sense of community belonging did not differ, feeling connected to the community was less common among people who were divorced, separated, or never married than among those who were married. Even when potentially confounding factors such as other structural health determinants (e.g., education, household income, and marital status) were taken into account, feeling socially connected continued to be strongly related to health. These findings show that social relationships are important for both healthy people and healthy societies.

Informal Care and Illness as Embodied Experience: Making Sense of Sickness and Maintaining a Healthy Self-Identity

Before ending our discussion of informal care, let's take a look at hidden components of the iceberg of health care in action by examining how people deal with the most prevalent symptom of ill health that we experience in daily life—that is, persistent pain. "Pain is one of the most common and potentially most disruptive experiences in people's lives" (Baszanger 1989, 425). In a commentary on the many challenges that people face in trying to live with chronic pain, Cowan (2011, 307) emphatically states that pain "can destroy our ability to function, maintain any kind of normal relationship or be a productive part of society." Good and colleagues (1992, 1) further emphasize this point by stating that "pain is a ubiquitous feature of human experience" and highlighting the fact that "acute pain, lasting minutes or hours is reported at some time by virtually all adults in North American society, across the span of ethnic groups and social classes, of age and gender. It is the single most frequent complaint brought to the offices of physicians in North America."

Bendelow and Williams (1995) argue that the physical sensation of pain (i.e., feelings of bodily discomfort) is inseparable from the social and emotional significance of this meaning-laden experience. In their words, "Mind and body are fully interfused in pain" (1995, 150). In discussing the dualisms of pain, they state that pain pervades every aspect of people's lives and call for an approach that understands pain as physical and socio-emotional, as biological and cultural. In fact, "the possible meanings of everyday pain in our culture are rich and varied" (Aldrich and Eccleston 2000, 1639). Bendelow and Williams (1995, 140) assert that "pain lies at the intersection between biology and culture" and is an important topic for sociological investigation. A number of researchers informed by the sociology of the body paradigm have commented critically on the medicalized conception of pain and the Cartesian split between mind and body and have challenged dualistic models of embodiment in their analyses of the ways in which people make sense of everyday pain (Bendelow 2006; Chandler 2013; Ojala et al. 2015). For example, Chandler (2013, 727) reports that the participants in her study "struggled to separate mind and body, emotion and physicality in their attempts to relate their pain experiences." Ojala and colleagues (2015) acknowledge that despite extensive research, the experience of living with chronic pain is still poorly understood. They argue that since it is now widely recognized that the pain experience is multi-dimensional and involves the interplay of physical, psychological, social, and other contextual factors, it is time to "shift from the traditional dualistic explanation to a holistic paradigm" that offers a better understanding of what it means to live with chronic pain.

To understand pain as a lived embodied experience, we need to recognize that while the sensation of pain may be based on physiological processes, pain expression and behavioural responses are shaped by socio-cultural factors (e.g., gender, ethnicity). Cultural values and norms and membership in various social groups influence whether we keep pain private or express it publicly. Without minimizing the importance of acute pain (resulting from an accident or injury), we are going to focus on the ways in which living with constant, unrelenting pain associated with long-term chronic conditions affects people's everyday lives and involves informal care.

Early in the book (Chapter 3), when we examined the meaning and measurement of health, we discussed the importance of digging deeper and using qualitative methods to enable people to describe, in their own words, their health and illness experiences. Illness narrative accounts have been recommended as the best method for discovering the explanatory beliefs that people hold about the onset of ill health, the ways in which they interpret the meaning of symptoms such as pain, and how they make sense of sickness (particularly chronic conditions) and meet the many challenges they face in their everyday lives to maintain a healthy self-identity (i.e., to continue thinking of themselves as a healthy person). As Medved and Brockmeier (2008, 469) explain, "Illness has meaning, and narrative is the language of meaning." Many studies have used an illness narrative approach (e.g., Buchbinder 2010; Frank 1995; Kleinman 1988) or a process of narrative reconstruction (Williams 1984) as a means of eliciting people's personal stories about their embodied illness experiences and gaining critical information about "the experiential side of how chronic illness and its treatment affect a person or family" (Gerhardt 1990, 1149). In fact, Frank (1995) argues that becoming seriously ill is a call for stories! Bury (2001, 265) suggests that in view of the increasing prevalence of chronic illness, personal narratives may tell us more about how people deal with common symptoms (such as persistent pain) in their everyday lives than the "grand narratives of science and medicine." Qualitative methods give people an opportunity "to voice and share their personal experiences" and provide critical insights into the daily lives of those living with chronic pain (Wallace et al. 2014, 296).

A Narrative Account: The Meaning and Management of Pain

Radley and Billig (1996) describe symptoms such as pain as inescapable facts of life and assert that enabling people to share their personal accounts or private stories gives voice to the lived experiences of people in pain. Furthermore, they argue, when people talk about their health, "as well as supplying information about the body, what they say also tells others about the status of the self" (1996, 220). Here are some questions about pain for you to consider.

- Do you experience constant pain?
- Do you hurt all over?
- Do you have multiple tender points on your body where even slight pressure causes pain?
- Do you frequently feel exhausted?
- Does pain interfere with your daily activities, including sleep?
- Is your doctor having trouble finding something specifically wrong with you?

If your answer is "yes" to these questions, then you may have a condition known as fibromyalgia. It has been estimated that fibromyalgia affects approximately 1 million Canadians (or about 3 per cent of the population). Canadian prevalence rates increase "with age, and female patients are affected at least 6 times more often than male patients. Although seen most often in middle-aged women, fibromyalgia has been described in men, children, teenagers and older people" (Fitzcharles, Ste-Marie, and Pereira 2013, E645). Widespread chronic pain is the main symptom of fibromyalgia and is often accompanied by fatigue and muscle weakness, sleep disturbance, cognitive dysfunction (such as memory loss and a lack of concentration), and mood disorders (such as depression and anxiety). Canadians living with fibromyalgia frequently report that they need help with heavy household chores (such as spring cleaning and yard work) and, to a lesser extent, with doing their routine housework and getting to appointments or running errands. Research shows that people living with fibromyalgia may experience a higher level of functional impairment and activity restrictions than people living with other types of chronic conditions. This raises a contentious issue, since "impairment in fibromyalgia, which may be greater than impairment in rheumatoid arthritis, is difficult to reconcile with a mostly healthy-looking individual" (Fitzcharles, Ste-Marie, and Pereira 2013, E650).

Most people suffer with fibromyalgia for many years before it is diagnosed. The symptoms of fibromyalgia may fluctuate over time, but they seldom disappear completely. A medical diagnosis is typically based on a physical examination and a thorough history. In this case, physicians attempt to assess the extent of pain experienced when slight pressure is applied to a number of areas known as trigger points located in the neck, shoulders, back, hips, arms, and legs. Blood tests may also be used to rule out other causes of pain, tenderness, or stiffness in muscles, tendons, and ligaments. However, there are no laboratory or imaging tests to confirm a diagnosis of fibromyalgia! "In the absence of physical findings or abnormal results from laboratory tests, clinicians must rely on the time-honoured art of medicine to diagnose fibromyalgia" (Fitzcharles, Ste-Marie, and Pereira 2013, E645). As a result, diagnosing the cluster of symptoms that make up this medically unexplained syndrome remains controversial, and there is continuing "debate within medicine regarding its legitimacy as a diagnosis" (Sim and Madden 2008, 57). This "contested" illness creates difficulties for patients in terms of their subjective experience of symptoms and their interaction with health-care professionals. The uncertainty regarding the cause of fibromyalgia and the lack of consensus on how best to treat the symptoms are also problematic for physicians (Fitzcharles, Ste-Marie, and Pereira 2013; Asbring and Narvanen 2003).

Along with conditions such as chronic fatigue syndrome and multiple chemical sensitivity, fibromyalgia has been characterized as a "non-disease." For example, in a discussion of "medically unexplained physical symptoms," or "MUPS," Park and Knudson (2007, 43) include those living with fibromyalgia among the substantial number of Canadians who "report symptoms of conditions that cannot be definitively identified through physical examination or medical testing." Kornelsen and colleagues (2015) argue that the type of prolonged diagnostic uncertainty experienced by patients and physicians in these cases has given rise to the label MUPS and seriously tests the credibility of doctors and the legitimacy of patients. They conclude that the lived experience of MUPS is rooted in uncertainty about what may be causing the symptoms, how they should be managed, and how they may affect the individual's future health and well-being. While Fitzcharles, Ste-Marie, and Pereira (2013, E650) contend that fibromyalgia is changing from a condition of "suspect validity" to being more widely accepted as a "true syndrome," they conclude that "until the pathogenesis of fibromyalgia has been more clearly established, scepticism about the condition will remain."

Until then, the underlying cause (or causes) of this chronic condition remains unknown, there is no cure, and physicians often encounter difficulties in diagnosing and treating fibromyalgia. Women presenting the symptoms of fibromyalgia may be told to relax, to learn how to manage stress better, or simply to pull themselves together. It is not uncommon to be told that the symptoms are all in your mind (Canadian Women's Health Network 2012). The reality, however, is that although the intensity of pain may vary, some degree of muscle pain is always present and has a profound effect on the quality of people's lives. In addition to the debilitating effects of persistent pain, fibromyalgia is associated with anxiety and depression that may stem from uncertainty about both the causes and consequences of this condition and the frustration of trying to find appropriate medical care. The condition presents untold opportunities for self-health management and active involvement of the informal health-care system as the affected individual struggles to make sense of her illness experience, perform her usual well roles, and maintain a healthy self-identity while searching for a diagnosis and effective treatment.

The illness and the individual's credibility may both be questioned, since fibromyalgia is basically an invisible condition and there may be a significant difference between the individual's appearance and her ability to meet the expectations of others. Asbring and Narvanen (2002) contend that since it is not possible to verify the illness using objective measures and resolve the uncertainty, people experiencing symptoms of fibromyalgia run the risk of being stigmatized. Their study indicates that "many women experienced having the reality of their symptoms called into question by those closest to them, by their caregivers, and by the staff at the social insurance office" (Asbring and Narvanen 2002, 157). Living with fibromyalgia typically entails engaging in a lengthy and "complicated process, which involves drawing on a range of resources, including health professionals and support groups, as well as individuals' own experience" (Madden and Sim 2006, 2970) to find a way to give meaning to the condition, manage its effects, and continue to participate fully in social life.

Let's explore this type of embodied illness experience by using a narrative case study and giving our fictional narrator a name, an identity, and an opportunity to tell her story. The following fictional example (Anna's story) is intended to illustrate what an illness narrative account can reveal about the process involved in making sense of sickness and the type of challenges encountered in trying to maintain a healthy self-identity. Box 9.7 presents Anna's narrative account of how her life has been affected by fibromyalgia. This condition is characterized by constant pain throughout the body, extreme exhaustion, and sleep disturbance and poses a number of serious challenges that are commonly encountered by people living with chronic illness. The major challenges that Anna faces are explanation (finding answers for questions such as: why is this happening to me, what does the pain mean, and what does the future hold?) and adaptation (figuring out the best way to carry on and not give up, managing the symptoms and adjusting to living with the condition, and maintaining a normal, healthy life).

The type of chronic pain reported by Anna gives rise to a search for meaning (i.e., a diagnosis or a way to interpret and understand what is happening to her body and health) and, at the same time, a search for ways to manage the experience (i.e., to find relief from the pain, gain some degree of mastery or control over her suffering, and carry on with life). Baszanger (1989, 428) explains that the chronic pain sufferer seeks to maintain control not only to lessen but if possible to eliminate the pain and also to preserve "both personal bodily integrity and the presentation of a competent self which the pain experience tends to destroy." This point is vividly illustrated by Anna's narrative account of her struggles to understand what was causing her pain and to find a way to minimize the disruption in her personal and social life. People living with conditions such as fibromyalgia typically struggle to keep up with the demands of everyday life, perform normal roles, and resist the loss of their previous identity while experiencing "numerous changes to their life situation, with regard to family and social relations, social responsibilities, employment or leisure" (Sim and Madden 2008, 63).

Box 9.7 Missing Voices: Narrating a Life in Pain—Anna's Story

Hi, my name is Anna. I'm 45 years old, married, and have two children—a 12-year-old son and a 10-year-old daughter. I used to be a healthy, active person. I worked full-time at a bank and coped well with a hectic family life. I was involved in activities at my children's school and frequently drove carpool so they could participate in recreational and sports programs after school. Plus, there were music lessons, birthday parties, and doctor's appointments to keep us busy . . . not to mention the usual demands of grocery shopping, meal preparation, and housekeeping. I even found time to go to the gym a couple of times a week. While life got stressful sometimes, I had lots of energy, and everything seemed to be going really well. That was until two years ago, when my life dramatically changed.

I started to experience pain when I performed many daily activities. It got progressively worse until I was unable to move any part of my body without pain. I couldn't even lie in bed comfortably, turning over was painful, and I woke up frequently during the night. I went to bed in pain . . . and I woke up with stiffness and pain that lasted all day! The lack of sleep and chronic fatigue made it more difficult for me to cope with the persistent pain. I developed tender spots on my body where even slight pressure caused excruciating pain. I didn't have the heart to tell my children that their hugs hurt mommy. The daily struggle to get up in the morning and look after my family, to keep up with the demands at work, and to try to meet all my other commitments became overwhelming, and I found myself becoming more and more depressed. I couldn't understand why I had so much pain and so little energy. Instead of being able to take care of my children and our family home, I started to feel that I needed someone to take care of me, but I wasn't sure where to turn for help. I found myself living on ever-increasing doses of pain medication. Eventually, I had to take sick leave from work and cut down on my usual activities.

I went to see my family doctor several times, but she couldn't offer a clear medical explanation for what I was going through. I also discussed my symptoms at length with my husband and my sister. They were very sympathetic and tried to offer emotional support and practical assistance with some of the daily activities that I could no longer manage. Several months ago, one of my co-workers told me that her sister experienced the same type of pain that I described and gave me the name of the specialist she had consulted. Fortunately, I was eventually able to get an appointment with the recommended rheumatologist. After a thorough physical examination my condition was diagnosed as fibromyalgia syndrome.

My first reaction was relief . . . now that I had a named condition, I was hopeful that there would be effective treatment. I had never heard of fibromyalgia, so I tried to learn as much as I could about the causes, symptoms, and treatment of the condition. I found a great deal of information on the Internet, including the name of a fibromyalgia self-help group in my city. Participating in a self-help group and sharing my story with others who are in the same situation helped me to feel less isolated. I have also learned how to manage the symptoms by modifying my lifestyle practices (e.g., listening more closely to my body and using heat therapy and rest). This has helped to alleviate some of the pain and suffering, and I now feel like less of a burden on my family. Even though I feel that my voice is finally being heard, I am still waiting for them to find a cure for fibromyalgia so that I can get back to being myself . . .

Persistent pain, particularly back pain, incapacitates millions of people in Canada and the United States, such as Anna, and can have serious consequences for the individuals and their family members (Roy 1992). West and colleagues (2012) describe the many ways in which chronic pain can have an extensive impact on the family, including life changes such as a reversal of roles, the loss of friendships, and emotional turmoil illustrated by Anna's narrative account. This study clearly demonstrates that "while pain is an individual experience, the effects of pain are far reaching into the family structure" (2012, 3355). *National Population Health Survey* (*NPHS*) data indicate that approximately 4 million Canadians over the age of 15 have chronic pain; it is the number one reason that people seek formal health care and accounts for about one-half of all physician visits; as well, 70 per cent of Canadians living with chronic pain rate it as moderate to severe and report interference with their normal daily activities. Roy (1992) characterizes chronic pain as an "enigmatic problem." It may be an ongoing, embodied aspect of the lived experience of many people, but at the same time, pain is a highly elusive concept that is difficult to define and even more difficult to measure. Roy argues that we need to focus on the social context of chronic pain sufferers such as Anna to be able to understand the process by which people interpret the meaning of this embodied experience and manage to carry on their daily lives. According to Bendelow (2006, 65), if we are going to be able to move beyond the medical understanding of pain, we need "to conceptualize pain sociologically and contextualize it as part of everyday life."

The sensation of pain is very real, particularly for those who are experiencing it (as illustrated by Box 9.8), but pain is subjective and, therefore, like other symptoms, cannot be directly observed or measured. Whelan (2003, 463) illustrates this in stating:

> When I experience pain, its reality is insistent and self-evident to me. But only to me. To others, my pain can be nothing more than my account of my pain. Not only can my account of my pain never capture fully my experience of it; my account can be neither verified nor disconfirmed by others. We attempt to defy pain's privacy by defining it, measuring it, theorizing about it and analyzing the accounts of the one in pain. But representations of pain—definitions, measurement, body language, theories—are not equivalent to pain itself. Only representations of pain are public objects; pains themselves are not.

At best, we have only indirect means of assessing the nature of people's pain experience. As you may recall, Anna said that even slight pressure on certain spots on her body caused excruciating pain. Her choice of terms suggests that her pain is extremely severe and, perhaps, at times unbearable. Regardless of how we interpret her language, it is apparent that pain disclosure is an important part of her embodied experience. Chronic pain sufferers (such as Anna) have to make choices every day about whether to keep pain private or to express it publicly. This is particularly problematic for people like Anna with conditions such as fibromyalgia. "Individuals living with chronic pain often struggle to present themselves as credible when seeking medical care because pain is invisible" (Wallace et al. 2014, 291). Living with an invisible chronic illness means that individuals like Anna can try "to maintain an image of a healthy self . . . and choose whether to disclose information about the illness" (Sim and Madden 2008, 64). The situation is further complicated by the fact that a diagnosis of fibromyalgia may be both a relief and a burden for the individual (Asbring and Narvanen 2002). In telling her story, Anna stated that her initial response to the diagnosis was relief but that she had never heard of fibromyalgia and did not know anything about the causes or treatment of this condition. Madden and Sim (2006, 2966)

Box 9.8 Pain: A Private Sensation Made Public

We draw on a cultural repertoire of behavioural responses to reveal to others that we are experiencing pain. The private sensation of pain is made public to others through our language and actions. Based on the things that we say and do, others then infer that we must be in pain and attempt to assess the nature and quality of the sensation (i.e., the location, duration, intensity, and severity of the pain) by asking questions such as the following: Where does it hurt? How long have you been in pain? What kind of pain is it? Pain becomes public when we express it to others through visual cues (e.g., facial expressions, such as a grimace, which we have learned to interpret as a "pained look" in our cultural context); vocal cues (e.g., sounds that we have learned may be indicative of pain, such as moaning or groaning); verbal cues (e.g., the language we use to describe the pain sensation); and bodily cues (e.g., clutching or grabbing the presumed pain site, such as holding your head, which may be interpreted by others to mean that you have a headache). We actually have a very rich pain vocabulary. To illustrate, pain can be described, for example, as sharp, dull, aching, stabbing, throbbing, burning, or pressing. Can you think of other common pain descriptors?

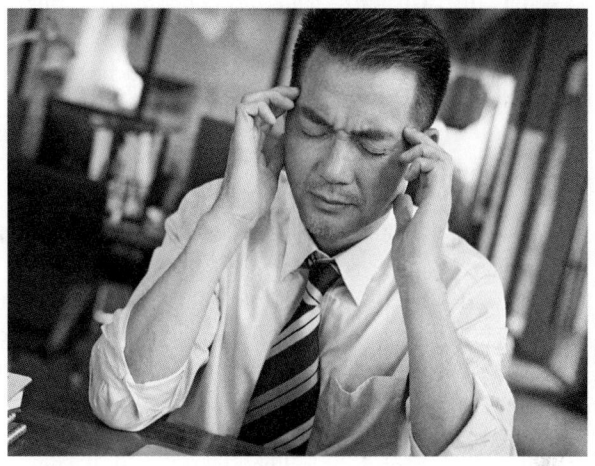

---

characterize fibromyalgia syndrome as "an empty diagnosis" that contributes little to people's "knowledge about their illness, and thus no basis for interpretation to reduce the uncertainty of the illness experience."

In an effort to resolve some of the uncertainty about whether to share the illness experience and diagnosis with others, individuals such as Anna try to find answers to questions such as the following: Whom should I tell? How much information should I disclose about my pain and suffering? Will revealing to others that I have a condition such as fibromyalgia change the way they view me? Will my employer and co-workers still see me as a healthy, capable person? It is clear that pain represents a threat to the legitimacy of self, and in the case of chronic pain "what is at stake is the self as rational and competent" (Aldrich and Eccleston 2000, 1640). In addition, Anna is faced with the ongoing struggle of dealing with competing demands of the social imperative to carry on despite the pain and the sometimes overwhelming physiological imperative to give in to the pain! For example, Anna struggled to fulfill all of her usual social roles for as long as she could, but eventually she had to take a leave from work and ask members of her informal social network for assistance with activities of daily living. Finally, as illustrated by Anna's story, living with chronic conditions (which are, by definition, long-term and irreversible) means working hard to adjust to a life permanently altered by sickness and trying to reconstruct your sense of self so that you can continue to consider yourself a healthy person. In fact, health sociologists (Corbin and Strauss 1985; 1988) use the term "chronic illness work" to highlight the fact that to deal with an assault on the self and the personal and social threats that accompany chronic illness, individuals such as Anna must work hard to reconstruct their identities and their lives.

Chronic Illness Work

Despite facing many challenges, the majority of chronically ill persons find a way to manage their chronic conditions and to lead meaningful lives. Corbin and Strauss (1985) use the concept of "work" (i.e., a set of tasks that must be performed) to analyze the ways in which people manage chronic illness at home. They identify three types of work related to the different challenges posed by chronic illness. First, they describe illness-related work. This entails taking care of long-term symptoms such as persistent pain and finding the best way to treat the chronic condition. A second type of work—everyday life work—involves responding to the demands created by the impact of chronic illness on activities of daily living (i.e., routine practical tasks) and maintaining social relationships (and giving meaning to a restructured social world). Finally, there is critically important biographical work, which is directed at cognitive and emotional components of chronic illness and the need to reconstruct the meaning of one's health status, sense of self-identity, and life circumstances.

Chronic illness has been characterized as a "biographical disruption" (Bury 1982, 1991; Williams 2000). As Anna's narrative shows, the onset of chronic illness results in changes not only to the body but also to the individual's general sense of identity and patterns of social interaction. According to Bury, chronic illness places past, present, and future meanings at risk and therefore can be understood as a **biographical disruption**, since it creates considerable uncertainty about the individual's health and social life. In many ways, learning to live with chronic illness means dealing with uncertainty and unpredictability. For example, the cause of the illness may be unknown (as in the case of Anna's experience with fibromyalgia), treatment may be a matter of trial and error, and the eventual outcome of the illness may be equally uncertain. As a result, chronic illness disrupts the shared meaning of everyday experiences and creates a great deal of social and emotional uncertainty for the individual in addition to pain and physical limitations. Bury (1982, 169) contends that chronic illness is the "kind of experience where the structures of everyday life and the forms of knowledge which underpin them are disrupted" along with the "explanatory systems normally used by people." In other words, chronically ill people (such as Anna) have to find a way to make sense of their sickness in terms of both physical functioning and psychosocial well-being.

In a related discussion, Charmaz (1983; 1991) described chronic illness as an assault on the body and the self (i.e., the person's feelings of self-worth and confidence in social situations) as well as on the social world of the individual and her family. The process of renegotiating the meaning of one's life as health status changes raises a variety of psychosocial challenges for the chronically ill person. Charmaz summarizes these social and psychological problems by describing the impact of chronic illness on the individual's sense of self, restrictions on everyday life, difficulties in maintaining social relationships, feelings of being discounted and discredited, and concerns about becoming a burden on others. All of these challenges are evident in Anna's story about how she endures a life of pain and suffering.

The physical pain and psychological distress that typically accompany chronic illness result in an assault on the body and the self. Past taken-for-granted assumptions about the self and the social world are placed at risk, and established behavioural patterns are disrupted. According to Charmaz, depending on the nature and severity of the condition, chronic illness may result in different levels of assault on the self. It may begin with disruption (as suggested by Bury) but then progress to intrusion as the chronic illness pervades more and more aspects of the person's life and eventually end in immersion as the chronically ill person is redefined in terms of her chronic condition. Living with the pain, discomfort, and limitations that may accompany chronic illness means that everyday life becomes increasingly restricted. As in Anna's account, the chronically ill person may no longer be able to perform previous normal well roles and, as a result, may experience a loss of independence as well as a loss of enjoyment associated with previously valued social and leisure activities. Chronic illness also threatens social relationships. The chronically ill person may require more assistance from others and be unable to live up to their expectations based on pre-illness performance, thus disrupting the reciprocal nature of social relationships. Living with a condition such as fibromyalgia may strain even supportive social networks. The loss of meaningful social relationships may, in turn, lead to feeling discounted (i.e., the perception that you are no longer a valuable contributing member of society) and discredited (i.e., a lack of self-worth). According to Charmaz (1983, 185), "When ill persons realize that significant others do not understand or accept the limitations inherent in their present physical conditions, they feel discounted." This is a highly problematic issue for Anna, since people suffering from fibromyalgia generally appear to be healthy and, consequently, the condition of their health is often misunderstood by family members, friends, and co-workers. Together, these factors may make chronically ill people feel that they have become a burden on others!

Researchers continue to use Corbin and Strauss' conceptual framework to guide their investigations of the everyday practices involved in chronic illness work (Clarke and Bennett 2012; Pickard and Rogers 2012; Lindsay 2009). In fact, this topic is increasingly important, since the majority of older adults live today with the social and physical realities of managing the symptoms and functional losses associated with having multiple chronic conditions. The gaps in our understanding of how older adults manage to adjust to living with chronic pain "is especially troubling given the greater prevalence of chronic pain with advancing age" (Chan et al. 2012, 192). Lindsay (2009, 984) argues that "relatively little is known about how patients self-manage multiple chronic conditions and especially how they *prioritize* which of their health problems will be given the greatest attention." What is well known, however, is that self-care is a major component of this complex and dynamic process and that most of the burden of managing multiple chronic illnesses and minimizing the extent of their disruption on life falls on the affected individuals and their families and takes place outside of the formal health-care system.

According to Clarke and Bennett (2012, 213), self-care practices have been shown to be an important means of managing biographical disruptions and retaining or regaining a sense of control over "unpredictable chronic illness experiences and trajectories." Most of the participants in Lindsay's (2009) study emphasized the importance of trying to keep their illnesses as stable as possible and maintaining an acceptable way of life within the limitations of their chronic conditions. Illness narratives offer health sociologists an opportunity to see these types of chronic illness work being done and to learn more about the hidden depths of health care.

Chapter Summary

This chapter explored hidden depths of the iceberg of health care by examining lay beliefs about health and illness, self-care behavioural practices, and the importance of supportive social networks. Health researchers are still in the process of learning about the health benefits of informal care and the ways in which self-health management and social support contribute to the pursuit of health and wellness. We do know, however, that lay conceptions of health and illness help "to make the world a stable, orderly and predictable place" (Furnham 1988, 9). Our personal ideas about what makes people healthy or sick serve a number of important functions. Beliefs about health maintenance and illness management help us to give personal meaning to both health and illness, deal with feelings associated with the onset of illness, and evaluate and select appropriate health-care practices. Lay beliefs help us to define the personal meaning of healthiness and to deal with the uncertainty often associated with sickness. In other words, they guide our search for meaning and our efforts to find answers to questions about our health status. In this way, lay beliefs shape what we think about the pursuit of health and the impact of illness on our lives.

Lay beliefs also help to shape the importance that we attach to good health and our feelings about illness experiences. For example, these beliefs may assist us in dealing with the emotional demands of serious illness (i.e., coping with the fear, anger, and anxiety that often accompany sickness). In other words, lay beliefs help us to deal with feelings about being sick and concerns about the impact health problems may have on our personal and social life. Finally, lay beliefs guide our behavioural responses to health-related matters. They shape our health-protective behaviour, the way we behave when we become sick, and our selection of health-care practices. In this way, lay explanatory beliefs help us to decide who is a relevant helper and what type of care is most appropriate.

We now have proof that people routinely engage in a wide variety of self-health management practices, including health-protective and illness treatment activities. In each case, the defining characteristic is that behaviours carried out to maintain health, achieve symptomatic relief, or manage chronic illness all reflect the individual's self-care capacity, autonomous participation in the decision-making process, and the exercise of personal responsibility for health care. Self-health management also includes mutual aid exchanges that occur when people informally come together with members of their social networks to offer each other practical assistance and emotional support. Informal helping networks have an extensive capacity to aid us in dealing with health maintenance and illness management. Research shows that good social relationships, strong supportive networks, and socially cohesive communities have a powerful protective effect on health.

We concluded the chapter by discussing a narrative case study demonstrating the link between informal care and illness as an embodied experience. Fibromyalgia, a chronic condition characterized by widespread persistent pain, was used to demonstrate the many social, psychological, and physical challenges facing chronically ill people and the ways in which informal care facilitates efforts to make sense of sickness and maintain a healthy self-identity. Chronic conditions and symptoms such as constant pain, not relieved by medical treatment, present vast opportunities for engaging in self-care practices. Self-health management is particularly important for people with long-term chronic health problems, because the formal health-care system is limited in its ability to offer assistance over the many years in which they have to manage chronic illness at home and its impact on their daily lives. Under these circumstances, informal care, personal health practices, and belonging to supportive social networks may play a more significant role in day-to-day life for chronically ill individuals than formal biomedical care.

Self-care tasks involved in managing chronic illness include self-monitoring, or the ongoing observation of changes in physical condition and level of functioning, managing drug therapy at home and deciding when to take prescribed and non-prescribed medications, and treatment activities to manage symptoms associated with the condition. Self-management of chronic illness also involves dealing with emotions (e.g., frustration, anger, and depression) that may be associated with chronic illness. As well, it may mean adjusting to a future that is permanently altered by long-term illness while working hard to maintain a normal way of life as well as maintaining a healthy self-identity. Overall, this chapter demonstrated that there is compelling evidence that self-health management (even though it is not readily visible) is a basic component of the health-care system. Continuing to learn more about the hidden depths of the iceberg of health care and the many health benefits of informal care should lead to increasing awareness that members of the lay community are active participants in the health-care process, primary providers of care, and producers of health (in addition to being consumers of professional health-care services). In the next two chapters, we will turn our attention to the formal part of the health-care system (the tip of the iceberg) and examine the contribution of biomedical and complementary and alternative health-care practitioners to the pursuit of health and wellness.

Study Questions

1. Summarize the features of lay conceptions of good health that emphasize positive aspects such as fitness, healthiness, and functional ability.
2. Comment on the relationship between popular and professional conceptions of health and illness.
3. Explain the relationship between lay beliefs about illness causation and controllability.
4. Describe the types of health-related behaviours included in the concept of self-health management.
5. Explain the difference between regulatory and preventive self-care health behaviour.
6. Comment on the relationship between social networks, social support, and health.
7. Explain the meaning of the statement that pain lies at the intersection between biology and culture.
8. Summarize the ways in which chronic illness involves a biographical disruption. What are the limitations of this concept?
9. Outline the different types of chronic illness work that are involved in making sense of sickness and maintaining a healthy self-identity.

Recommended Readings

Bendelow, G., and S. Williams. 1995. "Transcending the dualisms: Towards a sociology of pain." *Sociology of Health and Illness* 17: 139–65.

Bury, M. 2001. "Illness narratives: Fact or fiction?" *Sociology of Health and Illness* 23: 263–85.

Caulfield, T. 2015. *Is Gwyneth Paltrow Wrong about Everything? When Celebrity Culture and Science Clash*. Toronto: Viking.

Hughner, R., and S. Kleine. 2004. "Views of health in the lay sector: A compilation and review of how individuals think about health." *Health: An Interdisciplinary Journal for the Social Study of Health, Illness, and Medicine* 8: 395–422.

Lee, J., C. Dallaire, M.-P. Markon, L. Lemyre, D. Kewski, and M. Turner. 2014. "'I can choose': The reflected prominence of personal control in representations of health risk in Canada." *Health, Risk and Society* 16: 117–35.

Lupton, D. 2013. "The digitally engaged patient: Self-monitoring and self-care in the digital health era." *Social Theory and Health* 11: 256–70.

Radley, A., and M. Billig. 1996. "Accounts of health and illness: Dilemmas and representations." *Sociology of Health and Illness* 18: 220–40.

Smith, K., and N. Christakis. 2008. "Social networks and health." *Annual Review of Sociology* 34: 405–29.

Thoits, P. 2011. "Mechanisms linking social ties and support to physical and mental health." *Journal of Health and Social Behavior* 52: 145–61.

Ziguras, C. 2004. *Self-Care: Embodiment, Personal Autonomy and the Shaping of Health Consciousness*. New York: Routledge.

Recommended Websites

American Self-Help Group Clearinghouse:
www.selfhelpgroups.org

Holmes-Rahe Social Readjustment Rating Scale:
www.harvestenterprises-sra.com/The Holmes-Rahe Scale.htm

Self-Help Resource Centre:
www.selfhelp.on.ca

Medicalizing Beings and Bodies: The Link between Population Health and Biomedical Care

10

Learning Objectives

This chapter examines biomedicine as the dominant form of formal health care, considering such issues as

- the historical development of biomedical knowledge;
- basic ideas of the biomedical model;
- consequences of continued dominance of biomedicine in formal health care; and
- the tendency to understand aspects of human experience as medical issues requiring biomedical intervention.

In addressing these topics, we will critically assess contributions made by the formal biomedical health-care system to population health.

Biomedical dominance of the pursuit of health and wellness has been described as "The Greatest Benefit to Mankind" (Porter 1997). As Chapter 4 discussed, access to formal health care is one of the general determinants of health. We need ready access to doctors and hospitals when we are seriously ill. However, the extent to which formal biomedical health care contributes to improvements in population health remains an unanswered question. Industrialized nations, such as Canada, spend an increasing percentage of their gross domestic product on formal health care. The latest data show that total health expenditure in Canada was $205.4 billion in 2012 and was forecast to reach $214.9 billion in 2014 (Canadian Institute for Health Information 2014).

Total health spending accounted for 10.9 per cent of GDP in Canada in 2012, compared with an average of 9.4 per cent across Organisation for Economic Co-operation and Development countries (OECD 2013). The United States (16.9 per cent), The Netherlands (12.1 per cent), France (11.6 per cent), Switzerland (11.4 per cent), Germany (11.3 per cent), Austria (11.1 per cent), and Denmark (11.0 per cent) each had a higher share. In terms of health-care spending per capita, Canada was among the top 10 countries (and was comparable to Denmark and Luxembourg). There is a big difference, however, between the United States, the top spender, and the rest of the OECD countries.

For the most part, Canadians are proud of their health-care system; it consistently emerges as a top priority when polling companies ask citizens what issues they consider important. However, the data depicted in Figure 10.1 force us to consider whether spending more and more money on delivery of formal biomedical health care is the best way of improving population health. These data show that countries that spend the most on formal health care do not necessarily receive proportionate returns in terms of population health status. For instance, countries such as Japan and Italy have the highest life expectancy (82.7 years) and relatively low

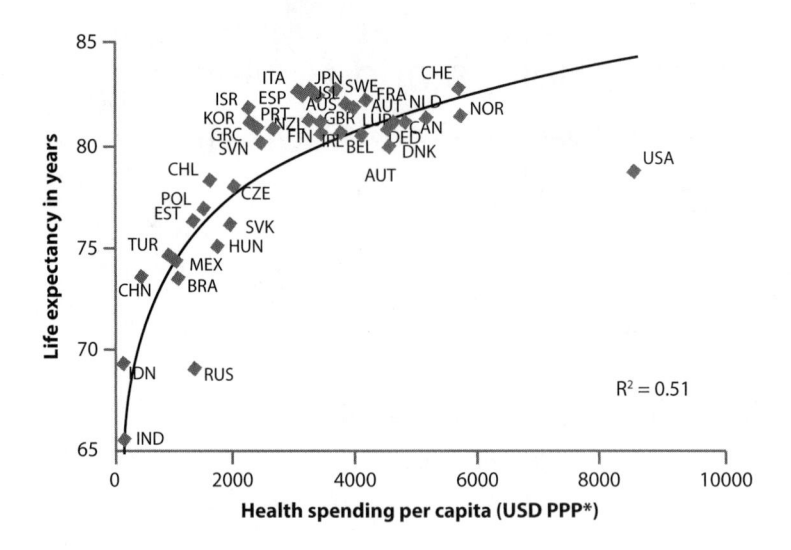

Figure 10.1 Life Expectancy at Birth and Health Spending per Capita, 2011.

Higher health spending per capita is generally associated with longer life expectancy, although this link tends to be less pronounced in countries with the highest expenditures.

* PPP = purchasing power parities

Source: OECD 2013.

health-care spending per capita (approximately $3000). In comparison, the United States ranks first in health spending per capita ($8508), but its life expectancy of 78.7 years is among the lowest.

Our formal health-care system is designed to care for us when we become ill rather than to promote health. Today we have primarily a medicalized health-care system focused on providing acute care for sick people within institutions such as hospitals. **Medicalization** is the term used by health sociologists to describe the tendency to understand aspects of life as medical issues requiring intervention and control on the part of medicine. The current formal health-care system is based on a biomedical model of care which promotes the medicalization of life rather than the pursuit of health and wellness. Furthermore, health care can be bad for your health, and the "creeping medicalization" of society comes with steep economic, social, and human costs (Wright 2009). Although health researchers have been investigating the process of medicalization for four decades and have described in detail how an increasing number of conditions have come under medical jurisdiction, few studies have systematically tried to estimate the costs of medicalization. Conrad, Mackie, and Mehrotra (2010, 1946) attempted to address the extent to which "medicalization has been a major driver of increased health care costs in the United States." Although their findings are limited, they make a strong case for further research on this topic to determine the extent to which medicalization contributes to the spiralling health-care expenditures cited earlier.

According to Conrad (2013, 195), "medicalization has become a central analytic theme in medical sociology" because this expanding global trend continues to affect society. This chapter explores the processes whereby human experiences have become medicalized. We will examine the social construction of ideas that have led to the dominance of biomedicine in both the formal health-care sector and society at large. We will begin by tracing the origins of the biomedical response to illness, considering the social construction of biomedical knowledge. This will set the stage for a look at major ideas that characterize the biomedical model and consequences of this way of pursuing health and wellness. The chapter concludes by exploring contemporary issues, such as the growing dominance of biomedicine in life and the role played by pharmaceutical companies, genomic medicine, and biotechnology in the increasing medicalization of beings and bodies. The focus throughout this chapter is on critically assessing the link between biomedicine and population health.

The Origins of the Biomedical Model

In an important early paper on the development of the biomedical model, Jewson (1976) explored how formal health care developed alongside changes in the mode of production of medical knowledge. Guided by a Marxist perspective, Jewson's argument was that as the social relations of healing changed so too did the ideas that make up medical knowledge. In Jewson's words, these changes culminated in "the disappearance of the sick-man [sic]," or the diminishing importance of the subjective experiences of the patient in biomedical health care. He argued that as medicine became more technical, the importance of the human element in health care declined. His sociologically informed history of medicine is very different from those produced by doctors and others with vested interests in the institution of medicine. Often, medical histories celebrate the triumphs of "great doctors" and "medical breakthroughs" (e.g., Porter 1997). Such accounts of "medical progress" downplay the point that medical knowledge is socially produced. Jewson, on the other hand, explored how changes in society prompted changes in medical knowledge. His analysis of the development of the biomedical model clearly demonstrates what was described in Chapter 2 as the social construction of medical knowledge.

Jewson drew on earlier histories of medicine to show how medicine moved through stages of "bedside medicine" to "hospital medicine" to "laboratory medicine," each stage characterized by a different way of understanding disease shaped by prevailing power relations in society at that time (see Box 10.1). Armstrong (1995) added another stage to Jewson's history, which he argued characterized the biomedical model at the turn of the century, and Nettleton (2004) added yet another stage to describe the manner in which biotechnological developments have propelled a further change in medical knowledge. Let's start with the stages described by Jewson, and, later in the chapter when we explore medicalization of social life, we will look at the most recent stages added by Armstrong and Nettleton. It is important to bear in mind that Jewson's argument is that changing social relations of healing produced changes in the structure of medical knowledge. In this way, he shows that medical knowledge, rather than being objective truth, is socially constructed and changes with social and cultural transformations.

Bedside Medicine

In the eighteenth century, the social relations of healing were characterized by a power imbalance in which doctors had lower social status than patients. Doctors offered services to patients of upper-class backgrounds who could afford private medical care. As the name suggests, during

> **Box 10.1** The Development of Medical Knowledge
>
> Bedside Medicine (the Middle Ages to the eighteenth century)
> "What is the matter with you?": Symptom
> ↓
> Hospital Medicine (Industrial Revolution onward)
> "Where does it hurt?": Pathological Lesion
> ↓
> Laboratory Medicine (mid-nineteenth century onward)
> "Let's wait and see what the tests say": Cellular Pathology
> ↓
> Surveillance Medicine (turn of the twentieth century)
> "What are your risks?": Risk Factor
> ↓
> E-scaped Medicine (twentieth century onward)
> "What communication breakdown in the human system has initiated disease?":
> Digitalized Body
>
> The development of medical knowledge can be understood as proceeding through these five stages based on the work of Jewson (1976), Armstrong (1995), and Nettleton (2004).

this period doctors attended to wealthy patients at their private bedsides. Freund, McGuire, and Podhurst (2003, 214) offer the following description of healing during this period:

> Several kinds of physicians, each having very different ideas about the causes and treatments of sickness, competed for patients and social legitimacy. Furthermore, physicians were only a small percentage of the total number of persons practicing various healing arts, who included, among others, midwives, bone setters, nurses, pharmacists, barbers (who performed minor surgery), herbalists, and folk and religious healers.

This competition produced a status difference in which "doctors had to compete with each other to please the patient" (Armstrong 2003, 85). In other words, patients were the dominant participants in medical encounters between doctors and patients! The result was that doctors had to impress patients with their medical knowledge and care as well as with their interpersonal skills. The doctors' goal was to develop close personal relationships with clients while, at the same time, setting their treatments apart from those of their competitors. In Jewson's words (1976, 232), this power imbalance profoundly shaped medical knowledge of the period: "In this situation the political and economic power of patrons insured that they retained ultimate control over medical investigators and the process of production of medical knowledge."

As depicted in Box 10.1, under such social relations doctors needed to pay close attention to patients' symptoms: "The model of illness that emerged from this relationship was one based on the interpretation of individual symptoms: doctors had no need to physically examine their patients; they only had to pay attention to their patients' demands and experiences (in the form of symptoms)" (Armstrong 2003, 85). White (2002, 121) explains that the culture of the period can be summarized in the question, "What is the matter with you?" He argues that this question illustrates a holistic orientation to the patient that characterized Bedside Medicine. Doctors retained the favour of their patients by focusing treatment on the symptom(s) that the patients reported. Jewson (1976, 228) describes how under Bedside Medicine, "disease was defined in terms of its external and subjective manifestations rather than its internal and hidden causes." In Bedside Medicine, symptoms and illness were considered the same thing.

Medical knowledge during Bedside Medicine was characterized by **humoral theory,** which understood disease as resulting from a unique lack of balance involving physical, environmental, and spiritual factors. According to humoral theory, the human body was composed of four basic substances known as the four humours (i.e., black bile, yellow bile, phlegm, and blood). Imbalance in one of these four humours produced illness. Health was restored by balancing the four humours through personalized treatment. As depicted in Box 10.2, treatment consisted of various invasive measures ("heroic medicine") intended to return balance to the humours, such as bloodletting and blistering. While humoral theory underpinned the cultural understanding of disease during the period of Bedside Medicine, medical knowledge was quite diverse. Each doctor offered an assortment of heroic cures tailored to patients' specific symptoms while demonstrating his techniques for balancing the humours. However, by the end of the eighteenth century, "a new system emerged that claimed that the symptom was no longer the illness but merely a pointer or indicator" (Armstrong 2003, 84).

Box 10.2 Heroic Medicine

James Gillray's 1804 English caricature, *Breathing a Vein,* depicts the common treatment of bloodletting that, according to humoral theory, characterized Bedside Medicine. The University of Virginia's historical collection notes, "The title suggests that the procedure was a pleasant way to allow the vein a little air. The reality of the procedure was something else, as the cartoon suggests. A tourniquet was placed above the elbow, the artery in the forearm was punctured by a lancet, and the blood, gushing like a geyser, was captured in a bowl."

Breathing a Vein. James Gillray, published by H. Humphrey, St James's Street, London, 28 January 1804.

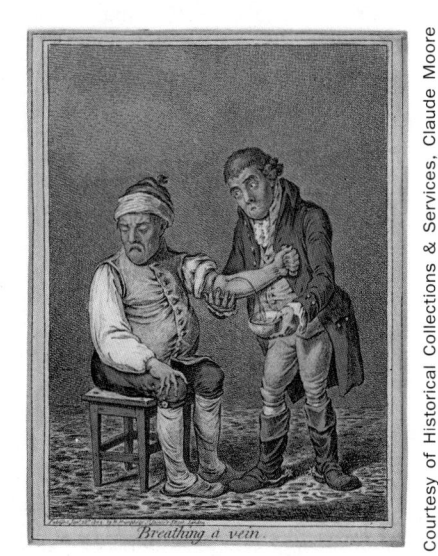

Courtesy of Historical Collections & Services, Claude Moore Health Sciences Library, University of Virginia.

Hospital Medicine

This new medical model emerged not because of scientific progress in medical knowledge but because social relations of healing changed along with wider social transformations, such as industrialization and urbanization. These changes turned the power imbalance between doctors and their patients on its head, with doctors gaining their now familiar position of dominance in medical encounters. First in Paris and later throughout Europe, large hospitals were built to treat the sick masses. Armstrong (2003, 85) describes how "doctors now found themselves treating (usually for charity) socially inferior and therefore more passive patients." The hospital setting resulted in the emergence of a way of understanding disease that was very different from the symptomatic focus of Bedside Medicine.

Rather than privileging patients' accounts of symptoms, a new model for understanding disease emerged in eighteenth-century hospitals. As depicted in Box 10.1, the goal of Hospital Medicine was identifying the underlying biophysical defect, or **pathological lesion** within the body, that caused disease. For example, the symptom of a headache could be caused by an underlying pathological lesion such as a brain tumour. White (2002, 121) explains that "the question directed by the doctor at the patient, 'Where does it hurt?' catches many of the characteristics of this period." According to this model, the physician's goal was to examine the patient's body by interpreting physical signs and symptoms in order to discover the pathological lesion. "Medical investigators concentrated upon the accurate diagnosis and classification of cases rather than upon the prognosis and therapy of symptom complexes.... Diagnoses were founded upon physical examination of observable organic structures rather than verbal analysis of subjectively defined sensations and feelings" (Jewson 1976, 229–30). With Hospital Medicine, the patient figuratively and literally is transformed into a "medical case"—a biophysical carrying case of signs and symptoms interpreted by the physician, whose job was to search for the underlying causes of disease (Prior 2009). These causes were discovered by examining human anatomy—either before or, often, after death.

Hospital Medicine also marked the emergence of medicine as an organized profession that could exercise both medical dominance over competing healers and autonomy over the conditions of medical education and practice. In 1908, the leading American charity of the time, the Carnegie Foundation, commissioned the educational expert Abraham Flexner to prepare a report on the state of medical education in North America. Flexner spent a year and a half visiting medical schools. In his groundbreaking report, published in 1910, Flexner chose the system of medical education at Johns Hopkins Medical School as the model other medical schools were to follow. The report argued that medical schools should be affiliated with universities and provide a science-based education together with clinical experience gained while treating patients in teaching hospitals. Eventually, this resulted in both a reduction in the number of medical schools and standardization of medical education along bioscientific lines. Freund, McGuire, and Podhurst (2003, 218) describe how "In defining the scope of its work, the medical profession also eliminated much of its competition. Some professional competitors, such as homeopaths and osteopaths, were co-opted; others, such as pharmacists, nurses, anesthetists, and X-ray technicians, were subordinated; whereas still others, such as midwives, clergy, and barber-surgeons, were driven from legitimate practice outright." The 1910 Flexner Report secured the dominance of biomedicine over competing health-care professions. Before Flexner, the medical profession was much less standardized in terms of medical education and who had the legal right to call themselves doctors. The Flexner Report provided the model for professional medicine and shaped social relations that characterized Hospital Medicine!

Consider Jewson's (1976, 235) description of Hospital Medicine and its effects on the social relations of healing:

> The thousands of poor and destitute sick housed within the hospitals had little opportunity to exercise control over the activities of the medical staff. The powerlessness of the patients, combined with an enormous size of the hospital system, provided the clinicians with an inexhaustible fund of acquiescent research material. Clinicians thus gained control over and autonomy within the technical process of production of medical knowledge.

It was these developments that Foucault (1973) detailed in *The Birth of the Clinic* (see Chapter 2). The physical setting of early hospitals provided doctors with the opportunity to examine bodies in large numbers and establish concepts of statistical normality and abnormality that allowed for the objectification of the human body. For example, we now know that "normal" blood pressure is 120/80 because of statistical analyses based on medical examination of large numbers of people's bodies. It was during the period of Hospital Medicine that many common medical instruments, such as the stethoscope and sphygmomanometer, designed to measure bodily and biophysical processes, were invented and first applied. Together with practices such as the dissection of human cadavers, this allowed physicians to objectify the bodies of the sick in the name of searching for pathological lesions. Foucault (1973) points out the irony that opening up corpses revealed inner mechanisms of life!

The "medical gaze" that originated as a result of social relations of healing in early teaching hospitals allowed for a new, objective way of understanding life. When we objectify something, we turn it into a thing, and this, according to Foucault, is exactly what the newly emerging hospitals of the eighteenth century facilitated with the development of the medical gaze. White (2002, 121) describes how "the patient became dependent on the now professional doctor, while disease becomes a problem of the pathology of a specific organ, distinct from the whole existence of the individual." Armstrong (2009, 644) concludes that "The emergence of pathological medicine was not therefore the result of 'scientific progress' or advancement, but rather the direct expression of a doctor–patient relationship that placed the doctor centre-stage." Hospital Medicine produced passive patients. However, as Jewson explains, the increasing technological sophistication of medicine eventually displaced both doctors and patients in medical encounters, leading to another change in social relations of healing, which again reshaped medical knowledge.

Laboratory Medicine

Jewson (1976, 237) notes that "Whereas Hospital Medicine had celebrated the interests and perceptions of clinicians, Laboratory Medicine was founded upon the world-view of the scientific research worker." As its name suggests, during the period of Laboratory Medicine the social relations of healing moved out of the hospital ward and into the research laboratory. Both doctors and patients took a back seat to scientific researchers in this mode of production of medical knowledge. The search for the cause of disease moved from the anatomical level of the pathological lesion to microscopic search for **cellular pathology**. In other words, scientific breakthroughs allowed disease to be understood at the cellular level as a biochemical process. Berliner (1984, 30–1) explains that "scientific medicine emerged in the late nineteenth century primarily from French and German laboratories. It based itself around the discovery of micro-biological agents (bacteria) as the cause of disease and around the theory of specific etiology as a mechanism for explaining the role of these agents." During the late 1800s, scientific discoveries were made, such as Pasteur's revelation that certain diseases were caused by microbial infection and Lister's development of advanced techniques for sterilizing operating procedures. White (2002, 121) explains how the interpersonal relationships between physicians and patients became less important in the context of these technological developments, noting that social relations of healing under Laboratory Medicine could be summed up by the phrase, "let's wait and see what the tests say." For the first time, health and illness were defined in terms of statistical measures of biochemical processes occurring at the cellular level.

In this way, Jewson (1976, 238) demonstrates how changes in social relations that produce biomedical knowledge are responsible for displacement of the human element in health care: "Thus whilst Hospital Medicine had dissolved the integrated vision of the whole man into a network of anatomical structures, Laboratory Medicine, by focusing attention on the fundamental particles of organic matter, went still further in eradicating the person of the patient from medical discourse." For example, instead of treating patients in a clinical setting, physicians specializing in pathology use sophisticated imaging technologies, such as the scanning electron microscope, to identify biological abnormalities at the cellular level, such as that depicted in Box 10.3. Such medical specialists may never see actual patients but instead analyze tissue samples.

Pickstone (2009, 646) summarizes the importance of Jewson's three-step history of the development of medicine by explaining that "For all three steps, he related knowledge production to patterns of professional work and power—from the eighteenth-century doctors' deference towards the 'philosophies' of their patrons, to early nineteenth-century professional competition over pathological novelties in Paris hospitals and museums, to the later University world of biomedical research projects." Nettleton (2009, 634) underscores the importance of Jewson's linking of the development of medicine to societal changes by stating that "The value of this revelation is the confirmation that medical knowledge, practices and technologies are socially contingent. They are shaped, constructed, influenced, prioritized and mediated by 'the social,' be that social interests, cultural preferences, economics or social hierarchies."

Jewson's sociological perspective on the development of the biomedical model shows that within a relatively short period of 100 years, the subjective importance of the individual patient (i.e., "the sick-man" [sic]) disappeared from medical knowledge to be replaced by the objectification of the patient as a biomedical case. What this demonstrates is that medical knowledge is socially constructed. That is, a culture's ideas about illness and healing are the product of its social history. This is the case for biomedicine in the West just as it is the case for other cultures' health belief systems (as we will explore in the next chapter). Thus, it is possible to define the **biomedical model** as a model of health care based on scientific understanding that, at the level of basic knowledge, sees health and illness in terms of biological processes and, at the applied clinical level, privileges individualized, biologically orientated, pharmacological, surgical, and other technological interventions. The medico-centric biases of Western culture often hide social factors involved in the construction of the biomedical model. Let's look at the basic ideas that comprise the biomedical model before moving on to consider consequences of medicalizing the pursuit of health and wellness.

Basic Ideas of the Biomedical Model

As the history of medicine demonstrates, biomedicine developed in relation to broader cultural changes occurring in Western society. As biomedicine developed, the mystery and awe

> **Box 10.3** Cellular Pathology
>
> This image of a skin cancer cell produced by a scanning electron micrograph illustrates the *cellular pathology* which is the focus of Laboratory Medicine.
>
> Steve Gschmeissner/Science Photo Library

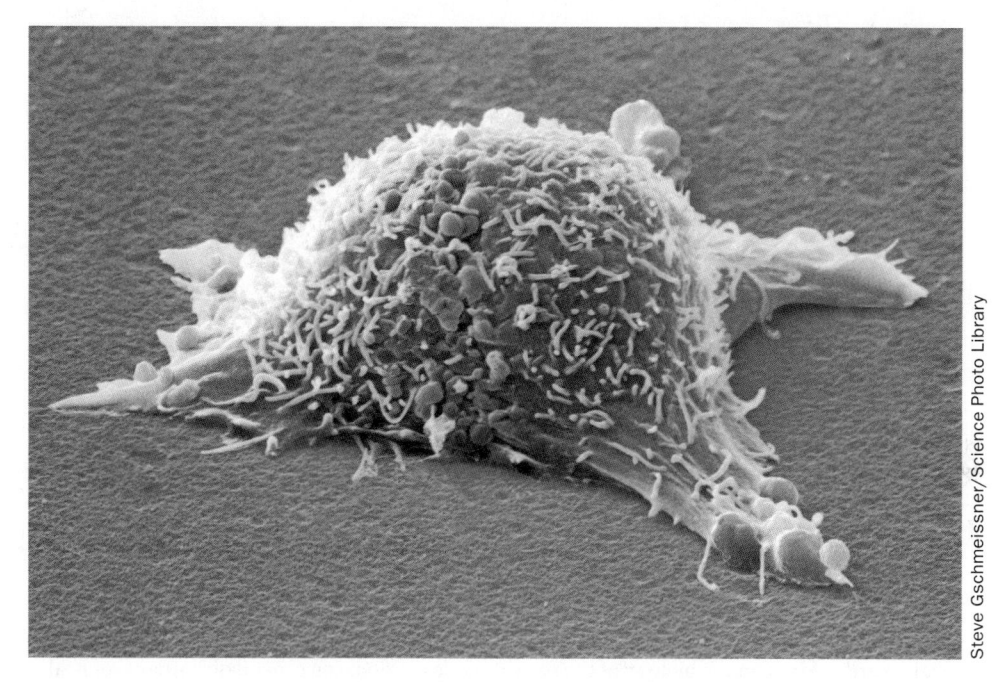

of human life gave way to scientific understandings of health, illness, and the body. This transformation parallels a more general change in Western society first described by Max Weber (1958). Weber noted that with the development of capitalism, behaviour came to be increasingly dominated by rational scientific thinking that swept away traditional ties to the past. He described this process as one of increasing "rationalization" that would eventually remove any sense of mystery from life and kill the human spirit. Building on Weber's ideas, Turner (1995) shows how this is the case with knowledge of the body and health. He argues that as science replaced religion as a way of understanding human experience, views of the body shifted from "sin to sickness" (1995, 18). Similarly, in an insightful criticism of medicalization, Hadler (2004, 101) explains that "our forefathers were frequently seduced by the pronouncements of the sages, particularly the religious sages, about the path to a good, if not longer, life. Today we wait for the next pronouncements of the biomedical establishment." The rational scientific approach to understanding the body and its illnesses that developed in the West is comprised of five basic ideas that characterize the biomedical model. Freund, McGuire, and Podhurst (2003, 220–2) outline these ideas in Box 10.4.

> **Box 10.4**   Five Ideas That Characterize the Biomedical Model
>
> - Mind–body dualism
> - Physical reductionism
> - Specific etiology
> - Machine metaphor
> - Regimen and control
>
> **Source:** Freund, McGuire, and Podhurst 2003.

Mind–Body Dualism

Descartes' (see Chapter 2) **mind–body dualism**, or philosophical separation of mind and body, provided a rationale for focusing solely on the individual biophysical body as a way to understand health and illness. As Sullivan explains, this philosophical separation has had serious consequences for how we understand and treat illness: "One of the most prominent reasons offered for medicine's inability to respond to the distinctively human dimensions of sickness is that it employs a dualistic image of the patient. The patient and his body are seen as composed of two radically different kinds of substance [*sic*]" (1986, 331). Influenced by Descartes' mind–body dualism, medicine adopted the scientific method of studying the human body as a physical object separate from social and psychological factors. The drawback of this separation is that it led health care to focus on the biology of the patient while overlooking other determinants of health. The mind–body dualism is closely related to the next basic idea of the biomedical model.

Physical Reductionism

Reductionism refers to an approach to understanding the world that breaks phenomena into smaller and smaller parts in order to understand them. According to reductionism, the best way to understand something is to reduce it to its constituent parts and examine these parts in isolation (Lewontin and Levins 2007). For example, if you wanted to understand how a clock works, reductionism would direct you to open up the clock and examine all the cogs and gears that make up the inner mechanism. Reductionism has its origins in Isaac Newton's belief that the entire universe could be understood as a cosmic clock! Launsø (1989, 240) provides the following description of the connection between physical reductionism and biomedicine: "The basis of modern biological and medical theory is the conviction that all aspects of living organisms can be understood, if we reduce them to their smallest part and thereby study the interrelationship between these components." As biomedical knowledge developed, health care became increasingly reductionist. This is nowhere more evident than in the inward-directed search for genetic causes of sickness. This type of reductionism individualizes illness to the microscopic level of DNA, diverting attention from social causes of illness. Switankowsky (2000, 571) explains that reductionism is problematic because it disregards social and psychological dimensions of sickness: "Viewing illness and disease reductionistically is misguided since it is a counterintuitive view of illness. Most individuals are quite aware that illness affects their ordinary lives and their well-being, and, therefore, recognize that illness affects the body as well as the mind." This underscores that health is multi-faceted and includes physical, psychological, and social dimensions. Physical reductionism is the opposite of the holistic, multi-dimensional view of health.

Specific Etiology

Following from reductionism, biomedicine understands disease in terms of observable biophysical changes in the body (i.e., signs) that are caused by pathogenic agents, such as germs or viruses. According to the principle of **specific etiology**, it is assumed that each disease has a particular cause. This assumption has important implications for the social organization of health care. For example, health care based on germ theory focuses on searching for detectable pathology in an effort to identify causal factors. This approach is based on the belief that discovering the cause will, in turn, lead to intervention and treatment that will hopefully cure the disease. McKee (1988, 776) contrasts the biomedical model with the definition of health offered by the World Health Organization, noting that "health tends to be defined in functional rather than experiential terms, as the absence of disease." This means that sickness is reduced to its biophysical dimension. Disease becomes reified or treated as a concrete biophysical reality, ignoring social dimensions of sickness. Berliner and Salmon (1979, 35) explain that "disease and its associated symptoms become the focus of attention, rather than the whole patient." Reifying disease as a biophysical process distracts attention from other determinants of health, making sickness seem natural and unavoidable, rather than locating the sources of illness within the structures of society.

Biomedical health care attempts to either control causes (through drug therapy), remove them (through surgery), or do both. Wolpe (1987, 170) explains how reductionism, along with the principle of specific etiology, "results in a concentration on parasites, bacteria, viruses, and toxins as the primary causes of disease, and therapy is an attempt to kill, eradicate, or remove the attacking agents from the body. The individual's body becomes a malfunctioning machine, a discrete environment in which a militaristic campaign against the agents must be waged by the physician." In other words, the principle of specific etiology leads to a form of health care in which physicians wage a war against pathogenic forces, such as germs and viruses that have invaded the body, while ignoring the social context of disease.

Gillet (1994, 1127) explains that this approach to health care "works most comfortably where there is a biochemical and/or structural defect that provides a simple key to understanding the disease being studied." This means that acute diseases, those that are of a finite duration and have a readily identifiable cause, can usually be treated by biomedicine. For example, a bacterial infection can often be treated with antibiotic medication. However, chronic diseases can't be cured in this way. Unfortunately, the most prevalent illnesses today in Western societies, such as Canada, are chronic conditions: "At least in the developed world, most medical conditions now are chronic ones, and the interventions are aimed at restoring the person's level of functioning, reducing disability and at the end, palliation" (Streiner 1997, 124–5).

Some six decades ago, Dubos (1959) made the point that the doctrine of specific etiology fails to account for how social circumstances shape biological vulnerability to pathogens. Individual susceptibility to pathogens is a function of biological factors as well as socio-environmental variables, such as stress levels, nutrition, and the experience of social exclusion. An illustration of this comes from a study of hepatitis C virus infection among Aboriginals in British Columbia. Researchers have known for some time that the hepatitis C virus causes liver disease. The disease is seven times more prevalent among Aboriginal peoples than non-Aboriginals. A team of BC researchers (Craib et al. 2010) showed that the experience of historical trauma associated with having a parent or grandparent who was forced to attend residential school is linked to higher rates of hepatitis C infection among Aboriginal young people. Risk factors such as injection drug use are an unhealthy way of coping with the legacy of social exclusion experienced by Canada's Aboriginal peoples. This shows that socio-environmental factors affect individual vulnerability to pathogens and illustrates the shortcomings of the doctrine of specific etiology.

The Machine Metaphor

The dominant metaphor by which the biomedical model has understood the human body is that of a machine. Freund, McGuire, and Podhurst (2003, 222) point out that this way of understanding health and illness is specific to Western culture, noting that other cultures have different metaphors by which they understand the human body: "Ancient Egyptian societies used the image of a river, and Chinese tradition refers to the balance of elemental forces (yin and yang) of the earth." In our culture, based on the biomedical model, most people tend to regard the human body as a biological machine made up of biophysical processes. Health is defined clinically by biophysical processes operating within predefined, scientifically measurable parameters. For example, according to the latest guidelines (which are periodically lowered in the interests of pharmaceutical corporations expanding the market for cholesterol-lowering drugs), if your ratio of total cholesterol to HDL cholesterol (i.e., HDL-C ratio) is less than 6.0, it is considered normal, whereas if it is higher, this is taken as evidence of the disease "high cholesterol" (Moynihan and Cassels 2005). Consider, as illustration of the machine metaphor, the following description of the "human being" offered in the 2010 edition of *Guyton and Hall Textbook of Medical Physiology*:

> In human physiology, we attempt to explain the specific characteristics and mechanisms of the human body that make it a living being. The very fact that we remain alive is the result of complex control systems, for hunger makes us seek food and fear makes us seek refuge. Sensations of cold make us look for warmth. Other forces cause us to seek fellowship and to reproduce. Thus, the human being is, in many ways, like an automaton, and the fact that we are sensing, feeling, and knowledgeable beings is part of this automatic sequence of life; these special attributes allow us to exist under widely varying conditions (Hall 2010, 3).

This excerpt reveals the deterministic metaphor through which medical students come to understand health. Science offers this machine-like view of humanity (i.e., "an automaton" following the "automatic sequence of life") and a health-care system based upon it, and we in the West have by and large accepted this medicalized approach to the pursuit of health.

Foucault links the machine metaphor to development of the medical gaze. He describes how the medical gaze facilitated the emergence of "*L'homme-machine*" (the human machine) and the idea that the body could endlessly be worked on to repair or replace defective parts (Foucault 1977, 136). Conceptualizing the body as a machine leads to health care oriented to treating biophysical malfunctions. Other machines are used to diagnose the nature of the malfunction and then used to fix the human machine. Friedman and DiMatteo (1979, 2) describe how "dialysis machines, CAT scanners, heart-lung bypass machines and similar technological marvels direct attention to specific problems and narrow mechanisms, and away from the other influences on the patient's health." Searight (1994, 226) reminds us that "while there are broadly trained physicians who are able to incorporate knowledge from psychology, sociology, as well as history and even philosophy into clinical care," we must also be aware that "this intellectual diversity rarely 'filters down' to daily practice" and that there exists a "pressure to acquire an ever-expanding technological base of diagnostic and treatment information [that] may prevent the reflective process of viewing patients from alternative vantage points." Just like other applied scientists such as engineers, physicians are expected to possess expert knowledge of the machines it is their job to repair. Indeed, as Wolpe points out, "The physician is trained in our society as a technician, an engineer, whose guiding principles are the results of objective measures of dysfunction first" (1987, 81).

In repairing the human machine, biomedical health care is based on the belief that physicians must remain objective if they are to effectively treat illness. In this way, Friedman and DiMatteo (1979, 7) point out that the machine metaphor reinforces the objectification of patients by biomedical health care: "With technological advances, it becomes ever easier for the health care provider to place the patient in the role of object or 'medical case.' The disease tends to be separated from the human being who has been struck down by it." Taylor (1984, 207) explains that "Both popular culture and firsthand accounts of serious illnesses and the health care personnel who try to conquer it are full of images of cold, abrupt professionals who are nevertheless superb technicians, men and women who acquire flawed personal styles perhaps because of the fact that they are dedicated to science." Box 10.5 provides an example of one such portrayal of physicians in popular culture.

Box 10.5 House, M.D.

Fox Television's Dr Gregory House (played by Hugh Laurie) of the medical drama "House, M.D." is perhaps an extreme example of the widespread cultural image of the cold and abrupt physician who nevertheless is a superb biomedical technician. While House has a terrible bedside manner, he has expert knowledge of the human machine, which allows him to diagnose and treat the most difficult of medical cases.

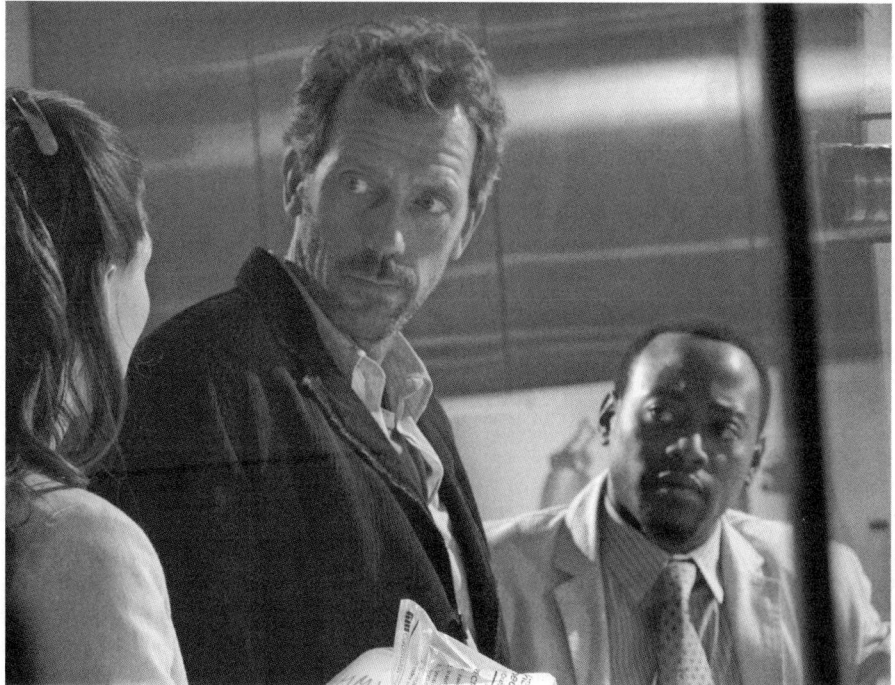

Rosch and Kearney (1985, 1407) describe how the machine metaphor is reflected in the vocabulary of physicians: "Patients are depersonalized in a vocabulary that reduces individuals to specific clinical conditions: 'the coronary in ICU,' 'the ulcer in Room 212.' Throughout the entire range of medical care, there is less and less evidence of the sensitive, caring, human touch and more and more reliance upon the regularized automated hum of computer chips and laser beams and the rhythmic staccato of computer printouts." Physicians speak about bodies in expert, technoscientific jargon. They describe the malfunctioning body part rather than the whole patient. Haas and Shaffir (1992, 407–8) offer the following excerpt from an interview with a medical student as illustration of the consequences of the machine metaphor for health care:

> Somebody will say, "Listen to Mrs. Jones' heart. It's just a little thing flubbing on the table." And you forget the rest of her. Part of that is the objectivity and it helps in learning in the sense that you can go in to a patient, put your stethoscope on the heart, and listen to it and walk out . . . the advantage is that you can go in a short time and see a patient, get the important thing out of the patient and leave.

The biomedical model facilitates an approach to health care that objectifies the body as a machine like any other, reducing patients to machine-like carrying cases of biophysical parts. This assumption meshes with other cultural values, resulting in the medical and social emphasis on standardized body disciplines of diets, exercise programs, routines of hygiene, and even sexual activity. The machine metaphor is related to the focus in preventive medicine and public health on individualized responsibility.

Therapeutic Focus on Individualized Regimen and Control

Each of us, as "owner" of our "biological machine," is personally responsible for care and maintenance of our bodies. An illustration of this is the title of one of television personality and popular medical authority Dr Oz's health and wellness how-to books: *YOU: The Owner's Manual: An Insider's Guide to the Body That Will Make You Healthier and Younger* (Roizen and Oz 2005). Disease is understood by the biomedical model as an occurrence that can be avoided, fought, or, at the very least, minimized through regimen and control (Freund, McGuire, and Podhurst 2003). Biomedical experts such as Dr Oz become icons of popular culture by instructing us in how to "discipline" (Foucault 1977) our bodies through bodily regimens such as diet and exercise. As Launsø (1989, 242) explains, "In the health-care system, disease is dressed in a 'language dress' characterized by viewing disease as something negative, something that must be denied as a part of life, and consequently, the disease has to be fought, removed, and controlled by experts." The individual is responsible for watching out for health risk factors and controlling them through regimens such as daily exercise, proper diet, managing stress levels, and submitting oneself to routine medical screening. This accounts for health experts advocating physical activity guidelines that, for most people, are an unworkable means of disciplining the body through regimen and control.

For example, the Canadian Society for Exercise Physiology's guidelines for adults recommends that people accumulate two-and-a-half hours of moderate-to-vigorous physical activity over the course of a week along with resistance training at least two days a week (Canadian Society for Exercise Physiology 2012). However, some biomedical researchers maintain that even more daily activity is a necessary part of the pursuit of health! In 2008, the United States updated its guidelines to recommend an astonishing 60 to 90 minutes of daily physical activity of moderate intensity to maintain weight loss and 60 minutes of activity of moderate to vigorous intensity to manage weight or prevent gradual weight gain in adulthood. How much physical activity do you get every day? Is it effective to promote health through such demanding regimen and control, or would biomedical experts be wise to pay attention to Dubos' (1959) warning about the mirage of perfect health?

The notion of regimen and control leads to cultural idealization of the perfectible body in which individuals are encouraged to obtain a state of perfect health through bodily deployments, such as physical exercise, diet and nutrition, and cosmetic and other enhancement surgeries. However, Dubos (1959, 1) dismissed perfect health and happiness as mirages, noting that "In reality, complete freedom from disease and struggle is almost incompatible with the process of living." Given the socio-cultural factors that undermine individuals' ability to exercise such high levels of regimen and control, the sociological perspective raises questions about the feasibility

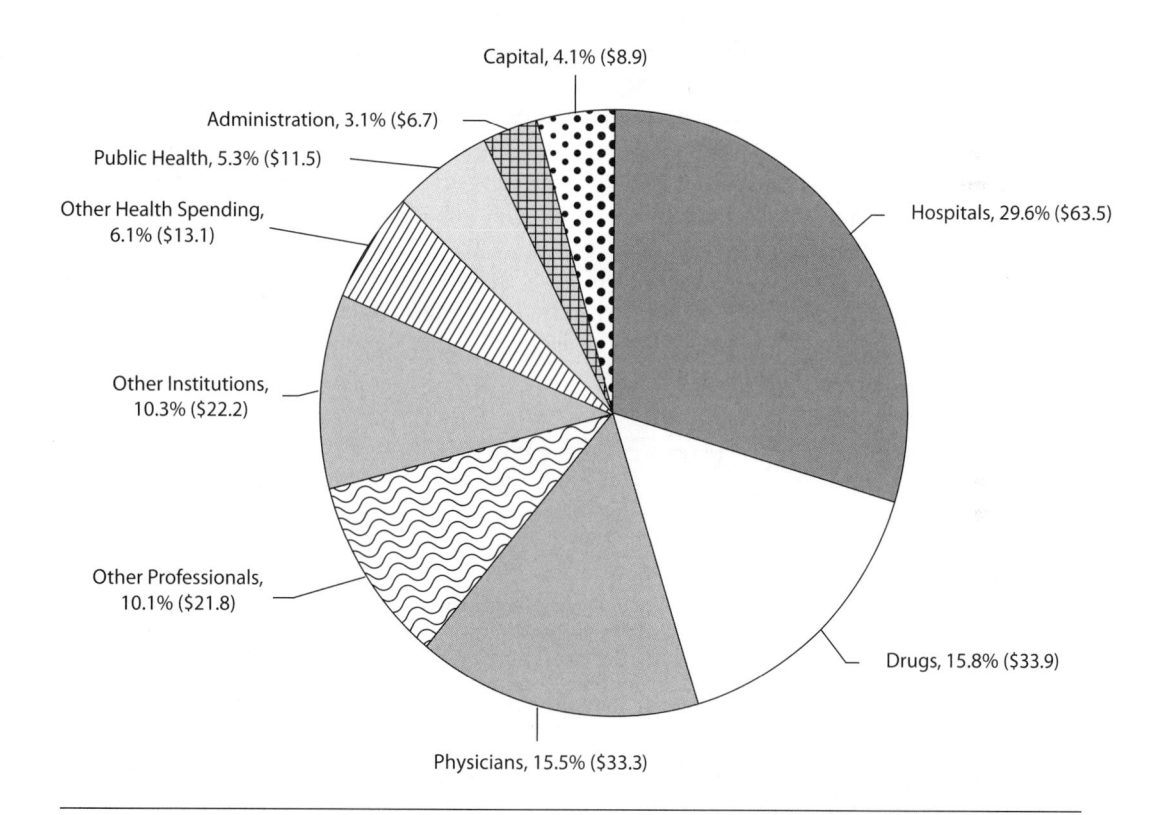

Figure 10.2 Total Health Expenditures by Use of Funds, Canada 2014 (Percentage Share and Billions of Dollars)

In 2014, Canada spent an estimated $215 billion on health care, and the bulk of this (more than 60 per cent) was spent on formal health-care services and products. Hospitals accounted for approximately 30 per cent of total health-care expenditures in 2014, followed by prescription medication and physician services. In contrast, only 5 per cent was spent on public health. This is evidence that Canada's health-care system medicalized!

Data Source: Canadian Institute for Health Information 2014.

of individualistic approaches to the pursuit of health and wellness. It is possible that, faced with these high standards of bodily discipline, many will give up altogether on the pursuit of health rather than trying to meet unobtainable expectations.

In summary, we have seen that biomedicine developed in response to general changes in social relations of healing in Western society and that the biomedical model is characterized by five interrelated ideas concerning how best to understand and treat illness. Together, these five ideas have exerted a powerful cultural influence on society and our health-care system. Furedi (2008, 98) explains the connection of these ideas to a medicalized pursuit of health and wellness by observing that "the promotion and celebration of health as the paramount values of western society have encouraged people to interpret a growing range of human activities through the vocabulary of medicine." Together, the ideas, images, language, and practices offered by biomedicine have led to the widespread cultural dominance of a medico-centric understanding of health that privileges biophysical factors in the provision of health care.

In our current formal health-care system, "health" is often equated with biophysical functioning, and "health care" is all too often reduced to the provision of biomedical products and services (such as pharmaceutical drugs and surgery) by the medical profession. In other words, as depicted in Figure 10.2, our health-care system is more aptly described as a medicalized system that treats biophysical disease and in which physicians exercise dominance. These data show that spending on hospitals, other institutions, physicians, and prescription drugs accounts for 71.2 per cent of all health expenditures, in comparison with 5.3 per cent spent on public health measures. Less than a tenth of what was spent on formal health care was spent on public health in Canada in 2014! The next section shows that while this way of caring for the health-care needs of Canadians has had benefits, it also has very high economic, social, and human costs.

Medical Dominance of the Health-Care System

Undoubtedly, biomedicine has made positive contributions to health. Wright (2009, 3) asks the provocative question, is it possible to have too much health care? and lists some of the ways that medicine has benefited humanity:

> The general health of the population today must be considered one of the greatest marvels of human civilization and ingenuity. Pregnant women no longer have to dread the 10 percent risk of death at childbirth that used to be usual; a newborn in Canada today can expect to live 80 years; death related to childhood infections is now rare; the long-term outcome of childhood leukemia has changed from 85 percent mortality to 85 percent survival; patients with cataracts, osteoarthritis and heart disease benefit from surgery that was unimaginable 40 years ago; many cancer patients can now be offered substantial relief and some even long-term survival.

The achievements of biomedicine are undeniable. Lives have been saved, relief from pain and suffering provided, and opportunities for a more rewarding life afforded by biomedical health care. Compassionate physicians and nurses care for us when we are sick, sometimes at great costs to their own pursuit of health and well-being (Wallace, Lemaire, and Ghali 2009). It cannot be denied that medicine has been a great benefit to humanity. However, there is evidence that shows that the contribution of biomedical care to population health is less than commonly believed. Improved health care is usually credited as the major cause of the modern decline in death rates and, hence, the primary factor related to the increased longevity enjoyed by people today. If this were indeed the case, then it would be a compelling justification for further expansion of biomedicine. However, detailed analyses in England and Wales by McKeown and associates (1975) and in the United States by Dubos (1959; 1968) and McKinlay and McKinlay (1977) have, for decades, shown otherwise.

McKeown (himself a physician) revealed that the decline in mortality at the end of the nineteenth century and during the twentieth century was due totally to the reduction of deaths from infectious diseases. Biomedical health care did not contribute to this decline other than by immunization for smallpox, where it accounted for only about one-twentieth of the reduction! The rise in medical-care expenditures started after almost all (92 per cent) of the modern decline in mortality had already occurred. This means that other factors besides formal health care were responsible for increases in longevity. McKeown attributed the decrease in mortality to public health measures, including rising standards of living, especially diet, improved hygiene, and increased natural immunity to some micro-organisms. He singles out availability of affordable nutritious food as the major factor contributing to the decline in mortality witnessed in the modern period.

In the United States, McKinlay and McKinlay agree that the decline in mortality rates can be attributed primarily to the control of infectious disease, in particular to the decrease in 11 major infectious conditions: typhoid, smallpox, scarlet fever, measles, whooping cough, diphtheria, influenza, tuberculosis, pneumonia, diseases of the digestive system, and poliomyelitis. These researchers identified the medical intervention believed to account for the decline in the occurrence of each disease and the date when treatment for that disease became available on a widespread basis and related these factors to mortality data that included cause of death. In many cases, the medical intervention was introduced several decades after major decline had occurred and revealed no detectable influence. There was a noticeable decline for only five of the diseases after the introduction of the medical intervention (influenza, pneumonia, diphtheria, whooping cough, and poliomyelitis). Even if the entire subsequent decline is attributed to medical treatment, at most 3.5 per cent of the total decline resulted from the medical measures introduced for the diseases considered. What this shows is that biomedicine's role in extending life expectancy has been modest. Hadler, himself a physician (2004, 12), explains the limited contribution medicine has made to longevity by noting that three-quarters of the hazards to longevity are due to social conditions, while only one-quarter are related to lifestyle behaviours and biological risk factors. He argues that the current health-care system is misguidedly preoccupied with individualized health promotion and biophysically based treatment, noting that in its current form, "Contemporary medicine nibbles at the fray of the other 25 per cent of mortal hazard." Despite evidence that questions its role in helping us live longer lives, biomedicine has continued to expand its boundaries in the twenty-first century.

Despite increasing medicalization of life, evidence suggests that biomedicine is not a cure-all. Indeed, it was not primarily responsible for much of the decline in mortality experienced over the past century. However, it has continued to expand its boundaries, enjoying tremendous public acceptance. Medical doctors are viewed as legitimate professionals when matters of health are of concern. Indeed, physicians are gatekeepers to our health-care system. Given the history of medicine, it is not surprising that physicians have attained and maintain a position of dominance in the formal health-care system. The many books written on the rise of the profession of medicine note that organized medicine has been successful in standardizing its workers and bringing cohesion to them. Medicine has also been able to convince the state to grant a monopoly so that, for example, one requires a medical licence in order to practise as a doctor and medical schools and the medical profession control what is taught and who receives licences. Furthermore, the public respects the doctors' role in healing and assumes they have expert knowledge. "Empirical studies point to the remarkable persistence of asymmetry" in the doctor/patient relationship (Pilnick and Dingwall 2011, 1374). For example, Benoit and colleagues (2010) studied the medicalization of human reproduction in Canada and Australia and conclude that despite neo-liberal reforms in these two countries, there have not been substantial changes in the historically hegemonic role medicine has played in the provision of maternity care (including pregnancy and childbirth).

Informed by the conflict paradigm, Freidson (1970a; 1970b) noted that medicine has achieved professional autonomy and dominance through a political process that has resulted in the medicalization of everyday life. That is, it is physicians themselves who define the scope of their work, define standards of practice, and maintain the right to enforce these standards. Part of doctors' ability to maintain professional dominance is their assumed expert knowledge, which patients do not have. In addition, the medical profession successfully eliminated or gained control of its competition. They control recruitment and training of new physicians as well as examining and licensing those who can become doctors. They are able to consolidate their control over the conditions of work through the organization of hospitals. They have a monopoly on defining illness through medical diagnosis, directing treatment, and deciding who can be admitted to hospital, who can receive prescription medications, and who can receive medical tests. In some provinces, they also control who can see a specialist and who can seek the care of allied health-care providers, such as massage therapists. They also control remuneration. Even in Canada, where we have universal medicare, we do not have socialized medicine. Doctors work primarily on a fee-for-service basis with a guaranteed third-party payer—in this country, the government and, ultimately, the taxpayer. That is, medicare guarantees that doctors will be paid for their work.

These factors mean that within the health-care system, doctors enjoy professional dominance reflecting their high social status within capitalist society. Not surprisingly, the majority of physicians are male, and most of the other health-care workers are female, reflecting the patriarchal structure of Canadian society even into the twenty-first century. While more women are entering the medical profession, there is a reinforcement of gender stratification. Women physicians tend to be at the bottom of the hierarchy among physicians. This trend has been demonstrated in England, the United States, Norway, and Canada (Armstrong and Deadman 2009; Elston 1993; Riska and Wegar 1993). Although women physicians no longer face formal discrimination that once denied them access to medical schools and residencies, they still do not occupy top positions in the profession. They are rarely heads of large, prestigious services, large teaching hospitals, or medical centres. Women are held back by a glass ceiling blocking their upward mobility, kept from top-level positions by subtle and informal processes, if no longer by explicit legal barriers. Women physicians tend to be in family practice and primary care, where they lack the kind of occupational autonomy and power that male physicians in other medical specialities typically possess.

Health-care workers other than physicians are predominantly female (Armstrong and Deadman 2009). They include nurses, who are structurally subordinated both to physicians and to hospital bureaucracies. Their work has changed considerably, with many no longer spending time in direct patient care other than distributing medication. They largely spend time co-ordinating staff, making notes on charts, and keeping records. Other nurse-related categories have emerged, such as the licensed practical nurse, the vocational nurse, and the nurse's aide. Most nursing responsibilities are under the direction of physicians. At a more advanced level, there are a variety of occupations, including the nurse practitioner, the certified nurse midwife, the certified registered nurse, and the physician assistant, often working in remote areas that are unable to attract physicians.

In addition, there are other categories of allied health workers, including, for example, physical therapists and medical technologists required for diagnosis and treatment. Many of these occupations developed around particular technologies or techniques requiring specialized knowledge and training. Even when these specialists perform diagnostic tests, the tests are usually ordered and interpreted by physicians. Thus, physicians control access to available medical technology. In summary, it is clear that biomedicine is the central player in formal health care and physicians continue to exercise professional dominance over the health-care system. As the next section shows, medical dominance has extended beyond the health-care system and into the wider society.

Medicalizing Beings and Bodies

More and more aspects of life are being transformed into medical issues requiring biomedical health care. What types of conditions or life events have been medicalized? While there is a long list, Conrad (2013) (See Box 10.6) suggests that we can conceptualize a number of general categories of medicalized conditions. In some cases, medicalization can be understood as a form of social control in which behaviour that departs from what is regarded as normal or socially acceptable (i.e., deviance) is understood as having biophysical causes. Conrad and Schneider (1992, 28) provide examples of "the medicalization of deviance," such as alcoholism and other addictions, mental illness, child abuse, hyperactivity, and obesity. These authors describe how "deviant behaviors that were once defined as immoral, sinful, or criminal have been given medical meanings," claiming that our culture has moved from "badness to sickness" as a way of understanding and coming to terms with deviance (1992, 1). For instance, alcoholism, once viewed as a moral issue, has been redefined as a disease. More recently, attention deficit hyperactivity

Box 10.6 Peter Conrad (1945–)

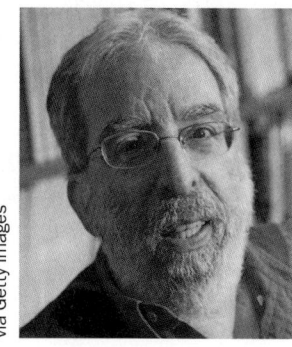

- Foremost North American medical sociologist specializing in medicalization
- Prolific author whose research shows how culture has moved from "badness to sickness" as a way of understanding and coming to terms with deviance

"Deviant behaviours that were once defined as immoral, sinful, or criminal have been given medical meanings" (1992, 28).

disorder (ADHD) has been defined as a disease experienced by persons who demonstrate short attention span, restlessness, and impulsivity. As Conrad's (2007) research shows, first difficult-to-handle schoolchildren and later adults came to be diagnosed with this illness and treated with pharmaceuticals, especially Ritalin. While ADHD was seen for many years as a disorder of children, it is now viewed "as a lifespan disorder" (Conrad 2013, 197). Once such behaviours are defined as illnesses, they are subjected to medical means of social control, since they apparently fall within the authority of health-care professionals.

Defining such behaviours as illness focuses on the biophysical dimension, framing causes and treatment in pathological terms (Carpiano 2001). Social aspects of deviance become obscured, as do moral issues. What social situations facilitate excessive drinking, for example, and what social modifications can be adopted to assist these individuals? Medicalization allows such questions to be disregarded. The individual is viewed not holistically but rather as a malfunctioning biophysical machine and frequently reduced to a defective body part as disease is reified and associated with particular aspects of the individual's physiology. The medicalization of ADHD, for example, individualizes the causes and consequences of disruptive behaviour by locating both within the individual's neurochemistry. Other ways of dealing with disruptive classroom behaviour, such as providing more teaching resources (i.e., more teachers and teachers' assistants), which would allow for smaller class sizes and individualized attention for disruptive children, are overlooked in favour of the medicalized response of psychotropic drugs that chemically engineer docility. Medicalization is, thus, a form of social control that focuses on biophysical factors.

Conrad (2013) explains that in other cases it is "natural life events" that have been redefined in terms of ideas, images, language, and practices offered by biomedicine. Here, notable examples include childbirth, a natural occurrence that has become medicalized to the point that in developed nations such as Canada, fully one-quarter of babies are delivered using the surgeon's scalpel (OECD 2009). As research oriented by the feminist paradigm has demonstrated, the treatment of pregnancy and childbirth is an area where physicians took over the responsibility of midwives. Women's reproductive lives, which used to be a part of normal life, have become part of pathology, falling under the definition of illness. Obstetrics and gynecology are male-dominated areas of specialization where medical knowledge is presumed necessary for healthy reproduction, viewed in physical and pathological terms (Oakley 2005). Feminist analysis casts doubts on the contention that medicalization of birth happened solely in the interests of health (Berenson, Miller, and Findlay 2009).

Other life events that have come to be understood in our culture as health issues requiring medical treatment include menstruation, menopause, aspects of aging such as baldness, and even death and dying (Conrad 2013; 2007; 1992). Illich (1976) and Zola (1972b) contend that this process actually involves the medicalization of life (and not just deviance). The basic argument is that more and more aspects of everyday life are being transformed into medical matters and as a result, health has been expropriated and our lives have become subject to medically based social control from "the womb to the tomb" (Illich 1976). In addition, "problems in everyday living" such as anxiety, shyness, sexuality (erectile dysfunction and lack of libido), and difficulty becoming pregnant have also become medicalized (Conrad 2013, 197). Most of these problems were previously considered to be part of life that had to be tolerated or accepted. Today, they have become medical diagnoses!

As depicted in Box 10.7, Conrad (1992, 211) explains that "Medicalization can occur on at least three distinct levels: the conceptual, the institutional, and the interactional levels." When a problem is defined in medical terms, medicalization is said to have occurred on the conceptual

> **Box 10.7** Conrad's Three Levels of Medicalization
>
> - Conceptual level—a medical vocabulary (or model) is used to define a problem.
> - Institutional level—organizations adopt a medical approach to treating a problem.
> - Interactional level—occurs as part of doctor–patient interaction.
>
> **Source:** Conrad 1992

level. At this point, medical professionals need not be involved directly in the problem, and medical treatments may not necessarily be applied. Conrad (1992, 211) notes that "On the institutional level, organizations may adopt a medical approach to treating a particular problem in which the organization specializes." He describes how physicians may act as gatekeepers to services offered by other health-care professionals working for organizations providing medically approved treatments such as physiotherapy. On the interactional level, medicalization occurs when physicians diagnose a problem as medical or respond to a social problem with medical treatment. Conrad's conceptualization illustrates the complexity of medicalization.

Recently, studies of medicalization have also focused on "enhancements of healthy people." According to Conrad (2013, 198), these are "biomedical interventions that are meant to improve an individual's life condition or performance" and include various forms of cosmetic surgery, pharmaceuticals (such as Viagra to improve normal sexual performance), and human growth hormones to increase height. Finally, the medical management of risk has been identified as an area of increasing medicalization. "With the development of many sophisticated technologies that can screen and scan the body, such as MRI, CAT scans or genetic screenings, physicians can identify risks for future disorders at increasingly earlier stages" (Conrad 2013, 204). Preventive medicine today means routinely having your blood pressure, cholesterol, or PSA levels monitored and having a mammogram or a colonoscopy to assess the risk (or probability) that you may develop a medical condition sometime in the future. "While the early detection of risk may be medically beneficial, it is also an expanding form of medicalization" (Conrad 2013, 204). We will explore this type of medicalization in more detail later in the chapter, but for now it is important to understand the key point—that the medical management of risk increases the amount of medical surveillance we experience in our everyday lives.

Sociological studies make it clear that medicalization is a socio-cultural process rather than a purely biophysical one. This is illustrated by the fact that some behaviours come to be defined in terms of medical issues, only to be later redefined as outside the domain of medicine. According to Conrad (2013), this process is bidirectional and includes both medicalization and demedicalization. Furthermore, medicalized conditions are "elastic" and can both expand and contract. Conrad (2007, 97) describes **demedicalization** as the situation in which "a problem is no longer defined in medical terms and the involvement of medical personnel is no longer deemed appropriate." He investigates homosexuality as a case study of a behaviour that was medicalized and later demedicalized, only to be now subject to possible efforts of remedicalization. Medical researchers are busily trying to find the biological basis of sexual orientation. The case of homosexuality illustrates the socially variable nature of medicalization—that is, medicalization is best understood as an ongoing process that is influenced by changes in the larger culture and society. While Halfmann (2011, 187) agrees that "there is probably more medicalization than demedicalization in western societies," he argues that there have been missed opportunities to do research on situations in which both aspects of this continuous process occur simultaneously (and uses abortion to illustrate his argument).

There are degrees of medicalization, and the extent to which non-medical problems come to be defined and treated as medical issues is, thus, an outcome of complex socio-cultural processes. A memorable example of this is the social construction of the disease "onanism," analyzed by Freund, McGuire, and Podhurst (2003, 198). These authors refer to a late nineteenth-century health and wellness how-to book's description of onanism:

> It retards the growth, impairs the mental faculties and reduces the victim to a lamentable state. The person afflicted seeks solitude, and does not wish to enjoy the society of his friends; he is troubled with headache, wakefulness and restlessness at night, pain in various parts of the body, indolence, melancholy, loss of memory, weakness in the back and generative organs, variable appetite, cowardice, inability to look a person in the face, lack of confidence in his own abilities.
>
> When the evil has been pursued for several years, there will be an irritable condition of the system; sudden flushes of heat over the face; the countenance becomes pale and clammy; the eyes have a dull, sheepish look; the hair becomes dry and split at the ends; sometimes there is a pain over the region of the heart; shortness of breath; palpitation of the heart . . . the sleep is disturbed; there is constipation; cough; irritation of the throat; finally, the whole man becomes a wreck, physically, morally and mentally (Stout 1885, 333–4, as cited in Freund, McGuire, and Podhurst 2003, 198).

The authors then reveal that "this serious disease was onanism, better known as masturbation. . . . The diagnosis of masturbation as a disease syndrome is no longer common; indeed, in many medical and lay conceptions it is now considered to be quite normal and healthy" (Freund, McGuire, and Podhurst 2003, 198). Health sociology is full of many such historical examples showing that medicalization is a socially relative process influenced by wider society and culture. As Freund, McGuire, and Podhurst (2003, 197) demonstrate, "The forces shaping the so-called discovery of disease categories are not purely objective, scientific factors; rather, value judgments, economic considerations, and other social concerns frequently enter the process." Depending on the prevailing cultural climate, some behaviours become defined as "disease," only to be later redefined as cultural values shift. How did medicalization emerge in the first place? Answering this question takes us back to the development of the biomedical model and the rationalization of society discussed earlier in the chapter.

Explanations for Medicalization

Furedi (2008, 102) argues that medicalization "has been underwritten by sociocultural processes that continually throw up a demand for medical definitions to make sense of existential problems." Biomedical ideas, images, language, and practices offer answers to basic questions of human existence posed by issues of embodiment, such as abnormality, illness, suffering, and disability. While spirituality and religion once offered answers to these questions, with rationalization and the rise of science we now turn to biomedicine to understand the meaning of sickness and suffering. Both Zola and Illich contend that medicalization is related to the rationalization of society. Zola (1972b, 487) argues that medicalization "is rooted in our increasingly complex technological and bureaucratic system—a system which has led us down the path of the reluctant reliance on the expert." Illich (1976) similarly suggests that medicalization is connected to wider processes of industrialization and bureaucratization.

Sociologists began to pay attention to medicalization in the 1960s as part of a critique of the medical profession and medical institutions. It was during this period that Goffman (1961) studied the social construction of mental disorder, the research of Laing (1961) and Szasz (1971) spurred the anti-psychiatry movement, Freidson (1970a; 1970b) wrote two books criticizing the professional dominance of medicine, Zola (1972b) pointed out the social control functions of medicine, Illich (1976) moved discussions of medical error into popular discourse, and Oakley (1980) began to publish research on the medicalization of childbirth. These studies provided the basis for "the medicalization thesis" (Ballard and Elston 2005, 231). Following these early studies, sociological efforts to understand medicine's increasing cultural influence in Western societies can be grouped into two general approaches to the study of medicalization. First came approaches associated with the original medicalization thesis that emerged from the conflict paradigm's critique of the professional power of organized medicine. Later, approaches that stemmed from the sociology of the body paradigm followed and, in particular, Foucault's ideas concerning the individualization and internalization of bodily surveillance in modern societies. Let's start with conflict approaches to understanding medicalization before moving on to consider the approach influenced by Foucault.

Conflict Approaches: Medicalizing from Above—Iatrogenesis

Early studies of medicalization focused on the social control aspects of organized medicine within capitalist society. As Zola (1972b, 487) puts it, "Medicine is becoming a major institution of social control, nudging aside, if not incorporating, the more traditional institutions of religion and the law." In keeping with the conflict paradigm's understanding of "health and illness as professional constructs," this approach understands medicalization as legitimating the capitalist system. This is what is meant by the term "medicalization from above" (Cornwall 1984, 119); medicalization is imposed on the whole of society in the self-serving interests of the powerful few.

Numerous researchers influenced by the conflict paradigm have characterized professional medicine as a system of social regulation and commented on the expanding boundaries of medical expertise (e.g., Conrad 1975; Conrad and Schneider 1980; Ehrenreich 1978; Illich 1976; Navarro 1976; Waitzkin 2000; Zola 1972b). According to these researchers, medicine has become a major institution of social control in capitalist society and has expropriated our health (i.e., by removing it from individual control through self-health management and making our pursuit of health increasingly dependent on professional health care).

As an illustration of this approach, conflict sociologists such as Navarro (1976) and Waitzkin (2000) explain the medical profession's conspiracy with the capitalist class with reference to the interest both groups have in convincing people that the causes of ill health reside in nature (e.g., disease-causing germs and viruses) rather than in social conditions of capitalist society. Acknowledging that illnesses are caused by economic and social factors would mean challenging medical dominance and questioning the claim that advances in organized medicine and medical technology have produced the greatest improvements in population health. Therefore, the alliance between the capitalist class and the medical profession serves the interests of both by maintaining professional dominance of biomedicine, by sustaining a reasonably healthy working population for capitalists to exploit, and by generating profit from the sale of medical goods and services. In fact, it is not difficult to think of "new diseases" that are constantly emerging to be treated with profitable pharmaceutical products—for example, premenstrual dysphoric disorder (PMDD), social anxiety disorder (SAD), attention deficit hyperactivity disorder (ADHD), and erectile dysfunction (ED). "Big Pharma" generates big profits through "selling sickness" in this way (Moynihan and Cassels 2005). Conrad (2013, 199) refers to this as "disease mongering" and characterizes the pharmaceutical industry as a driving force behind medicalization "as drug companies seek to expand the markets for their products by creating new medical categories."

Ivan Illich (1976) contends that by making medicine applicable to an ever-increasing part of human existence, the medicalization process enabled the profession of medicine to claim control over anything that can be labelled an illness, regardless of its ability to deal with it effectively. Illich's work (see Box 10.8) epitomizes the conflict approach to explaining medicalization and its consequences. Wright (2003, 185) describes the concept of **iatrogenesis** as "the centrepiece" of Illich's work on medicalization. Illich popularized the term "iatrogenesis," which is based on the Greek word *iatros*, for physician, and *genesis*, meaning origin, to describe sickness and injury caused by the health-care system. He identified three interrelated types of iatrogenesis: clinical iatrogenesis, social iatrogenesis, and cultural iatrogenesis:

> A professional and physician-based health-care system that has grown beyond tolerable bounds is sickening for three reasons: it must produce clinical damages which outweigh its potential benefits (i.e., *clinical iatrogenesis*); it cannot but obscure the political conditions which render society unhealthy (i.e., *social iatrogenesis*); and it tends to mystify and to expropriate the power of the individual to heal himself and to shape his or her environment (i.e., *cultural iatrogenesis*) (Illich 1976, 16; emphasis added).

As Illich (1976) carefully documented, despite the "do no harm" mantra of the Hippocratic Oath, medical care frequently harms patients with ineffective, toxic, and unsafe treatments. Doctors make mistakes, drugs are improperly administered, medical treatments may have unforeseen or unintended risks, and some surgeries are unnecessary, inappropriate, or botched. Even when there aren't errors, there is the possibility of medical treatment causing unnecessary suffering. For example, in some cases medical treatments come with harmful side effects and

---

Box 10.8   Ivan Illich (1926–2002)

- Argued that modern medicine is the major threat to health in *Medical Nemesis: The Expropriation of Health* (1976)
- Popularized the term "iatrogenesis" to describe illness caused by doctors and the health-care system

"The medical monopoly over health care has expanded without check and has encroached on our liberty with regards to our own bodies" (1976, 13).

Photo by Sigfrid Casals/Cover/Getty Images

yet do little to either extend or improve quality of life. Illich described these kinds of medical harm as **clinical iatrogenesis**, writing that "Clinical iatrogenic disease comprises all clinical conditions for which remedies, physicians, or hospitals are the pathogens, or 'sickening' agents" (1976, 36). In other words, clinical iatrogenesis is illness or injury caused directly by the health-care system.

When we go to see the doctor or enter the hospital as patients, we surrender our autonomy to health-care professionals. We do this because we are seeking help with issues of embodiment that confront us, such as pain, illness, or suffering. The implicit deal we make is that when we give our bodies and ourselves over to medical authority, in return we expect our health to be cared for by compassionate and competent health-care professionals. As Lupton (1996) has shown, the encounter with medicine is a supreme act of interpersonal trust, since the patient literally places her "life in their hands." However, studies of medical error show that not only is the encounter with medicine a supreme act of trust, it is often an act of supreme danger, which all too often ends as an encounter with disability or death.

While the full extent of clinical iatrogenesis is unknown, there is evidence that the health-care system is a considerable source of morbidity and mortality. Research into harm caused by medical care typically uses methods such as analyzing administrative data produced by health-care organizations, tracking the rate of malpractice lawsuits and claim settlement amounts, conducting reviews of patient charts, and surveying patients and their families about the experience of medical error. All of these types of research face the challenge posed by under-reporting to estimate the scope of clinical iatrogenesis. For instance, a report prepared for Health Canada (2004) shows that more than 70 per cent of health-care professionals surveyed in 2003 admit that under-reporting of adverse drug reactions is a very or somewhat serious problem. The Canadian Institute for Health Information (2004, 17) adds that "many other types of events are also typically under-reported by medical personnel." Despite such under-reporting, research has demonstrated the devastating effects of medical error in Canada and in other countries.

The Institute of Medicine in the US (2000) reports that as many as 98,000 Americans die each year from medical errors that occur in hospitals, more than the number who die from motor vehicle accidents, breast cancer, and AIDS, making the health-care system the fifth leading cause of death in the United States! Canadian data on medical errors in hospitals (which are euphemistically labelled in biomedical jargon as "adverse events," "critical incidents," and "nosocomial infections") show that as many as 24,000 Canadians die each year because of preventable medical errors. This statistic is based on the first-ever Canadian Adverse Events Study (Baker et al. 2004). The study reviewed the medical records of 3745 patients in 20 acute-care hospitals in five provinces and found that in 2000–1, adverse events occurred in 7.5 per cent of admissions in non-specialized acute-care hospitals. This statistic omits errors that occur in specialized care settings, such as pediatric, mental health, and rehabilitation centres and smaller hospitals. It also omits psychiatric, obstetric, and short-stay patients and, therefore, significantly underestimates the prevalence of medical error. Thirty-seven per cent of the mistakes analyzed in the study were judged by the researchers to be preventable.

In an international survey, one in four respondents from Australia, Canada, New Zealand, and the United States reported that they had experienced either a medical or medication error in the past two years (Blendon et al. 2003). A similar study undertaken for the Canadian Institute for Health Information (2004) found that 24 per cent of Canadians surveyed reported that either they or their family members had experienced an adverse event. About half of these individuals said that the most recent event had serious consequences. Another Canadian study found that

37.3 per cent of Albertans surveyed reported that either they or their family members had experienced a medical error (Northcott et al. 2007).

The most common adverse events are medication errors, followed by nosocomial (i.e., health care–associated) infections and patient falls. A national study (Baker et al. 2004) found that "drug-and-fluid"-related (i.e., medication) errors accounted for one in four adverse events occurring in hospitals. While the full extent of medication errors occurring outside of hospital settings is unknown, a US study of outpatient clinics found that drug complications occurred in 18 per cent of patients (Gandhi et al. 2000). Preliminary Canadian estimates are that 110 nosocomial infections occur per 1000 adult patients in hospital (89 per 1000 child patients). Staff shortages and ineffective medical care can also lead to harm caused by falls while in the hospital. In particular, seniors are at risk of injury caused by in-hospital falls, with one in-patient hip fracture for every 1124 hospitalizations. While less common, for every 6667 surgeries performed, one patient has a foreign object, such as a sponge or an instrument, left accidently in his or her body (CIHI 2004).

Patients suffering clinical iatrogenesis sometimes resort to legal action to seek redress for medical harm. Between 1971 and 1987, the number of malpractice claims increased sevenfold, with the rates stabilizing in the range of 1.7 to 2.5 claims per 100 physicians (CIHI 2004). Data from the *Alberta Patient Safety Survey* (Northcott et al. 2007) show that 42 per cent of Albertans who reported that either they or their family members had experienced medical error felt that more lawsuits for malpractice were a possible deterrent, compared with 33 per cent of those with no experience of medical error.

What this adds up to is that clinical iatrogenesis has exceedingly high economic, social, and human costs, with more than 60 Canadians dying each day in hospitals because of preventable medical errors. The Canadian Institute for Health Information (2004, 42) notes that "that's more than the number who die from breast cancer, motor vehicle and other transport accidents, and HIV combined." The scope of clinical iatrogenesis is as disturbing today as it was more than 40 years ago when Illich first drew widespread public attention to the problem.

In addition to biophysical injury, patients suffering medical error are harmed in at least two other ways. First, there is the injury done to their sense of coherence when they suffer bodily harm at the hands of people they placed their trust in to act as compassionate and competent health-care professionals. Second, they, or their surviving relatives, often endure additional trauma from the manner in which medical professionals respond to errors. An illustration of this is the case of homeless Winnipeg man Brian Sinclair (detailed in Box 7.3 in Chapter 7), who died after spending 34 hours in the Health Sciences Centre waiting room being repeatedly overlooked by the doctors, nurses, and medical aides at the emergency triage desk. Not only did Brian Sinclair's family suffer the harm of having a loved one's death caused by 34 hours of medical neglect, but they also had to endure the medical system's attempts to at first conceal and then obscure the negligence of the hospital staff. The medical profession's unchallenged authority in defining and responding to medical error is the clearest example of medical dominance (Rosenthal 1995).

Biomedical proponents (e.g., McCarthy and Blumenthal 2006; Reason 2000) argue that clinical iatrogenesis can be reduced through a focus on developing a "safety culture" within the health-care system. The hallmark of such an approach is the conviction that medical errors cannot be prevented by focusing on negligent actions of individual health-care staff who commit errors. Rather, it is suggested that medical errors emerge as a result of the complexity of the health-care system. In its report on medical error, the Canadian Institute for Health Information

(2004, 15), for example, attempts to draw an analogy with the risks encountered in the nuclear energy and aerospace industries, stating that "Like nuclear energy and aerospace, health care is a complex environment where errors can maim or kill." In other words, it is argued that in a highly complex system that involves the use of potentially dangerous, high-tech treatments, such as pharmaceutical and surgical interventions by many different people, mistakes are bound to happen. "Safety culture" proponents believe that such mistakes cannot be prevented by what they term the "naming, blaming, and shaming" approach, which focuses on individual responsibility for errors (Reason 2000, 768).

What is overlooked by those who wish to draw analogies between health care and the nuclear power or aviation industries is that the rate of adverse events in health care is 10 thousand times greater than the rates in these other complex, highly technical systems (Evans, Cardiff, and Sheps 2006; Sheps and Cardiff 2005). However, blaming the system does serve sociological functions. Waring's (2007, 41) research shows that "systems thinking can therefore be invoked to protect against professional blame and responsibility when patient care is threatened or substandard." This means that a "systems thinking" approach to patient safety relieves negligent hospital staff of responsibility for their actions while minimizing potential legal fallout in the form of lawsuits for medical malpractice. In other words, by scapegoating "the system," the current patient safety system safeguards medical dominance as much as it does patients' pursuit of health and wellness!

The "safety culture" hypothesis, which assumes that "as health professionals are actively watching for safety hazards and are encouraged to share information about things that go wrong, they may become more aware of adverse events and near misses, and also be more likely to report them" (CIHI 2004, 17), is consistently disproved by social and behavioural science. There is no clearer illustration of this than research showing that approximately one-half of health-care workers in Canadian hospitals can't seem to be persuaded to wash their hands in the interests of the safety of their patients (CIHI 2004). Health-care professionals are well aware of risks posed to patients by nosocomial infections, and still as many as half of them don't take straightforward actions to prevent such iatrogenesis. So-called systems thinking approaches, such as awareness raising and educational campaigns, have proved unsuccessful in affecting cultural change that would promote patient safety through basic infection control measures such as handwashing (Lee et al. 2009). Waring's (2007) research shows that rather than learning from mistakes blamed on "the system," physicians tend to cope with them with resigned acceptance. The reluctance of physicians to participate in "safety culture" initiatives through reporting their mistakes has been well documented (e.g., Waring 2005).

Patient safety lessons can, however, be learned from regulatory measures that have met with success in reducing rates of nosocomial infections by holding non-compliant health-care professionals and the hospitals they work for accountable for their actions (Gardam et al. 2009). The notion that patient safety can be secured through the simplistic introduction of a "safety culture" is naive from a sociological standpoint. Such "safety culture" discourse has been effectively used in defence of medical dominance over the patient safety system (Mizrahi 1984; Waring 2007). For example, it allows medical officials to explain away instances of iatrogenesis, such as that which resulted in Brian Sinclair's death, with reference to "system frailties" (Winnipeg Regional Health Authority CEO Dr Brian Postl, quoted in the *Winnipeg Free Press*, 7 February 2009). By scapegoating the system, medical officials attempt to explain medical error in a manner that doesn't challenge the profession's control over defining and responding to medical mishaps. The problem is that "systems thinking" treats the medical system as if it were a closed system in which only medical professionals have the ability or right to decide what counts as medically inappropriate, harmful, or negligent behaviour. Further, the agency of individuals involved in the system is overlooked. The "safety culture" argument holds that the behaviour of health-care professionals cannot be judged without considering the systemic context of their conduct. In this way, blaming the system actually safeguards medical dominance over the health-care system.

The sociological imagination enables us to realize that behavioural change occurs through changing the structural context that makes that behaviour possible in the first place. One of the most effective and straightforward means of accomplishing structural change is with regulatory measures that govern individual behaviour. Indeed, this is one of the lessons from the sociological study of the social determinants of health. It hasn't been smoking risk awareness campaigns that have reduced the incidence of this health-adverse behaviour; it has been a series of interrelated regulatory measures. Individuals avoid the adverse events associated with smoking not because they suddenly learn that such behaviour is bad for their health; they quit smoking when it became stigmatized, expensive, and, as with the case of smoking in public places or in automobiles with children in them, illegal. That is, a population health version of "name, blame, and shame" lowered smoking rates!

Similarly, industries such as nuclear power and aviation have been more successful in preventing errors than the health-care system because they employ a blend of systemic and regulatory measures. The sociological lesson is that patient safety from clinical iatrogenesis will only be achieved when regulatory models from other high-risk technical systems (such as aviation) are adopted to offset the dominance of the medical profession. A cornerstone of this type of safety management system is an impartial agency set up to investigate the cause of accidents and find fault (Sheps and Cardiff 2005).

> Health care is a decade or more behind other high-risk industries in its attention to ensuring basic safety. Aviation has focused extensively on building safe systems and has been doing so since World War II. Between 1990 and 1994, the U.S. airline fatality rate was less than one-third the rate experienced in mid century. In 1998, there were no deaths in the United States in commercial aviation. In health care, preventable injuries from care have been estimated to affect between three to four percent of hospital patients. Although health care may never achieve aviation's impressive record, there is clearly room for improvement (Institute of Medicine 2000, 5).

The aviation industry's success in reducing catastrophic errors was achieved through a mix of safety measures focused on identifying and rectifying both proximate causes (such as individual pilot error) and distal causes (such as system complexity). Rather than allowing the aviation industry or pilot associations to investigate errors, this function is performed by an industry-independent agency (in the United States, the Federal Aviation Administration, and in Canada, the Transportation Safety Board). Such industries provide a model for the type of patient safety system that needs to be put in place to minimize the threat to health posed by clinical iatrogenesis. However, medical error is not the only or even the most dangerous type of iatrogenesis Illich warned against.

Illich (1976, 49) argued that medicalization also perpetuates what he termed **social iatrogenesis** in which people become dependent on medical interpretations of reality:

> Social iatrogenesis is at work when health care is turned into a standardized item, a staple; when all suffering is "hospitalized" and homes become inhospitable to birth, sickness,

and death; when the language in which people could experience their bodies is turned into bureaucratic gobbledegook; or when suffering, mourning, and healing outside the patient role are labelled a form of deviance.

Illich was critical of the manner in which medicalization of troubling aspects of life obscures the reality that it is capitalist society that causes sickness and suffering. Social iatrogenesis refers to the indirect harm medicalization causes to society in general by defining more and more aspects of life, from birth through sorrow, suffering, and sickness, to death, as medical issues. When biomedical ideas, images, language, and practices become the lens through which our culture understands questions of life and morality, we have reached the point of social iatrogenesis.

However, what worried Illich most about medicalization was what he termed **cultural iatrogenesis**. He feared that the increasing medicalization of life would eventually compromise people's abilities to look after their own health without professional medicine's help (as illustrated by the cartoon). While evidence presented in the previous chapter shows that self-health management makes up the bulk of health care, there is equally compelling evidence that biomedical conceptions of health and health care have had the type of deskilling effect on self-care behaviour forewarned by Illich. In a culture preoccupied with what Crawford (1980, 371) describes as "healthism," "a medicalized perception sets boundaries on ways of thinking and channels consciousness and behaviour." This means that much self-care, while deprofessionalized, is imbued with the ideas, images, language, and practices offered by biomedicine. For example, in 2004 the British government decided to make cholesterol-lowering statin drugs available without a doctor's prescription in an effort to encourage this form of self-care for the treatment of cardiovascular disease while reducing the strain on government finances. This demonstrates, as Ballard and Elston (2005, 233) point out, that "medical dominance and medicalization are not synonymous."

Despite the contributions of those working within the conflict paradigm, Ballard and Elston (2005, 230) argue that medicalization is a multidimensional concept that extends beyond the dominance of the medical profession and speculate that "medicalization might be a much more complex, ambiguous, and contested process than the 'medicalization thesis' of the 1970s implied." Let's turn our attention to what more recent research on medicalization and its consequences, guided by Foucault's ideas, has taught us about medicalizing beings and bodies.

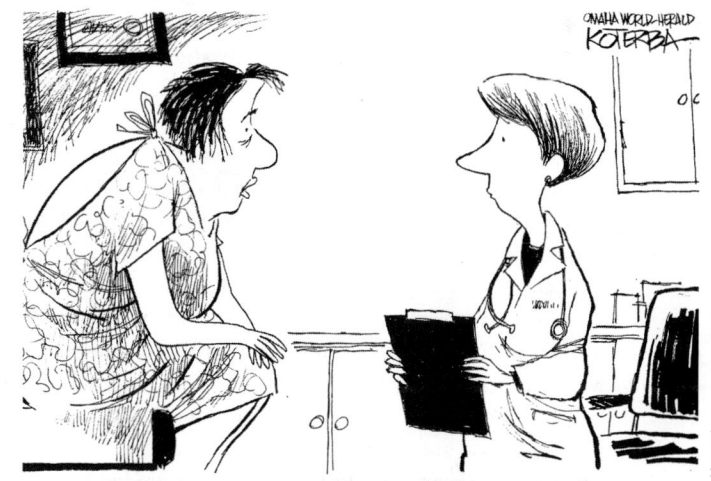

"AMBIEN MAKES MY HUSBAND EAT IN HIS SLEEP. RITALIN GIVES MY SON HALLUCINATIONS. WHAT DO YOU HAVE FOR DEPRESSION?"

Jeffrey Koterba, cartoonist

Given the rise in medical consumerism, perhaps Illich's concerns over the medicalization of life were prophetic?

Foucauldian Approaches: The Web of Medicalization—Surveillance and E-scaped Medicine

Reviewing explanations of the causes and consequences of medicalization, Conrad (2005; 2007; 2013) suggests that "the engines of medicalization are shifting." At an earlier stage, medicalization may have been driven by dominance of the medical profession or, in some cases, activities of social movements (such as Alcoholics Anonymous), which sought to define deviant behaviours in terms of disease. However, Conrad claims that since the 1980s, the primary engines or social forces underlying medicalization are health-conscious medical consumers and the pharmaceutical and biotechnological corporations that market health-care products and services (often directly to consumers). In other words, he argues that the sources of medicalization are decentralizing beyond the scope of the medical profession. Conrad (2013, 201) points out that "there is abundant evidence that the pharmaceutical industry has a more dominant and powerful impact on health affairs than it did four decades ago when the first studies of medicalization were published." Today, drug interventions are increasingly used for a wide range of human conditions and, to a great extent, physicians have been relegated to the role of gatekeepers for the expansion or contraction of medicalization. Clarke and Shim (2011, 176) similarly state that while "the professional autonomy of physicians has certainly been eroded, the dominance of medical technosciences and interventions, and of the sociocultural and economic sector of medicine, remain powerful." Along with this "shift in the engines of medicalization," there has been a parallel change in how health sociologists understand the ever-increasing scope of the "medical gaze" on everyday life.

Studies inspired by Foucault's social theories concerning the role of the "medical gaze" in the development of "biopower" (see Chapter 2) offer an image of "a sticky web of medical power" that characterizes the growing medicalization of life (Lupton 1997a, 101). Unlike conflict approaches to understanding medicalization, researchers informed by Foucault's approach understand medicalization as a process that proceeds through a complex set of social relations rather than being imposed from above by an expansionistic medical profession. Nye (2003, 117) distinguishes Foucauldian approaches from the medicalization thesis of conflict researchers by explaining that, rather than being viewed as "a nefarious collaboration of experts and state authority imposed from above," medicalization is seen as "a process whereby medical and health precepts have been embodied in individuals who assume this responsibility for themselves." This understanding of medicalization is in line with the focus of the sociology of the body paradigm on the importance of embodiment as a basis of identity. According to this approach, it is individuals' internalization of the ideas, images, language, and practices offered by biomedicine that drives medicalization.

Carpiano (2001) terms the role that individual action plays in promoting medicalization "passive medicalization." As Parsons (1951) showed many years ago with the sick role, accepting medical interpretations of reality brings with it certain social benefits. For example, the professor who routinely shows up drunk for his classes is likely to welcome the medicalized label of "alcoholic," or someone who is suffering from the disease of "alcoholism," over other interpretations that his dean or students might have for such deviant conduct! This illustrates that the Foucauldian view understands medical knowledge as productive, not repressive. In this perspective, the power of medicine stems from its ability to offer productive ways of understanding health and behaviour and delivering on the promise of health.

In this way, Nye (2003, 115) argues that "current assessments of medicalization are far more nuanced, and somewhat more optimistic, than they were 35 or 40 years ago." Whereas earlier analyses tended to focus on the dangers and harm caused by medicalization, recent studies explain how medicalization may represent "the positive utilization of medicine to improve the way in which problematic social experiences and forms of deviance have previously been managed" (Ballard and Elston 2005, 234). For example, Berenson, Miller, and Findlay (2009, 251) argue that medicalization increased public visibility of issues such as "woman abuse, or PMS" by framing them in medical terms and helped place them on the "political agenda." It seems that medicalization isn't always such a bad thing! Conrad (2005, 9) observes that "individuals' self-medicalization is becoming increasingly common, with patients taking their troubles to physicians and often asking directly for a specific medical solution." Notable examples of this type of self-medicalization include people's increasing desire to submit themselves to technologies of medical surveillance (such as medical screening) and the growing use of pharmaceutical technologies to reshape mood and emotion. Let's return to the history of medicine to examine the latest stages in the development of medical knowledge reflected by the growing influence of pharmaceutical and biotechnological industries in medicalizing beings and bodies: "the rise of Surveillance Medicine" (Armstrong 1995) and "the emergence of E-scaped Medicine" (Nettleton 2004).

Armstrong (1995) picks up on Jewson's history of medicine to suggest that during the twentieth century the social relations of healing changed once again, marking the emergence of a new stage in the development of biomedicine, which he calls Surveillance Medicine. Drawing upon Foucault's ideas of the surveillance and control of bodies, Armstrong argues that social relations of healing no longer occur in terms of the bodies of hospitalized patients (i.e., Hospital Medicine) or of tissue samples in the laboratory (i.e., Laboratory Medicine) but instead moved into the general population through widespread medical screening as an aspect of population health promotion. Contrasting Hospital Medicine with Surveillance Medicine, Armstrong (1995, 395) claims that "Hospital Medicine was only concerned with the ill patient in whom a lesion might be identified, but a cardinal feature of Surveillance Medicine is its targeting of everyone." With the rise of Surveillance Medicine, the question becomes, "What are your risks?" and the medical goal becomes identifying hidden risk factors (such as those depicted in Box 10.9) that embody potential threats to everyone's health.

As illustrated in Box 10.9, **risk factors** are factors believed to lead to diseases that often are treated as diseases in their own right. Skolbekken (1995) notes that cholesterol is only one of 300-plus risk factors that have been associated with heart disease. However, thanks in large measure to the marketing efforts of pharmaceutical companies, "high cholesterol" is mistaken in its own right for a disease condition (Moynihan and Cassels 2005). Wright (2009, 4) criticizes such "disease mongering," arguing that "Health risks that in many cases are insignificant, such as raised cholesterol or lowered bone density, are now categorized as diseases and the relevant drugs are marketed vigorously, even though they at best cause only very marginal benefits, again at huge cost to the public purse." The "prevalence and contagiousness" of the term "risk" within medical research literature led Skolbekken (1995, 296) to describe biomedical preoccupation with risk as a "risk epidemic"! He highlights factors such as the development of increasingly sophisticated statistical techniques for modelling probability, the new public health, and breakthroughs in computer-based technologies for processing medical information as causes of the risk epidemic and warns that this may lead to further iatrogenesis.

By focusing on lifestyle behaviours, this type of "risk factor epidemiology" individualizes causes of disease (Forde 1998; Link and Phelan 1995; Skolbekken 1995). Forde (1998, 1157) criticizes epidemiology together with the new public health movement for "imposing risk awareness as a form of cultural imperialism" by claiming that "a healthy lifestyle has become in our language

> **Box 10.9** Hidden Risk Factors
>
> Pfizer Canada's "Making the Connection" campaign illustrates the "tangled web" of medicalization described by Foucauldian researchers. The campaign is aimed at raising public risk awareness via a partnership between the number one supplier of cholesterol-lowering statin drugs and organizations such as the Heart and Stroke Foundation and the Canadian Football League. (A prominent advertising campaign featured Wally Buono, the coach of the British Columbia Lions, sharing his own illness narrative of being diagnosed with angina and urging football fans to "Make the Connection.")
>
> Research has shown that through such "direct to consumer" advertising and the use of celebrity spokespersons, what Moynihan, Heath, and Henry (2002) describe as "disease mongering," corporate interests capitalize on raising risk awareness. This type of "disease mongering" is so prevalent in our culture that often it is difficult to tell the difference between state-sponsored health promotion (e.g., the Cancer Care Manitoba campaign discussed in Chapter 8) and medical consumerism encouraged by corporate interests.
>
> The difference between health promotion and medical consumerism is that, unlike health promotion (from which no party directly benefits financially), medical consumerism is intended to generate profit from the marketing of health. In this case, Pfizer wants the public to make a connection between the risk of heart disease, cholesterol, and products they make billions selling, such as Lipitor, the top-selling prescription drug of all time.
>
> ---
>
> **www.makingtheconnection.ca/en/interactive_tools__f/multimedia**
>
> Visit Pfizer Canada's Making the Connection campaign, and spend some time exploring the site. Note the strategic placement of partner organization logos at the bottom of the home page and the use of celebrity endorsements. Without prior knowledge of the medicalization of health and wellness, would these strategies of using organizational partnerships and celebrity spokespeople have made you more or less inclined to consider a drug as a first course of action toward achieving better heart health?

almost synonymous with a lifestyle characterised by risk evasion." Explaining the connections among risk awareness, medicalization, and medical consumerism, she states that "By increasing anxiety regarding disease, accidents and other adverse events, the risk epidemic enhances both health care dependence and health care consumption" (1998, 1155). Similarly, Nettleton (2009, 635) notes that "responsibility, and increasingly culpability for health status, lies with the 'person' who is impelled to become aware of, and act upon, the wealth of health information and advice to be found not only in the health clinic, but also throughout various forms of popular media, on supermarket shelves, the Internet and so on." In this way, Surveillance Medicine is connected with the growth of health consciousness and medical consumerism introduced in the first chapter. Medicalization spreads throughout culture as everyone is encouraged to keep close watch on potential risks to health by being active, health-conscious medical consumers. This expansion of health risk awareness is the defining feature of Surveillance Medicine.

In this way, Foucauldian health researchers argue that Surveillance Medicine blurs the lines between ill and healthy as everyone becomes a "pre-patient" (Rose 2007, 20), with susceptibility for future disease lurking within our bodies or behaviour. Armstrong (1995, 398) explains how "the blurring of the distinction between health and illness, between the normal and the pathological, meant that health care intervention could no longer focus almost exclusively on the body of the patient in the hospital bed. Medical surveillance would have to leave the hospital and penetrate into the wider population." To focus on population health, Surveillance Medicine uses techniques such as epidemiological surveys, medical screening, and individualized health promotion campaigns. According to Armstrong (1995, 399), Surveillance Medicine represents the "realization of a new public health dream of surveillance in which everyone is brought into the vision of the benevolent eye of medicine through the medicalization of everyday life." A good illustration of this comes from the regulatory control achieved through medical screening.

The goal of **medical screening** is to assess individuals for the presence of disease that has not yet appeared symptomatically (Raffle and Gray 2007). Examples of screening programs run from annual physical exams, blood and Pap tests, through PSA (prostate) and mammography (breast) screening, to high-tech imagining (such as CT and MRI scanning) and advanced genetic testing. In this sense, these screening tests are different from diagnostic tests that are performed on patients who already feel ill or are exhibiting symptoms of disease. In other words, medical screening is a form of preventive medicine focused on healthy individuals to identify chances of future disease.

The common wisdom is that medical screening saves lives by catching diseases before they become symptomatic (Welch 2004). The mantra "early detection saves lives" has become a cliché in our overly medicalized society (Wright 2009). Despite such common sense beliefs, research shows that early detection is not always healthful. In fact, medical screening can actually be bad for your health! For example, in a book that asks the provocative question, "Should I be tested for cancer?" Welch (2004) highlights dangers associated with medical screening such as "false negatives" (when a test fails to find disease in a person in whom it is actually present), "false positives" (when a test finds evidence for a disease in a person who does not have the disease), and "overtreatment." Using the example of "pseudo-disease," Welch shows that many screening tests find evidence for the presence of cancer where the disease progresses so slowly (if at all) that people die of other causes long before the cancer produces noticeable symptoms. He explains that technologically sophisticated medical screening can find evidence of pathology that would have otherwise remained undetected for the person's entire life. As over-diagnosis results in over-treatment, this leads to what Raffle and Gray (2007, 68) describe as "the popularity paradox": "The greater the harm through over diagnosis and overtreatment from screening, the more people there are who believe they owe their health or even their life to the programme." In other words, the widening web of medical surveillance supports an increasing medicalization of life as more and more healthy people come to understand themselves as "at risk" and unquestioningly accept the moral obligation to submit their bodies and behaviours to medical attention.

The blurring of the lines between health and illness characteristic of Surveillance Medicine is nowhere more evident than in the growing influence the pharmaceutical industry has in health care. Expenditures on pharmaceuticals are the fastest-growing cost to the Canadian health-care system, having increased about 136 per cent since 1998 (CIHI 2009). Moynihan and Cassels (2005, 171) offer the following commentary on the unhealthy influence the medical-industrial complex has on the medicalized pursuit of health and wellness:

> The extent of the pharmaceutical industry's influence over the health system is simply Orwellian. The doctors, the drug reps, the medical education, the ads, the patients

groups, the guidelines, the celebrities, the conferences, the public awareness campaigns, the thought-leaders, and even the regulator's advisers—at every level there is money from drug companies lubricating what many believe is an unhealthy flow of influence.

Here we see a vivid example of the web of medicalization described by researchers influenced by Foucault's approach. Conrad (2005, 5) argues that the extent of involvement of corporate interests in the health-care system sets contemporary medicalization apart from that described by earlier conflict paradigm researchers such as Illich: "Drugs or technologies were not the driving force in the medicalization process; facilitating, yes, but not primary. But this is changing. The pharmaceutical and biotechnology industries are becoming major players in medicalization." Through a diversity of mechanisms, the medical-industrial complex both profits from and encourages medicalization of life. For instance, several researchers have documented the numerous techniques pharmaceutical companies have employed to socially construct diseases and disorders in order to make huge profits by offering pharmaceutical fixes for biomedically defined issues (e.g. Abraham 2010; Padamsee 2011). Studies of the intersection between medicalization and the ever-increasing role of pharmaceuticals and the pharmaceutical industry in modern life in the twenty-first century have even led to the use of the term **pharmaceuticalization** to describe "the process by which social, behavioural or bodily conditions are treated, or deemed to be in need of treatment/intervention, with pharmaceuticals by doctors, patients, or both" (Bell and Figert 2012, 775–6).

While it is unclear whether pharmaceuticalization represents an extension of medicalization or is better understood as a fundamentally new phenomenon, what does seem clear is that pharmaceutical-driven medicalization proceeds through a complex process involving many different participants. First, disease is often socially constructed by enrolling concerned patient groups in the process. Furedi (2004, 99–100) explains how "one of the most important ways in which medicalization has evolved during the second half of the twentieth century has been through 'discovering' diseases that are nonphysical and are to do with emotional problems. Increasingly, psychological problems associated with stress, rage, trauma, low self-esteem or addiction provide a medical label for interpreting every human experience." Moynihan and Cassels (2005, 62) provide the illustration of how "partnering with patient groups," such as concerned parents, facilitated the medicalization of attention deficit disorder (ADD) as a medical condition: "With ADD, as with other medical conditions, company-funded consumer groups provide a service to their sponsors by helping to paint a picture of an underdiagnosed medical disorder best treated with drugs and by giving a human face to that disorder." In this way, a crucial step in pharmaceutical-driven medicalization is the creation of widespread public belief in the biomedical roots of illness and disorder.

Once troubling aspects of life, such as deviant behaviour and unpleasant emotional states, are redefined as biophysical issues that require medical and pharmacological fixes, they are then sold to the public, governments, and other third-party payers. Rose (2003, 46) has gone as far as describing contemporary developed societies as "**psychopharmacological societies**" in which "the modification of thought, mood and conduct by pharmacological means has become more or less routine." He offers a Foucauldian understanding of medicalization, explaining that "in such societies, in many different contexts, in different ways, in relation to a variety of problems, by doctors, psychiatrists, parents and by ourselves, human subjective capacities have come to be routinely re-shaped by psychiatric drugs." Rose argues that medicalization has been extremely successful because it has managed to redefine life itself in biochemical terms.

Perhaps the most powerful means by which the pharmaceutical industry has been able to define the reality of illness is through the co-optation of medical research. Quite simply, most of the funding for medical research comes from industry sources, with pharmaceutical companies sponsoring clinical studies into the safety and effectiveness of their products, funding medical conferences where paid researchers ("thought-leaders") promote the use of drug treatments to other health professionals, and even secretly paying medical experts to lend their names to research papers that have been "ghostwritten" by the companies themselves! For example, a team of researchers (Lexchin et al. 2003, 1168) conducted a systematic review of studies investigating the relationship between researchers' financial ties to pharmaceutical companies and the likelihood that they reported positive results and found that "research sponsored by the drug industry was more likely to produce results favouring the product made by the company sponsoring the research than studies funded by other sources." In another instance, the *New York Times* (Singer 2009) broke a story about pharmaceutical companies paying medical researchers to "ghostwrite" (i.e., to lend their names and credentials to reports they did not write) studies that were, in fact, written by private contractors hired by the companies. Physicians rely on medical journals to provide them with up-to-date information regarding pharmaceutical treatments for their patients but may not be aware of the extent of industry bias. Murray, Brophy, and Palepu (2010) report preliminary results of a study that show that as many as 10 per cent of articles published in leading medical journals had ghost authors. Such conduct has led to many medical journals requiring that authors detail their role in the preparation of research and disclose conflicts of interest. However, research by Sismondo (2015) shows that the pharmaceutical companies' influence over the conduct of medical research goes beyond ghostwriting to what he refers to as "ghost management" of the entire research process.

A final illustration of the increasing influence of the pharmaceutical industry in medical research comes from the appointment of a senior executive of Pfizer Canada as a member of the governing council of the Canadian Institutes of Health Research (CIHR; see Box 10.10). CIHR is the largest health research funding council in the country and is supported by tax revenue. As a publicly funded institution, CIHR has a mandate is to serve the public interest by providing the knowledge base required to make societies and people healthy. The central issue is whether it is possible for a long-time drug company executive and active lobbyist for the private sector to act in the best interests of the public and give priority to improving the health of the population over a corporate obligation to make money for shareholders (Lewis 2010).

Research has revealed complicated relationships between pharmaceutical companies and physicians. Studies of pharmaceutical sales practices have shown how drug sales are facilitated through pharmaceutical representatives working in conjunction with direct-to-consumer advertising (Oldani 2004). For example, when patients enter clinics asking about drugs and conditions they have seen advertised, doctors are likely to contact drug representatives for product information. In this way, direct-to-consumer advertising complements the marketing efforts of pharmaceutical representatives. Oldani (2004, 327) provides dramatic accounts of how gifts that pharmaceutical companies give to doctors, ranging from free coffee and meals to sponsored travel, help to establish a "three-way gift cycle" between doctors, salespersons, and patients. While physicians often deny that pharmaceutical gifts influence their prescribing, Oldani's research shows that gifting establishes a normative relationship in which physicians are expected to reciprocate by prescribing certain drugs to patients. Whether it is through shaping public beliefs about the nature of health and illness, co-opting medical research, or direct contact with physicians, it is clear that the pharmaceutical industry has contributed significantly to creating a medicalized society.

Box 10.10 The Medical-Industrial Complex's Growing Influence over Medical Research

The Man from Pfizer: Should Big Pharma Help Steer Health Research?

"The appointment of a Pfizer Canada vice-president to the governing council of the Canadian Institutes of Health Research raises issues" (Picard 2009).

Should a senior executive of a large pharmaceutical company sit on the governing council of an institution whose role is to fund health research on behalf of taxpayers? That is a fiercely debated question in the corridors of health research, and one that belongs in the public realm. Bernard Prigent is vice-president and medical director of Pfizer Canada, a division of the world's largest pharmaceutical company, Pfizer Inc. On Oct. 5, he was appointed to the governing council of the Canadian Institutes of Health Research. The CIHR, which funds more than 13,000 health researchers and trainees, has a budget of $973-million, money it gets from the federal government.

For some, Dr. Prigent is the personification of evil, a Big Pharma operative who has infiltrated a body that Canadians depend on to finance unbiased, independent health research in the public interest. For others, the Pfizer Canada vice-president will bring a much-needed private-sector voice to the table and help ensure that CIHR invests tax dollars wisely in innovative and beneficial research and gets more bang for the buck. The truth probably lies somewhere between those extremes, but the reality is that the underlying issue matters to researchers and, by extension, to the public that benefits (or should) from health research.

Like all members of the CIHR governing council, Dr. Prigent has impeccable credentials, with a distinguished career in international health before joining the pharmaceutical industry. His particular area of specialty—and what led the CIHR to recruit him—is the management of research and development of commercial products.

"In Canada, we have some of the best health researchers in the world," Dr. Prigent said at the parliamentary committee that is reviewing his appointment. "Where we are less successful is in moving health research results out of the lab and into hospitals and clinics where they can improve health outcomes."

While it is hard to argue with that statement, the concern is that, by appointing a pharmaceutical company executive, the CIHR is sending a message that it is going to overtly and aggressively promote research that is profitable ahead of research that is merely useful. (All other members of the board are eminent researchers and health-care administrators in the public sector.)

The governing council of the CIHR does not actually dole out research funds. There is a complex system of open competition and peer-review for that function. But the governing council sets the strategic direction of the CIHR and that affects what is funded.

The overriding mission of the CIHR is "to improve the health of populations and promote health equity in Canada and globally through research and its applications to policies, programs and practice in public health and other sectors."

Continued

The legislation governing the institutes, the CIHR Act, also sets out that one of its objectives should be ". . . to excel, according to internationally accepted standards of scientific excellence, in the creation of new knowledge and its translation into improved health for Canadians, more effective health services and products, and a strengthened health care system, by . . . encouraging innovation, facilitating the commercialization of health research in Canada and promoting economic development through health research in Canada."

The president of CIHR, Alain Beaudet, said that Dr. Prigent's experience in innovation and commercialization will "fill a major expertise gap" on the board. While that gap needs to be filled, how it is done matters. Perceptions matter a whole lot, too.

The perception over this appointment was perhaps best enunciated by NDP health critic Judy Wasylycia-Leis, who said: "Having drug companies advise the government is like having the big bad wolf advising the three little pigs on how to build their homes."

Critics of the appointment have also underscored some of the major ethical transgressions of Pfizer in recent years. In September, for example, Pfizer Inc. was ordered to pay a record $2.3-billion (US) in fines and penalties because it marketed four drugs for conditions for which they were not recommended. While there is no suggestion Dr. Prigent was personally involved in the malfeasance, ethicists argue that his association with the company could breed cynicism and compromise the scientific integrity of the CIHR.

For its part, Rx&D, the organization representing research-based pharmaceutical companies, argues that the attacks on Dr. Prigent are spurious and "threaten to derail Canada's efforts to improve health research in this country." There are serious allegations and legitimate concerns at both ends of the spectrum. At the very least, there should be public discussion and debate about the role of private-industry representatives on government bodies and about the wisdom of government-funded institutions jumping on the commercialization bandwagon. But the parliamentary committee has, to date, heard only two witnesses on this appointment: Dr. Prigent and Dr. Beaudet. By hearing only one side of the debate, they are hardly carrying out their watchdog function as elected representatives. However accomplished Dr. Prigent may be, his appointment should not be a *fait accompli*.

Source: Andre Picard. "The man from Pfizer: Should Big Pharma help steer health research?" December 3, 2009. © The Globe and Mail Inc. All Rights Reserved.

As discussed in this article, there is a controversy regarding a conflict of interest involving the pharmaceutical industry and health research in Canada. Do you believe that the appointment of a senior executive of a major pharmaceutical company as a member of the governing council of the Canadian Institutes of Health Research (CIHR) is a conflict of interest?

Conrad (2013, 210) offers "a glimpse at the future" and identifies a number of areas where he anticipates that medicalization will exert even greater influence in the coming years. In his opinion, "pharmaceutical companies, when they don't have blockbuster drugs like Viagra or Lipitor, will attempt to find new uses for their already existing drugs. A current example is the repackaging of Prozac as Serifem (sic), the same drug under a new name now marketed for premenstrual dysphoric disorder." Consequently, he concludes that pharmaceutical medicalization will continue to be a strong force that will shape formal health care in the future.

A final element considered part of the sticky web of medicalization is the development of biomedical technologies, such as genomic medicine, that combine with breakthroughs in information technology to transform medicine and medical care. Clarke et al. (2003, 162) argue that breakthroughs in medical technology, such as practices in genetics (e.g., genetic diagnosis and population screening for genetic illness), computer-assisted imagining, telemedicine, and electronic medical information systems, have changed medicalization into "**biomedicalization**": "the increasingly complex, multisided, multidirectional processes of medicalization that today are being both extended and reconstituted through the emergent social forms and practices of a highly and increasingly technoscientific biomedicine." They contend that both the organization and practice of biomedicine have changed dramatically as a result of the implementation of technoscientific modes of intervention. As a result, Clarke and Shim (2011, 176) state that "medicine is now so much more than the profession, or the clinical provision of treatments, or even the health care system." Hallin, Brandt, and Briggs (2013) provide some interesting evidence to illustrate the transformations associated with biomedicalization. Based on a content analysis of health-related articles in two major US newspapers (the *New York Times* and the *Chicago Tribune*), they conclude that biomedical researchers have eclipsed physicians and public health officials as important sources of information about health and medicine.

Rose (2007, 11) agrees that because of technological innovation, medicine "has become technomedicine, highly dependent on sophisticated diagnostic and therapeutic equipment." He argues that rather than seeking to cure or prevent disease, the aim of many biomedical technologies is optimization and enhancement of "life itself." Indeed, "biomedicine has magnified the reach of modern medicine beyond the medical profession, the health system, or the provision of medical treatment" and has in fact made "its way into the life course and into everyday life" (Sulik 2011, 464). While Conrad (2005, 5) doesn't believe medicalization is "morphing into a qualitatively different phenomena" (as implied by the term "biomedicalization"), he does agree that biotechnology has brought about major changes that have produced an expansion of medicalization.

Nettleton (2004, 673) goes as far as to suggest that these developments represent the emergence of an additional stage in the development of medical knowledge, which she terms "E-scaped Medicine" to denote how "health and medical knowledge are being metamorphosed into information and it is circulating beyond the walls of medical schools, hospitals, and laboratories." Just as the doctors of Hospital Medicine were displaced by the scientists of Laboratory Medicine, who then gave way to the epidemiologists of Surveillance Medicine whose job it was to place the entire population under surveillance for hidden risk factors, they too have been displaced by information scientists who analyze the communicative systems that comprise the digitized body of E-scaped Medicine. Nettleton contends that the twentieth century's dominant metaphor of the body as machine is giving way to a new understanding of the body as an information system, alongside technoscientific breakthroughs in information and communication technologies, such as Internet-based communication, telecare, telemedicine, telesurgery, and health informatics and the collection, storage, and retrieval of health-related information made possible by computers. In her words, Nettleton (2004, 666) explains that "biology is becoming an information science, mapping information at the level of cells, proteins and genes. Medicine more generally is becoming information-based in terms of its delivery and management." The ethos of the e-scaped stage in the development of medical knowledge may be summarized by the question, "what communication breakdown in the human system has initiated disease?" focused on the human body understood as an assemblage of data that is represented in digital forms, such as sequences of DNA. As Nettleton (2004, 668) explains, within the era of E-scaped Medicine, "disease becomes a form of information malfunction or a 'communication pathology'; accordingly the prime pathology is stress—communications breakdown—which depresses the immune system."

Nettleton goes on to suggest that in contrast to the collection of risk factors characteristic of Surveillance Medicine, E-scaped Medicine places the individuality of the patient at centre stage, but this time in the form of the expert patient characteristic of today's health-conscious medical consumer: "Unlike the classic sick role relationship where the doctor told the patient what was wrong and what s/he had to do or 'take' to get better, in the information age the doctor is just as likely to tell the patient what might be wrong and outline a range of possible risks, treatments or therapies" (2004, 672). This shift is exemplified by the promised appearance of "**personalized medicine**" wherein medical knowledge of each person's genome serves as the basis for tailoring medical interventions designed specifically for the individual's unique biology (Cullis 2015). What makes personalized medicine so potentially revolutionary, however, is that it promises to move beyond treatment to prevention tailored to each person's unique genomic risk profile (Rose 2013). Commenting skeptically on the promise of personalized medicine, Tutton (2012, 1721) cautions that "Personalized medicine should be understood as a 'rhetorical entity' used by actors from industry, government, regulation, academia, patient advocacy, clinical practice to not only describe a future state but to bring it into being." Similarly, Rose (2013, 342) remarks on the affinities personalized medicine shares with prevailing cultural values of neo-liberal society: "In contemporary Western culture, at least, it seems obvious that no-one would want 'impersonal' services, or 'one size fits all' provisions; surely everyone wants to be treated as an individual, wants to have freedom of choice, their own decisions respected, to be treated as a whole, unique person responsible for their own life and their own health." Despite these cultural affinities, Rose (2013, 350) concludes by reminding us that

> The major advances in healthcare outcomes in the developed world—to the extent that they cannot simply be attributed from poverty reduction and increasing education—have not come about through personalization and individualization, but from the reverse—from interventions that have been addressed to all—clean air, water, effective sewage systems, pure food, programmes of population wide vaccination and so forth.

While such criticisms of personalized medicine may be valid, it does seem that biotechnological developments may well be prompting yet another stage in the development of medical knowledge, aptly characterized as E-scaped Medicine.

Together, the factors described in this section represent what in Foucault's terms would be called an expansion of biopower and the widespread internalization of the medical gaze. As part of the transformation of medicalization into biomedicalization, it has been suggested that there has been a shift in the meaning of this concept from "the clinical gaze" (which focuses on acute and chronic illnesses/diseases and associated risk factors) to "the molecular gaze" (which focuses on the microbiological level and genomics and the management of risk through technoscientific means, such as human cloning and stem cell research) (Clarke and Shim 2011). While the next chapter focuses on the ways in which individuals are "moving beyond biomedicine" by using alternative types of formal health care, it is worth noting that according to some researchers (e.g., Lowenberg and Davis 1994; Fries 2008), it is possible to interpret the resurgence of medical pluralism as further evidence of increasing medicalization!

Chapter Summary

The purpose of this chapter was to critically assess the link between biomedicine and population health. The discussion started by tracing stages in the historical development of the biomedical model and explored ways in which formal health care reflects changes over time in the social construction of biomedical knowledge. The argument presented was that as social relations of healing changed, so too did basic ideas that make up medical knowledge. Initially, doctors provided medical services in the homes of wealthy patients who could afford to pay for private care (Bedside Medicine). The primary focus at this stage was on diagnosing and treating patients' symptoms. As social relations of healing changed, medical care was institutionalized (Hospital Medicine). At this stage in the development of the biomedical model, a new way of understanding disease emerged, and patients were transformed into medical cases requiring treatment in hospital settings. Hospital-based medicine allowed physicians to objectify the bodies of the sick in the process of trying to identify underlying pathology that causes disease. This stage marked the emergence of medicine as an organized profession that was able to exercise medical dominance over competing healers. Eventually, the increasing technological bases of biomedicine led to another change in medical knowledge and practice. During the period of Laboratory Medicine, healing moved out of hospital wards and into research laboratories as the search for causes of disease changed from the anatomical level to cellular pathology. What this quick look back at the historical development of the contemporary biomedical model demonstrates is that medical knowledge is socially constructed.

The chapter then reviewed five basic ideas that comprise the biomedical model today: mind–body dualism, physical reductionism, specific etiology, the machine metaphor, and regimen and control. Together, these ideas exert a powerful cultural influence on formal health care and our increasingly medicalized society. More and more aspects of everyday life are being transformed into medical matters requiring biomedical health care. In fact, it has been argued that the medicalization process has enabled the profession of medicine to claim control over any aspect of human existence that can be labelled an illness (regardless of its ability to deal with it effectively). Two alternative explanations for the process of medicalization were reviewed: the conflict paradigm's critique of the professional power of organized medicine as an instrument of social control and the sociology of the body paradigm's ideas concerning the individualization of health care and the role of surveillance medicine and medical screening in modern societies. To illustrate the consequences of living in a medicalized society, a number of contemporary issues were considered, such as the role played by pharmaceutical and biotechnology companies in marketing health-care products and services and contributing to the increasing medicalization of beings and bodies.

The most damaging thing about medicalization is that it makes us forget the lessons learned from the history of the development of biomedicine. As we have seen, the dramatic gains in population health experienced by developed nations such as Canada were not simply the result of medical care. The reason we began to live longer and healthier lives during the twentieth century was because it was during this period that social policies were introduced that had direct positive impacts on population health status, such as universal education, housing policies, child and mother welfare policies, labour laws, civil rights, and redistributive taxation policies. Our over-medicalized society has forgotten the salutary lesson that medical care cannot and should not be equated with health care. As a result of medicalization, attention has focused primarily on the consumption of health-care products and services rather than the production of population health (Evans and Stoddart 1990).

In questioning the relationship between the formal health-care system and population health, the point of this chapter has not been to raise doubts about the necessity of biomedical care. As McKeown (1979, viii) argued decades ago, "The conclusion that medical intervention is often less effective than has been thought in no way diminishes the clinical function. When people are ill they want all that is possible to be done for them and small benefits are welcome when larger ones are not available." However, if medical care is to realize its full potential in helping us to pursue health and wellness, we need to critically evaluate the relative contribution of biomedicine compared to the significant part played by social determinants of health in the formation of healthy societies and healthy people.

Study Questions

1. In what way is the current formal health-care system actually a "sick-care system" that promotes the medicalization of life?
2. Outline the economic, social, and human costs associated with medicalized societies.
3. With direct reference to Jewson's "history of medicine," explain the connection between changing social relations of healing and basic ideas that make up medical knowledge.
4. Outline the major ideas that characterize the biomedical model, discussing how they have been socially constructed.
5. Summarize the evidence that shows that biomedicine's contribution to population health is less than is commonly believed.
6. Describe the dominance of the medical profession in the formal health-care system.
7. Compare and contrast explanations given for the causes and consequences of medicalization provided by researchers informed by the conflict and sociology of the body paradigms.
8. Outline the three types of iatrogenesis described by Illich, providing specific examples of each.
9. How are the new public health movement, medical screening, and the growing influence of the pharmaceutical industry illustrations of Surveillance Medicine?

Recommended Readings

Abraham, J. 2010. "Pharmaceuticalization of society in context: Theoretical, empirical and health dimensions." *Sociology* 44: 603–22.

Canadian Institute for Health Information. 2004. *Health Care in Canada 2004*. Ottawa: CIHI.

Clarke, A., and J. Shim. 2011. "Medicalization and biomedicalization revisited: Technoscience and transformations of health, illness and American medicine." In B. Pescosolido, J. Martin, J. McLeod, and A. Rogers, eds, *Handbook of the Sociology of Health, Illness, and Healing: A Blueprint for the 21st Century*, 173–99. New York: Springer Science.

Conrad, P. 2007. *The Medicalization of Society: On the Transformation of Human Conditions into Treatable Disorders*. Baltimore: John Hopkins University Press.

——— 2013. "Medicalization: Changing contours, characteristics, and contexts." In W. Cockerham, ed., *Medical Sociology on the Move*, 195–214. Dordrecht, NY: Springer Science.

Hadler, N.M. 2004. *The Last Well Person: How to Stay Well despite the Health-Care System*. Montreal: McGill-Queen's University Press.

Moynihan, R., and A. Cassels. 2005. *Selling Sickness: How the World's Biggest Pharmaceutical Companies Are Turning Us All into Patients.* Toronto: Greystone Press.

Recommended Websites

Health Canada–Current Patient Safety Initiatives:
www.hc-sc.gc.ca/hcs-sss/qual/patient_securit/index-eng.php

OECD **Health at a Glance 2013:**
http://dx.doi.org/10.1787/health_glance-2013-en

Recommended Audiovisual Sources

"At war with death," *"The Nature of Things"* with David Suzuki, CBC TV, 1985.

Hospital City. Directed by Rosemary House, produced by Kent Martin and Mary Sexton, National Film Board of Canada, 2004.

"Killed by care: Making medicine safe," *"The Nature of Things"* with David Suzuki, CBC TV, 2004.

"White coat, black art," hosted by Dr Brian Goldman, CBC Radio, 8 September 2010, www.cbc.ca/whitecoat

Moving beyond Biomedicine: Medical Pluralism

11

Learning Objectives

This chapter explores medical pluralism by looking at people's use of alternatives to biomedicine in pursuit of health and wellness, considering

- cultural origins of medical pluralism and the need for sociologists studying alternative health belief systems to pay close attention to the language used to describe types of medical knowledge and practice;
- explanations provided by sociologists for the growing popularity of alternative medicine;
- how medical consumerism and cultural diversity are factors in alternative medicine's increasing popularity; and
- the compatibility of biomedical and alternative health-care systems and prospects for developing "integrative medicine" as part of a future formal health-care system.

Biomedicine is at the height of its success, delivering more health-care products and services to more people, at greater expense, than ever before (Jonas 2002). Despite the widespread success of biomedicine in treating illness and influencing how we understand health in Western societies such as Canada, for a growing number of people the pursuit of health and wellness is moving beyond biomedicine. As humorously depicted in the cartoon, some think the use of alternative medicine means people are "losing faith in Western medicine"! The editors of the *New England Journal of Medicine* summarize the situation in this way: "Now, with the increased interest in alternative medicine, we see a reversion to irrational approaches to medical practice, even while scientific medicine is making some of its most dramatic advances" (Angell and Kassirer 1998, 840). While there is no indication that people are losing faith in biomedicine, more and more people are turning to alternative medicine in an effort to deal with illness and maintain health.

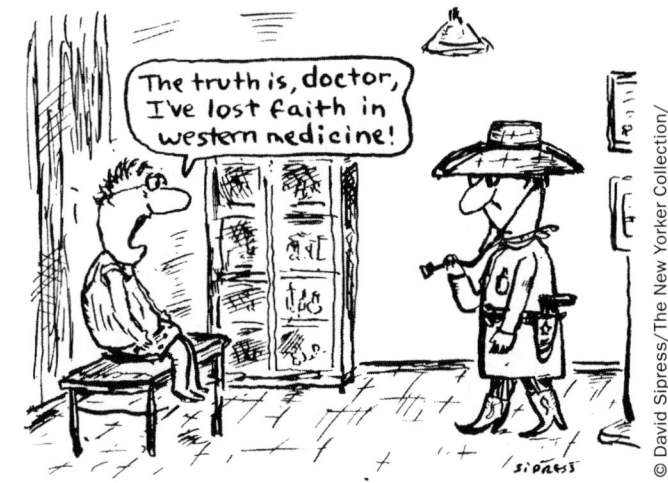

This chapter explores **medical pluralism**, or "the co-existence in a society of differing medical traditions, grounded in different cultural principles or based on different worldviews" (Cant 2004, 183). We will learn that alternative medicine has historically been controversial and continues to be characterized by heated debate with strong language. We will review research that seeks to explain the revival of medical pluralism alongside the dominance of biomedicine, summarizing various explanations that have been put forward to account for alternative medicine's growing popularity. We will also examine the role cultural diversity plays in explaining why many people are using alternatives to biomedicine in pursuit of health and wellness. The chapter concludes by taking a critical look at recent efforts to merge alternative medicine and biomedicine into a new form of medicine called "integrative medicine."

The Social Construction of Healing: A Sociological Perspective on Medical Pluralism

In the introductory chapter, we learned that in a sociological perspective, health is understood as a social construction, meaning that social factors influence health and the manner in which we interpret the meaning of health, illness, and the body. Understanding health as a social construction is necessary in sociological studies of medical pluralism, because this avoids ethnocentrism and medico-centrism; not privileging one health belief system above others. Health and wellness are socially constructed and are therefore understood differently by different people. The sociological perspective also helps us to appreciate conceptions of health and illness; ideas about what it means to "be healthy" and the nature of "healing" are shaped by location and experiences in the social world. In other words, just as definitions of health are socially constructed, so too are definitions of healing! Different cultures have different ways of understanding health and the body and offer different healing systems. Box 11.1 illustrates the social construction of healing.

While healing practices such as moxibustion are part of traditional Chinese culture, in other cultural contexts they may be regarded as harmful or even torturous. This shows that different cultures have various ways of understanding the body and forms of healing! This example illustrates that a sociological perspective on health belief systems recognizes the cultural relativity of medical knowledge. As discussed in Chapter 9, a **health belief system** can be defined as a systematic set of ideas and generally accepted practices with regard to health, healing, and self-care that varies by culture and social location.

As O'Connor (1995) explains, health belief systems provide a basis for interpreting causes and consequences of illness and for selecting a course of action to manage sickness. In other words, they shape what counts as appropriate treatment. Importantly, health belief systems originate within particular cultural contexts and reflect norms and values of the culture that give rise to them. Depending on a person's health belief system, practices such as balancing chi energy through moxibustion might be viewed as healing by some individuals, while others with different social locations might regard these practices as ineffective, illegitimate, or even fraudulent. Consequently, in a sociological perspective medical knowledge is culturally relative!

Box 11.1 Healing as Socially Constructed

In Traditional Chinese Medicine, healing is intimately connected with ancient Chinese spirituality, which contains conceptions of an elemental life force or "chi" (pronounced "chee") energy that flows through the body. Illness results from energy imbalance. Healing is achieved by balancing this cosmic energy. Once imbalance is detected through a variety of diagnostic techniques, such as measuring pulses and observing the tongue, eyes, and skin, the Traditional Chinese Medicine practitioner may employ several techniques to restore balance and, consequently, health (Shealy 1999). These techniques include acupuncture (in which small needles are inserted at points along the body's energy pathways, called "meridians"), herbal medicines, manual therapies, the exercises and breathing techniques of tai chi, special diets, or, as depicted here, moxibustion—the burning of dried herbs over the skin. In the context of traditional Chinese culture, such a practice is considered a form of healing. Would you use alternative medicine as a healing practice? How does your social location influence your health care choices?

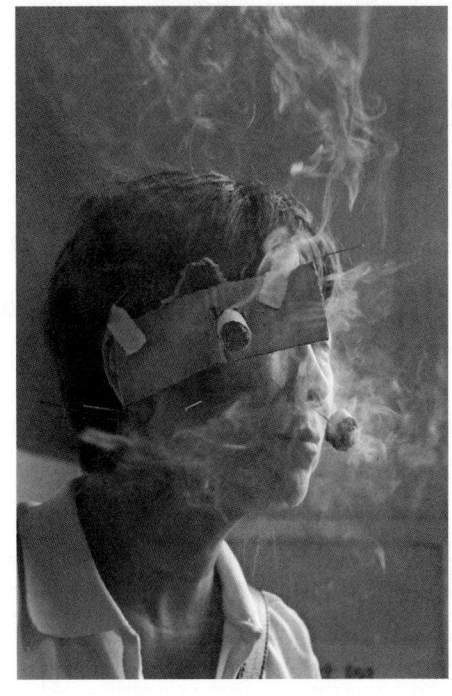

© PANBING/Cpressphoto/Corbis

In Chapter 2 we learned that Foucault explains that it is possible to understand health as a "cultural fact" "that is tied to a certain state of individual and collective consciousness" (2000, 379). Foucault means that culture influences people's ideas about what counts as appropriate medical treatment and healing. Importantly, in a sociological perspective this is true for all health belief systems: Western and non-Western, biomedical and alternative. Wolpe (1987, 194) uses the example of appendicitis to illustrate how culture influences knowledge of the body: "Though the physician may insist that having appendicitis has little symbolic content, the acceptance of that label, and not that the devil has your innards, or that you are a victim of witchcraft, or that you have an imbalance in your humours, was a meaningful and symbolic act." Depending on an individual's health beliefs, acute pain in the side might be caused by inflammation of an organ known as the appendix, or it might be because "the devil has your innards," or because of "witchcraft," or because of "an imbalance in the humours." Health belief systems define the nature of health problems and guide the course of action taken by sufferers to find relief.

The implication of the cultural relativity of health belief systems is that sociologists studying medical pluralism must be careful to avoid medico-centric bias: seeing biomedical knowledge as indisputable scientific truth and dismissing other health belief systems as false. Summarizing the value of understanding biomedicine as a health belief system alongside other health belief systems, O'Connor (1995, 22) notes that "Its protestations to the contrary notwithstanding, modern biomedicine is, like [other] health belief systems, profoundly culturally shaped." As we saw in the previous chapter, biomedical knowledge reflects the culture of the Western societies in which it originated. While the scientific world view has dominated Western culture, medical pluralism has remained a persistent feature of all societies, Western and non-Western.

The Historical Persistence of Medical Pluralism

In the West, biomedicine has become the dominant health-care system. However, a variety of health beliefs and health-care systems have existed throughout history and across the globe. As we learned in the previous chapter, biomedicine achieved dominance in the West largely because of historical events, such as the Medical Act of 1858 in England and the 1910 Flexner Report, *Medical Education in the United States and Canada,* and is a rather recent development. This means that biomedical dominance in the West is an "exception" to the historical "rule" of medical pluralism. Conrad (1995, 479–80) notes that "Anthropological writers have provided the evidence that suggests that all human cultures, Western and non-Western, ancient and modern, display certain beliefs about bodies, food, and the environment, that pre-date the successful development in Western medicine of the so-called biomedical model." He describes the history of Western medicine as "the journey away from this world, one that earlier had been shared with non-European cultures" and adds that even in the West, this model was preceded by a "balanced," "interactionalist" perspective that saw humanity as more than "materialist," as having "environmental" and "supernatural" elements.

Over "centuries of time" (Conrad 1995, 481), biomedical conceptions of health, illness, and healing displaced earlier holistic perspectives. Salmon (1984, 266) describes how healing was connected to the development of science: "The loss of a spiritual dimension in health and healing came with the elevation of science over religion across the last century and a half. When the body became viewed more as a machine with the natural occurrence of disease located in the individual, treatment logically was extended to individualized biomedical intervention to fight disease." This marked the beginning of the dominance of biomedicine in health and healing discussed in the previous chapter.

Despite the dominance of biomedicine since the nineteenth century, a range of alternative health belief systems have persisted. Anyinam (1990, 69) offers the following description:

> Alternative therapies are derived from diverse geographical, cultural, social, and philosophical backgrounds, as well as from different historical periods. These systems are, however, linked by the fact that they are different from biomedicine, or what is usually referred to as modern scientific medicine. While some have persisted from the nineteenth century (e.g., chiropractic, naturopathy, osteopathy, and homeopathy), others are of fairly recent origin (e.g., biofeedback and Rolfing). A few have diffused from the Far East (e.g., acupuncture, reflexology, and yoga); and others are traditional or folk remedies which have existed for a long time (e.g., herbalism).

Beck, Giddens, and Lash (1994) describe the ironic process whereby technological development has undermined public confidence in expert knowledge. As depicted in Box 11.2, they explain that the downsides of scientific and technological development, such as environmental pollution and climate change, have led many people to become distrustful of science. Combined with the risks of iatrogenesis, these cultural and social developments have undermined confidence in biomedicine, contributing to the resurgence of medical pluralism. As O'Connor (1995, 1) explains, the assumption that "folk and popular systems of health beliefs and practices would inevitably decline in modern and industrialized societies, falling away before the forces of modernization and progress to be replaced by modern, Western medicine," has proved to be wrong.

Box 11.2 Rise of the Health Truthers: Medical Skeptics and Conspiracists in Search of Certainty in a Confusing World

From a major measles outbreak at Disneyland in California to the revelation Queen's University has for years incorporated anti-vaccine misinformation in a health course, and from the rise of "pet anti-vaxxers" to "pox parties" and "flu flings," in which diseases are deliberately spread to create immunity, the power of alternative views about infectious disease control is deeply established and resistant to mainstream criticism and scientific evidence. All these cases show how decisions about health are rarely like scientific judgments. Rather, they can be esthetic choices, personal and subjective, based as much on intuition and emotion as reason and evidence.

In Canada, the vaccine controversy follows the outcry over the death of Makayla Sault, the First Nations' girl who pursued alternative therapy for leukemia. This raised the question of how much society should defer to alternative views of health and well-being, and whether the answer is different in the Aboriginal context.

But health trutherism is broader than medicine. It spans many aspects of modern life, from grocery shopping to energy policy. Adherents have many bugaboos: wind turbines, vaccines, some environmental illnesses, perfume sensitivity, toxins, gluten, pesticides, fluoride, cellphone radiation . . .

These issues are connected by skepticism about mainstream science, usually for its links to industry. Often the underlying fear is of a departure from the natural or the pure, although this romantic vision glosses over its more destructive aspects, like killer viruses. Just as often, there is a resistance to changing one's views even in the face of strong evidence or authoritative advice.

"Part of this is about how people navigate a complex, uncertain world," says Herbert Northcott, interim chair of sociology at the University of Alberta. "In the past, I think people had less information, there weren't as many experts making pronouncements. They trusted the priest, they listened to the priest, then they prayed to God. That's how they managed risk." Health trutherism, then, "functions like religious faith used to function." Like religion, it mixes fear and hope into a single motivation, and like religious faith, it is

Continued

impervious to worldly arguments. Prof. Northcott cites the "Thomas Theorem," a principle of sociology that says whatever people believe to be real is real in its consequences.

"It's mostly a class-based thing," says Jacqueline Low, who studies the use of alternative therapies at the University of New Brunswick. These treatments "cost money, so it tends to be people who have the money to purchase them." "The common thing I've found was that they were solving health problems that they could not solve in any other way," she says.

"Far from being scientifically illiterate, these individuals have a well-developed understanding of both the principles and practices of science," says Christopher J. Fries, a health sociologist at the University of Manitoba. "However, it is actually this understanding that leads them to be suspicious of scientific knowledge. They understand that technoscientific knowledge, while at times valuable, is shaped by commercial and economic interests. . . . This leads many to be skeptical of science as a way of knowing." The result is many people "shop around and pick and choose diverse elements with which to construct [their] lay beliefs about health and illness—a little science here, a little ethnic and indigenous knowledge there."

"A lot of the anti-scientific movements are attempts for people to get control over their lives in a world that seems increasingly out of our control," says Stephen Kent, who studies alternative religions at the University of Alberta. "As we lose faith in people in power, a lot of people believe they can only rely upon themselves." Pop culture taps this vein of suspicion nicely, he said, with movies about "vaccinations run amok," such as World War Z. "It's not that people think they are real, but their constant presence wears down people's remembrance that they are fictions. They think this could have happened."

Source: Excerpted from Joseph Brean, "Rise of the health truthers: Medical skeptics and conspiracists in search of certainty in a confusing world," 6 February 2015. © The National Post. All Rights Reserved.

As discussed in this article, alternative approaches to health and healing have made a big comeback in the West, with many people skeptical about science and biomedicine. What do you think accounts for the resurgence in popularity of alternative health belief systems and practices such as that described in this article?

A casual glance through the *Yellow Pages* telephone directory of any Canadian metropolitan area reveals that Canadians are offered a wide variety of alternatives to the scientifically based treatments offered by biomedicine. Economic data indicate that Canadians spend significant amounts of money making use of these practices. According to the Fraser Institute (Esmail 2007), Canadians spend approximately $5.6 billion out of pocket on visits to alternative health-care providers in a year. "If the additional money spent on books, medical equipment, herbs, vitamins, and special diet programs is included, the estimated total out of pocket spending on alternative medicine in Canada increases to an estimated $7.84 billion" (Esmail 2007, 4–5). Clearly, Western countries such as Canada have experienced a revival in the popularity of alternatives to biomedical definitions of healing.

The return of popular interest in alternatives to biomedical treatment is unprecedented in its sheer magnitude, if not its occurrence. The *Canadian Community Health Survey* (*CCHS*) shows that an estimated 20 per cent of Canadians, or 5.4 million people over the age of 12, consulted an alternative medical practitioner in the months prior to the survey and that use of such health-care practices is growing (Park 2005). In the face of this resurgence of alternative medicine, social and behavioural scientists are attempting to understand this health-care behaviour. As the next section shows, in conducting research sociologists need to avoid the medico-centric temptation to explain the growing popularity of alternative medicine in terms of a presumed scientific ignorance or gullibility on the part of those who use these forms of health care.

Avoiding the "Stereotypes of Marginality" in Social Studies of Alternative Medicine

In the midst of a technoscientific culture in which biomedicine has had such success in treating disease and illness, why would anyone use alternative types of formal health care? Criticizing attempts to answer this question, O'Connor (1995, 2) notes that "Too often, these studies have been plagued with prejudgments and value-laden terminology, which have in some cases, entirely precluded accurate presentation of information about the systems being studied." She (1995, 15–16) points out that research concerning medical pluralism is filled with "stereotypes of marginality," implying that people who use alternative medicine are in some way marginal to mainstream Western society:

> The stereotypes of marginality typically include one or more of the following features: geographic remoteness or isolation . . . ; recent immigration or minimal acculturation to core American culture; ethnic minority membership or strong ethnic self-identification or group affiliation; poverty or low socioeconomic status; low formal educational attainment; mental or emotional imbalance; or desperation induced by grave illness or poor outcomes of conventional therapeutic efforts. These factors are interpreted as producing ignorance of the existence or availability of modern medical strategies and technologies, lack of understanding of disease processes and their relationship to conventional therapeutic responses, lack of physical or financial access to conventional care, or failure or inability to exercise judgment.

Such stereotypes of marginality assume that people who use alternative medicine must be socially excluded in a way that makes them ignorant of the fact that, in the West, biomedicine is the most accepted form of health care. Their presumed ignorance is attributed to a number of potential factors: Perhaps they are from poor rural areas far removed from health care provided by physicians and nurses. Maybe they are newcomers to our society and don't know what biomedical health care has to offer, or then again, they may be poor, or uneducated, or suffer from mental disorder, and these factors explain the use of alternative medicine. Finally, it is possible that they suffer from illnesses that biomedicine can't cure, so they turn to alternative medicine out of desperation. All of these explanations for the revival of medical pluralism rest on stereotyping people who use alternatives to biomedicine as marginal in some way to mainstream society.

O'Connor goes on to point out that what is overlooked by such medico-centric explanations is that people who use these therapies may do so not because they are marginal but simply because they have health belief systems that differ from those of the dominant culture: "These factors are defined as 'barriers' to use of biomedicine, and are perceived to be located in the specific populations they are used to describe—rather than in the *relationship* between differing worldviews (biomedical and non-biomedical), and differing ways of defining and preferring to address matters of health, illness, and care" (1995, 15–16; original emphasis). She points out that such explanations for the use of alternative medicine are medico-centric and ethnocentric—they are biased in favour of Western biomedical treatment. However, as data show, the use of alternative medicine, far from being marginal, is becoming increasingly mainstream! In order to understand the revival of medical pluralism, sociological explanations for the use of alternative medicine need to move beyond such stereotypes. One of the main ways of avoiding bias is to pay close attention to language used to label alternative forms of medical knowledge and practice.

Labelling Alternative Medicine

In order to understand medical pluralism, health sociologists need to first define what "alternative medicine" means. This has proved to be a challenging task. In their worldwide review of the "legal status of traditional medicine and complementary/alternative medicine," the World Health Organization (2001, 1–2) offers the following commentary on the difficulty associated with defining alternative medicine:

> The terms "complementary medicine" and "alternative medicine" are used interchangeably with "traditional medicine" in some countries. Complementary/alternative medicine often refers to traditional medicine that is practised in a country but is not part of the country's own traditions. . . . The comprehensiveness of the term "traditional medicine" and the wide range of practices it encompasses make it difficult to define or describe, especially in a global context.

In other words, "alternative medicine" can mean different things to different people. The National Center for Complementary and Alternative Medicine (2007, 2) in the US notes that "The list of what is considered to be complementary/alternative medicine changes continually, as those therapies that are proven to be safe and effective become adopted into conventional health care and as new approaches to health care emerge." Quah (2008, 420) points out that many researchers studying medical pluralism have uncritically used culturally loaded labels: "It is unfortunate that the discussion of healing options in the social science literature has incorporated terms from the mass media and introduced new labels without rigorous scrutiny of their meaning and consistency." She argues that researchers need to pay careful attention to the language used to describe medical pluralism.

Why are words so important? After all, they're just labels, aren't they? In a sociological perspective, words and phrases that come into use to describe the social world are never "just labels." Labels used by everyday people, researchers, and policy-makers are important because they carry meaning and thereby structure human experience (Becker 1963). The centrality of culture in health belief systems means that sociological analysis of medical pluralism must begin by understanding differences between the labels used to describe alternatives to biomedicine (Fries 2009). In other words, cultural norms and values are often hidden in the labels used to describe the social world. This is why both individuals and groups "fight" over labels and why health sociologists studying medical pluralism need to be aware of power relations inherent in labels and labelling. An example of the importance of labels attached to medical knowledge and practice comes from a 1902 guide for physicians concerned with positioning

"Regular Medicine" (i.e., biomedicine) in opposition to a form of alternative medicine known as "Homeopathic Medicine":

> Remember that the term "Allopath" is a false nickname not chosen by regular physicians at all, but cunningly coined, and put in wicked use against us, in his venomous crusade against Regular Medicine by its enemy, Hahnemann, . . . and ever since applied to us by our enemies with all the insinuations and derisive use the term affords. "Allopathy" applied to regular medicine is both untrue and offensive and is no more accepted by us than the term "Heretics" is accepted by Protestants . . . or "Niggers" by the Blacks (*Transactions of the New Hampshire Medical Society*, 1902, as cited in Whorton 1985, 34).

"Allopath" is a term referring to the treatment of disease using remedies whose effects differ from those produced by the disease, which was applied by the founder of homeopathy, Samuel Hahnemann (1755–1843), to differentiate biomedicine from homeopathic medicine. In this quotation, you can see how strongly early biomedical physicians reacted against this label, which they viewed as amounting to the equivalent of a racial slur.

The use of biased language in the debate over medical pluralism remains prevalent. Consider the strong language used by editors of the *Journal of the American Medical Association* almost a century later: "There is no alternative medicine. There is only scientifically proven, evidence-based medicine supported by solid data" (Fontanarosa and Lundberg 1998, 1618). Sociologists studying medical pluralism must realize that cultural values are embedded in the labels people use to describe the social world. "Thus, all general descriptive terms for health belief systems, to be useful as descriptions rather than opinions, must be considered to be relative terms whose complete meaning can be derived only from an understanding of their contexts of use and their relationships to one another" (O'Connor 1995, 3). This means that in order to be unbiased, the sociological study of alternative medicine needs to be aware of ongoing power struggles between biomedical and alternative health belief systems.

In research concerning medical pluralism, it is now common to use the term **alternative medicine** to describe forms of health care that are used instead of biomedical care. For example, an individual might decide to treat her heart disease with homeopathic medication instead of using common medications such as cholesterol-lowering statin drugs. The term **complementary medicine** is applied to describe treatments that are used alongside biomedical care. As illustration, a person undergoing chemotherapy to treat cancer might also use aromatherapy to help control side effects such as nausea. Researchers commonly use the acronym CAM (complementary/alternative medicine) as a general term to describe alternative and complementary medicines without necessarily differentiating between them. Each of these labels has meanings attached to them that are important in struggles over health beliefs and healing practices. In her review of the sociology of CAM, Gale (2014, 816) points out that "the challenge to avoid reproducing biomedical dominance in terminology and analysis is vital."

Three Streams of Complementary Alternative Medicine Research

As Fries (2009) argues, research on alternative medicine, like alternative medicine itself, is a complex cultural activity and a diverse undertaking. He explains that "It is possible to think of research on CAM as proceeding along three different, but not necessarily incompatible, streams":

the medical stream, the epidemiological stream, and the social scientific stream (2009, 333). Furthermore, "within the medical sciences, there is a stream of research that is primarily concerned with establishing the safety and effectiveness of particular" CAM practices (2009, 333). Fries also points out that the main research method in this stream is the randomized control trial (RCT), and persons conducting this research are biomedical researchers whose work is guided by scientific thinking. The RCT is a scientific experiment that compares one group of patients who have received a treatment (i.e., the experimental group) with a group of patients who have not received the treatment (i.e., the control group). Fries (2009) explains that closely related to the medical stream of CAM research is a stream of epidemiological studies of CAM. In these studies, the focus is on using statistical methods to determine who uses which practices and with what results in order to begin the "plausibility-building process" (Hoffer 2003) that allows for scientific testing of the safety and effectiveness of CAM by medical researchers. The potential integration of CAM therapies into biomedical treatment is a central concern of these two streams of research (Fries 2008).

According to Fries (2009), the third stream of alternative medicine research involves researchers from the social and behavioural health sciences. He argues that the central concern here is with broader socio-cultural and psychosocial issues, such as the social and policy consequences of alternative medicine. While epidemiology is limited to describing who uses CAM, social scientists tackle the more difficult questions of why people use CAM and what are the consequences of medical pluralism for the pursuit of health and wellness. Outlining the usefulness of the social sciences in addressing these questions, Kelner and Wellman (2000, 3) describe the research agenda of social sciences regarding CAM as seeking "to clarify the social context in which CAM has created such popular interest. This includes explanations of who uses these therapies, why they choose to consult CAM practitioners and how they find their way to their offices [and] encompasses the key issues of research and policy in response to user demands." Gale (2014, 807) summarizes this growth of social scientific research concerning medical pluralism by describing how "In the last 15 years, there have been substantial empirical developments, including both quantitative studies exploring patterns of CAM usage and qualitative studies exploring patient experiences of using CAM."

Fries (2009) contends that data generated by any one of these research streams flow into a common pool of health information and are likely to have a bearing on research undertaken by the other two streams. However, he cautions that one should not assume the compatibility of research methods, goals, or perspectives. Much research conducted within the medical stream regards CAM with suspicion. Medical researchers, for instance, use scientific methods such as the RCT to question the safety and effectiveness of particular CAM treatments. Additionally, as we will learn at the end of this chapter, much research carried out in the medical and epidemiological streams has the ultimate goal of assimilating scientifically based alternative therapies within integrative medicine. Once a CAM treatment has been scientifically shown to be safe and effective, it is likely that the therapy will be adopted by biomedicine as part of clinical practice. For example, once acupuncture was found to be a safe and effective alternative for treatment of arthritic pain, biomedical physicians and allied health professionals, such as physiotherapists, began offering acupuncture stripped of its connections to traditional Chinese spirituality (Frank and Stollberg 2004). In summary, it is important to recognize that there are important differences between the three streams of alternative medicine research. The next section reviews explanations that the social scientific stream of CAM research has provided for the revival of medical pluralism.

Explanations for the Revival of Medical Pluralism

The revival of medical pluralism prompted the Institute of Medicine in the US to write that "To provide a rational, effective, efficient, and personally satisfactory health care system, it is important and useful to know who is using alternative therapies and why" (2005, vii). It has been relatively straightforward for researchers to conduct studies that identify the demographic characteristics of users of CAM. Typically, such research uses data from population health surveys to profile the users of CAM. Using data from the CCHS, Fries (2012) reports that 11.6 per cent of Canadians, or about 2.7 million people, had at least one consultation with chiropractors, the most popular CAM practice. Seven per cent of Canadians, or about 1.6 million people, used massage therapy. An estimated 2.3 per cent of Canadians, or approximately half a million people, consulted homeopaths or naturopaths. Acupuncturists were visited by 2.1 per cent of Canadians, or about half a million people. Other, lesser-known CAM practices in Canada include spiritual/religious healers (used by about 41 thousand Canadians), relaxation therapists (used by about 34 thousand Canadians), and biofeedback practitioners (used by about 6 thousand Canadians). Less than one-tenth of 1 per cent of Canadians consulted CAM practitioners such as Feldenkrais or Alexander technique teachers, Rolfers, herbalists, or reflexologists.

In general, social scientists also know how aspects of social location, such as gender, social class, and health status, influence the use of alternative medicine (Fries 2009; 2012). Fries (2012, 114) summarizes existing research findings by noting that "women marginally outnumber men as users; usage peaks in the West of North America; users are slightly more affluent, better educated, and have more chronic diseases than the general population; and the use of CAM is supplemental to biomedical health care." He argues that further research is needed to understand how these factors intersect to motivate the use of CAM. Simply stated, it has been much more difficult to explain why people use alternatives to biomedical health care than it has to describe who uses CAM. Social and behavioural scientists provide a wide range of plausible explanations for the revival of medical pluralism. These explanations can be grouped into four categories that we will summarize before presenting a sociological perspective on medical pluralism that synthesizes existing research findings (see Box 11.3).

The Demographic Transition and Population Aging

One explanation given for CAM's increasing popularity "has to do with a demographic transition underway in Western, industrialized societies" (Fries 2009, 334). More people are living to older

---

Box 11.3 Explanations for the Revival of Medical Pluralism

- The demographic transition and population aging
- Dissatisfaction with biomedicine
- The postmodern condition
- Individualization and consumerism

Source: Fries 2009.

ages, and as a result, there is increasing prevalence of chronic diseases, such as arthritis, rheumatism, and back and neck problems. Researchers argue that "biomedicine has insufficiently alleviated the pain and misery that goes along with chronic illness" and, consequently, "people are seeking health-care alternatives" (Fries 2009, 335). Fries goes on to note that "several studies report a connection between the use of these practices and prevalence of chronic illness, providing some evidence that the use of CAM is often an act of 'desperate pragmatism' (Fries and Menzies 2000) for those faced with debilitating effects of chronic disease" (Fries 2009, 335). In a more recent study of how older Canadians use CAM therapies to resist "the biomedicalization of aging," Fries (2014) found that his participants expressed a belief that CAM therapies are based on a more optimistic view of health and aging than biomedical approaches, which they felt often reduced aging to a process of inevitable deterioration.

Dissatisfaction with Biomedicine

A second, related explanation is the hypothesis that a general dissatisfaction with biomedicine is responsible for the increasing popularity of CAM (e.g., Furnham and Forey 1994; Ruggie 2004). According to this line of thought, people are increasingly dissatisfied with the impersonal and technological nature of the doctor–patient relationship, which under biomedicine is producing harmful effects. As Ruggie (2004, 45–6) explains:

> Scholarly studies and mass media reports tell us that patients have become dissatisfied with the quality of health care. Treatments are intrusive and overmedicalized; physicians speak in the fragmented and fragmenting language of biomedicine; and the disjuncture between medicine, which is oriented toward curing illness, and health care, which is oriented toward wellness and the prevention of illness, is deep and wide.

Central to this explanation is the idea that people are attracted to the preventive aspects of CAM, which focus on wellness rather than illness. However, Fries (2009) cautions that in evaluating this explanation, it must be remembered that dissatisfaction with the biomedical outlook should not be confused with disuse of biomedical health care. He points out that numerous studies (Astin 1998; Eisenberg et al. 1998; Fries and Menzies 2000) have shown that most often the use of CAM is supplemental to biomedical treatment. That is, most CAM users combine both alternative and biomedical health-care practices as part of their pursuit of health and wellness. Two recent Canadian studies (Fries 2013; 2014) found evidence that indicates users of CAM are dissatisfied with biomedicine. For instance, participants in Fries' (2014) narrative study told stories about how their parents suffered as they aged poorly under the care of biomedicine, relating this to their own use of CAM, while expressing concern regarding the potential harm caused by biomedical treatments. CAM therapies were valued as providing what was viewed as a more natural and less risky way of caring for health issues.

The Postmodern Condition

A third explanation for the growing popularity of CAM is connected to a cultural suspicion of expert knowledge (such as biomedicine). It is argued that cultural skepticism toward expert knowledge, theorized to be characteristic of the "postmodern condition" (Lyotard 1979, xxiii) of contemporary societies, is linked to rejection of science and the underlying system of belief upon which biomedicine is based. "Researchers argue that under such postmodern cultural conditions, people view nature and natural as holistic, spiritual, and safe in contradiction to what are perceived as the scientific and technological risks associated with biomedicine" (Fries 2009, 335). An early study by Astin (1998) found that patients report similarity between their beliefs and the philosophy of alternative medicine as a reason for using such therapies. In his words, Astin (1998, 1548) explains that "Alternative medicine users appear to be doing so not so much as a result of being dissatisfied with conventional medicine but largely because they find these health care alternatives to be more congruent with their own values, beliefs, and philosophical orientations toward health and life." Fries' (2013, 42) study of a group of users of CAM whom he, following the comments of one of his participants, terms "high performance humans," finds support for this explanation: "The disposition of the high performance human habitus is to assume personal responsibility for the co-production of health and distinguishing oneself as healthy in a postmodern sense that transcends Cartesian boundaries of body and mind; a work of art fully realised in body, mind, and spirit."

Individualization and Consumerism

Finally, other researchers (e.g., Cant and Sharma 1999; Lupton 1997b; Kelner and Wellman 1997) have explained CAM's "increasing popularity by pointing to expansion of capitalist consumer society that, in a neoliberal context, is producing more individually oriented" medical consumers who "seek out health-care products and services from a wide market of" health-care choices (Fries 2009, 335). The idea is that consumers of CAM have accepted individual responsibility for their health and, while distrustful of biomedicine, find CAM reassuring. "At a macro level, the capitalist state supports these cultural transformations in the hopes of containing escalating health-care costs and as a means of demonstrating its legitimacy in culturally diverse societies by granting a degree of recognition to medical pluralism" (Fries 2009, 335). According to this explanation, the increasing popularity of CAM may, at least in part, be connected to the medicalization critique discussed in the previous chapter in that people use CAM in an effort to take back control of their bodies and lives. In a cultural context that encourages individual patient empowerment and medical consumerism, the use of CAM may be attributable to what Beck, Giddens, and Lash (1994) have outlined as the "reflexive project of the self."

Beck (1992) argues that scientific development has produced wealth and prosperity, but at the cost of risk. Calculation of the probability of risk has become an essential feature of contemporary social life: according to Beck, we are living in the "risk society." Faced with this risk, people begin to exhibit "reflexive modernization" (Beck, Giddens, and Lash 1994) in which they question scientific authority. As part of reflexive modernization, people actively seek out alternative knowledge and technologies (such as CAM) to counter the insecurities brought about by scientific modernization. In a "network society" (Castells 1996), it is easier than ever before for people to gain information concerning their health and learn about various forms of treatment, using the Internet to shop for health-care alternatives.

As Lupton (1997b) has demonstrated, medical consumerism is a good fit with the reflexive project of the self in that people use health-care choices to help construct their sense of body and self. According to this explanation, this environment of individual responsibility, consumerism, and an overload of information combines with an increasing emphasis on wellness (Sointu 2005) and not health care to explain why so many are turning toward CAM. In trying to live up to the cultural pressure to be healthy, consumers seek out CAM.

In summary, the question "why do people use alternatives to biomedical care?" is a complex sociological question with many possible answers. Further, as the World Health Organization (2001) points out, CAM is an increasingly global phenomenon. This suggests that the revival of medical pluralism can be explained in reference to the cultural diversity of contemporary societies. The next section describes how the revival of medical pluralism is related to the growth of cultural diversity in countries such as Canada.

Crossing Cultures in Pursuit of Health and Wellness: Choosing Healing Practices

According to Quah (2008, 419), the pursuit of health takes people on a journey that crosses cultures in search of wellness:

> When disease strikes the most immediate reaction is to seek a solution: How to stop this? How to get well again? Then comes the intriguing part: How did I get this problem, and why me? Research findings in medical sociology and anthropology over the past five to six decades show these to be virtually primordial questions, irrespective of geographical location, lifestyle, and ethnic, religious, linguistic or other background. While the questions tend to be the same, the answers vary widely, as they are fashioned precisely by people's location, way of life, socio-cultural, religious, linguistic, and other differences. More importantly, amidst the rainbows of healing options and solutions, one trend predominates: people do cross cultural boundaries in search of a cure or in their quest for the proverbial fountain of youth.

Quah calls this crossing of cultures "**pragmatic acculturation**," which she defines as "the borrowing of ideas, ways of thinking or ways of doing things from a culture that is not your own, for the purpose of solving a particular problem" (2008, 419). In the case of medical pluralism, the particular problem requiring solution is the mystery of health, and evidence is mounting that increasing cultural diversity means that people are able to cross cultures in search of healing in ways never before possible. Box 11.4 provides an example of the cultural mixing and matching that characterizes some people's pursuit of health and wellness.

Health sociologists have long recognized that aspects of social location, such as socioeconomic status, gender, ethnicity, and stage of the life course, work together to inform people's choices of health-care practices. We also know that some people have social locations that present them with a wide diversity of cultural beliefs and practices. Perhaps they are wealthy and can afford to travel to far-off destinations or have a social network of friends from different ethnic backgrounds who share aspects of other cultures with them. Maybe they have a taste for foreign art, cinema, literature, music, clothing, or food. As a result of experience with other cultures, they might learn about health belief systems that originate within different cultural traditions and diverse ethnic heritages. It follows that cultural diversity is particularly important to examine as a factor in the revival of medical pluralism, because the context of alternative medicine's rising popularity is a global society characterized by increasing intermingling of cultures. Such cultural exchanges play an important part in the revival of medical pluralism in Western society (Fries 2006). The next section explains how cultural diversity offers people a way to cross cultures in pursuit of health and wellness.

Box 11.4 Crossing Cultures in Pursuit of Health and Wellness

On 8 October 2009, three people died and 18 more were hospitalized after participating in a healing practice led by alternative medicine and spiritual guru James Ray. The victims participated in a New Age version of a traditional Native American healing ceremony known as a "sweat lodge." Each paid $9000 USD for a five-day retreat called "Spiritual Warrior," which ended tragically when Ray crowded approximately 60 already dehydrated participants into the makeshift sweat lodge, with temperatures inside reaching 53 degrees Celsius. Why would anyone participate in such an extreme healing practice? Contrary to stereotypes of marginality, James Ray's clients were not uneducated or in some other way underprivileged or ignorant of modern biomedicine. Rather, the participants were financially well-off and well educated, with successful occupations, such as financial advisor, real estate agent, and rancher. Despite their privileged social locations (or perhaps because of them), these people placed their health and wellness in the hands of an alternative healer, and some lost their lives as a result. The question for health sociologists is, what is it about their social locations that led these individuals to cross cultures and participate in a blend of New Age mysticism and traditional practices, which James Ray has become rich and famous marketing as healing?

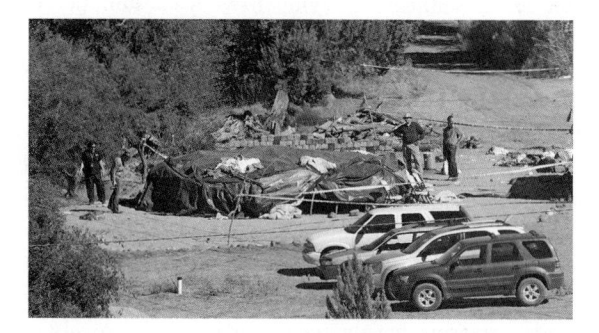

Investigators examine the sweat lodge at Ray's retreat.

From *The Arizona Republic* © Gannett-Community Publishing. All rights reserved. Used by permission and protected by the Copyright Laws of the United States. The printing, copying, redistribution, or retransmission of this Content without express written permission is prohibited.

Medical Consumerism, the Marketing of Ethnicity, and the Revival of Medical Pluralism

We have learned that our society is characterized by consumer culture and medical consumerism. In consumer culture, goods and services are used as expressions of personal identity. This is especially the case for health-care products and services because they are so closely connected with embodiment. We saw how individualized health promotion encourages people to become health-conscious medical consumers who accept personal responsibility for fashioning healthy lifestyles. Medical consumerism encourages people to shop around for ways to look after their health while also expressing their personal identity. Meanwhile, living in the "risk society"

(Beck 1992) leads people to become distrustful of science and preoccupied with global health risks and how they can protect themselves (e.g., Beck, Giddens, and Lash 1994). As part of cultural distrust of science and technology, biomedical treatments such as surgery and pharmaceutical drugs are increasingly regarded with suspicion. For example, many drugs have serious side effects and seem "unnatural" and, hence, dangerous. These factors motivate people to search for alternative ways of pursuing health and healing.

At the same time, cultural diversity exposes people to a vast range of products and services connected to other cultures. Halter (2000, 12) describes how cultural diversity has led to an "ethnic revival" in which ethnicity offers a way of anchoring a sense of self-identity "amid the vast and chaotic landscapes of consumption." She explains how "the marketing of ethnicity" has become commonplace in the consumer culture of culturally diverse societies: increasingly, we are sold goods and services on the basis of their connection to particular cultures. Think, for example, of cultural beliefs such as "the best cars are German-engineered," "the French produce the best red wines," or "rich Italian leather." Cultural diversity allows people to shop for a sense of identity by purchasing goods and services that are "authentic" and rooted in "tradition." In this process of "shopping for identity" (Halter 2000), "authentic" is symbolized by consumption of products and services linked to ethnocultural traditions.

This is also the case for alternative medicine. Much has been made of the promise of alternative medicine and the holistic approach to health that its supporters contend it represents to reconnect us with forgotten spiritual dimensions of humanity. We're always hearing how alternative medicine is supposed to be more "holistic," "natural," and "authentic" than biomedical treatment. As illustrated by Box 11.5, those marketing alternative medical products and services are aware of the desirability that ethnic tradition has in multicultural societies.

From the global trade in culture, we learn that different cultures offer alternative ways of understanding health, illness, and the body. We also learn about alternative forms of healing originating within other cultures. It stands to reason that the increasing cultural diversity of multicultural societies exposes people to medical knowledge and health beliefs from other cultures. Some choose to use these cultural traditions in pursuit of health and wellness. In this way,

Box 11.5 Medical Consumerism and the Marketing of Ethnicity

Marketers for Lakota™ herbal medicines realize the appeal of combining traditional ethnic knowledge with science. The advertisements for Lakota™, which feature Native American actor Floyd Red Crow Westerman of *Dances with Wolves* fame, state, "Based on traditional native remedies, and supplemented with modern science, Lakota is effective, natural source medicine for arthritis pain." As the media backgrounder for Lakota™ explains, "Lakota is a key Canadian player in the burgeoning health and wellness industry. Health and wellness is differentiated from the 'sickness' industry due to its focus on preventative medicine from natural sources versus manufactured medicine designed to only treat existing sickness and disease" (available online at www.lakotaherbs.com/PDF/backgrounder-e.pdf). Ethnicity is used as a way to market products and services, including health care.

the revival of medical pluralism is connected to multiculturalism. Fries (2013) shows that some individuals in multicultural societies such as Canada are fashioning a secure sense of self by employing non-Western cultural traditions in their pursuit of health. Ruggie (2004, 73) speculates that "perhaps modern individuals are better equipped to recognize that both medicine and CAM have special roles in treating their bodies. Perhaps people are responding to their options by picking and choosing for themselves the therapies they believe will best satisfy their needs." The picking and choosing of healing practices that Ruggie describes has become a definable feature of contemporary social life in multicultural societies.

People's beliefs about health, illness, and the body draw upon the cultural diversity associated with contemporary global society. Consider the following from an interview conducted by one of your authors (Fries 2006) with a young woman whose pursuit of health includes CAM:

> Chinese Medicine is amazing in terms of their depth of knowledge and of the body system . . . anything coming from China and the Indian therapy I believe in. . . . Because they have a history, thousands and thousands of years of doctors and professionals working in that area. And, because they look at the mind, body, and spirit connection, and because they're very sophisticated. They work; they're very effective. I have done a bit with the Chinese, acupuncture worked. Chinese Medicine totally worked for me for instance in helping me quit smoking. I also went to see an Ayurveda doctor from India who works with the idea of looking at what and how much you eat and when, and your activities, and your blood pressure. It's very holistic! (Christine, 32, adult educator)

For such individuals, ethnicity is a source of cultural capital used in constructing cultural meanings, such as what counts as healing. In his study of ethnoculture as a symbolic resource used in the negotiation of alternative medicine as cure, Fries (2005) draws upon Appadurai's (1996) post-colonial theory and Bourdieu's concept of the habitus to argue that in multicultural societies, people creatively use ethnoculture to shape their habitus. He (2005, 94) explains how "cultural changes attending the emergence and development of contemporary, consumer society in the West have facilitated the emergence of new identities surrounding health and illness issues. Due to the centrality of ethnicity in the development of these new societal forms, one of the sites at which the effects of this identity construction can be readily observed is in the differing symbolic constructions of those therapeutic practices viewed as legitimate, efficacious, or cure." This symbolic process provides individuals with "a strategy that serves as an anchor in coping with health risks in an evolving postmodern environment" (Cockerham, Rütten, and Abel 1997, 338). Postmodern health belief systems exhibit a blend of beliefs and healing practices derived from both biomedical and alternative health-care systems in pursuit of health and wellness.

Astin (1998) found that those described as "cultural creatives" were significantly more likely to use CAM. In describing social practices of cultural creatives, Ray (1997, 31) highlights development of a "Trans-Modern world view" associated with the development of cultural diversity, listing spirituality and love of the exotic among the values held by these individuals (Ray and Anderson 2000). This is further evidence that the revival of medical pluralism may be explained by increasing cultural diversity associated with global consumer culture. Data from the *Ethnic Diversity Survey* (Statistics Canada 2003) show that just over half of Canadians report the importance of their ethnic ancestry and about 63 per cent of these people, or 6.5 million Canadians, say that maintaining ethnic customs and traditions is important. The current context is clearly one in which the increasing cultural diversity described by Appadurai (1996) is an important element in people's crossing cultures in pursuit of health and wellness. As the next section discusses, efforts to create a new medicine that integrates CAM and biomedicine are motivated by these cultural developments.

Integrative Medicine: Prospects for a New Medicine

Given that different cultures offer different ways of understanding health, illness, and the body, perhaps it makes sense to combine various health belief systems in pursuit of health and wellness. This is the basic rationale behind efforts to develop integrative medicine. **Integrative medicine** is a form of health care that brings together CAM treatments that have been scientifically proven safe and effective with conventional biomedical treatments. Lambert (2002, 46, original emphasis) offers the following explanation of the significance of the changing labels applied to CAM: "In the last few years, the term 'alternative,' suggesting something done *instead of* conventional medicine, has been giving way to 'complementary,' a therapy done *along with* mainstream treatment. Both words may ultimately be replaced by 'integrative medicine'—the use of techniques like acupuncture, massage, herbal treatments, and meditation in regular medical practice." As Baer and Coulter (2008, 331) explain, "Whereas alternative medicine is often defined as functioning outside biomedicine and complementary medicine beside it, integrative medicine purports to combine the best of both biomedicine and CAM." Supporters of integrative medicine argue that biomedicine would benefit from incorporation of some of CAM's ideas and practices. Integrative medicine rests upon three central beliefs:

- Health is a holistic phenomenon.
- Healing relationships should be patient/client–centred.
- Treatments must be evidence-based.

The first belief is that health is a holistic phenomenon that includes not only biophysical elements but also psychological, social, and even spiritual aspects. **Holism** is an approach to understanding the world that views whole entities as made up of more than the sum of their parts. Integrative medicine is a holistic approach that considers health to be produced by complex interaction of biological, psychological, social, and spiritual factors. According to the holistic philosophy of integrative medicine, health can't be understood by looking at one of these elements in isolation from the others. The holism of integrative medicine distinguishes its conception of health from the reductionism that underlies the biomedical approach. As supporters of integrative medicine explain, "Integrative medicine represents a higher-order system of systems of care that emphasizes wellness and healing of the entire person (bio-psycho-socio-spiritual dimensions) as primary goals, drawing upon both conventional and CAM approaches in the context of a supportive and effective physician–patient relationship" (Bell et al. 2002, 133). In this way, supporters of integrative medicine maintain that physicians need to consider the whole patient: mind, body, and spirit, as well as environment and society. There is a belief in the **mind–body connection**—the idea that biophysical health is linked to mental states such as emotions and stress. This holistic approach to healing is one of the main characteristics that define integrative medicine.

The second central belief of integrative medicine is that healing relationships between physicians and patients should be "client-centred." Boon and colleagues (2004, 51) explain that in "integrative health care," "there is an emphasis on the role and responsibility of the patient for her/his own health, as well as a need to include patient participation, preferences and self-knowledge when designing any treatment plan." In the integrative medical vision, it is the individual medical consumer who directs the healing relationship; gone are the days of the passive patient giving herself over blindly to medical authority. Explaining the centrality of the individual medical consumer for integrative medicine, Fries (2008, 361) claims that "The autonomous individual of neoliberalism is the focal point for emerging integrative therapies." According to the model proposed by integrative medicine, physicians are to act as expert guides to patients/clients, who make their own treatment decisions on the basis of information provided by their doctors.

The third defining belief of integrative medicine is a commitment to an "evidence-based" approach to incorporating CAM therapies within biomedicine (e.g., Jonas 2002). This means that only therapies tested by scientific methods associated with the RCT are considered suitable for integration. Only when CAM therapies have been scientifically demonstrated to be safe and effective are they considered "evidence-based"—despite the irony remarked upon by Baer (2004, 155) that "it is important to note that many biomedical procedures and techniques have not been subjected to RCTs and that aspirin and penicillin were widely used before research scientists determined how they work." Fries (2005, 93) draws upon Bourdieu's theoretical perspective to demonstrate how the RCT has been used by biomedicine for the purposes of the "symbolic domination of the medical field." He points out that CAM therapies that can be readily evaluated by scientific methods are most suitable for incorporation into integrative medicine, while those that rest on non-scientific belief systems are likely to be rejected by biomedicine. In this way, biomedicine uses the standards of science to determine what counts as legitimate healing and which practices should be integrated with biomedical health care.

Integrative medicine seems to present a positive vision of the new medicine. This is because, like a sociological perspective on health, integrative medicine seems well suited to understanding the multi-dimensional nature of health. However, as Fries (2008, 353) explains, "From a sociological perspective, 'integrative medicine' is a term as politically charged as it is culturally loaded." The integration of CAM therapies into biomedical practice is a contentious subject. While CAM is regarded with suspicion by some biomedical researchers and physicians, others suggest that it makes sense to integrate medical knowledge from alternative and complementary health belief systems into Western biomedical practice. As illustration, supporters of integrative medicine, such as Snyderman and Weil (2002, 396), argue that integrative medicine offers a way to "bring medicine back to its roots" through "restoration of the focus of medicine on health and healing" rather than focusing on treatment of biophysical disease. In contrast, other physicians, such as Relman, argue that "Integrating alternative medicine with mainstream medicine would not be an advance but a return to the past, an interruption of the remarkable progress achieved by science-based medicine over the past century" (Relman and Weil 1999, 2122). Given this ongoing debate, what are the prospects for the future of integrative medicine?

In a critical analysis of integrative medicine, Hollenberg (2006) uses a theoretical perspective grounded in the sociology of Max Weber to study interactions between biomedical and CAM practitioners in integrative health-care settings. Based on ethnographic and document analysis, he reports that, contrary to ideals of integration, in reality biomedical physicians exercise professional dominance over CAM practitioners in such settings through monopolizing medical records, referrals, and diagnostic testing; selectively appropriating CAM therapies; and using biomedical jargon as a means of excluding CAM practitioners. Hollenberg (2006, 742) concludes that "Western biomedicine continues to maintain its dominance in Integrative Health Care settings." Baer and Coulter (2008, 337–8) reach a similar conclusion, noting that "It appears that biomedicine, governments, and various corporate entities have domesticated holistic health as a popular movement and transformed it initially into CAM and more recently integrative medicine, a system in which certain heterodox therapies often function as adjuncts to the arsenal of high-tech approaches." Baer (2004, 149) concludes that "despite the best efforts on the part of proponents of holistic health to develop an alternative to biomedicine, what in reality has occurred has been in large part the co-optation of alternative medicine under the rubrics of CAM and integrative medicine or integrative health care." In other words, it seems clear that biomedicine continues to dominate CAM in the formal health-care system.

Numerous factors support the continued dominance of biomedicine in health care. Among these factors is that while governments fund biomedical health care, consumers have to pay for CAM therapies either out of their own pocket or with private health insurance. For example, Hollenberg (2007) notes that while biomedical care in Canada is funded through medicare, CAM remains a private service paid for by the patient/client. He contends that this financial reality poses a significant obstacle to further development of integrative medicine. Another factor in the dominance of biomedicine has to do with the power of provincial Colleges of Physicians and Surgeons to safeguard their monopoly in formal health care. Based on interviews with integrative health-care clinicians, Gaboury and colleagues (2009) report that this inhibits collaboration between biomedical and CAM practitioners. Cant and Sharma (1999, 432–3) conclude that "biomedicine is still the most powerful single health-care profession and is unlikely to cease to be so: those forms of alternative medicine that have been most successful in terms of gaining greater public recognition and legitimacy are, on the whole, those that had the approval of a sizeable section of the medical profession."

Additionally, Lupton (1997b) points out that not all patients are willing to give up the security that comes with the role of passive patient in favour of adopting a more client-centred approach that places them in charge of health care. She argues that the highly emotional nature of illness means that some patients are more than willing to happily accept the authority of biomedical experts. Finally, Ruggie (2004, 197) explains that despite consumer demand for alternatives to biomedical treatment, "directors of integrative clinics admit . . . that their ventures are not money making enterprises." As a business model, the integration of CAM and biomedical therapies is rarely profitable—a fact attested to by the many integrative health-care clinics in both the United States and Canada that go out of business. For integrative medicine to become a fully realized vision of a new medicine, governments will have to be convinced to foot the bill. This is unlikely, given the efforts governments in both countries have made to slow health-care spending. Factors such as these limit prospects for integrative medicine.

The extent to which supporters of integrative medicine achieve their stated goal of "transforming healthcare by returning the soul to medicine" (Bravewell Collaborative 2009) will be related to how such a transformation fits with broader social and cultural changes. Indeed, with more than 100 integrative health-care clinics in the United States and 31 in Canada, some success in the development of integrative medicine has taken place (Gaboury et al. 2009). Supporters of integrative medicine are quick to point out that this vision of future health care fits with demands made by a growing number of medical consumers. As illustration, Snyderman and Weil (2002, 396) explain that "integrative medicine is the term being used for a new movement that is being driven by the desires of consumers." However, in a critical sociological analysis, Fries (2008, 354) views integrative medicine in Foucauldian terms as an aspect of medicalization—in his words, "integrative medicine represents an expansion of medical rationality into all domains of human life: biological, psychological, sociological and spiritual. This proposed expansion of medical influence rests not upon domination but rather, through enabling the autonomous individual at the centrepiece of neoliberal governance." He argues that although integrative medicine appears to have initially emerged in the United States and the United Kingdom, it has spread to other countries as a "consequence of transnational cultural flows." From a sociological perspective, rather than viewing sources of disease or illness as rooted in social structural forces, integrative medicine reflects the cultural value of individual responsibility for health, thus contributing to turning health care into a commodity, consistent with a growing global neo-liberal agenda.

Chapter Summary

In this chapter, a sociological perspective on health and healing allowed us to explore the issue of medical pluralism. We saw that just as health can be understood as a social construction, so too can healing. An individual's understanding of what counts as healing is shaped by location and experiences in the social world. Similarly, different cultures give rise to varying ways of understanding health and healing. In a sociological perspective, health belief systems are seen as shaped by culture. Although biomedicine has become the dominant health-care system in the West, globally and historically a diversity of health beliefs and health-care systems has persisted. There are numerous healing traditions and health-care systems that were not displaced by modern medicine and have been used for centuries to prevent and treat illness. Despite the dominance of biomedicine in the West, people are increasingly using alternative therapies in pursuit of health and wellness. Power struggles over alternative medicine underscore the importance of paying close attention to the labels used to describe forms of medical knowledge and practice. It makes clear the need for critical social studies of medical pluralism to avoid relying on "stereotypes of marginality" in explaining the growing popularity of alternative medicine.

Scientists study alternative medicine from a number of different perspectives that can be grouped into three research streams: medical science, epidemiology, and social science. Each of these streams has its own research goals and methods. A review of the explanations that social scientists have provided for the revival of medical pluralism shows that alternative medicine is a complex sociological issue whose understanding requires the application of sociological theory. Theories that explore increasing cultural diversity help us to understand why some individuals are more likely to cross cultures in pursuit of health and wellness and are therefore attracted to alternative medicine. As part of their exposure to other cultures, some people learn about different health belief and healing systems. Multiculturalism means that it is becoming easier for people to cross cultures. Globalization and migration have the effect of moving diverse forms of medical knowledge and practice all over the globe. In this way, trends toward medical consumerism and "the marketing of ethnicity" help to explain the popularity of alternative medicine. Alternative medicine is increasingly being marketed on the basis of its connection to ethnocultural traditions as an option to biomedical health beliefs and practices. Thus, cultural diversity is contributing to the revival of medical pluralism.

In a multicultural context, supporters of integrative medicine argue that it makes sense to use medical knowledge and practices of other cultures to help create a new medicine combining the best features of various health belief systems within biomedicine. They are trying to integrate the holism of other belief systems with the scientific ethos of biomedicine. However, efforts to develop integrative medicine are hotly debated. There are powerful indications that biomedicine will remain the culturally dominant formal health-care system in the West. Further, health sociologists have pointed out that there are drawbacks associated with development of integrative medicine, including the way it encourages individualization of the pursuit of health and wellness. The vision that integrative medicine offers for a new medicine directs our attention to questions of health-care policies and practices intended to achieve healthy futures.

Study Questions

1. Why is the idea that health is a social construction particularly useful for sociological studies of medical pluralism?
2. Explain how healing is socially constructed.
3. Explain "stereotypes of marginality" and why they must be avoided in social studies of alternative medicine.
4. Why do health sociologists studying medical pluralism need to pay attention to language used to describe forms of medical knowledge and practice?
5. Explain the different research streams that investigate CAM.
6. What explanations have been given by social scientists for the revival of medical pluralism?
7. Comment critically on the relationship between medical consumerism, the marketing of ethnicity, and the use of CAM.
8. Explain the three central beliefs of integrative medicine.
9. Critically evaluate the development of integrative medicine from a sociological perspective.

Recommended Readings

Baer, H. 2004. *Toward an Integrative Medicine: Merging Alternative Therapies with Biomedicine.* Walnut Creek, CA: AltaMira Press.

Fries, C.J. 2009. "Bourdieu's reflexive sociology as a theoretical basis for mixed methods research: An application to complementary and alternative medicine." *Journal of Mixed Methods Research* 3: 326–48.

Kelner, M., and B. Wellman. 2000. *Complementary Alternative Medicine: Challenge and Change.* New York: Harwood Academic Publishers.

Low, J. 2004. *Using Alternative Therapies: A Qualitative Analysis.* Toronto: Canadian Scholars Press.

O'Connor, B. 1995. *Healing Traditions: Alternative Medicine and the Health Professions.* Philadelphia: University of Pennsylvania Press.

Ruggie, M. 2004. *Marginal to Mainstream: Alternative Medicine in America.* New York: Cambridge University Press.

Recommended Website

National Center for Complementary and Alternative Medicine (US):
http://nccam.nih.gov

Recommended Audiovisual Sources

"The Alternative Fix," "Frontline." PBS video, 2003.
"The New Medicine," "Frontline." PBS video, 2006.

"Vaccines - Calling the Shots," "Nova." PBS video, 2014.

Achieving Healthy Futures

12

Learning Objectives

This final chapter summarizes key issues discussed throughout the book and critical components of a sociological analysis of healthy societies and healthy people, concluding with a discussion of unresolved issues regarding the prospects for achieving healthy futures. The first section includes a summary of

- alternative sociological paradigms for studying health;
- an intersectional model of health across the life course;
- a mixed-methods approach to measuring the dimensions of health;
- social determinants of health; and
- sources of social inequality and health disparities.

The chapter then comments critically on personal, professional, and public responsibility for health, briefly considering examples of policy initiatives that have the goal of improving population health and wellness. The chapter ends with a cautionary note regarding the importance of understanding the whole iceberg of health care and the complex multi-dimensional process involved in the pursuit of health and wellness and raises some unanswered questions about the differences between

- the vision of a healthy society and the reality of health-care reform;
- understanding the social reproduction of health inequalities and reducing them;
- formulating and implementing healthy public policies that address the social determinants of health;
- health as a personal and societal value and wellness as a virtue; and
- the medicalized society and a salutogenic society.

Toward a Sociological Understanding of Healthy Societies and Healthy People

The pursuit of health and wellness is a fundamental aspect of everyday social life and is, consequently, an important topic for sociological analysis. Throughout the book, it was argued that it is essential to recognize that health is a social construct if we hope to be able to unravel the mystery of good health and gain a greater appreciation of salutary factors that contribute to population health and wellness. A salutogenic model of health was introduced to focus attention on exploring the meaning of good health and social conditions that influence the pursuit of health and wellness. The discussion highlighted the need to learn more about social determinants of health and ways in which people manage to protect health and stay well. From a sociological perspective, health is understood not merely as a biophysical state experienced in the same manner by all people in all times and places but, rather, as a socially constructed life course experience varying over time according to different social, cultural, and economic life circumstances.

Developing a sociological imagination was recommended as a way of gaining insight into the relationship between healthy societies and healthy people. A sociological imagination helps us to understand the dual process by which societal structures (such as health-care institutions and professional providers of formal care) influence individual behaviour (such as personal health practices and informal self-health management) and, in turn, how social behaviours reproduce structural components of society. The idea that society shapes and is shaped by human behaviour is a basic aspect of sociological theory. An improved sociological understanding of the connection between healthy societies and healthy people requires not only more theoretically oriented approaches to studying the pursuit of health and wellness but also careful elaboration of an intersectional life course model that captures the complex, multi-dimensional nature of health as well as the application of mixed methods that take into account both quantitative and qualitative factors when measuring the dimensions of health.

Studying Health: Alternative Sociological Paradigms

Dunn (2006) argues that there is still a need to develop a better social theoretical foundation to guide population health research. He contends that a theoretically informed approach is necessary if population health research is to meet the many challenges it faces, including explaining how people manage to stay well and the systematic differential distribution of health and illness based on social location. There are a number of theoretical paradigms that sociologists employ to guide studies of health and illness. Depending on the paradigm selected, sociologists make certain assumptions about how the social world works and the basic relationship between the individual and society, focus on selective aspects of social life, formulate specific research questions, and use particular methods to investigate behaviour.

For example, they can draw on traditional theoretical perspectives. According to the structural functionalist paradigm, health and illness can be understood as social roles (e.g., the sick role). For the conflict paradigm, health and illness are viewed as professional constructs that result from power struggles between competing interest groups. Symbolic interactionists understand health and illness as interpersonal meanings, since people socially construct the reality of their lived experience in society through interaction with others. Alternatively, research may be guided by more contemporary theoretical perspectives such as: feminist social theory and a focus on health and illness as gendered experience; the sociology of the body paradigm, which highlights the importance of understanding health and illness as embodied cultural facts; or the life course perspective, which understands health and illness as unfolding across time.

All of these theoretical paradigms contribute in different ways to our understanding of connections between healthy societies and healthy people. Each paradigm provides a unique conceptual framework or way of thinking and methodological guidelines for applying the sociological imagination to the study of health and illness. It is important to recognize, however, that they are not mutually exclusive and that population health is too complex to be explained by any one theoretical paradigm. Consequently, this book has adopted an eclectic approach for examining the pursuit of health and wellness. Despite differences in the central concepts emphasized by each paradigm, it is possible to build theoretical links between constructs, such as social roles, power, conflict, inequality, and interpersonal meanings, and engage in a comprehensive intersectional analysis of the gendered and embodied experience of health and illness across the life course. In other words, greater theoretical integration is required to account for the many interacting social factors that over time influence the pursuit of health and wellness.

Developing an Intersectional Model of Health across the Life Course

To unravel the mystery of health, we need to formulate an intersectional model reflecting the fact that health disparities result from the dynamic interplay of life chances and life choices across the life course. Better understanding of the complex, dynamic processes by which differing social locations intersect with aspects of individual lived experience to shape population health requires an expanded theoretical framework. The evidence clearly demonstrates that social location affects life chances, including chances of being healthy or becoming sick. One's position in society, based on the combined effects of factors such as socioeconomic status, gender, ethnicity, and age, can have positive or negative impacts on health depending on the ways in which these structures of inequality intersect with other determinants of health, such as lifestyle behaviours. From the perspective of intersectional analysis, health-related lifestyles and life choices provide a conceptual link between societal factors, such as social location, and individual behaviours that collectively influence population health.

An intersectional model of health across the life course, such as that outlined in this book, highlights the ways that individual differences in health are socially produced over time by wider sources of inequality within society. The central component of this model is a conception of health as a biosocial reality that emerges from intersecting biological and social contexts. To illustrate, biological development occurs in a particular socio-cultural environment, and these factors collectively shape our health. The intersectional life course model of health also emphasizes the theoretical importance of understanding the direct effects that life chances associated with structures of inequality have on health, the part that habitus plays in mediating effects of social structure (life chances) and agency (life choices), health lifestyles as a collective rather than an individual phenomenon and a vital mechanism through which structure and agency together contribute to health, and the interaction effects of social structural, behavioural, and psychosocial factors.

Adding a life course perspective to the intersectional model helps us to unravel the mystery of health and gain greater insight into the impact of various intersecting determinants on health disparities. An intersectional life course approach enables researchers to better understand ways in which social determinants of health (such as socioeconomic status, gender, and ethnicity) function at every stage of development and to explain the ways these intersecting forces operate over time to shape population health. In other words, adopting a life course perspective in health research makes it possible to gauge time lags that occur between cause and effect and to identify causal factors that result in both immediate and long-term health outcomes. For example, the socioeconomic life circumstances we experience during childhood or gender differences in smoking during adolescence may not have immediate negative effects on health, but they may be related to chronic health problems in later life. Similarly, the healthy immigrant effect changes over time. An increasing number of researchers are using a life course approach in their studies of social inequalities (e.g. Halfon 2012; Pavalko and Caputo 2013). Several decades of research have documented the ways in which SES disparities in health unfold over time and how social inequalities in health persist across the life course. Consequently, "it is now well understood that life course factors affect a diverse range of outcomes, from general well-being to physical functioning and chronic diseases" (Hertzman and Power 2006, 87).

Thus, it is important to recognize that the contribution of structural factors to disparities in health varies at different stages of the life course. Evidence suggests that people experience structures of social inequality, such as class, gender, and ethnicity, differently depending on their age. An intersectional life course analysis (of longitudinal data) clarifies the causal linkages between social location and health disparities and facilitates a better understanding of the cumulative impact on health that results from experiences across the life course and the multiple pathways through which social determinants intersect over time and influence healthy societies and healthy people. An important next step in the process of unravelling the mystery of health is undertaking studies guided by an intersectional life course model to gain greater insight into the complex pathways involved in the social production of health.

Measuring the Dimensions of Health: A Mixed-Methods Approach

Each of the alternative sociological paradigms provides methodological guidelines that influence ideas about the best measures to use in collecting evidence to help unravel the mystery of health. For example, if we consider health to be an objective state of being that is primarily the outcome of biophysical factors, we tend to rely on quantitative methods recommended by the structural functionalist paradigm to assess population health (e.g., official statistics and population health surveys). In contrast, if health is viewed as part of an ongoing process with socially constructed subjective meanings, as suggested by the symbolic interactionist and sociology of the body paradigms, then we generally rely on qualitative methods to measure the dimensions of health (e.g., health diaries and illness narrative accounts). In each case, the central concepts that exemplify the paradigms have to be theoretically specified in order to be able to assess the health of the population.

This book recommends a salutogenic approach to measuring the dimensions of health to ensure that the salutary factors that protect and promote good health are included (as well as the risk factors that contribute to the onset of diseases and illness). Looking at the dimensions of health through a salutogenic lens focuses attention on the meaning of good health and measurement of social factors that influence the pursuit of health and wellness. If we are to be successful at defining and measuring good health (wellness) and ill health (sickness) as separate entities, we need to acknowledge that although these two dimensions are related, they represent different aspects of health. Recognizing that separate movement in either direction on the good health and ill health dimensions is possible and that health status is the result of dynamic social processes enables us to better solve the mystery of health. However, the multi-dimensional nature of health raises a number of methodological challenges that need to be addressed when it comes to measurement.

An improved sociological understanding of population health requires mixed-methods approaches to measurement, incorporating various types of information and multi-level analysis of the many interconnected aspects of society and individual behaviour that shape health. In other words, intersectional analysis calls for the use of mixed-methods research designs, employing both qualitative and quantitative measures, to assess the intersecting dimensions of social location, behavioural patterns, and health across the life course.

There are a number of sources of information that reflect the health of the population, including surveys, statistics, and stories. For example, population health surveys collect extensive details regarding personal practices such as smoking and physical activities, administrative databases contain hospital and medical use statistics, and census and vital statistics include information on death rates. While these sources reveal a wealth of quantitative information about the health status of the population, counting prevalence and incidence of disease or calculating morbidity and mortality rates or even smoking rates and daily energy expenditure is not the same as giving people the opportunity to account for their health and illness experiences and to explain in their own words how they maintain good health and manage ill health. The quantitative approach to measuring dimensions of health provides little insight into subjective meanings of good health. Population health surveys and statistics don't tell us the whole story!

We need to dig deeper to be able to unravel the mystery of health. This means giving "voice" to study participants and enabling them to detail the ways health and illness are given meaning and experienced in daily life. It has been suggested that people's views about health and illness are best understood as accounts shared with others as public statements (what we might tell an interviewer in a health survey) or as private stories (what we might tell a close friend during a conversation). Qualitative methods have been used to gather in-depth health information and enable people to tell personal stories about health and illness experiences. Health diaries have been used to learn about the ways people interpret the meaning of symptomatic conditions and give them an opportunity to record information about informal (and often hidden or taken-for-granted) daily health-related activities and self-care practices. The health diary method has potential for collecting valuable information (that is not captured by population health surveys or statistics) about the ongoing decision-making process involved in maintaining good health and managing ill health. Illness narrative accounts enable people, particularly those living with chronic illness, to recount their stories and to share ideas about the onset of conditions, perceived seriousness of symptoms, personal strategies for managing illness, and their efforts to make sense out of sickness. Embodied stories told by people reveal the personal and social significance of health and illness. In this way, illness narrative accounts provide valuable insights into people's understanding of the relationship among bodies, behaviour, and society.

No single methodology can completely unravel the mystery of health in all of its dimensions (just as there is no single theoretical paradigm that provides a complete explanation). It should be apparent that population health assessment requires a comprehensive, inclusive approach to measurement and greater access to longitudinal data. In other words, health needs to be measured with mixed methods over time to gain a more complete picture. We need to combine quantitative and qualitative studies and make concerted efforts to synthesize population health information derived from diverse sources. By integrating surveys, statistics, and stories, we will be better able to assess determinants of population health and gain a thorough understanding of the complex intersecting factors involved in the pursuit of health and wellness across the life course.

Social Determinants of Health: Reflections on What We Have Learned

The extensive body of research that has been accumulated over the past few decades has refined our knowledge of the wide range of determinants that influence the health of individuals and societies. Although we have learned a great deal about general determinants of population health, unfortunately we still know much more about what makes people sick than about what makes them healthy. We need to learn more about determinants of good health, or salutary factors that foster a sense of healthiness, physical fitness, and general social capacity for the performance of well roles. Once we have an improved understanding of the factors that contribute to the pursuit of health and wellness, we will be in a better position to solve the mystery of health and explain how some people manage to stay well. The challenge facing researchers is to expand the scope of studies to incorporate determinants of good health as well as complex interactions between social environments and individual behaviour in search of an explanation of the factors that make societies and people healthy.

Structural and Personal Determinants of Health

There is widespread agreement that population health is shaped by many different factors and that social determinants play a critical part in this process. Initially, key determinants of health were identified as human biology, lifestyle, environment, and health care. Over time, the search for causal factors has become broader. Currently, "even a partial listing of such factors would include influences as disparate as genetic endowment, gender, personal health practices, early childhood development, coping skills, health care, housing, employment and working conditions, education, social status, income, social support, cultural environment, and physical and natural environments" (Stoddart et al. 2006, 327). Other factors that could be added to this list of health determinants include age, life course transitions, income and wealth inequality, and social inclusion/exclusion.

Regardless of the length of the list, most studies of health determinants distinguish between personal (or individual) factors and structural (or societal) factors. The major determinants of health are typically divided into two broad categories: personal determinants such as health beliefs and self-care practices, which are evident at the individual level; and structural determinants, which include aspects of the social environment, such as income distribution and living and working conditions, and are evident at the societal level. While these determinants operate at different levels, they interact with each other, and, together, intersections of history and biography have combined effects on population health. For example, structural factors, such as living and working in health-protective social environments, provide the societal context within which personal factors, such as lifestyle behaviours and self-care practices, take place. It is important to recognize that personal and structural factors not only influence health, they also influence each other and have both direct and indirect effects on health. A thorough understanding of what makes societies and people healthy requires the application of a sociological imagination in an intersectional life course analysis of mutually reinforcing effects that various structural and personal determinants have on the pursuit of health and wellness.

Sources of Social Inequality and Health Disparities: Intersections of Socioeconomic Status, Gender, and Ethnicity

Determinants of health intersect to compound the root causes of health disparities. The conventional approach to investigating determinants of health has been to conceptualize them as separate categories. However, in reality determinants of health are not reducible to single categories.

Major determinants of health are better understood as complex social locations that together shape the experience of health and illness. From the perspective of intersectional analysis, health outcomes are produced by combined and overlapping structures of inequality. A key challenge for researchers is to gain a better understanding of the pathways through which these intersecting forces affect population health over time if they are to be more successful at addressing the link between sources of social inequality and health disparities and unravelling the mystery of health.

Sociologists argue that social inequality or unequal life circumstances exist because opportunities are differentially distributed in society, based on factors such as socioeconomic status, gender, ethnicity, and age. These sources of social inequality are associated with enduring patterns of advantage and disadvantage that get under the skin, shaping the ways people interact and engage in the pursuit of health and wellness. The common denominator in each of these intersecting sources of social inequality is that living in poverty or experiencing sexism, racism, or ageism may result in social exclusion. The consequences of this process of marginalization include unequal power relationships between groups in society and unequal access to social, cultural, economic, and political resources. In other words, social inequality has important implications for all aspects of people's lives, including disparities in their health!

Many of the studies that have explored the link between social inequality and health conclude that we need an intersectional model to understand the complex interacting determinants of population health and health disparities. For example, it has been recommended that future research critically examine the intersection of socioeconomic status, gender, ethnicity, and age, since these multiple social locations collectively contribute to the creation of health disparities. Structures of inequality, such as socioeconomic status, act upon women and men differently and pattern behaviours (including health and illness behaviour) differently according to socially constructed gender roles. Consequently, it is important to recognize the gendered nature of health and illness and to examine the relationship between sources of social inequality and health disparities through a gender lens.

In addition to socioeconomic status and gender, there is another intersecting social location—ethnic group membership—that affects the pursuit of health and wellness. Ethnicity is an important basis of an individual's identity that works in concert with aspects of social location, such as socioeconomic status, gender, and age, to shape health. The fact that certain ethnocultural groups (such as Aboriginal peoples) are socially excluded highlights the need to conduct intersectional analyses of overlapping health disparities. To understand the intersectionality of health, researchers have to move beyond studying ethnic diversity and health or carrying out class- or gender-based analyses. The challenge for future research is to make a concerted effort to assess the multiple and interconnected pathways through which various social locations intersect with each other over time to produce specific outcomes such as disparities in health.

Life Chances and Health Choices: The Structure–Agency Question

"Understanding and reducing social inequalities in health have been key issues and a central challenge in public health. Both structural conditions and individual agency have been identified for their roles in influencing these inequalities" (Abel and Frohlich 2012, 236). The relative importance of social determinants of health, however, is still a matter of debate. Although this issue has been the focus of considerable sociological inquiry, research has not yet provided a definite answer to the structure–agency question. We still don't know the extent to which health-related actions that people undertake with respect to exercise, diet, and smoking are a matter of individual choice or the result of life chances that are shaped by factors such as socioeconomic status and gender. How this question is answered and whether agency or structure is seen as the most important factor in explaining health disparities depends on the theoretical paradigm that guides researchers. For example, structural functionalist and conflict paradigms attach more significance to structural factors, while the symbolic interactionist paradigm emphasizes agency of individuals in explaining health outcomes. In contrast, the feminist and sociology of the body paradigms view health as a consequence of interaction between structure and agency. In other words, researchers guided by these paradigms contend that health is the outcome of complex social processes that combine effects of life choices, or decisions that people make in their selection of personal practices, and life chances, or the probabilities of translating choices into action. The choices we make throughout life are constrained by structural conditions, such as socioeconomic status, gender, ethnicity, and age. If good health were simply a matter of personal choice, then who wouldn't choose health? As we have seen, however, good health is not just a matter of making the right choices in life. Chan (2009) uses the term "constrained choices" to make the point that disadvantaged life circumstances resulting from different sources of social inequality limit people's opportunities over the life course to make healthful choices and to actively engage in the pursuit of health and wellness. There is widespread recognition today that efforts to reduce social inequalities in health must take into account both social structure and individual agency (Abel and Frolich 2012; Frolich and Abel 2014).

Shared Responsibility for Making Societies and People Healthy

Health is a multi-dimensional concept embodying social, psychological, and physical components. Achieving health and wellness requires a co-ordinated approach to population health promotion. Lundell, Niederdeppe, and Clarke (2013, 1124) refer to "layers of responsibility for health" to reflect the fact that in addition to feeling personally responsible for their own health, people also assign responsibility for health to others such as "the workplace, the local community, the state, and the country." In other words, individuals, their families, schools, employers, communities, informal and formal health-care providers, governments, and society share responsibility for maintaining and promoting health. Unfortunately, responsibility for health does not mean the same thing to various stakeholders. The following discussion summarizes the meaning of personal, professional, and public responsibility for health.

Personal Responsibility: Informal Care and Health

Our exploration of the hidden depths of health care clearly demonstrated that the essence of self-health management is control by individuals (and their family members) of the decision-making process and resources used in maintaining good health and managing ill health. Self-care health and illness behaviour and other types of informal care, such as social support or mutual aid, are firmly rooted in the cultural values of Western liberal democratic societies, such as individualism and self-reliance. In other words, in our cultural context, members of society expect to be able to exercise personal responsibility in the conduct of their lives (e.g., in choosing their own career path and raising their children). The same is equally true of health choices. For the layperson, the critical issue is not whether care is self- or other-provided but whether health care is self-managed (i.e., ultimately within the control of the individual and her social network). Self-care health behaviour became a popular topic after Illich (1976) called attention to the expropriation of health and challenged the public to demystify and overcome professional dependency and re-establish personal control of health. Among the proponents of self-health management, Green (1985, 326) has argued that "self-care brings with it the possibilities of reducing chronic illness, promoting wellness, and raising the level of well-being." Levin (1976) portrayed self-care as a force for helping people to make decisions for themselves, to take initiative in dealing with their health and responding to their illnesses, and to use professional resources in a self-protecting manner.

Clarke and Bennett (2012) point out that self-health management takes place in a social and political context in which responsibility for health has essentially shifted from the state to the individual, who is increasingly expected to be an active consumer of health care. Self-health management "requires individuals to monitor their symptoms, adhere to prescribed treatments and medication regimens, cope with physical limitations and emotional consequences of disease, discipline their bodies through diet, exercise, and other lifestyle modifications, and seek expert advice and intervention only where appropriate" (Clarke and Bennett 2012, 212). In other words, self-care has become a socially valued means of demonstrating that you are actively pursuing health and wellness. Higgs and colleagues (2009) use the term "will to health" to reflect the fact that health has become a required goal for individual behaviour (comparable to a "will to live"). They contend that personal responsibility for health translates at the individual level into a "will to health" and has become a defining feature of successful aging!

It is important to note that self-care has its critics (e.g., Crawford 1977, 1980, 1986; Knowles 1977). The basic criticism of self-care behaviour is that increased emphasis on personal responsibility for health brings with it the potential for victim-blaming. Self-care is based on the assumption that individuals and members of their informal social networks have the power to control conditions that shape health. Critics argue that this is more apparent than real. A danger of highlighting self-care as an important health promotion mechanism is that individuals are often held responsible for things that are not within their control (e.g., environmental and occupational health hazards). Crawford (1980) characterizes the preoccupation with personal responsibility for health and self-care behaviour as **healthism**. He argues that healthism promotes heightened health consciousness as well as the importance of personal responsibility for health. Healthism portrays lifestyle behavioural changes (e.g., getting more exercise) as a matter of choice. As a result of this perspective, ill health may be equated with personal failure, and the individual may be blamed and, in this way, victimized. In other words, this approach individualizes broad social issues involved in population health promotion and leads to a course of action that focuses on changing individual behaviour rather than addressing sources of social and economic inequality related to disparities in health. Furthermore, critics contend that self-care may be used as a justification for decreasing the level of formal health-care services and, perhaps more important, that an extreme emphasis on individualized responsibility for health distracts attention from a critical analysis of social, economic, and political factors that make societies and people healthy.

Although the increased emphasis on personal responsibility for health may have "created a greater sense of agency for the individual, it has also been accompanied by the redefining of poor health as a signifier of moral laxity and personal failure" (Clarke and Bennett 2012, 214). For example, many of the Canadian older adults who participated in Clarke and Bennett's study claimed that proactive and reactive self-care behaviour is an individual's moral responsibility. They interpret this finding to mean that people have internalized healthist beliefs and the expectation that they must be active consumers of health care. Clarke and Bennett (2012, 226) conclude that "given population aging, the increasing prevalence of chronic conditions, and the emphasis on demonstrating one's morality through healthy lifestyles and body investments, reactive and proactive self-care will become ever more important, if not expected, in later life." Overall, healthism obscures the extent to which health and illness are socially determined and, consequently, a shared responsibility.

Professional Responsibility: Formal Care and Health

Turning to professional responsibility for health, the essence of formal medicalized health care, as described in the earlier examination of biomedicine, is legitimate, organized autonomy based on specialized knowledge and technical expertise. The power of the medical profession to control health-related matters leads to the tendency to equate the exercise of personal responsibility for health with compliance with professionally prescribed treatment regimens of medication and behavioural change. This limited conception of self-care health behaviour is based on the assumption that professionals are ultimately responsible for health and reflects biomedical dominance of the health-care system. The dominant position of the medical profession within the division of labour in the health-care sector has led to the tendency to overestimate the therapeutic impact of physicians and institutional care while underestimating the part played by individuals, families, and informal social support networks in the provision of community-based health care. As discussed in Chapter 9, the nature of the health-care system changes dramatically when it is organized on the basis of self-care (as the primary form of care) rather than medical care and when we take the whole iceberg of health care into account.

While informal lay health care and formal professional health care coexist, personal and professional responsibilities for health are certainly not well co-ordinated. The biomedical health-care system has not yet acknowledged the prevalence and potential of informal care (and the other hidden components of the iceberg of health care) and tends to view self-care as a challenge to physicians' professional authority. There is little evidence that formal health-care professionals are actively involved in promoting and supporting informal health care in a way that is consistent with the principles of self-determination and self-health management. In contrast, there is evidence that self-care is being medicalized (i.e., increasingly controlled by health professionals). In the context of a formal health-care system that is dominated by biomedicine, sharing responsibility for health essentially means that the individual is expected to accept responsibility for her health care when it is delegated by a health professional rather than show personal initiative by taking responsibility for the management of health care.

Public Responsibility: The Governance of Health

Finally, in the case of public responsibility for health, the essence of government involvement in health care is regulation based on rational–legal authority. Elected officials exercise regulatory power by enacting legislation regarding delivery of formal health-care services and the conduct of informal health-related activities. For example, governments regulate the formal health-care system, including the producers of health goods, such as pharmaceutical companies and biotechnology manufacturers, and providers of health services (i.e., health-care professionals such as physicians and nurses). Government involvement in health care, however, most frequently takes the form of regulating informal health practices by codifying in law individualized health promotion strategies, such as seat belt use and anti-smoking legislation. According to Kickbusch (2007, 147), modern governance of health has expanded "the role of the state in health through new types of regulations which influence the behavior of individuals and their role in the production of health." For example, government policies now regulate where it is permissible to smoke, who can buy tobacco products, where (and at what price) they are sold, and even access to images and messages about smoking through restrictions on advertising tobacco products.

The prevailing government approach to promoting population health combines providing individuals with information to guide their health choices and legislating public adoption of health risk avoidance and/or health-protective behaviours. In other words, the exercise of public responsibility for health through government action typically concentrates on personal determinants of health (i.e., the so-called lifestyle behavioural practices) rather than critical structural determinants of health (i.e., social and economic inequality). This overemphasis on personal responsibility for maintaining health once again deflects attention from the need to improve living and working conditions in order to reduce upstream social inequalities in the production of health. Governments have a responsibility not only to promote individual health-protective behaviour but also to bring about the type of changes that will alter the impact of structural determinants of health and, ultimately, make both societies and people healthier.

To date, the major structural intervention in the health-care field undertaken by the Canadian government was the introduction of comprehensive, universal health insurance (known as **medicare**) more than 40 years ago. Based on findings that many Canadians did not have access to adequate medical care, the final report of the Hall Royal Commission on Health Services recommended in 1964 that provincial and federal governments introduce a health-care program that would remove economic barriers preventing people from seeking physicians' services. It took several years of debate before the federal government passed legislation in 1968 establishing a national medicare program. The implementation of this program also took time, since health (like education) is under provincial jurisdiction and it was up to each province to decide on the format for introducing medicare at the provincial level. The federal health-care plan was finally implemented by all provinces in 1972, and medicare provided all Canadians with coverage for medical services provided by physicians.

To participate in the cost-sharing arrangement that was established, each province was required to meet the five fundamental principles of medicare:

- **accessibility**—reasonable access to medical care is guaranteed for all Canadians;
- **comprehensiveness**—all necessary medical services are guaranteed without dollar limit and are available solely on the basis of medical need;
- **universality**—all Canadians are eligible for coverage based on uniform terms and conditions (regardless of ability to pay);
- **portability**—benefits are transferable from province to province; and
- **public administration**—the health-care program is administered by a non-profit agency or commission.

The basic assumption underlying the introduction of medicare was that adequate medical care must be viewed as a fundamental human right and not as a privilege for those who can afford to pay for physician and hospital services. Even though the medicare program has been in place for several decades, this basic assumption is still not universally accepted today. Many of the original issues continue to be debated. For example, there is ongoing controversy regarding the right of physicians to extra-bill or charge user fees, the legitimacy of private clinics, the existence of a two-tiered (public/private) system, the definition of medically necessary services and the deregulation of insured services, and the financing of medicare (the funding formula and transfer payments from the federal government to provincial governments have changed over time).

The primary objective of medicare was to remove the economic barrier between patients and physicians (i.e., direct payment for services at the time they are received) and to provide all Canadians with equal access to adequate medical care. The hope was that assured access to physicians would translate into increased utilization, which, in turn, would eventually influence lay beliefs and health-protective behaviours and, ultimately, result in improvements in the health of all Canadians. We will return to this point in the concluding section of the chapter when we take a critical look at the link between universal health insurance and reduction of disparities in population health.

A number of researchers have addressed the challenges facing a human rights–based approach to health-care planning and policy development. For example, McPherson (2012) contends that Canadians' right to health means that our government and public authorities have an obligation to develop policies and implement action plans that will lead to available and accessible health care for all. Unfortunately, this approach focuses on the consumption of health care and not on the production of health. McGibbon and Shebib (2012) emphasize the importance of distinguishing between the right to health care and the right to healthiness. They state that this basic human right "embraces the following two areas: 1) elements related to health care; and 2) elements concerning the underlying preconditions for health, including a healthy environment, safe drinking water and adequate sanitation, occupational health and access to health information" (2012, 188). In other words, governments also have a responsibility to ensure that public policies address the full range of social determinants of population health. Has the Canadian government fulfilled this key responsibility? The following discussion provides a brief historical overview of policy initiatives in Canada intended to make society and people healthy.

Health Policy Initiatives: Lalonde and Beyond

Canada has a rich tradition in terms of health policy. Bryant (2012) describes health policy as a type of public policy that focuses on the allocation and management of resources within the health-care system. In addition, she points out that health policy is also intended to improve and maintain the health of the population "by ensuring access to social and economic resources of health and social well-being" (2012, 139). In other words, health policy should address the upstream social determinants of health such as income, education, and employment. The Canadian government has been working for many years on the development of a framework for action to promote population health that takes into account general determinants of both good health and ill health. The primary purpose of most of these policy initiatives has been to formulate a model of population health promotion that reflects a broader definition of health (as more than the absence of disease and illness), a broader approach to health determinants, and an explicit focus on health promotion (in addition to disease prevention). The model goes beyond conventional medical care by incorporating an expanded view that includes formal and informal health care. The ultimate objective in each case is to provide guidelines for improving the overall health and well-being of the population. The following discussion critically summarizes the way in which several key national policy documents, introduced over a 40-year span, depict determinants of health and the recommendations they offer for reducing social inequalities in health (see Box 12.1).

> **Box 12.1** History of Key Health Policy Initiatives in Canada
>
> - *A New Perspective on the Health of Canadians* (1974)
> - *Achieving Health for All: A Framework for Health Promotion* (1986)
> - *Ottawa Charter for Health Promotion* (1986)
> - *Strategies for Population Health: Investing in the Health of Canadians* (1994)
> - *Building on Values: The Future of Health Care in Canada* (the Romanow Royal Commission) (2002)
> - *The Integrated Pan-Canadian Healthy Living Strategy* (2005)

Lalonde (1974), as previously discussed, is credited with introducing one of the most influential health policy documents. His report, entitled *A New Perspective on the Health of Canadians*, was innovative at the time it was written and changed the basic understanding of determinants of health. The Lalonde report argued that health is influenced by a broad range of factors, including human biology, lifestyle, the organization of health care, and the social and physical environments in which people live. Today, this perspective on population health is widely endorsed, and it should be acknowledged that, to a great extent, it was the Lalonde report that helped to legitimize the development of health policies and practices that reflect an approach to determinants of health that goes beyond access to formal health-care services. This policy document received international acclaim for identifying non-medical factors that contribute to population health (Hancock 1986).

In 1986, Canada hosted the First International Conference on Health Promotion. Two key policy documents resulted from this conference—*Achieving Health for All: A Framework for Health Promotion* and the *Ottawa Charter for Health Promotion*. Both documents called attention to underlying societal conditions that determine health and, consequently, were instrumental in focusing policy discussions in the following decades on processes by which health is created (or produced) and how good health can be achieved equitably by all members of society. The policy document entitled *Achieving Health for All: A Framework for Health Promotion*, distributed by the Canadian minister of health, was related to an earlier WHO (World Health Organization) initiative intended to achieve health for all by the year 2000. While this was a commendable goal, it was obviously not accomplished! Consequently, in their policy document, the Canadian government omitted a target date for achieving health for all. According to the Canadian framework for health promotion, health may be conceptualized as a resource that gives people the ability to manage their lives. This framework is consistent with a salutogenic approach and portrays health as a part of everyday living that "emphasizes the role of individuals and communities in defining what health means to them" (Epp 1986, 3). Without explicitly using the term "self-health management," the framework also recognizes informal care as a vital component of health promotion.

The population health framework consists of three health challenges, three health promotion mechanisms, and three implementation strategies. The three health challenges identified include: finding ways to reduce inequities between the health of high- and low-income groups of Canadians; becoming more effective at preventing injuries, illnesses, chronic conditions, and their resulting disabilities; and enhancing people's ability to manage and cope with chronic health problems by providing them with needed skills and community supports. In the context of discussing people's capacity for effectively managing their health, the report highlighted "the importance of ensuring that informal care-givers have access to the support they need. Many people, especially women, care for others on a regular basis. The health and capacity of these individuals to manage is no less important than the health of those for whom they care" (Epp 1986, 5).

The three health promotion mechanisms described include: self-care, or the decisions and actions that individuals take in the interest of preserving their health (i.e., the regulatory and preventive self-care practices discussed earlier); mutual aid, or the actions people take to help each other deal with their health concerns by sharing ideas, information, and experiences and providing practical and emotional support (again, as previously discussed); and healthy environments, or creation of social, economic, and physical surroundings that not only preserve but also enhance good health. This means "ensuring that policies and practices are in place to provide Canadians with a healthy environment at home, school, work or wherever else they may be. It means communities and regions working together to create environments which are conducive to health" (Epp 1986, 9). This framework explicitly acknowledges that population health promotion involves self-care behaviours that protect health and reduce the risk of illness as well as the need to improve living and working conditions. In other words, both personal and structural determinants of health must be addressed to ensure that individual health practices take place in healthy environments. Furthermore, by recognizing that informal supportive social networks are a fundamental aspect of health promotion, this policy document acknowledges the vital role played by hidden parts of the iceberg of health care in achieving health for all.

Finally, three implementation strategies outlined include: fostering public participation to ensure that Canadians are able to "take responsibility" and act in ways that improve their own health; strengthening community health services to provide a continuum of care, including short- and long-term care, respite care, and home care, plus institutional care; and co-ordinating healthy public policy that provides people with opportunities for health. This means more than just ensuring that people have equal access to formal health-care services. All policies that have a bearing on health, such as employment, income security, education, and housing, need to be co-ordinated. On the one hand, this policy document characterizes community health services as "an agent of health promotion, assuming a key role in fostering self-care, mutual aid and the creation of healthy environments," but on the other hand, it casts doubt on the feasibility of this implementation strategy successfully addressing the health challenges facing Canadians, since "adjusting the present health care system in such a way as to assign more responsibility to community-based services means allocating a greater share of resources to such services" (Epp 1986, 10). Such a move would threaten biomedical dominance of the health-care system.

The *Ottawa Charter for Health Promotion* also describes health as a resource for everyday life and a positive concept emphasizing social and personal resources as well as physical functioning. The underlying philosophy and core health promotion principles embodied in the *Ottawa Charter* are related to the salutogenic health framework (Lindstrom and Eriksson 2009; Eriksson and Lindstrom 2008). The type of health promotion actions advocated once again include building healthy public policy, creating supportive environments, strengthening communities, developing personal skills, and reorienting health services. The *Ottawa Charter* took a comprehensive view of health determinants and described fundamental prerequisites for good health: food, shelter, education, income, a stable ecosystem, sustainable resources, peace, social justice, and equity. It recognized that equal opportunities to acquire these prerequisites cannot be assured by the formal health-care sector alone but require co-ordinated action on the part of government, health-care providers, non-government organizations, the private sector, and the public. According to this policy document, health promotion is a process of enabling people to increase control over their health, reducing differences in health status, and ensuring equal opportunities and resources to enable all people to achieve health. In other words, rather than individualizing health, population health promotion focuses on achieving equity in health! Eriksson and Lindstrom (2008, 190) contend that as a result of the *Ottawa Charter*, "community and policies leading to a healthy society became central, thus expanding the focus from individuals and groups to the context of life." The *Ottawa Charter* has been described as "the key policy document of the international health promotion movement" (Lindstrom and Eriksson 2009, 17) and has influenced health promotion policy and programs around the world (e.g., Hills and McQueen 2007; Porter 2007).

In 1994, the Federal, Provincial and Territorial Advisory Committee on Population Health prepared a discussion paper entitled *Strategies for Population Health: Investing in the Health of Canadians*. This policy document intended to identify interprovincial and national health promotion strategies on which governments could collaborate to achieve significant results in making and keeping people healthy. Once again, the now-familiar broad range of health determinants was summarized in terms of five major categories: social and economic environment, physical environment, personal health practices, individual capacity and coping skills, and health services. A framework for action on population health was then developed to provide a more balanced approach to the many factors that influence health, with less of a medicalized preoccupation with formal health care. This was based on the realization that "there is mounting evidence that the contribution of medicine and health care is quite limited, and that spending more on health care will not result in further improvements in population health. On the other hand, there are strong and growing indications that other factors such as living and working conditions are crucially important for a healthy population" (Health Canada 1994, 11–12). While this was not a new point of view, it was forcefully expressed in this policy document.

Furthermore, it was argued that adopting a national population health strategy would strengthen understanding of determinants of health, build public support for and involvement in actions to improve the health of the overall population, and reduce health disparities experienced by some groups of Canadians. To achieve these objectives, however, the report acknowledged that a number of complex issues would first have to be addressed, including finding a new approach to deal with the link between health and factors such as unemployment, poor economic opportunities, and environmental pollution; building support for the population health approach among government partners outside of health (e.g., education, labour, housing, and social services); and making difficult decisions about reallocation of resources to tackle the full range of health determinants. Although there are potential benefits from implementing this framework, there are also serious challenges that have to be met to gain support for investing in actions that will improve the health of the entire population.

Approximately a decade later, in 2002, the Romanow Royal Commission released its final report, titled *Building on Values: The Future of Health Care in Canada*. This is an extremely lengthy report containing numerous recommendations that focus almost exclusively on changes necessary to ensure the long-term sustainability of Canada's formal health-care system. The basic premise of the report is that the pursuit of good health and access to universal health care are important social values for the majority of Canadians. In a later publication, Romanow (2006, 2) contends that "medicare is based on Canadian values—fairness, equity, compassion, and solidarity"—and while reform may be needed, medicare "remains one of the single greatest symbols of our uniqueness as Canadians." The pride that Canadians have in their health-care system is reflected by the fact that elections have been won or lost on the success of political parties at persuading the public that they are the best ones to protect medicare. In many ways, medicare has become a national symbol or a "sacred trust." Romanow (2002) characterizes Canadians' relationship with their health-care system as a "health covenant" and asserts that we all share the responsibility for keeping the Canadian health-care system functioning. What about the responsibility to keep Canadians healthy and the long-term sustainability of a healthy society? The Romanow report contains little information on health promotion and simply reiterates a rather limiting individualized approach by encouraging Canadians to make healthy lifestyle choices to prevent physical and mental illnesses (e.g., smoke less and lose weight). It overlooks any discussion of structural determinants of health or the importance of reducing social inequalities in health (other than a recommendation regarding the funding of Aboriginal health services). The report deals with funding issues at length and concentrates on identifying what needs to be done to repair and preserve the fundamental features of the Canadian health-care system (e.g., universal accessibility, public funding). Despite this, the Romanow report did little to heal the health-care system.

In 2005, *The Integrated Pan-Canadian Healthy Living Strategy* was released. This report outlines the key elements of a healthy living strategy at all stages of the life course and a framework for action. Unfortunately, the strategy is limited to the conventional approach to the prevention of prevalent chronic diseases (e.g., cardiovascular disease, cancer, and diabetes) and the reduction of common modifiable risk factors (e.g., physical inactivity, unhealthy diets, and tobacco use). The report fails to provide novel ideas about population health promotion or implementation strategies. The primary components of the recommended healthy living strategy are individualized lifestyle choices, such as healthy eating and physical activity! The report acknowledges that structural determinants underlie these personal health practices, including income, employment, education, and social exclusion, but does not deal with them in a meaningful way. The upstream "root causes" that lead to poor health outcomes (i.e., the living and working conditions and life chances that enable people to make healthy choices) are not a part of the healthy living strategy. Furthermore, the issue of health disparities is relegated to footnotes that state that the most prominent health disparities in Canada are related to factors such as SES, Aboriginal identity, gender, disability, culture, and geographic location (isolation). There is no discussion of possible actions to reduce social inequalities in health!

While it is not possible to examine them all in detail, Canadian health policy documents continue to be released (e.g. National Collaborating Centre for Healthy Public Policy 2010). What can we conclude about health policy initiatives in Canada based on this review? First, it appears that the Canadian government believes that the best approach to population health promotion is extensive study! Second, it seems that, with the experience we have gained over the past 40 years, we are getting better at collaborating on the formulation of health policy documents. It is still not clear, however, how much longer it will take to become more effective at implementing policies and population health promotion strategies that will significantly improve the health and well-being of all Canadians. Finally, even though we know a good deal about the relative importance of social determinants of health, policy initiatives remain preoccupied by the never-ending debate about reforming the formal health-care system. "Mainstream public health policy research and development is still focused on the development of health policy within the health sector" (Eriksson and Lindstrom 2010, 347). Koh and colleagues (2011) argue that improving health is too multi-faceted to be left to those working in the health sector and that a social determinants focus should be used to reframe the way the public, health care professionals, and policy-makers think about healthy societies and healthy people. Unfortunately, policy initiatives seldom offer concrete action plans for addressing the systemic sources of social inequality that contribute to continuing health disparities and limit opportunities of certain societal groups to experience life circumstances that support the pursuit of health and wellness. Although their focus is on the US, Woolf and Braveman (2011) suggest that current policies that concentrate on downstream determinants such as medical care may be making matters worse. They strongly recommend a "health in all policies" approach for dealing with the upstream social determinants of health. This would entail governments taking health consequences and health disparities into account when developing public policies in areas such as education, child care, employment, housing, transportation, and taxation. This expanded approach might ultimately lead policy-makers to fully recognize that "social policy and health policy are intimately linked" (Woolf and Braveman 2011, 1856).

The Ongoing Pursuit of Health and Wellness: Some Unanswered Questions

Lindstrom and Eriksson (2009) combine Antonovsky's salutogenic framework for studying health with many of the factors included in the intersectional model of health and core principles of the *Ottawa Charter* in their call for making healthy public policy at a national level. They argue that it is time to engage in the type of salutogenic policy process that will "create a nurturing culture, physical and social environment, prevent injustice, create working and living conditions that are enriching, provide opportunities for individual and communal flourishing, provide social support," as well as provide the other resources required to achieve a good quality of life and a healthy future (2009, 23). Eriksson and Lindstrom (2010, 340) assert that existing evidence shows the effectiveness of the salutogenic model as a positive and health-promoting construct for guiding research and practice, as well as being "valuable and useful in the making of healthy public policy." They go on to point out that "one of the most important challenges now is to implement the salutogenic approach on all societal levels in all policies, i.e. building healthy public policy the salutogenic way" (2010, 341). This is an essential step in the process of ultimately creating a salutogenic society! If we hope to achieve this goal, it means combining the sociological imagination with a theoretically informed critical analysis of intersecting factors that shape population health across the life course and addressing a number of unanswered questions. Furthermore, we need to keep in mind the fundamental distinction between producing health and consuming health care, as well as the difference between:

- the vision of a healthy society and the reality of health-care reform;
- documenting and reducing social inequalities in health;
- formulating and implementing healthy public policy;
- health as a personal and societal value and wellness as a virtue; and
- the present medicalized society and a future salutogenic society.

Achieving healthy futures depends on our recognition of the importance of the whole iceberg of health care and our success at answering the following questions.

How Does the Vision of a Healthy Society Differ from the Reality of Health-Care Reform?

What do you imagine a healthy society would look like? The vision of a salutogenic society that emerges from population health promotion research is one that commits appropriate resources to the production of health, reduces health disparities that result from intersecting sources of social inequality across the life course, and achieves health equity through action on social determinants of health (Friel et al. 2009). A critical component in this vision of a healthy society is taking action to deal with structures of social inequality and reduce health disparities based on socioeconomic status, gender, ethnicity, and age and, ultimately, to flatten the social gradient in health. As previously discussed, the *Final Report* released in 2008 by the WHO Commission on Social Determinants of Health calls on governments to lead global action to close the gap in health disparities within a generation. However, the authors of the report acknowledge that this is only possible if political will exists to bring about major societal changes, although they admit that since the disparities in health that exist today are so great, it may not be feasible to realistically expect to achieve this vision of a healthier society in a generation. In a follow-up discussion paper entitled *Closing the Gap: Policy into Practice on Social Determinants of Health* (2011b, 2), they state that the lack of progress in implementing a social determinants approach to reducing health inequities "reflects in part the inadequacy of governance at the local, national, and global levels to address the key problems of the 21st century."

The reality is that attention continues to focus on formal health-care reform and the apparent need to commit additional resources to improve the consumption of health care (i.e., repair the medicare system). As we have seen, for decades now Canadian governments have been engaged in a never-ending debate about health reform and the best way to fix medicare. Considerable resources have been devoted to trying to identify ways to improve the formal health-care system rather than taking action to address social determinants that contribute to the production of health and sources of inequality that limit opportunities for certain groups to achieve health and wellness. To illustrate this point, the Canadian prime minister established a select committee in the mid-1990s to review the need for health reform and to advise the federal government on innovative ways to improve the health of the population. After gathering extensive information and producing several reports, the National Forum on Health (1997) concluded that being healthy requires a clean, safe environment, good housing, adequate income, education, nutrition, meaningful roles in society, and social support in the community.

This conclusion should sound familiar because it essentially restates what we have known for years about social determinants of health. Since these are the critical factors that make societies and people healthy, what specific course of action was proposed? The National Forum recommended a restructuring and reorganization of Canada's health-care system while preserving the features of medicare that Canadians value (e.g., public funding for services). Macdonald and colleagues (2009, 526) comment that continued neglect of broad social determinants of health "is especially important as income inequality continues to grow in Canada and poverty levels remain very high in comparison with many European nations." International evidence indicates that health disparities between people at the top and those at the bottom of the social gradient are getting larger. In other words, the reality is that the social and economic gap is actually getting wider and the social gradient in health is becoming steeper!

By comparison, as summarized in Box 12.2, the elements that comprise the vision of a healthy future include improving population health through promotion strategies aimed at developing healthy communities as well as targeting personal health practices, strengthening the health benefits of informal care, and providing equal opportunities to achieve health equity by addressing the upstream structural determinants.

However, as summarized in Box 12.3, the reality is that the overriding belief that the best way to achieve a healthy future is by repairing the medicare system continues to dictate what

Box 12.2 The Vision: Achieving a Healthy Future by Creating Healthy Societies and Healthy People

Improve Population Health through Upstream Health Promotion
- develop healthy communities and better living and working conditions
- enhance self-care capacity and health-protective behaviour

Shift Health-Care Resources to the Community
- strengthen health benefits of social support and informal care
- reorient formal health-care services
- reallocate resources to sustain an expanded health-care system

Increase Health Expectancy
- postpone disability and dependency
- foster active living and improved quality of life
- ensure equal opportunities for all to achieve health
- close the gap in health disparities

Box 12.3 The Reality: Achieving a Healthy Future by Repairing the Medicare System

Improve Population Health through Disease Prevention and Early Intervention
- recruit and train health professionals
- balance public and private health services

Improve the Efficiency of Institutional Health Care
- rationalize the health services delivery system
- regionalize responsibility for health care
- commit additional resources to formal care

Increase Life Expectancy
- postpone disease onset and premature death
- improve medical management of chronic disease
- ensure equal access for all to medical care

has actually taken place in the health sector. This includes improving population health through the traditional disease prevention strategies, improving efficiency of institutionally based formal health care, and ensuring equal access for all to biomedical care.

Chappell (1993) points out that there have been changes in the Canadian health-care system. However, for the most part these changes have involved cutbacks to the institutional component of the formal health-care system (e.g., hospital closures, nursing layoffs) without a corresponding reallocation of resources to community-based care (e.g., the establishment of an often-promised national home care plan). Even though there is some evidence that government funding has been restored to pre-1990 levels, the system is still underfunded due to budget cuts and economic recession. Does spending more money on formal health-care services necessarily mean healthier societies and people? Despite decades of discussion about the need for health-care reform and increasing health-care expenditures, it appears that improvements to the health-care system have been limited and health disparities continue to persist across the country (Health Council of Canada 2013).

While fixing the medicare system may be necessary to increase the supply of health-care professionals and reduce wait times for diagnostic procedures and surgery, it is not sufficient to improve the health and well-being of the overall population. Creating healthy societies and healthy people requires adopting a salutogenic approach and addressing social factors that make people healthy as well as sources of social inequality that result in health disparities. For this to become a reality, the focus has to shift from the consumption of health care to the production of health, social and economic resources have to be reallocated, and concrete action has to be taken to implement the proposed health promotion strategies repeatedly described in the policy documents we have reviewed.

Is It Possible to Redress Social Inequalities in Health?

Based on our lengthy discussion of studies that have explored the relationship between sources of social inequality and health disparities, it could be argued that we don't need more research evidence or further policy analysis. The importance of structural determinants of health has been well documented. For example, research on income inequality and health has shown that "reducing disparities in the income distribution is the key to creating healthier societies" (Pop, van Ingen, and van Oorschot 2013, 1026). Not all Canadians have an equal opportunity to be healthy, since they do not all have equal access to the social and economic prerequisites needed for achieving health and wellness. Reducing disparities in health requires the implementation of policy-level social change and introduction of programs at a societal level that intervene in the relationship between key social determinants and health outcomes. Structural interventions are necessary to reduce social exclusion if we hope to equitably improve population health.

The process of redressing social inequalities in health involves bridging the gaps between research, policies, and programs. The first step in this process is translating research findings into public policy. As illustrated by our earlier look at health policy initiatives, this has largely been accomplished. Reducing social inequalities in health has become a major public policy priority internationally, and "most senior public health policy-makers agree that specific interventions are needed to reduce social inequalities in health" (Smith et al. 2014, 384). Population health research has influenced the process of public policy-making in a number of different ways. For example, research results have served a conceptual function and shaped the political agenda by providing new perspectives (e.g., Lalonde's report) and altered the way policy-makers and the public think about particular social issues (such as the major determinants of health). Research can also serve an instrumental function by helping policy-makers address a particular problem that is already on their agenda (e.g., who to target in smoking cessation campaigns). Finally, research can be used in a symbolic way "to neutralize opponents, convince undecided parties, and provide ammunition for supporters of a policy alternative" (Earle, Heymann, and Lavis 2006, 384–5). We now have a long list of policy documents that focus on social determinants of health and population health promotion. Indeed, Evans and Stoddart (2003) contend that we have become expert at consuming research and producing policy. While this step is necessary, it is not sufficient. We also need to translate policies into health outcomes. To reduce social inequalities in health, we have to both formulate and implement healthy public policy! According to Smith and colleagues (2014, 388):

> A gap exists between the descriptive and analytic evidence demonstrating social inequalities in health and the knowledge of which population health interventions are most likely to reduce the observed health inequalities. This mismatch of problems and solutions is not surprising, given the complexity of factors that are responsible for causing social inequalities in health. These factors can interact in non-linear ways, may only manifest over long periods of time and may change depending on the context and time period.

While Canada may be recognized as a world leader in developing healthy public policy, unfortunately, the government has not taken the next step and implemented these policies in a way that effectively addresses sources of inequality and produces a salutogenic society.

Given the importance of structures of social inequality as health determinants, there is reason to criticize the widespread tendency for governments to translate health policies into programs that focus on individualized health promotion. As we have seen, there are limited gains in population health associated with an individualized lifestyle approach to health promotion. This is true for the general population and even more so for those living in disadvantaged social and economic circumstances. For example, smoking cessation campaigns are important, but what health benefits are achieved if you quit smoking but have to go on living in poverty? These types of changes in personal health practices must be accompanied by significant changes in life circumstances (e.g., living and working conditions) to make societies and people healthy. This is certainly not a new idea. Almost 30 years ago, Epp (1987) explored the relationship between socioeconomic factors, such as education, employment, and income, and inequalities in health and questioned whether there are ways in which these life circumstances could be altered to make them more supportive of health. Even though this report highlighted the fact that health is affected by social and environmental factors (in addition to lifestyle behaviour and access to medical services), it came to the rather unsatisfactory conclusion that "whether or not inequities in health can ever be completely eliminated may be, to some, a matter of debate. Nevertheless, pursuing the elimination of inequities by enabling informed self-care, by strengthening mutual aid and by creating healthy environments must be considered a priority" (Epp 1987, 39). This means doing a better job of bridging the gap between policy analysis and social programs and taking action to address health disparities.

One of the few examples of a structural intervention undertaken in this country, based on the assumption that it would have a bearing on the social gradient in health, was the introduction of a universal health insurance program: medicare. Have disparities in health based on socioeconomic factors been reduced (if not eliminated) since the introduction of medicare? According to Badgley (1991), it was widely assumed that medicare would result in a progressive redistribution of health benefits to all Canadians regardless of their position on the social gradient and that a high level of equity would be achieved. Based on an analysis of available evidence at the time,

Badgley contends that social and economic inequalities in health have not levelled off since the introduction of medicare. In fact, he concludes that "the perception of greater equity having been realized rests more upon assumptions of how Canadian national health insurance is presumed to operate in principle than upon appraisals of how it actually functions in practice" (1991, 660). While all Canadians have benefitted to some extent from medicare in terms of access to biomedical care, Badgley points out that there has been little significant change in health disparities. In fact, evidence suggests that rather than decreasing, social inequalities in health may actually be increasing. Furthermore, Bryant (2012, 141) contends that "during the past two decades, Canada's capacity to address health inequalities by way of their underlying social determinants has weakened."

This leaves us wondering—does medicare matter? A limited number of studies have tried to answer this question by comparing medicare in Canada, the National Health Service in Britain, and the health-care system in the United States. For example, Adler and colleagues (1993) examined socioeconomic inequalities in health and conclude that countries such as England that have universal health insurance show the same type of social gradient in health as found in the United States. They assert that the evidence indicates that socioeconomic differences in health actually increased (rather than decreased) after the introduction of the National Health Service. Marmot and colleagues (1997) confirm that social inequalities in health have been increasing in both the United States and Britain. They analyzed the results of several studies carried out in these two countries and documented the fact that 30 years after the introduction of the National Health Service, "inequalities in health had widened, despite universal access to medical care, because the determinants of inequalities in health lay elsewhere" (1997, 901).

Researchers have explored the link between factors such as universal health insurance, access to medical care, and health disparities by carrying out comparative analyses of Canada and the United States. For example, Lasser, Himmelstein, and Woolhandler (2006) analyzed cross-national population-based survey data and found evidence of health disparities in both countries, although they were more pronounced in the United States. They conclude that universal health insurance does not entirely mitigate disparities in health based on factors such as income, race, and immigrant status. Willson (2009) provides further evidence that health disparities associated with socioeconomic status exist in Canada and the United States. In fact, the existence of a social gradient in health in both Canada and the United States has been well documented.

Birch and Gafni (2005) provide a critical overview of the achievements and challenges of medicare in Canada. They argue that it might be more meaningful to compare the Canadian health-care system to the system in a country in which the organization and funding of health-care services is similar rather than comparing it to the private health-care system in the United States. However, even though the results of such a comparison might be more revealing than Canadian–American comparisons, they would "still focus attention on how we are doing compared with (some) others rather than how we are doing in relation to what we set out to do" (Birch and Gafni 2005, 444). As previously described, the primary objective of introducing medicare was to enable Canadians to access formal health care without direct payment at the point of delivery and to remove ability to pay as a constraint on accessing physician services. The somewhat naive hope was that eliminating inequities in the distribution of formal biomedical care would eventually lead to improvements in overall population health.

We have now had medicare in place in Canada for more than 40 years and therefore should be able to determine whether public financing of universal health-care services has changed the link between socioeconomic status and health status and improved population health. Medicare has been successful at achieving its primary objective of removing the economic barrier between Canadians and the formal health-care system (i.e., access to physicians). Medicare, however, has not reduced social inequalities in health or addressed major social determinants of health (and cannot be expected to do so). Adler and colleagues (1993, 3140) argue that health insurance coverage alone cannot significantly reduce socioeconomic differences in health and that debate regarding health insurance as a means of improving population health deflects "attention from other factors that contribute to social inequalities in health status." In addition to providing equality of access to biomedical care, healthy societies and healthy people require social policies that provide equality of opportunity in terms of living and working conditions. Lasser, Himmelstein, and Woolhandler (2006, 1306) agree that universal health insurance is not sufficient to eliminate all health disparities and argue that "policies to address unfavourable social conditions that impact health are sorely needed. Such policies could include reduction of income inequality through tax reform, improved housing, and expanded educational and employment opportunities for the poor." In other words, healthy societies provide equal opportunities for people to pursue health and wellness.

Redressing social inequalities in health cannot be accomplished by continuing to engage in the never-ending debate about reforming the formal health-care system and modifying medicare (i.e., pointless arguments about the consumption of health care). While Canadians may "cherish their health care system and use it as a source of demarcation between themselves and the United States," the health-care system continues to be "a major focus of debate between those who adhere to a neoliberal market economy and those who believe in social justice, egalitarianism, and health care as fundamental human rights" (Nakhaie, Smylie, and Arnold 2007, 562). While the debate goes on, social inequalities endure, and the gap in health disparities continues to grow. Improvements in population health ultimately depend on resolving the debate and finding the political will to address social factors that influence the production of health and the structures of social inequality in Canadian society that perpetuate health disparities.

Why Is It So Difficult to Implement Healthy Public Policy?

Whitehead and Popay (2010) provide part of the answer to this question by pointing out that taking action on the social determinants of health inequalities involves swimming upstream. They argue that meaningful improvements in population health require action on the wider social determinants operating outside of the health care system and that "without political action on forces that are widening inequalities the impact of future health equity efforts will be seriously muted" (2010, 1235). Effective population health promotion requires implementation of policies that establish a balance between personal, professional, and public responsibility for health. This means that efforts to enhance self-care capacity, strengthen informal care, and foster healthy living by promoting individual behavioural changes must be co-ordinated at the structural level, with changes in the professional health-care sector and in government programs intended to produce healthy social and physical environments. Healthy public policy must support the exercise of personal responsibility for health by ensuring that the public has the knowledge and skills necessary to engage in self-health management, public access to formal health-care services including biomedical care and safe and effective forms of complementary and alternative care, and the creation of healthy living and working environments. To summarize, sharing responsibility for making societies and people healthy means that

- individuals must be supported in positive and practical ways in their efforts to exercise personal responsibility in the pursuit of health and wellness;
- formal health-care providers must find ways to exercise professional responsibility for health care that is consistent with public demand for self-direction of health-related matters; and
- public policies and programs must be implemented that reflect social responsibilities of governments to improve the health of the population through the creation of healthy living and working environments in addition to promoting health-protective behaviours.

There is evidence that the social determinants of health intersect and have a cumulative effect across the life course. In addition, as we discussed, the factors that shape health are not always immediately apparent. Consequently, the impact of health determinants cannot be adequately explained by simple cause-and-effect models but requires a complex intersectional life course explanatory model that recognizes the health outcomes of intersecting social locations. Unfortunately, due to the complexity and relative newness of this conceptual model, policy analysis based on the intersectionality framework is still quite underdeveloped. According to Hankivsky and Cormier (2011), the application of intersectionality to policy-making is at the very early stages of development. However, they go on to state that "the promise of intersectionality policy analysis is great: it does make available a novel way of understanding inequity as both experienced and systematically structured" (2011, 228). Despite its potential for informing public policies intended to address social determinants of health, McGibbon and McPherson (2011, 75) agree that "intersectionality remains a relatively unknown and underdeveloped concept in policy discussions and applications." There are ongoing efforts to refine this conceptual model and to develop an intersectionality-based framework for policy analysis and for tackling health inequities and creating more just and equitable societies (Hankivsky 2012c). Similarly, McDaniel and Bernard (2011) make a compelling case that the life course perspective also offers an important (but underutilized) policy lens. They suggest that the life course perspective "can open new policy approaches" and "can make visible policy options and interventions previously hidden" (2011, S10). As illustrated by the intersectional life course model of health presented in Chapter 8, these two perspectives have been integrated in an effort to provide a more comprehensive way of understanding the many factors that shape the pursuit of health and wellness.

According to Kickbusch (2007, 151), "a broad understanding of health determinants beyond the classic determinants of income and poverty—ranging from social support to the hierarchical structures of society, from gender to race, the organization of work to the social cohesion and social capital of communities" expands health policy into a wide range of sectors. An intersectional model of health calls for development and implementation of intersectoral health policies (i.e. the "health in all policies" approach described earlier). To be effective at achieving meaningful societal reform that will result in improvements in population health, policy initiatives intended to address social determinants of health need to involve several different sectors simultaneously (such as education, labour, housing, transportation, social services, and recreation). To illustrate, an **intersectoral approach** to formulating and implementing healthy public policy requires co-ordinated changes in the health-care sector (for example, physician and hospital services as well as home care) along with social service sectors such as child and family services, job creation and employment programs, community development, and housing.

Kickbusch (2007) describes this approach as the "deterritorialization" of health and cautions that it has significant consequences for the formulation of health policies and the way in which responsibility for healthy societies and healthy people is interpreted. While policy-makers outside of the traditional health sector are starting to understand that policies they develop can have important health consequences, implementing this type of intersectoral policy faces enormous challenges. Earle, Heymann, and Lavis (2006, 382) comment that

> policy makers need little or no prompting to examine relationships between health care financing policy and health outcomes or between occupational health and safety policy and health outcomes. However, they may well need prompting to examine relationships between tax policies and health, between labor-market policies and health, or between early childhood development policies and health.

Intersectoral collaboration across many different sectors is essential for successful population health promotion. As we have seen, many key determinants of health fall outside of the mandate of government departments of health. Consequently, the health sector cannot act alone to produce healthy societies and healthy people!

The implementation of healthy public policy requires not only an estimate of benefits (or risks) associated with social determinants but also a means of intervening to promote health and wellness. In other words, we still face the challenge of finding ways to accurately assess the relative contribution of structural and personal health determinants and identify those factors most amenable to intervention. Commentary by numerous health researchers over the past decade contends that despite Canadian leadership in drawing attention to the importance of social determinants of health, public policy in this country has been slow to respond with concrete actions designed to address these factors in a way that would reduce disparities and foster meaningful improvements in population health. For example, Glouberman and Millar (2003) state that although Canada has been among the countries leading the world in health promotion, there has been no co-ordinated national plan to deal with social inequality issues (such as family and child poverty) that have an upstream impact on population health. Despite some successes at modifying personal health-related practices (for example, through anti-smoking legislation and smoking cessation campaigns), Glouberman and Millar (2003, 391) contend that the population health approach, "while providing a deeper understanding of socioeconomic gradients in health status, has not yet resulted in adequate corresponding policy development to effectively reduce inequalities in health."

Macdonald and colleagues (2009, 527–8) echo this sentiment, stating that although Canada has been a leader in conceptualizing social determinants of health and has influenced policy developments around the world, "there is increasing evidence that Canada is failing to apply its own population health concepts in health research." They argue that social determinants, such as income and income distribution, are often treated as individual-level variables that are risk factors for disease and that many studies fail to identify the structural mechanisms that mediate pathways between income and health (such as the way in which society distributes social and economic resources among the population). In addition, they point out that life course analyses of the ways in which advantage and disadvantage accumulate across the lifespan and affect health are rare. Macdonald and colleagues (2009) conclude that it is not just government inaction that is to blame but also researchers' underdeveloped conceptualization of social determinants that make policy change unlikely.

Raphael (2003b, 398) makes essentially the same point, arguing that despite Canada's reputation as a world leader in health promotion and population health research and policy and the accumulated body of knowledge detailing the importance of social determinants of health and the limited impact of individualized health promotion, "public health practice emphasizes downstream—usually behavioural—strategies rather than addressing the broader societal determinants of health." Raphael (2003a; 2008) highlights the continuing discrepancy between what is known about social determinants of population health and government action on these issues and suggests that, as a consequence of failing to address sources of social inequality and health disparities, Canada has gone from being a policy leader to having a "policy vacuum." Based on a review of Canada's track record at addressing the social determinants of health and reducing health inequalities, Bryant and colleagues (2011) characterize this country as a "land of missed opportunity." They go on to state that Canadian public policy has not reduced inequalities in health and that "Canada's recent performance in numerous key policy areas suggests a bleak prognosis" (2011, 44). Raphael (2011) reinforces this point by concluding that Canada's current economic and political structures and the influence of corporate and business sectors upon public policy make it highly unlikely that we will achieve significant progress in reducing existing inequalities and improving overall population health.

There are a number of barriers facing the implementation of healthy public policies. Raphael (2003a, 37) asserts that "the reasons for governmental inaction on the social determinants of health are relatively easy to ascertain but much more difficult to redress." One of the major challenges is finding a way to put into practice the intersectoral approach to population health promotion recommended for making society and people healthy. This is a complex and difficult undertaking involving changes in government portfolios, co-ordination of various ministries' policy-making strategies, and reallocation of resources (such as funding and staff). In other words, making society healthy means remaking government. At present, very few policy mechanisms exist to facilitate this type of integrated approach to population health promotion.

Finally, there are conflicting interest groups within society and vested interests that resist efforts to bring about significant change. A number of years ago, Alford (1975) commented on the ideological and interest group barriers to reform and suggested that those who have a direct stake in the health-care system are unlikely to favour change, since their interests are well served by current arrangements. This situation has not changed, and such groups include health-care practitioners, such as physicians, hospitals, pharmaceutical companies, private laboratories, and medical equipment manufacturers, as well as self-employed health-care providers such as dentists and optometrists. In many respects, the pharmaceutical industry exemplifies the type of conflict of interest that arises in health care. Drug companies have an obvious profit motive and a huge financial stake in safeguarding the dominant medicalized approach to health care. According to Evans and Stoddart (2003, 378), one of the major challenges facing population health promotion is that these types of "well-defined, though narrowly based, economic interests will be threatened by any serious efforts to act on the nonmedical determinants of health." Vested interests in the health-care sector that are tied to a biomedical conception of disease and are limited to only one determinant of health (i.e., access to formal biomedical services) are unlikely to support implementation of healthy public policies that highlight the need to take action on social determinants of health. Returning to Whitehead and Popay (2010, 1236), swimming upstream is difficult because you are going against the current or, in their terms, you are swimming against "countervailing forces," since "some individuals and groups benefit from perpetuating inequalities." Consequently, there are substantial constraints on implementing policies explicitly intended to improve living and working conditions that have a major impact on population health.

Is Wellness Always Good for Your Health?

Kickbusch (2007, 147) claims that the salutogenic "promise that health can be created, managed and produced by addressing the determinants of health as well as by influencing behavior and lifestyles" has led to the widespread belief that "more health is always possible" and that every choice we make in life has a potential impact on our health. At the same time, we have witnessed the growth in the marketplace of an increasingly long list of products and services to which the added value of health has been attached. She argues that the "wellness revolution" has effectively linked the market, personal choice, and health. In her words, "Health translates into a product that can be bought on the market, promises wellbeing and changes the citizen into a consumer" (2007, 152).

The ideal of well-being that is vigorously promoted in today's consumer culture emphasizes proactive agency and responsibility for one's self and body. According to Sointu (2005), personal health and well-being have become popular notions and are actively embraced by the discerning consumer. In our overly medicalized health-conscious consumer culture, it is difficult to resist purchasing products and services that promise us benefits of good health as well as the possibility of achieving wellness. However, Hanlon and Carlisle (2009) caution that modern culture, with its extreme emphasis on "individualized consumerism" and materialism, may be bad for our health. They argue that the way in which wellness is marketed today is potentially damaging for all members of society, although the greatest impact is on the disadvantaged, and contributes to increasing social inequality, perpetuating disparities in health.

Health is an important human value. We place a high priority on good health compared to other aspects of our daily lives. People often comment that there is nothing more important than good health, which is valued for a number of different reasons. For example, it involves a feeling-state and a level of functioning that are inherently desirable. At the same time, good health is valued at both personal and societal levels because it facilitates achievement of individual objectives (e.g., a successful career, prosperity) and contributes to a dynamic and productive society. Eiser and Gentle (1988) suggest that values, such as health, should be understood as goals that define our behavioural intentions (e.g., I intend to eat better food) and health behaviour as goal-directed action (e.g., I have changed my dietary practices to improve my health). Although staying healthy is an important life goal, it is not a good basis for predicting future behaviours.

In fact, the value that we attach to good health does not necessarily translate into health-protective behaviour. This contradiction between health beliefs and health behaviours is hard to explain. We are growing increasingly health-conscious and are now better informed about health risks, but we continue to be inconsistent in our health behaviour (e.g., trading off healthful and harmful practices in our daily lives). "Indeed, individuals may make behavioral choices that appear inconsistent with respect to their value of health; for example, an individual may exercise regularly, but not wear seat belts, or adhere to dietary restrictions, but smoke cigarettes" (Bruhn 1988, 81). It is very difficult to convince people to change or give up routine personal practices and adopt behaviours that promise uncertain health benefits. Bruhn (1988, 80) argues that "one reason for the difficulty in getting people to change their health behaviors is that preserving health is not our society's highest value. It competes with many other values, including wealth, power, security, knowledge, and social acceptance." The list of competing values is actually much longer (e.g., we also value privacy and liberty). Furthermore, to repeat a point made earlier, we tend to take good health for granted and only become concerned about our health when we experience illness. As a result, when symptomatic conditions or life-threatening disease confronts us, the importance of health and the value placed on health care increase dramatically. It seems that protecting and enhancing good health is still not one of our highest values!

It is also important to recognize that health choices and behavioural practices take place in the context of broader moral and evaluative judgments about everyday life. Backett (1992) agrees with the assertion that good health is simply one of many competing priorities that affect our daily behaviour and that choices among these priorities typically involve wider social and moral evaluations. To explore these issues, she carried out a qualitative study of families and examined the role of moral evaluations in individuals' accounts of health and in their everyday health-related decisions and personal health practices. In Backett's (1992, 256) words, the focus of the research was "on how health-relevant decisions and behaviours can be understood as part of the everyday fabric of family interaction and prioritising, and that this in turn reflects and affects lay moralities about appropriate social behaviour."

This study suggests that the pursuit of health and wellness is embedded in moral judgments that we make in our everyday lives. For example, participants defined healthiness in moralistic terms that involved judgments about good and bad behaviour (and in some cases judgments about good and bad individuals). Furthermore, the majority of respondents "felt the need to apologise for and justify aspects of their lives which they thought might seem to be unhealthy" (Backett 1992, 261). In contrast, when respondents commented on their health-promoting practices, they described themselves as self-righteous. Backett concludes that to achieve good health, we have to deal with considerable uncertainty about the health benefits of our wellness-oriented life choices and, at the same time, make our way successfully through a moral minefield. This study highlights the fact that lay beliefs about healthy and unhealthy behaviour are closely connected to notions of good and bad and that health invariably involves moral evaluations of socially appropriate behaviour. With the growing emphasis on health promotion and the current wellness movement, we are likely to feel increasing pressure to demonstrate to others that we are taking steps (i.e., doing the "right" things) to maintain and improve both our health and wellness.

In a discussion of morality and the pursuit of health, Conrad (1994) suggests that wellness seekers live in a moral world of good and bad and engage in a moral discourse about health promotion. As discussed earlier in the book, wellness is a much broader concept than health. It includes the components of good health (i.e., a sense of healthiness, fitness, and functional ability) as well as satisfying living and working conditions, economic security, and meaningful social relationships. Although the meaning of wellness remains a bit vague and the precise health benefits of wellness activities have not been thoroughly documented, we have embraced the "wellness revolution." According to Conrad (1994, 385), "For more than two decades there has been a virtual explosion in interest in health promotion and wellness in American society." This statement was made some time ago, but it is still true of both the United States and Canada today. Our culture has become increasingly preoccupied with the pursuit of health and wellness.

Conrad characterizes wellness as a virtue. As previously described, health as a value refers to a desirable life goal that inadvertently becomes enmeshed in moral judgments as part of daily living and is reflected, to some extent, by our health choices and personal practices. In comparison, wellness explicitly embodies notions of moral superiority, uprightness, and goodness. You are probably familiar with the expression that "virtue is its own reward." Does this mean that the pursuit of wellness is also its own reward? If pursuing wellness is an end in itself, then we may feel better about ourselves simply because we engage in certain morally correct behaviours (e.g., joining a fitness club). Alternatively, we may worry ourselves sick over the pursuit of health and wellness. The lesson is that it is important to distinguish between lifestyle behavioural changes that have known health benefits (e.g., engaging in vigorous exercise to improve cardiovascular health) and wellness activities that are essentially moral actions intended to demonstrate to others that you lead a healthy life (e.g., purchasing home exercise equipment that you seldom use).

Leichter (1997) describes the wellness movement and lifestyle correctness as a new secular morality; it has become our culture's new religion. As such, it is viewed as the path to personal and social redemption and affirmation of a life lived virtuously. According to Leichter (1997, 359), by embracing "low-fat, high-fiber diets, metabolic workouts, aerobic stepping, stress management, fitness centre memberships, and at least eight glasses of designer-label water a day," we hope to achieve a secular state of grace. In many respects, health promotion has achieved the status of a moral imperative, and certain types of healthful behaviour have been equated with virtue (while other, health-harmful behaviours, such as smoking, have been equated with vice). The current wellness movement is based on lifestyle correctness and the belief that there are critical health-protective behaviours over which the individual has considerable control. Unfortunately, biomedicine remains ambivalent about the exact impact that practices such as jogging and eating heart-smart choices in restaurants have on our health. As a result, Leichter (1997, 361) cautions that "the new secular morality is only partly about health and a good deal about individual and collective social position, status and image."

Kirkland (2014a) points out that the term wellness has been around for some time now and combines ideas about health, morality, and responsibility. Wellness emphasizes personal responsibility for making lifestyle choices and self-care decisions that will improve health and well-being. Kirkland argues that the wellness movement suggests that the era of combating diseases has been replaced by an even more complex problem facing societies today—that is, the challenge of living well! To illustrate this point, Kirkland goes on to state that "striving for wellness is a personal responsibility that an individual can achieve if she really wants to, and if she fails to undertake it, it must be because she lacks information, access, or incentive" (2014b, 977).

She agrees with earlier critics such as Conrad and Leichter that wellness promotes a "single-minded and detailed view of what kind of life is worth living" (2014b, 975) as well as a "conservative, individualistic health ideology" (2014b, 976) that distracts us from focusing on the upstream structural determinants of health. Furthermore, Kirkland (2014a, 957) argues that wellness has become a popular buzzword today and the use of this term has spread dramatically to include "wellness programs, wellness centres, wellness contests, wellness conferences, wellness journals, wellness administrators, wellness awards, wellness tourism, and even a Wellness brand cat and dog food." This has led to the appearance of articles in major newspapers (such as the one in Box 12.4) questioning whether wellness has become a dangerous ideology. According to this article in *The Globe and Mail*, the danger stems from the fact that the wellness ideology places too much emphasis on personal responsibility for health, obscures the fact that structural determinants play a greater role in shaping population health, and perpetuates a moralistic ideal of well-being that may not only be unattainable but also does not necessarily have clearly established health benefits. This suggests that a critical sociological analysis would be helpful in evaluating the behavioural practices advocated by the wellness movement to identify salutary factors that have positive health benefits and actually contribute to the goal of making societies and people healthy.

Box 12.4   Has "Wellness" Become a Dangerous Ideology?

Wellness is prized these days. We want to balance our work and life, ensuring a healthy lifestyle. We try to carve out time for exercise, avoid fatty foods, and shun smoking (and smokers). Positivity is considered a virtue.

But Stockholm business school professor Carl Cederstrom believes we have gone overboard with our walking meetings, treadmill desks, and meditation classes. "Wellness has become an ideology," he says during an interview—a dangerous ideology because not all of us can live up to the wellness creed and there can be intolerance towards smokers and people with weight issues, for example. But it's also dangerous because it obscures the fact that economic and social factors—and political decisions—can have a much greater determinant on overall health than the individual actions of the higher income folk.

If you're unhealthy and unhappy, Prof. Cederstrom says, the implication is that you have failed morally in some fashion. Not only is that a heavy burden to bear but it's purely individual when good health has social-economic implications. People are now adding their exercise successes to resumes, noting the marathons or triathlons they have participated in, as our wellness obsession implies that means they will make better employees: More vigorous, more disciplined. If you are a healthy person exercising you are assumed to be a committed, effective employee. If you smoke or are overweight, beware. "We have shifted from the work ethic to the work-out ethic," he says.

Source: Excerpted from Harvey Schachter, "Has 'wellness' become a dangerous ideology?" 4 September 2015. Special to *The Globe and Mail*.

What Is Required to Remake the Medicalized Society into a Salutogenic Society?

It should be apparent that health and wellness are complicated topics that defy simple explanation. We still have a long way to go before we will be able to fully explain the multiple pathways through which social determinants shape health and the complex social processes involved in the pursuit of health and wellness across the life course. Achieving healthy futures requires a reduction in social inequalities in health, improvements in living and working conditions, and involvement of well-informed community members in pursuit of this common goal. Earlier in the book, we commented on the fact that members of the public are primary providers of health care and active participants in the production of health. The critical difference between producing health and consuming health care was effectively described a number of years ago by Evans and Stoddart (1990). Their framework questions the widespread belief that availability and use of medical care are central to the health of individuals and populations. This thought-provoking paper influenced the development of current Canadian policies on population health promotion and a broader approach to health by highlighting the distinction between producing health and consuming health care. Evans and Stoddart argue that modern societies devote too many resources to the delivery of formal health care and that determinants of health go beyond the marginal contribution of these types of services. Their extended framework acknowledges the many intersecting behavioural, environmental, and biological determinants of health and encourages researchers to recognize that the goal of health care cannot simply be the prevention of disease (as defined by the formal health-care system). Acknowledging that we are active producers of health (and not just passive consumers of biomedical care) requires shifting the focus to enhancing positive health actions and supporting daily management of health as a resource for living.

Remaking the medicalized society into a salutogenic society requires that decisions be made with respect to the reallocation of resources. We need to question whether investing more in medicalized responses to illness, such as pharmaceutical and biotechnological innovations, is the most effective way of producing population health. One of the prerequisites for healthy societies is a clear distinction between biomedical care and health care. Resources directed toward provision of medical care undeniably save lives and lessen suffering. These benefits, however, come at the cost of resources that could be directed toward the "indirect societal factors that are mainly responsible for making and keeping people healthy" (Wright 2009, 3). Simply stated, money spent on responding to illness in the form of biomedical care is money that can't be directed to making society healthy. Cross-national research (Leon, Walt, and Gilson 2001) shows that population health status returns from per capita spending on medical care drop off sharply after $1000. (Currently, in Canada we spend more than five times this amount.) This demonstrates that there are limits to how much population health can be produced by investing in formal health care and sustaining medicalized societies.

In order to make societies and people healthy, governments and citizens alike need to face the reality that there is more to producing health than providing access to biomedical care. Medicine does not equal health! Research discussed throughout this book provides evidence that investments in policies intended to make society more salutogenic succeed in making people healthier. If formal health-care services are to make a meaningful contribution to improvements in the health of the overall population, they must be designed to maintain and promote health and wellness for all members of society. Services such as prenatal care and well baby clinics play an important part in risk reduction and disease prevention related to maternal and child health, but at the same time, additional health promotion services are required that provide people with the knowledge and skills to lead healthier lives. As Wilkinson and Marmot (2003) point out in their discussion of health determinants, there is clear evidence that coping skills and personal practices acquired early in life have a major impact on lifelong health and wellness. Consequently, health services that are explicitly intended to help people (from an early age) to engage in health-protective behaviours are much more consistent with a salutogenic society's approach to producing long-term population health benefits.

Investing in a salutogenic society has payoffs in terms of both individual and population health. The difficulty, however, is that the benefits of committing additional resources to making societies and people healthy take years, and sometimes even decades, to be realized. In contrast, spending more money on biomedical care—for example, to reduce surgical wait times—provides almost immediate (although temporary) improvement in delivery of formal care, as well as the type of short-term public recognition on which politicians make their reputations and win elections. Reallocating resources upstream to create a salutogenic society through investing in childhood development programs such as daycare, early life nutrition, and literacy will make children healthier as adults, but such health benefits have a distant horizon. For a salutogenic society to emerge as a viable alternative to the medicalized society, we need political leadership and the collective societal will to pursue long-term changes that will make both societies and people healthy.

The ongoing pursuit of health and wellness is a lengthy process, and there are many obstacles to overcome. The basic premise of this book is that sociological theory and methods have important parts to play in supporting efforts to achieve healthy futures. For example, in-depth sociological analysis can contribute to a better understanding of the relationship between health as a societal value and the organization of formal health care, as well as the link between the personal value of health and routine self-care health and illness behaviours. Sociology has the potential to help foster development of effective strategies for making societies and people healthy.

If health is largely influenced by the social environment in which we live and work, then life circumstances and the social context in which health and illness are experienced should be the major focus of future population health promotion initiatives. Walters (2003, 6) emphatically underscores this point by stating that in the past,

> the dominant emphasis has been on biomedical interventions in relation to the individual, and these have been guided by a disease-based model. But if the targets for intervention are socio-economic, then we have to take features of social life as a starting point. We must place a primary emphasis on fighting poverty, social exclusion, unemployment, poor working conditions and gender inequalities, each of which can influence lifestyles and prompt or exacerbate a range of different health problems.

This is not to dismiss the role of biomedicine and formal health care, since we need to understand how the social is embodied and the ways in which we respond to ill health. It does, however, offer an alternative, less medico-centric vision of future health-care policy and programs. This perspective highlights the need for major changes in the way we think about the meaning of good health and the structural and personal factors that make societies and people healthy. Furthermore, it draws attention to the fact that improvements in population health depend on initiatives to tackle sources of social inequality that result in health disparities and to create salutogenic societies that provide individuals with necessary opportunities to achieve healthy futures.

Is there any reason to be optimistic about the prospect of achieving a healthy future? There are continuing calls for global upstream action on the social determinants of health and for renewed efforts to reduce inequalities in health (e.g. Friel and Marmot 2011; Lee 2010; Marmot, Bell, and Goldblatt 2013; Marmot, Allen, and Goldblatt 2010). These researchers point out that we now have global evidence of the impact of social determinants on population health and that it is time to act on the unequal distribution of social and economic resources and inequalities in the conditions of everyday life. Marmot, Bell, and Goldblatt (2013, S127) call for cross-government commitment to act on the "toxic combination of poor policies and programmes, unfair economic arrangements and bad governance" that are responsible for producing and reinforcing health inequalities. They go on to state that "the circumstances in which people are born, grow, live, work, and age" lead to health inequalities "between groups defined by socioeconomic position, ethnicity or geographic residence" (2013, S127). Friel and Marmot (2011, 232–3) believe that "the launch of a global movement that perceives equitable health as a societal good, at the heart of which lies social policy and action" can lead to significant social change. The political strategy guiding the movement is to make health equity a priority in global, national, regional, and local public policies. While there has been some progress and there may be reason to be optimistic, it seems quite unlikely that the health gap will be closed in a generation (as suggested by the WHO in 2008). Overall, the general opinion is that a growing global social movement calling for action on the social determinants of health and health equity has the potential to transform social and economic policies in a way that will ultimately result in a fairer society and healthier lives (Marmot and Bell 2012).

In the Canadian context, Meili (2012) echoes this sentiment in his discussion of the types of democratic reforms that could help to shape public policy on the social determinants of health and create a truly healthy society. Keon and Pepin (2009) make a strong case for taking action in their report on building a healthy, productive Canada. After examining the impact of multiple factors on the health of the Canadian population, they conclude that it is unacceptable for a wealthy country such as Canada to continue to tolerate extreme disparities in health. The report includes a long list of recommendations, starting with implementation of a population health policy at the federal level. It also recommends establishing intergovernmental mechanisms for collaboration and intersectoral action and assigning priority to social determinants of health, such as parenting and early childhood learning, education, housing, and economic development. The report stresses the importance of developing the longitudinal research capacity needed to monitor the health and well-being of Canadians across the life course. It is time to take bold and innovative action to achieve greater health equity. Labonte (2012) recommends a health equity approach to public policy but cautions that one of the major challenges facing global action on the social determinants of health is the willingness of governments to make policy choices that will address rapidly escalating income and wealth inequalities. While the challenges ahead on the road to health and wellness are daunting and the task of finally implementing the type of actions that have been repeatedly recommended will be difficult, there is reason to believe that it is possible to do a better job of creating healthy societies and healthy people.

Study Questions

1. Describe the ways in which making society and people healthy is a shared responsibility.
2. Comment critically on the strengths and weaknesses of the Canadian health policies reviewed.
3. Summarize the main obstacles facing the implementation of healthy public policies.
4. Outline the major differences between the vision of a healthy society and the reality of health-care reform that has taken place.
5. Comment on the relationship between universal health insurance, access to medical care, and health disparities.
6. Describe the types of public policy initiatives you feel would be effective in reducing disparities in health related to social inequality.
7. How can the pursuit of wellness be hazardous to your health?

Recommended Readings

Birch, S., and A. Gafni. 2005. "Achievements and challenges of medicare in Canada: Are we there yet? Are we on course?" *International Journal of Health Services* 35: 443–63.

Bryant, T., D. Raphael, T. Schrecker, and R. Labonte. 2011. "Canada: A land of missed opportunity for addressing the social determinants of health." *Health Policy* 101: 44–58.

Conrad, P. 1994. "Wellness as a virtue: Morality and the pursuit of health." *Culture, Medicine and Psychiatry* 18: 385–401.

Evans, R.G., and G.L. Stoddart. 1990. "Producing health, consuming health care." *Social Science and Medicine* 31: 1347–63.

Friel, S., and M. Marmot. 2011. "Action on the social determinants of health and health equities goes global." *The Annual Review of Public Health* 32: 225–36.

Hankivsky, O., and R. Cormier. 2011. "Intersectionality and public policy: Some lessons from existing models." *Political Research Quarterly* 64: 217–29.

Hanlon, P., and S. Carlisle. 2009. "Is 'modern culture' bad for our health and well-being?" *Global Health Promotion* 16: 27–34.

McDaniel, S., and P. Bernard. 2011. "Life course as a policy lens: Challenges and opportunities." *Canadian Public Policy* 37 (2011 Supplement): S1–S13.

Whitehead, M., and J. Popay. 2010. "Swimming upstream? Taking action on the social determinants of health inequalities." *Social Science and Medicine* 71: 1234–6.

Willson, A. 2009. "'Fundamental causes' of health disparities: A comparative analysis of Canada and the United States." *International Sociology* 24: 93–113.

Recommended Websites

National Collaborating Centre for Healthy Public Policy
www.ncchpp.ca

Wellness Checkpoint:
www.wellnesscheckpoint.com

Glossary

accessibility The fundamental principle of medicare that reasonable access to medical care is guaranteed for all Canadians.

agency The ability of individuals to act as self-conscious, willful social agents and to make free choices about behaviour.

age stratification The unequal distribution of wealth, power, and privilege among people at different stages in the life course, which has both direct and indirect effects on health.

age structure A demographic term used to describe the age composition of a population.

alternative medicine Forms of health care that are used instead of biomedical care.

androcentric A way of thinking that privileges the masculine perspective when trying to understand social life.

biographical disruption The understanding of chronic illness as interference in an individual's life story, since it creates considerable uncertainty about the ill person's health and social life.

biological determinism The belief that human behaviour can best be explained in terms of the innate biological properties of individuals, such as genes and biochemical processes.

biomedicalization The extension of medicalization brought about through technoscience.

biomedical model A model of health care based on scientific understanding that, at the level of basic knowledge, sees health and illness in terms of biological processes and, at the applied clinical level, privileges individualized, biologically oriented, pharmacological, surgical, and technological interventions.

biopower Foucault's term explaining how medical knowledge provides a basis for power and control in modern societies.

body projects Shilling's term describing the manner in which bodies act as mediums for the expression of identity and social status.

built environment Aspects of the physical environment that affect health, such as housing and the design of cities.

CAM The acronym for complementary/alternative medicine used as a general term to describe alternative and complementary medicines without necessarily differentiating between them.

causality The illness belief dimension that assumes that every identified disease has a specific underlying cause or combination of causal factors.

cellular pathology A microscopic biophysical defect within the body that, according to Laboratory Medicine, is believed to cause disease.

chronic disease A long-term physical health problem that lasts for more than six months and has been diagnosed by a health professional.

clinical iatrogenesis Harm caused directly by health care.

co-morbidity The presence of one or more additional diseases occurring at the same time as a primary disease.

complementary medicine Forms of health care that are used alongside biomedical care.

comprehensiveness The fundamental principle of medicare that all necessary medical services are guaranteed without dollar limit and are available solely on the basis of medical need.

conflict paradigm A theoretical perspective that argues that the distinctive feature of capitalist society is that it is composed of a number of competing interest groups. The conflict paradigm focuses on group power struggles (e.g., social class, gender, ethnic relationships) and interprets social relations primarily in terms of political and economic dimensions of social inequality.

consumer culture A dominant characteristic of advanced capitalist society is that the consumption of goods and services makes statements about self-identity and location in the social world.

controllability The illness belief dimension that refers to the extent to which individuals believe that illness is controllable and can be managed by either the sick person or another person such as a health-care professional.

cultural capital Symbolic and informational resources for action, such as values, normative beliefs, knowledge, and skills, that are acquired through socialization in particular socio-cultural contexts.

cultural competency A form of intercultural care in which health-care providers are expected to understand how ethnocultural diversity affects the behaviour of specific patient subpopulations such as ethnic groups and to tailor care accordingly.

cultural iatrogenesis The manner in which the medicalization of life compromises people's abilities to look after their health without professional medicine's help.

cultural safety An approach to intercultural care that gives the patient the power to judge whether a particular health-care professional or treatment is safe from the perspective of their culture.

cultural sensitivity An approach to intercultural care that emphasizes an awareness on the part of health-care providers that patients may come from different cultural backgrounds.

culture The totality of ideas, beliefs, values, knowledge, and way of life of a group of people who share a certain historical, religious, racial, linguistic, ethnic, or social background.

demand–control model A model that focuses on the ways in which a low level of control over work schedules and job conditions and the psychological demands of work negatively affect health.

demedicalization When an aspect of social life is no longer defined in medical terms and the involvement of medical personnel is no longer deemed appropriate.

differential exposure hypothesis The suggestion that the higher number of health problems among lower-SES groups can be explained by greater exposure to psychosocial stressors, such as financial insecurity, neighbourhood issues, and social isolation.

differential vulnerability hypothesis The suggestion that the higher number of health problems among lower-SES groups can be explained by harmful behavioural practices, such as smoking, used to cope with environmental stressors.

disease An objective, biophysical phenomenon that is characterized by altered functioning of the body as a biological organism.

effort–reward imbalance model A model that emphasizes the importance of social reciprocity in our work lives and the ways that health is adversely affected if the time and effort devoted to work are not matched by adequate rewards.

e-health The application of communication and information technologies in health care, such as websites offering health information.

embodiment Ways in which human perception and experience of society and culture happen through the body.

emotional support Supportive social relationships that contribute to feelings of being cared for and valued, which help us to feel part of a meaningful network or group of people.

ethnic ancestry/origin The place where an individual or her ancestors were born.

ethnic density effect Health benefits associated with living in a neighbourhood with a high concentration of others from one's own ethnic group.

ethnic groups Social groupings that exist within a particular cultural framework.

ethnic identity A social characteristic by which a person locates and understands herself within the world based on ethnic group membership.

ethnicity A shared (whether perceived or actual) group identity that is rooted in cultural elements, such as custom, language, religion, or history, or some mixture of these factors.

ethnic stratification The unequal distribution of wealth, power, and privilege based on ethnic group membership, which has both direct and indirect effects on health.

ethnoculture Cultural features associated with ethnic groups, which support patterns and processes of ethnic identification.

feeling-state orientation The belief that good health means a sense of well-being.

feminist paradigm A theoretical perspective that comprises many diverse waves of feminist thought that have in common a focus on historical oppression of women.

fitness The physical dimension of good health that refers to biophysical function, such as aerobic capacity or muscle strength.

gender The socio-cultural expression of sex in terms of personal identity and role performance (e.g., being feminine), shaping the ways in which health and illness are experienced.

gender stratification The unequal distribution of wealth, power, and privilege between men and women, which has both direct and indirect effects on health.

habitus Bourdieu's concept explaining the embodiment of social location and culture.

health A socially constructed, multidimensional life course experience that varies over time according to different social, cultural, and economic life circumstances.

health as a resource for living A conception of health that combines the social, psychological, and physical dimensions and understands health as an asset to be managed.

health as a sense of well-being A conception of health that emphasizes positive psychosocial aspects of health, such as feelings of healthiness and happiness along with rewarding relationships.

health as fitness A conception of health that understands health to mean being physically active and having a healthy body with psychological energy and vitality.

health as functional ability A conception of health that emphasizes the individual's ability to carry out daily tasks and cope with the demands of everyday life and social roles.

health assets Factors that enhance the ability of individuals or populations to maintain health and well-being, including social, economic, and environmental resources.

Glossary

health as the absence of illness and disease A negative conception of health-in-a-vacuum that understands health in terms of what is absent from the individual's life: illness.

health behaviour Routine health-protective activities, including personal self-care regulatory and preventive practices (e.g., exercise, nutrition), risk reduction, and disease prevention (e.g., smoking cessation).

health belief system A systematic set of ideas with regard to health, healing, and self-care that are shaped by aspects of culture and social location.

health consciousness The degree to which an individual is aware of and attentive to her own health, which involves monitoring health status, assessing and interpreting the condition of her mind and body, and engaging in a wide variety of health actions.

health diary A data collection method used to gather detailed information about ongoing health and illness behaviours that is well suited for obtaining records of symptomatic conditions that do not restrict daily activities or prompt medical care and for gaining a more complete picture of population health.

health expectancy (or **health-adjusted life expectancy**) A comprehensive indicator reflecting the average number of years one can expect to live in good health.

health inequities A term used to describe avoidable health inequalities that are unnecessary and unjust.

healthism A preoccupation with personal responsibility for health and self-care behaviour.

health lifestyles Collective patterns of health-related behaviour based on choices (i.e., agency) from options available to people according to their life chances (i.e., structure).

health literacy The ability to access, understand, and evaluate information as a way to maintain and improve health across the life course.

health promotion A state-sponsored process aimed at getting individuals to take control over and improve their health by providing them with health-related education and information.

health reserve The concept of health as an asset to be managed.

health sociology Sociological analysis of social structures and behavioural practices that influence both personal and population health. This perspective focuses on good health as well as ill health and critically evaluates the link between sources of social inequality and health disparities.

health status designation Twaddle's term for the complex, ongoing social process involved in adapting to changing demands of life and responding to health concerns.

health trajectory Changes in the patterns of health experienced over time.

healthy immigrant effect The finding that immigrants to Canada typically have better health than those born in Canada.

hegemonic masculinity The culturally dominant ideal of what it means to be male and how masculine men are supposed to behave within patriarchal society.

holism An approach to understanding the world that views whole entities as made up of more than the sum of their parts.

horizontal structures Raphael's term describing immediate factors that have a direct impact on health, such as family environment, the nature of work and workplace conditions, quality of housing, and availability of neighbourhood resources (e.g., recreational facilities).

humoral theory An ancient understanding of illness as resulting from imbalance involving physical, environmental, and spiritual factors reflected in four substances known as the humours.

iatrogenesis Sickness and injury caused by the health-care system.

illness A subjective, psychosocial phenomenon in which individuals perceive themselves as not feeling well and engage in different types of behaviour in an effort to overcome their ill health.

illness behaviour Perception and evaluation of the meaning of daily symptoms (e.g., perceived seriousness, causal attributions) and reactive self-care practices, including self-medication and illness-related activity restrictions (e.g., sick days).

illness narrative accounts Stories told by people, particularly those living with chronic conditions, regarding the meaning and management of illness experiences.

incidence rate The number of new cases of a specific disease identified over a period of time, such as a year. This information tells us whether more people are now affected by a particular condition than in the past.

income adequacy A calculation based on total household income and number of people in the family, measuring financial capacity to meet needs.

income inequality The uneven distribution of income within a society or community, which is linked to disparities in population health.

income inequality hypothesis The hypothesis originated by Richard Wilkinson that greater inequality in income distribution within a population increases social problems, including a social gradient in health.

informational support Supportive social relationships that are an important source of information about health-related matters.

instrumental support Supportive social relationships that provide individuals with practical assistance with the activities of daily living.

integrative medicine A form of health care that brings together CAM treatments that have been scientifically proven safe and effective with conventional biomedical treatments.

intercultural care An approach to health care that recognizes the cultural uniqueness of individual patients from different ethnic backgrounds.

intergenerational trauma Negative emotional effects stemming from an initial terrible experience felt throughout the life course and reproduced through subsequent generations as a legacy of suffering.

intersectional analysis An approach that studies the interaction of factors such as gender, socioeconomic status, ethnicity, and age, which together shape behaviour and life chances, such as health outcomes.

intersectoral approach An approach to improving population health that involves co-ordinated policy initiatives across several different government sectors simultaneously.

lay beliefs Ideas and perspectives employed by ordinary people to make sense of and find meaning in their everyday life experiences, such as health and illness.

life chances Aspects of the social structure that provide a social context for individual life choices.

life choices The decisions that individuals make in their selection of lifestyle behaviours, which affect health outcomes.

life course An age-graded sequence of multiple stages or phases and roles embedded in a network of social relationships.

life course perspective The view that current and future health is the dynamic outcome of past experiences.

life expectancy The estimated number of years that people can expect to live.

lifestyle A collective way of life reflecting beliefs, attitudes, and values, as well as patterns of behaviour, that are shaped by life circumstances and socio-cultural context.

medical consumerism The view of health as a commodity that can be preserved and improved through purchasing health-care products and services.

medical dominance The power exercised by the profession of medicine over the health-care system.

medical gaze Foucault's term describing the development of the modern medical view of the human body as a biophysical object.

medical ideology The belief system of the profession of medicine used to justify the position of physicians as the ultimate authorities on health matters.

medical-industrial complex A term used by Navarro to describe the development of a huge, profit-driven health-care industry.

medicalization The tendency to understand aspects of social life as medical issues requiring intervention and control on the part of medicine.

medical pluralism The coexistence in a society of differing medical traditions grounded in different cultural principles or based on different world views.

medical screening A process that assesses individuals for the risk of disease that has not appeared symptomatically.

medicare The system of universal health insurance introduced by the Canadian government in 1968.

medico-centric bias A way of thinking about health, illness, and the body that privileges the norms and values of biomedicine and the dominance of the medical profession in the health-care sector.

mind–body connection The idea that biophysical health is linked to mental states such as emotions and stress.

mind–body dualism Descartes' seventeenth-century philosophical separation of mind and body, which provided a rationale for focusing solely on the individual biophysical body as a way to understand health and illness.

morbidity The distribution of disease in populations.

mortality The number of deaths in a population within a prescribed time, expressed as either crude rates for the overall population or rates specific to diseases or to age, sex, or other attributes (e.g., age-specific mortality rates).

mutual aid Ways people informally come together to offer each other mutually beneficial forms of support or reciprocal assistance.

natural environment Aspects of the physical environment that affect health, such as air and water quality.

normal health A unique combination of aspects of good health and ill health blending feelings of healthiness, physical fitness, and performance of one's usual well roles together with the routine experience of symptomatic conditions.

optimum capacity The social dimension of good health that refers to individual ability to fulfill personal goals and perform socially defined roles in a way that meets cultural expectations.

pathogenesis The origins of disease as defined by biomedicine.

pathological lesion An underlying biophysical defect within the body that, according to hospital medicine, is believed to cause disease.

perceived susceptibility The illness belief dimension that reflects the degree to which a person believes that she is vulnerable to or might experience health problems.

performance orientation The belief that good health means being able to carry out one's usual daily activities.

personalized medicine A form of formal health care in which medical knowledge of each person's genome serves as the basis for tailoring medical interventions designed for the individual's unique biology.

personal determinants Factors specific to the individual that exert an internal influence on health, such as genetic makeup, beliefs, attitudes, and behavioural practices.

personal health status An approach to assessing health that focuses on individuals who have a health problem or are at risk of developing one.

pharmaceuticalization The process by which social, behavioural, or bodily conditions are treated, or deemed to be in need of treatment, with pharmaceuticals.

physical capital Resources for action tied to particular expressions of embodiment.

political economy An interdisciplinary field of social science that critically analyzes the political, economic, and social relations of the capitalist social system.

population aging A trend whereby the proportion of people over the age of 65 is expected to accelerate in the future.

population health status An inclusive approach to assessing health that focuses on the general population or specific subpopulations.

portability The fundamental principle of medicare that benefits are transferable from province to province.

pragmatic acculturation The borrowing of ideas, ways of thinking, or ways of doing things from a culture that is not one's own for the purpose of solving a particular problem such as illness.

prevalence rate The proportion of people in the general population who have a diagnosed disease at a given point in time. This information tells us how widespread the selected condition is.

preventive self-care Deliberate health actions undertaken to reduce the risk of illness.

primary determinants Factors that have a direct effect on health, such as household income, education level, and employment status.

psychopharmacological societies Rose's term to describe societies in which the modification of thought, mood, and conduct by pharmacological means has become more or less routine.

public administration The fundamental principle of medicare that the health-care program is administered by a non-profit agency or commission.

race A scientifically discredited concept that nonetheless is an important social construction that has significant consequences for people's lives, bodies, and health in that it is a major basis of social exclusion.

racialization Processes by which people are systematically categorized and socially excluded according to perceived racial differences.

racism Prejudicial treatment of groups and individuals according to subjective understandings of race.

reactive self-care Self-initiated responses to symptoms that have not been diagnosed by a physician.

reductionism An approach to understanding the world that breaks phenomena into smaller and smaller parts in order to understand them.

regulatory self-care Daily habits of living that affect health but may not be viewed as actions that are explicitly intended to improve health and well-being.

religiosity The degree of adherence to and participation in religious belief and practice.

residential schools Government-funded and church-operated boarding schools that removed Aboriginal children from their families and communities with the goal of assimilating them into mainstream Canadian culture.

restorative self-care Actions intended to overcome health problems in the case of acute disease or to adjust one's daily life to achieve an optimum level of functioning in the case of chronic disease.

risk factors Factors that are believed to lead to disease and are often treated as diseases in their own right.

risk-taking hypothesis The suggestion that men are socialized to take health risks while women are socialized to be cautious and concerned about taking care of health.

role accumulation hypothesis The suggestion that multiple roles contribute to better health because they provide a variety of benefits, such as greater self-esteem, life satisfaction, more sources of social support, and improved financial resources.

role strain hypothesis The suggestion that increased stress and excessive demands on time and energy associated with performing multiple roles result in poorer health outcomes for women.

salutogenesis Antonovsky's term describing the origins of positive health, which was introduced to encourage researchers to pay attention to the factors that protect and enhance good health.

salutogenic model of health A conceptual model introduced by Antonovsky to provide a guide for identifying and understanding salutary factors that make populations healthy. The model contributes to an improved understanding of the origins of good health and social conditions that facilitate health-protective behaviours.

secondary determinants Factors that reflect our living and working conditions and play an important intervening role between social status and health status, such as daily behavioural practices (e.g., smoking) and psychosocial well-being (e.g., sense of coherence).

self-care The many everyday health-care activities that lay people informally undertake to manage personal and family health concerns as a fundamental part of self-health management.

self-health management A term that reflects the fact that members of the public routinely engage in personal health practices, including health-protective and illness treatment activities, that are an expression of personal autonomy and active involvement in a complex decision-making process.

self-help groups Organizations that help people deal with specific common health-related problems by bringing them together to fill a gap that may exist between informal caregiving networks and formal professional health care.

self-rated health Individuals' self-reported health status as excellent, very good, good, fair, or poor.

sense of coherence Antonovsky's concept describing a way of seeing the world that consists of three core components: comprehensibility, manageability, and meaningfulness.

sense of healthiness The psychological dimension of good health expressed as emotional well-being or life satisfaction.

seriousness The illness belief dimension that reflects whether a person believes the condition is long-lasting, difficult to cure, and requires medical attention.

sex Physiological attributes of the person (i.e., being female), which are important biological determinants of health.

sex- and gender-based analysis (SGBA) A systematic approach to research, policies, and programs that explores biological (sex-based) and socio-cultural (gender-based) similarities and differences between women and men.

sickness A concept that includes both the presence of disease and the experience of illness.

sick role A concept used by Parsons to describe the set of behavioural expectations about how a sick person should behave (and be treated), which is built into the social system and is a patterned part of culture.

sick role behaviour Informal and formal help-seeking behaviour, such as lay consultation and the use of formal health-care services.

signs Observable indicators of bodily change that serve as the basic evidence used by biomedicine for diagnosing the presence of disease.

social acceptability hypothesis The suggestion that because of socialization into traditional gender roles, women are more willing to adopt the sick role (i.e., they are more willing to admit to being sick and to accept help in dealing with their health problems).

social capital Resources for action tied to interpersonal relations and group membership.

social class A social grouping based on a combination of socioeconomic factors, such as income, occupation, and education, which has significant impacts on health.

social determinants of health Societal factors, such as life circumstances in which people are born, live, work, and age, that affect health.

social epidemiology The study of social factors that place individuals and populations at risk for disease and illness.

social exclusion A process of marginalization reflecting unequal power relationships between groups in society that involve unequal access to social, cultural, political, and economic resources and have adverse health effects.

social gradient The graded association between socioeconomic status and population health.

social iatrogenesis The indirect harm medicalization causes society in general by defining more and more aspects of life, from birth, through sorrow, suffering, and sickness, to death, as medical issues.

social inequality Relatively stable differences between individuals and groups of people in the distribution of power and privilege that exist because opportunities are differentially distributed in society based on factors such as social class, gender, ethnicity, and age, which have a significant impact on health.

social medicine The view that health and illness are consequences of the social structural organization of capitalist society and that addressing social inequalities can improve the health of the population.

social structure Relatively stable patterns of behaviour that are learned from a society's culture and are observable.

social support The sense of self-worth and resources available for dealing with life's challenges that are part of belonging to a social network and result in health benefits.

socioeconomic status An individual's relative social and economic position in society based on personal factors such as income, occupation, and education.

sociology in medicine The application of sociological perspectives and research methods to solve medically defined problems, such as finding ways to improve the effectiveness of patient care.

sociology of medicine The critical application of sociological perspectives and research methods to improve theoretical understanding of social factors that affect health, such as the organizational structure in which patients and health-care professionals interact.

sociology of the body paradigm A theoretical perspective that adopts as its focus embodiment and the relationship between the body and society.

specific etiology The biomedical principle according to which it is assumed that each disease has a particular cause.

structural amplification A life course perspective that emphasizes the process by which parental education, occupation, and income structure many of our life experiences, including health.

structural determinants Factors evident at the societal level that exert an external influence on health, including aspects of social and economic environments such as income distribution, rates of unemployment, living and working conditions, and the organization of health care.

structural functionalist paradigm A theoretical perspective that views society as a harmonious social system made up of a number of interconnected parts or institutions that function to maintain order and stability.

structure–agency issue A complex sociological and philosophical debate about the extent to which human free will (i.e., agency) exists in the face of society's systems of social control (i.e., social structure).

structures of inequality Factors such as social class, gender, ethnicity, and age that are associated with enduring patterns of advantage (and disadvantage) and shape health outcomes.

symbolic interactionist paradigm A theoretical perspective that views society as the socially constructed product of everyday interactions of individuals. According to this perspective, society is made up of selves (i.e., unique individuals) who make their lives meaningful through social interaction.

symptom orientation The belief that good health means an absence of symptoms of illness.

symptoms Illness indicators that cannot be directly observed but are inferred based on indirect evidence, such as individuals reporting that they are in pain.

theoretical paradigm A conceptual framework or school of thought in which interrelated ideas and concepts about an aspect of reality are formulated.

universality The fundamental principle of medicare that all Canadians are eligible for coverage based on uniform terms and conditions (regardless of ability to pay).

urban health penalty The finding that those who live in urban centres have worse health than those who live in rural areas.

vertical structures Raphael's term to describe distant, macro-level factors that indirectly influence health, such as social, political, and economic policies regarding social welfare or taxation (e.g., child tax benefits).

wellness An inclusive concept that incorporates not only good health but also quality of life and satisfaction with general living conditions.

References

Abbott, S. 2007. "The psychosocial effects on health of socioeconomic inequalities." *Critical Public Health* 17: 151–8.

Abel, T. 1991. "Measuring health lifestyles in a comparative analysis: Theoretical issues and empirical findings." *Social Science and Medicine* 32: 899–908.

——— 2007. "Cultural capital in health promotion." In D. McQueen, I. Kickbusch, L. Potvin, J. Pelikan, L. Balbo, and T. Abel, eds., *Health and Modernity: The Role of Theory in Health Promotion*, 43–73. New York: Springer.

——— 2008. "Cultural capital and social inequality in health." *Journal of Epidemiology and Community Health* 62, doi: 10.1136/jech.2007.066159.

——— and K. Frohlich. 2012. "Capitals and capabilities: Linking structure and agency to reduce health inequalities." *Social Science and Medicine* 74: 236–44.

Abelsohn, A., R. Bray, C. Vakil, and D. Elliott. 2005. *Report on Public Health Urban Sprawl in Ontario*. Ontario College of Family Physicians.

Aboriginal Affairs and Northern Development. 2012. *Aboriginal Women in Canada: A Statistical Profile from the 2006 Census*. Catalogue no. 978-1-100-20156-6. Ottawa: Aboriginal Affairs and Northern Development.

Abraham, J. 2010. "Pharmaceuticalization of society in context: Theoretical, empirical and health dimensions." *Sociology* 44: 603–22.

Adams, T., J. Bezner, and M. Steinhardt. 1997. "The conceptualization and measurement of perceived wellness: Integrating balance across and within dimensions." *American Journal of Health Promotion* 11: 208–18.

Adelson, N. 2000. *Being Alive Well: Health and the Politics of Cree Well-Being*. Toronto: University of Toronto Press.

——— 2005. "The embodiment of inequity health disparities in Aboriginal Canada." *Canadian Journal of Public Health* 96: S45–61.

Adler, N., T. Boyce, M. Chesney, S. Cohen, S. Folkman, R. Kahn, and L. Syme. 1994. "Socioeconomic status and health: The challenge of the gradient." *American Psychologist* 49: 15–24.

Adler, N., T. Boyce, M. Chesney, S. Folkman, and L. Syme. 1993. "Socioeconomic inequalities in health: No easy solution." *Journal of the American Medical Association* 269: 3140–5.

Agriculture and Agri-food Canada. 2011. *Health and Wellness Trends for Canada and the World*. Ottawa: Agriculture and Agri-food Canada.

Aguinaldo, J.P. 2008. "The social construction of gay oppression as a determinant of gay men's health: 'Homophobia is killing us.'" *Critical Public Health* 18: 87–96.

Ahnquist, J., S. Wamala, and M. Lindstrom. 2012. "Social determinants of health—A question of social or economic capital? Interaction effects of socioeconomic factors on health outcomes." *Social Science and Medicine* 74: 930–9.

Albert, C., and M. Davia. 2010. "Education is a key determinant of health in Europe: A comparative analysis of 11 countries." *Health Promotion International* 26: 163–70.

Aldrich, S., and C. Eccleston. 2000. "Making sense of everyday pain." *Social Science and Medicine* 50: 1631–41.

Alexander, C., and F. Fong. 2014. "The case for leaning against income inequality in Canada." Special Report, TD Economics.

Alfonso, H., C. Beer, B. Yeap, G. Hankey, L. Flicker, and O. Almeida. 2012. "Perception of worsening health predicts mortality in older men: The health in men study (HIMS)." *Archives of Gerontology and Geriatrics* 55: 363–8.

Alford, R. 1975. *Health Care Politics: Ideological and Interest Group Barriers to Reform*. Chicago: University of Chicago Press.

Ali, S.H. 2009. "The political economy of environmental inequality: The social distribution of environmental injustice." In J. Agyeman, P. Cole, P. O'Riley, and R. Haluza-DeLay, eds., *Speaking for Ourselves: Environmental Justice in Canada*, 97–110. Vancouver: University of British Columbia Press.

——— and R. Keil, eds. 2008. *Networked Disease: Emerging Infections in the Global City*. Oxford: Wiley-Blackwell.

Allan, B., and J. Smylie. 2015. *First Peoples, Second Class Treatment: The Role of Racism in the Health and Well-Being of Indigenous Peoples in Canada*. Toronto: The Wellesley Institute.

Alwin, D. 2012. "Integrating varieties of life course concepts." *The Journals of Gerontology: Series B: Psychological Sciences and Social Sciences* 67: 206–20.

Anaya, J. 2014. *Report of the Special Rapporteur on the Rights of Indigenous Peoples, James Anaya, on the Situation of Indigenous Peoples in Canada*. United Nations General Assembly A/HRC/27/52/Add.2.

Andreev, K. 2000. "Sex differentials in survival in the Canadian population, 1921–1997: A descriptive analysis with focus on age-specific structure." *Demographic Research* 3: 1–19.

Angell, M., and J.P. Kassirer. 1998. "Alternative medicine—The risks of untested and unregulated remedies." *New England Journal of Medicine* 339: 839–41.

Annandale, E. 1998. *The Sociology of Health and Illness.* Cambridge: Polity Press.

——— 2009. *Women's Health and Social Change.* London: Routledge.

Antonovsky, A. 1979. *Health, Stress, and Coping.* San Franciso: Jossey-Bass.

——— 1987. *Unraveling the Mystery of Health: How People Manage Stress and Stay Well.* San Francisco: Jossey-Bass.

——— 1996. "The salutogenic model as a theory to guide health promotion." *Health Promotion International* 11: 11–18.

Anyinam, C. 1990. "Alternative medicine in Western industrialized countries: An agenda for medical geography." *The Canadian Geographer* 34: 69–76.

Appadurai, A. 1996. *Modernity at Large: The Cultural Dimensions of Globalization.* Minneapolis: University of Minnesota Press.

Arber, S., and H. Cooper. 1999. "Gender differences in health in later life: The new paradox?" *Social Science and Medicine* 48: 61–76.

Archer, M. 2003. *Structure, Agency, and the Internal Conversation.* Cambridge: Cambridge University Press.

Arluke, A., L. Kennedy, and R. Kessler. 1979. "Re-examining the sick-role concept: An empirical assessment." *Journal of Health and Social Behavior* 20: 30–6.

Armstrong, D. 1987. "Bodies of knowledge." In G. Scambler, ed., *Sociological Theory and Medical Sociology,* 59–76. London: Tavistock.

——— 1995. "The rise of surveillance medicine." *Sociology of Health and Illness* 17: 393–404.

——— 2003. *Outline of Sociology as Applied to Medicine.* New York: Oxford University Press.

——— 2009. "Indeterminate sick-men—A commentary on Jewson's 'Disappearance of the sick-man from medical cosmology.'" *International Journal of Epidemiology* 38: 642–5.

Armstrong, P. 2010. "Gender, health and care." In D. Raphael, T. Bryant, and M. Rioux, eds., *Staying Alive: Critical Perspectives on Health, Illness, and Health Care,* 2nd edn, 331–46. Toronto: Canadian Scholars Press.

——— C. Amaratunga, J. Bernier, K. Grant, A. Pederson, and K. Wilson. 2002. *Exposing Privatization: Women and Health Care Reform in Canada.* Aurora, ON: Garamond.

Armstrong, P., and J. Deadman. 2009. *Women's Health: Intersections of Policy, Research and Practice.* Toronto: Women's Press.

Arnett, J. 2006. "Psychology and health." *Canadian Psychology* 47: 19–32.

Asbring, P. 2012. "Words about body and soul: Social representations relating to health and illness." *Journal of Health Psychology* 17: 1110–20.

——— and A.-L. Narvanen. 2002. "Women's experiences of stigma in relation to chronic fatigue syndrome and fibromyalgia." *Qualitative Health Research* 12: 148–60.

——— 2003. "Ideal versus reality: Physicians' perspectives on patients with chronic fatigue syndrome (CFS) and fibromyalgia." *Social Science and Medicine* 57: 711–20.

Ashida, S., and C. Heaney. 2008. "Differential associations of social support and social connectedness with structural features of social networks and the health status of older adults." *Journal of Aging and Health* 20: 872–93.

Aspinall, P.J. 2001. "Operationalising the collection of ethnicity data in studies of the sociology of health and illness." *Sociology of Health and Illness* 23: 829–62.

Association of Faculties of Medicine of Canada. 2015. "Health inequalities." AFMC Primer on Population Health: A Virtual Textbook on Public Health Concepts for Clinicians. http://phprimer.afmc.ca/Part1TheoryThinkingAbout Health/Chapter2Determinants OfHealthAndHealthInequities/ Healthinequalities.

Astin, J.A. 1998. "Why patients use alternative medicine: Results of a national study." *Journal of the American Medical Association* 279: 1548–53.

Auger, N., and C. Alix. 2009. "Income, income distribution and health in Canada." In D. Raphael, ed., *Social Determinants of Health: Canadian Perspectives,* 2nd edn, 61–74. Toronto: Canadian Scholars Press.

Auger, N., D. Hamel, J. Martinez, and N. Ross. 2012. "Mitigating effect of immigration on the relation between income inequality and mortality: A prospective study of 2 million Canadians." *Journal of Epidemiology and Community Health* 66(6): e5–e5, doi 10.1136/jech.2010.127977.

Auger, N., G. Zang, and M. Daniel. 2009. "Community-level income inequality and mortality in Quebec, Canada." *Public Health* 123(6): 438–43.

Aukst-Margetić, B., and B. Margetić. 2005. "Religiosity and health outcomes: Review of literature." *Collegium Antropologicum* 29(1): 365–71.

Avison, W. 2010. "Incorporating children's lives into a life course perspective on stress and mental health. *Journal of Health and Social Behavior* 51: 361–75.

Ayo, N. 2012. "Understanding health promotion in a neoliberal climate and the making of health conscious citizens." *Critical Public Health* 22: 99–105.

Babones, S. 2010. "Income, education, and class gradients in health in global perspective." *Health Sociology Review* 19: 130–43.

Backett, K. 1992. "Taboos and excesses: Lay health moralities in middle class families." *Sociology of Health and Illness* 14: 255–74.

Badgley, R., ed. 1976. "Social science and medicine in Canada." *Social Science and Medicine* Special Issue 10: 1.

——— 1991. "Social and economic disparities under Canadian health care." *International Journal of Health Services* 21: 658–71.

Baer, H. 1989. "The American dominative medical system as a reflection of social relations in the larger society." *Social Science and Medicine* 28: 1103–12.

——— 2004. *Toward an Integrative Medicine: Merging Alternative Therapies with Biomedicine*. Walnut Creek, CA: AltaMira Press.

——— and I. Coulter. 2008. "Taking stock of integrative medicine: Broadening biomedicine or co-optation of complementary and alternative medicine." *Health Sociology Review* 17: 331–41.

Baer, R., S.C. Weller, J.G. de Alba Garcia, and A.L. Salcedo Rocha. 2008. "Cross-cultural perspectives on physician and lay models of the common cold." *Medical Anthropology Quarterly* 22(2): 148–66.

Baeten, S., T. Van Ourti, and E. van Doorslaer. 2013. "The socioeconomic health gradient across the life cycle: What role for selective mortality and institutionalization?" *Social Science and Medicine* 97: 66–74.

Bailis, D., A. Segall, and J. Chipperfield. 2003. "Two views of self-rated general health status." *Social Science and Medicine* 56: 203–17.

Baker, D. 2006. "The meaning and the measurement of health literacy." *Journal of General Internal Medicine* 21: 878–83.

——— M. Wolf, J. Feinglass, J. Thompson, J. Gazmararian, and J. Huang. 2007. "Health literacy and mortality among elderly persons." *Archives of Internal Medicine* 167: 1503–9.

Baker, G.R., P.G. Norton, V. Flintoft, R. Blais, A. Brown, J. Cox, E. Etchells, et al. 2004. "The Canadian Adverse Events Study: The incidence of adverse events among hospital patients in Canada." *Canadian Medical Association Journal* 170: 1678–86.

Baliunas, D., J. Patra, J. Rehm, S. Popova, M. Kaiserman, and B. Taylor. 2007. "Smoking-attributable mortality and expected years of life lost in Canada 2002: Conclusions for prevention and policy." *Chronic Diseases in Canada* 27: 154–62.

Ballard, K., and M. Elston. 2005. "Medicalisation: A multi-dimensional concept." *Social Theory and Health* 3: 228–41.

Baltes, M.M., H. Wahl, and U. Schmid-Furstoss. 1990. "The daily life of elderly Germans: Activity patterns, personal control, and functional health." *Journal of Gerontology: Psychological Sciences* 45: 173–9.

Bambra, C., M. Gibson, A. Sowden, K. Wright, M. Whitehead, and M. Petticrew. 2010. "Tackling the wider social determinants of health and health inequalities: Evidence from systematic reviews." *Journal of Epidemiology and Community Health* 64: 284–91.

Baranowski, T. 1981. "Toward the definition of concepts of health and disease, wellness and illness." *Health Values* 6: 246–56.

Barkwell, D. 2005. "Cancer pain: Voices of the Ojibway People." *Journal of Pain and Symptom Management* 30: 454–64.

Barofsky, I. 1978. "Compliance, adherence and the therapeutic alliance: Steps in the development of self-care." *Social Science and Medicine* 12: 369–76.

Bartley, M., and J. Ferrie. 2010. "Do we need to worry about the health effects of unemployment?" *Journal of Epidemiology and Community Health* 64: 5–6.

——— and S. Montgomery. 2006. "Health and labour market disadvantage: Unemployment, non-employment, and job insecurity." In M. Marmot and R. Wilkinson, eds., *Social Determinants of Health*, 2nd edn, 78–96. Oxford: Oxford University Press.

Baszanger, I. 1989. "Pain: Its experience and treatment." *Social Science and Medicine* 29: 425–34.

Baudrillard, J. 1998. *The Consumer Society*. London: Sage.

Bauer, G.R. 2012. "Making sure everyone counts: Considerations for inclusion, identification, and analysis of transgender and transsexual participants in health surveys." In *The Gender, Sex and Health Research Casebook: What a Difference Sex and Gender Make*, 59–67. Vancouver: CIHR Institute of Gender and Health.

——— 2014. "Incorporating intersectionality theory into population health research methodology: Challenges and the potential to advance health equity." *Social Science and Medicine* 110: 10–17.

Bauldry, S., M. Shanahan, J. Boardman, R. Miech, and R. Macmillan. 2012. "A life course model of self-rated health through adolescence and young adulthood." *Social Science and Medicine* 75: 1311–20.

Baum, E. 2009. "More than the tip of the iceberg: Health policies and research that go below the surface." *Journal of Epidemiology and Community Health* 63: 957.

Baum, F., and M. Fisher. 2014. "Why behavioural health promotion endures despite its failure to reduce health inequities." *Sociology of Health and Illness* 36(2): 213–25.

Baumann, B. 1961. "Diversities in conceptions of health and physical fitness." *Journal of Health and Human Behavior* 2: 39–46.

Baur, C. 2010. "New directions in research on public health and health literacy." *Journal of Health Communication* 15: 42–50.

Beck, U. 1992. *Risk Society: Towards a New Modernity*. London: Sage.

——— A. Giddens, and S. Lash. 1994. *Reflexive Modernization: Politics, Tradition and Aesthetics in the Modern Social Order*. Stanford, CA: Stanford University Press.

Becker, H.S. 1963. *Outsiders: Study in the Sociology of Deviance*. London: Free Press.

Beiser, M. 2005. "The health of immigrants and refugees in Canada." *Canadian Journal of Public Health* 96: S30–44.

Beland, F., S. Birch, and G. Stoddart. 2002. "Unemployment and health: Contextual-level influences on the production of health in populations." *Social Science and Medicine* 55: 2033–52.

Bell, I.R., O. Caspi, G.E.R. Schwartz, K.L. Grant, T.W. Gaudet, D. Rychener, V. Maizes, and A. Weil. 2002. "Integrative medicine and systemic outcomes research: Issues in the emergence of a new model for primary health care." *Archives of Internal Medicine* 162: 133–40.

Bell, S., and A. Figert. 2012. "Medicalization and pharmaceuticalization at the intersections: Looking backward, sideways and forward." *Social Science and Medicine* 75: 775–83.

Bendelow, G. 2006. "Pain, suffering and risk." *Health, Risk and Society* 8: 59–70.

——— and S. Williams. 1995. "Transcending the dualisms: Towards a sociology of pain." *Sociology of Health and Illness* 17: 139–65.

Benoit, C., D. Carroll, and M. Chaudhry. 2003. "In search of a healing place: Aboriginal women in Vancouver's Downtown Eastside." *Social Science and Medicine* 56: 821–33.

Benoit, C., and L. Shumka. 2009. *Gendering the Health Determinants Framework: Why Girls' and Women's Health Matters.* Vancouver: Women's Health Research Network.

——— K. Vallance, H. Hallgrimsdottir, R. Phillips, K. Kobayashi, O. Hankivsky, C. Reid, and E. Brief. 2009. "Explaining the health gap experienced by girls and women in Canada: A social determinants of health perspective." *Sociological Research Online* 14(5): 9.

Benoit, C., S. Wrede, I. Bourgeault, J. Sandall, R. De Vries, and E. van Teijlingen. 2005. "Understanding the social organization of maternity care systems: Midwifery as a touchstone." *Sociology of Health and Illness* 27: 722–37.

Benoit, C., M. Zadoroznyj, H. Hallgrimsdottir, A. Treloar, and K. Taylor. 2010. "Medical dominance and neoliberalism in maternal care provision: The evidence from Canada and Australia." *Social Science and Medicine* 71: 475–81.

Benyamini, Y. 2011. "Why does self-rated health predict mortality? An update on current knowledge and a research agenda for psychologists." *Psychology and Health* 26: 1407–13.

——— and E. Idler. 1999. "Community studies reporting association between self-rated health and mortality." *Research on Aging* 21: 392–401.

Berenson, C., L.J. Miller, and D.A. Findlay. 2009. "Through medical eyes: The medicalization of women's bodies and women's lives." In B.S. Bolaria and H.D. Dickinson, eds., *Health, Illness and Health Care in Canada*, 239–58. Toronto: Nelson Education.

Berger, P. 1963. *Invitation to Sociology: A Humanistic Perspective.* Markham, ON: Penguin.

——— and T. Luckmann. 1966. *The Social Construction of Reality: A Treatise in the Sociology of Knowledge.* Markham, ON: Penguin.

Berkman, N., T. Davis, and L. McCormack. 2010. "Health literacy: What is it?" *Journal of Health Communication* 15: 9–19.

Berkman, N., S. Sheridan, K. Donahue, D. Halpern, and K. Crotty. 2011. "Low health literacy and health outcomes: An updated systematic review." *Annals of Internal Medicine* 155: 97–107.

Berliner, H.S. 1984. "Scientific medicine since Flexner." In J.W. Salmon, ed., *Alternative Medicines: Popular and Policy Perspectives*, 30–56. New York: Tavistock.

——— and J.W. Salmon. 1979. "The holistic health movement and scientific medicine: The naked and the dead." *Socialist Review* 9: 31–52.

Bhatt, B., and M. Seema. 2012. "Occupational health hazards: A study of bus drivers." *Journal of Health Management* 14: 201–6.

Biderman, A., and A. Antonovsky. 1988. "The submerged part of the iceberg and the family physician." *Family Practice* 5: 174–6.

Bierman, A. 2006. "Does religion buffer the effects of discrimination on mental health? Differing effects by race." *Journal for the Scientific Study of Religion* 45(4): 551–65.

Birch, S., and A. Gafni. 2005. "Achievements and challenges of medicare in Canada: Are we there yet? Are we on course?" *International Journal of Health Services* 35: 443–63.

Bird, C., P. Conrad, and A. Fremont. 2000. Preface. In C. Bird, P. Conrad, and A. Fremont, eds., *Handbook of Medical Sociology*, 5th edn, viii. Upper Saddle River, NJ: Prentice-Hall.

——— and S. Timmermans. 2010. Preface. In C. Bird, P. Conrad, A. Fremont, and S. Timmermans, eds, *Handbook of Medical Sociology*, 6th edn, viii. Nashville: Vanderbilt University Press.

Bird, C., and P. Rieker. 2008. *Gender and Health: The Effects of Constrained Choices and Social Policies.* New York: Cambridge University Press.

Bishop, F., and L. Yardley. 2010. "The development and initial validation of a new measure of lay definitions of health: The wellness beliefs scale." *Psychology and Health* 25: 271–87.

Blais, R., and A. Maiga. 1999. "Do ethnic groups use health services like the majority of the population? A study from Quebec, Canada." *Social Science and Medicine* 48: 1237–45.

Blane, D. 2006. "The life course, the social gradient, and health." In M. Marmot and R. Wilkinson, eds, *Social Determinants of Health*, 2nd edn, 54–77. New York: Oxford University Press.

——— P. Higgs, M. Hyde, and R. Wiggins. 2004. "Life course influences on quality of life in early old age." *Social Science and Medicine* 58: 2171–9.

Blaxter, M. 1983. "The causes of disease: Women talking." *Social Science and Medicine* 17: 59–69.

——— 1990. *Health and Lifestyles.* London: Tavistock/Routledge.

——— 1997. "Whose fault is it? People's own conceptions of the reasons for health inequalities." *Social Science and Medicine* 44: 747–56.

——— 2000. "Medical sociology at the start of the new millennium." *Social Science and Medicine* 51: 1139–42.
——— 2003. "Biology, social class and inequalities in health: Their synthesis in 'health capital.'" In S. Williams, L. Birke, and G. Bendelow, eds, *Debating Biology: Sociological Reflections on Health, Medicine and Society*, 69–83. New York: Routledge.
Blendon, R.J., C. Schoen, C. DesRoches, R. Osborn, and K. Zapert. 2003. "Common concerns amid diverse systems: Health care experiences in five countries." *Health Affairs* 22: 106–21.
Bloom, S.W. 2000. "The institutionalization of medical sociology in the United States, 1920–1980." In C. Bird, P. Conrad, and A. Fremont, eds, *Handbook of Medical Sociology*, 5th edn, 11–31. Upper Saddle River, NJ: Prentice-Hall.
——— 2002. *The Word as Scalpel: A History of Medical Sociology*. New York: Oxford University Press.
Blumhagen, D. 1980. "Hypertension: A folk illness with a medical name." *Culture, Medicine and Psychiatry* 1: 197–227.
Bocock, R. 1993. *Consumption*. London: Routledge.
Bombak, A.E., and S.G. Bruce. 2012. "Self-rated health and ethnicity: Focus on indigenous populations." *International Journal of Circumpolar Health* 71: 18538, doi: 10.3402/ijch.v71i0.18538.
Boon, H., M.J. Verhoef, D. O'Hara, B. Findlay, and N. Majid. 2004. "Integrative healthcare: Arriving at a working definition." *Alternative Therapies in Health Medicine* 5: 49–56.
Borg, V., and T. Kristensen. 2000. "Social class and self-rated health: Can the gradient be explained by differences in life style or work environment?" *Social Science and Medicine* 51: 1019–30.
Bottorff, J., J. Carey, R. Mowatt, C. Varcoe, J. Johnson, P. Hutchinson, D. Sullivan, W. Williams, and D. Wardman. 2009. "Bingo halls and smoking: Perspectives of First Nations women." *Health and Place* 15: 1014–21.
Bourdieu, P. 1977. *Outline of a Theory of Practice*. Stanford, CA: Stanford University Press.
——— 1984. *Distinction: A Social Critique of the Judgement of Taste*. Stanford, CA: Stanford University Press.
——— 1990. *The Logic of Practice*. Stanford, CA: Stanford University Press.
——— 1992. "Doxa and Common Life: An Interview." *New Left Review* 191: 111–21.
——— 2001. *Masculine Domination*. Stanford, CA: Stanford University Press.
——— and L. Wacquant. 1992. *An Invitation to Reflexive Sociology*. Chicago: University of Chicago Press.
Bourgeault, I., R. Sutherns, M. MacDonald, and J. Luce. 2012. "Problematising public and private work spaces: Midwives' work in hospitals and in homes." *Midwifery* 28: 582–90.
Bowen, M., and H. Gonzalez. 2010. "Childhood socioeconomic position and disability in later life: Results of the health and retirement study." *American Journal of Public Health* 100: S197–203.
Brandt, M., C. Deindl, and K. Hank. 2012. "Tracing the origins of successful aging: The role of childhood conditions and social inequality in explaining later life health." *Social Science and Medicine* 74: 1418–25.
Brannlund, A., A. Hammarstrom, and M. Strandh. 2013. "Education and health-behaviour among men and women in Sweden: A 27-year prospective cohort study." *Scandinavian Journal of Public Health* 41: 284–92.
Braveman, P. 2006. "Health disparities and health equity: Concepts and measurement." *Annual Review of Public Health* 27: 167–94.
——— and C. Barclay. 2009. "Health disparities beginning in childhood: A life-course perspective." *Pediatrics* 124: S163–75.
Braveman, P., S. Egerter, and D. Williams. 2011. "The social determinants of health: Coming of age." *Annual Review of Public Health* 32: 381–98.
Bravewell Collaborative. 2009. "Major initiatives." http://www.bravewell.org/transforming_healthcare.
Brennenstuhl, S., A. Quesnel-Vallée, and P. McDonough. 2012. "Welfare regimes, population health and health inequalities: A research synthesis." *Journal of Epidemiology and Community Health* 66: 397–409.
Breton, R. 1991. *The Governance of Ethnic Communities: Political Structures and Processes in Canada*. Westport, CT: Greenwood Press.
——— 2005. *Ethnic Relations in Canada: Institutional Dynamics*. Montreal: McGill-Queen's University Press.
——— 2012. *Different Gods: Integrating Non-Christian Minorities into a Primarily Christian Society*. Montreal: McGill-Queen's University Press.
Bringsen, A., H. Andersson, and G. Ejlertsson. 2009. "Development and quality analysis of the salutogenic health indicator scale (SHIS)." *Scandinavian Journal of Public Health* 37: 3–19.
Broadbent Institute. 2012. *Towards a More Equal Canada: A Report on Canada's Economic and Social Inequality*. Ottawa: Broadbent Institute.
Brown, P. 2000. "Environment and health." In C. Bird, P. Conrad, and A. Fremont, eds, *Handbook of Medical Sociology*, 5th edn, 143–58. Upper Saddle River, NJ: Prentice-Hall.
——— 2013. *Toxic Exposures: Contested Illnesses and the Environmental Health Movement*. New York: Columbia University Press.
Bruhn, J. 1988. "Life-style and health behavior." In D. Gochman, ed., *Health Behavior: Emerging Research Perspectives*, 71–86. New York: Plenum Press.
——— B. Chandler, C. Miller, and S. Wolf. 1966. "Social aspects of

coronary heart disease in two adjacent ethnically different communities." *American Journal of Public Health* 56: 1493–506.

Bruhn, J., F. Cordova, J. Williams, and R. Fuentes. 1977. "The wellness process." *Journal of Community Health* 2: 209–21.

Bruhn, J., and S. Wolf. 1979. *The Roseto Story: An Anatomy of Health*. Norman, OK: University of Oklahoma Press.

Bryant, T. 2012. "Oppression, health and public policy in Canada." In E. McGibbon, ed., *Oppression: A Social Determinant of Health*, 138–49. Halifax: Fernwood.

——— D. Raphael, T. Schrecker, and R. Labonte. 2011. "Canada: A land of missed opportunity for addressing the social determinants of health." *Health Policy* 101: 44–58.

Buchbinder, M. 2010. "Giving an account of one's pain in the anthropological interview." *Culture, Medicine and Psychiatry* 34: 108–31.

Bulgar, R.J., and A.L. Barbato. 2000. "On the Hippocratic sources of Western medical practice." *Hastings Center Report* 3(4): S4–7.

Burdon, R. 2003. *The Suffering Gene: Environmental Threats to Our Health*. Montreal: McGill-Queens' University Press.

Burnham, J. 2014. "Why sociologists abandoned the sick role concept." *History of the Human Sciences* 27: 70–87.

Burton, N., and R. Ariss. 2014. "Diversity in midwifery care: Working toward social justice." *Canadian Review of Sociology* 51: 262–87.

Bury, M. 1982. "Chronic illness as biographical disruption." *Sociology of Health and Illness* 4: 167–82.

——— 1991. "The sociology of chronic illness: A review of research and prospects." *Sociology of Health and Illness* 13: 451–68.

——— 2001. "Illness narratives: Fact or fiction?" *Sociology of Health and Illness* 23: 263–85.

Butler-Jones, D. 2012. *The Chief Public Health Officer's Report on the State of Public Health in Canada, 2012:*
Influencing Health—The Importance of Sex and Gender. Catalogue no. HP2-10/2012E. Ottawa: Public Health Agency of Canada.

Buzzelli, M. 2007. "Bourdieu does environmental justice? Probing the linkages between population health and air pollution epidemiology." *Health and Place* 13: 3–13.

Calhoun, C., C. Rojek, and B. Turner. 2005. *Handbook of Sociology*. Thousand Oaks, CA: Sage.

Calnan, M. 1987. *Health and Illness: The Lay Perspective*. London: Tavistock.

——— 1989. "Control over health and patterns of health-related behaviour." *Social Science and Medicine* 29: 131–6.

——— and S. Williams. 1991. "Style of life and the salience of health." *Sociology of Health and Illness* 4: 506–29.

Cameron, E., and J. Bernardes. 1998. "Gender and disadvantage in health: Men's health for a change." *Sociology of Health and Illness* 20: 673–93.

Campbell, C.M., and R.R. Edwards. 2012. "Ethnic differences in pain and pain management." *Pain Management* 2(3): 219–30.

Canadian Cancer Society. Advisory Committee on Cancer Statistics. 2014. *Canadian Cancer Statistics 2014*. Toronto: Canadian Cancer Society.

——— 2015. *Canadian Cancer Statistics 2015*. Toronto: Canadian Cancer Society.

Canadian Index of Wellbeing. 2012. *How Are Canadians Really Doing? The 2012 CIW Report*. Waterloo, ON: Canadian Index of Wellbeing and University of Waterloo.

Canadian Medical Association. 2008. *No Breathing Room: National Illness Costs of Air Pollution*. Technical Report. www.cma.ca/multimedia/cma/content_Images/Inside_cma/Office_Public_Health/ICAP/CMAICAPTec_e-29aug.pdf.

——— 2013. *Policy on the Built Environment and Health*. http://cma.ca/Assets/assets-library/document/en/advocacy/PD14-05-e.pdf.
Canadian Society for Exercise Physiology. 2012. *Canadian Physical Activity Guidelines*. http://www.csep.ca/CMFiles/Guidelines/CSEP_Guidelines_Handbook.pdf.

Canadian Women's Health Network. 2012. "Fibromyalgia." www.cwhn.ca/en/node/40784.

Cant, S. 2004. "Medical pluralism." In J. Gabe, M. Bury, and M. Elston, eds, *Key Concepts in Medical Sociology*, 183–7. London: Sage.

——— and U. Sharma. 1999. *A New Medical Pluralism? Alternative Medicine, Doctors, Patients and the State*. London: UCL Press.

Carlisle, S., and P. Hanlon. 2008. "'Well-being' as a focus for public health? A critique and defence." *Critical Public Health* 18: 263–70.

Carpentier, N., P. Bernard, A. Grenier, and N. Guberman. 2010. "Using the life course perspective to study the entry into the illness trajectory: The perspective of caregivers of people with Alzheimer's disease." *Social Science and Medicine* 70: 1501–8.

Carpiano, R. 2001. "Passive medicalization: The case of Viagra and erectile dysfunction." *Sociological Spectrum* 21: 441–50.

——— 2008. "Actual or potential neighborhood resources and access to them: Testing hypotheses of social capital for the health of female caregivers." *Social Science and Medicine* 67: 568–82.

——— and D. Daley. 2006. "A guide and glossary on postpositivist theory building for population health." *Journal of Epidemiology and Community Health* 60: 564–70.

Castañeda, H., S.M. Holmes, D.S. Madrigal, M.E.D. Young, N. Beyeler, and J. Quesada. 2015. "Immigration as a social determinant of health." *Annual Review of Public Health* 36: 375–92.

Castells, M. 1996. *The Rise of the Network Society*. Malden, MA: Blackwell.

Caulfield, T. 2015 *Is Gwyneth Paltrow Wrong about Everything? When Celebrity Culture and Science Clash*. Toronto: Viking.

CDC (Centers for Disease Control and Prevention). 2008. "Injuries resulting from car surfing—United States, 1990–2008." *Morbidity and Mortality Weekly* 57: 1121–4.

Chan, C. 2009. "Choosing health, constrained choices." *Global Health Promotion* 16: 54–7.

Chan, S., T. Hadjistavropoulos, R. Carleton, and H. Hadjistavropoulos. 2012. "Predicting adjustment to chronic pain in older adults." *Canadian Journal of Behavioural Science* 44: 192–9.

Chandler, A. 2013. "Inviting pain? Pain, dualism and embodiment in narratives of self-injury." *Sociology of Health and Illness* 35: 716–30.

Chappell, N. 1993. "The future of health care in Canada." *Journal of Social Policy* 22: 487–505.

—— and L. Funk. 2011. "Social support, caregiving, and aging." *Canadian Journal on Aging* 30: 355–70.

Charmaz, K. 1983. "Loss of self: A fundamental form of suffering in the chronically ill." *Sociology of Health and Illness* 5: 168–95.

—— 1991. *Good Days, Bad Days: The Self in Chronic Illness and Time.* New Brunswick, NJ: Rutgers University Press.

Chen, Y., and T. Feeley. 2014. "Social support, social strain, loneliness, and well-being among older adults: An analysis of the health and retirement study." *Journal of Social and Personal Relationships* 31: 141–61.

Cheng, S., and A. Chan. 2006. "Social support and self-rated health revisited: Is there a gender difference in later life?" *Social Science and Medicine* 63: 117–22.

CIHI (Canadian Institute for Health Information). 2004. *Health Care in Canada 2004.* Ottawa: CIHI.

—— 2006. *How Healthy Are Rural Canadians? An Assessment of Their Health Status and Health Determinants.* Ottawa: CIHI.

—— 2007. *Health Care in Canada.* Ottawa: CIHI.

—— 2008. *Health Indicators 2008.* Ottawa: CIHI.

—— 2013a. *National Health Expenditure Trends 1975 to 2013.* Ottawa: CIHI.

—— 2013b. *Primary Health Care Voluntary Reporting System.* Ottawa: CIHI.

—— 2014. *National Health Expenditure Trends 1975 to 2014.* Ottawa: CIHI.

Cingano, F. 2014. "Trends in income inequality and its impact on economic growth." OECD Social, Employment and Migration Working Papers no. 163, OECD Publishing. http://dx.doi.org/10.1787/5jxrjncwxv6j-en.

Clarke, A., and J. Shim. 2011. "Medicalization and biomedicalization revisited: Technoscience and transformations of health, illness and American medicine." In B. Pescosolido, J. Martin, J. McLeod, and A. Rogers, eds, *Handbook of the Sociology of Health, Illness, and Healing: A Blueprint for the 21st Century*, 173–99. New York: Springer Science.

——, L. Mamo, J.R. Fosket, and J.R. Fishman. 2003. "Biomedicalization: Technoscientific transformations of health, illness, and U.S. biomedicine." *American Sociological Review* 68: 161–94.

Clarke, J.N. 2008. *Health, Illness and Medicine in Canada.* 5th edn. Don Mills, ON: Oxford University Press.

——, S. Arnold, M. Everest, and K. Whitfield. 2007. "The paradoxical reliance on allopathic medicine and positivist science among skeptical audiences." *Social Science and Medicine* 64(1): 164–73.

Clarke, L., and E. Bennett. 2012. "Constructing the moral body: Self-care among older adults with multiple chronic conditions." *Health* 17: 211–28.

Clarke, P., J. Morenoff, M. Debbink, E. Golberstein, M. Elliott, and P. Lantz. 2014. "Cumulative exposure to neighborhood context: Consequences for health transitions over the adult life course." *Research on Aging* 36: 115–42.

Clow, B., A. Pederson, M. Haworth-Brockman, and J. Bernier. 2009. *Rising to the Challenge: Sex and Gender-Based Analysis for Health Planning, Policy and Research in Canada.* Halifax: Atlantic Centre of Excellence for Women's Health.

Coburn, D. 2000. "Income inequality, lower social cohesion, and the poorer health status of populations: The role of neo-liberalism." *Social Science and Medicine* 51: 135–46.

—— 2004. "Beyond the income inequality hypothesis: Class, neo-liberalism, and health inequalities." *Social Science and Medicine* 58: 41–56.

——, K. Denny, E. Mykhalovskiy, P. McDonough, A. Robertson, and R. Love. 2003. "Population health in Canada: A brief critique." *American Journal of Public Health* 93: 392–6.

Coburn, D., and J. Eakin. 1993. "The sociology of health in Canada: First impressions." *Health and Canadian Society* 1: 83–110.

Cockerham, W.C. 2000. "The sociology of health behavior and health lifestyles." In C. Bird, P. Conrad, and A. Fremont, eds, *Handbook of Medical Sociology*, 5th edn, 159–72. Upper Saddle River, NJ: Prentice-Hall.

—— 2005. "Health lifestyle theory and the convergence of agency and structure." *Journal of Health and Social Behavior* 46: 51–67.

—— 2007. *Social Causes of Health and Disease.* Cambridge: Polity Press.

—— ed. 2013. *Medical Sociology on the Move: New Directions in Theory.* New York: Springer.

Cockerham, W.C., A. Rütten, and T. Abel. 1997. "Conceptualizing contemporary health lifestyles: Moving beyond Weber." *Sociological Quarterly* 38: 321–42.

Cockerham, W.C., and G. Scambler. 2010. "Medical sociology and sociological theory." In W.C. Cockerham, ed., *The New Blackwell*

Companion to Medical Sociology, 1–26. Oxford: Blackwell.

Cohen, D., T. Huynh, A. Sebold, J. Harvey, C. Neudorf, and A. Brown. 2014. "The population health approach: A qualitative study of conceptual and operational definitions for leaders in Canadian healthcare." *SAGE Open Medicine* 2: 2050312114522618.

Cohen, M.M., and H. Maclean. 2003. "Violence against women." In M. DesMeules, D. Stewart, A. Kazanjian, H. Maclean, J. Payne, and B. Vissandjée, eds, *Women's Health Surveillance Report: A Multidimensional Look at the Health of Canadian Women*, 1–31. Ottawa: Canadian Institute for Health Information.

Cohen, S. 2005. "The Pittsburgh common cold studies: Psychosocial predictors of susceptibility to respiratory infectious illness." *International Journal of Behavioral Medicine* 12(3): 123–31.

——— W.J. Doyale, R.B. Turner, C.M Alper, and D.P. Skoner. 2004. "Childhood socioeconomic status and host resistance to infectious illness in adulthood." *Psychosomatic Medicine* 66: 553–8.

Cohen, S., D. Janicki-Deverts, E. Chen, and K. Matthews. 2010. "Childhood socioeconomic status and adult health." *Annals of the New York Academy of Sciences* 1186: 37–55.

Cohen, S., D.A. Tyrrell, and A.P. Smith. 1991. "Psychological stress in humans and susceptibility to the common cold." *New England Journal of Medicine* 325: 606–12.

Colley, R.C., D. Garriguet, I. Janssen, C.L. Craig, J. Clarke and M.S. Tremblay. 2011. "Physical activity of Canadian adults: Accelerometer results from the 2007 to 2009 Canadian Health Measures Survey." *Health Reports* 22(1). Catalogue no. 82-003-X. Ottawa: Statistics Canada.

Collins, F. 2004. "What we do and don't know about 'race,' 'ethnicity,' genetics and health at the dawn of the genome era." *Nature Genetics* 36 (Supplement): S13–15.

Conference Board of Canada. 2013. "Income inequality." http://www.conferenceboard.ca/hcp/details/society/income-inequality.aspx.

Connell, R.W. 1995. *Masculinities*. Berkeley: University of California Press.

——— 2012. "Gender, health and theory: Conceptualizing the issue, in local and world perspective." *Social Science and Medicine* 74: 1675–83.

Conrad, L.I. 1995. *The Western Medical Tradition*. Cambridge: Cambridge University Press.

Conrad, P. 1975. "The discovery of hyperkinesis: Notes on the medicalization of deviant behavior." *Social Problems* 23: 12–21.

——— 1992. "Medicalization and social control." *Annual Review of Sociology* 18: 209–32.

——— 1994. "Wellness as a virtue: Mortality and the pursuit of health." *Culture, Medicine and Psychiatry* 8(3): 385–401.

——— 2005. "The shifting engines of medicalization." *Journal of Health and Social Behavior* 46: 3–14.

——— 2007. *The Medicalization of Society*. Baltimore, MD: Johns Hopkins University Press.

——— 2012. "Against health: How health became a new morality review." *Sociology of Health and Illness* 34(3): 479–80.

——— 2013. "Medicalization: Changing contours, characteristics, and contexts." In W. Cockerham, ed., *Medical Sociology on the Move*, 195–214. Dordrecht, NY: Springer Science.

Conrad, P., and K. Barker. 2010. "The social construction of illness: Key insights and policy implications." *Journal of Health and Social Behavior* 51(S): S67–79.

Conrad, P., T. Mackie, and A. Mehrotra. 2010. "Estimating the costs of medicalization." *Social Science and Medicine* 70: 1943–7.

Conrad, P., and J.W. Schneider. 1980. *Deviance and Medicalization: From Badness to Sickness*. St Louis: C.V. Mosby.

——— 1992. *Deviance and Medicalization: From Badness to Sickness*. Expanded edn. Philadelphia: Temple University Press.

Conroy, K., M. Sandel, and B. Zuckerman. 2010. "Poverty grown up: How childhood socioeconomic status impacts adult health." *Journal of Developmental and Behavioral Pediatrics* 31: 154–60.

Cooper, H. 2002. "Investigating socio-economic explanations for gender and ethnic inequalities in health." *Social Science and Medicine* 54: 693–706.

Corbin, C.B., and R.P. Pangrazi. 2001. "Toward a uniform definition of wellness: A commentary." *President's Council on Physical Fitness and Sports Research Digest* 3: 1–8.

Corbin, J., and A. Strauss. 1985. "Managing chronic illness at home: Three lines of work." *Qualitative Sociology* 8: 224–47.

——— 1988. *Unending Work and Care: Managing Chronic Illness at Home*. San Francisco: Jossey-Bass.

Cornwall, J. 1984. *Hard-Earned Lives: Accounts of Health and Illness from East London*. London: Tavistock.

Cotten, S.R., and S.S. Gupta. 2004. "Characteristics of online and offline health information seekers and factors that discriminate between them." *Social Science and Medicine* 59: 1795–806.

Courtenay, W.H. 2000a. "Behavioural factors associated with disease, injury, and death among men: Evidence and implications for prevention." *Journal of Men's Studies* 9: 81–142.

——— 2000b. "Constructions of masculinity and their influence on men's well-being: A theory of gender and health." *Social Science and Medicine* 50: 1385–401.

——— 2011. *Dying to Be Men: Psychosocial, Environmental, and Biobehavioral Directions in Promoting the Health of Men and Boys*. London: Routledge.

Cowan, P. 2011. "Living with chronic pain." *Quality of Life Research* 20: 307–8.

Cowen, E. 1991. "In pursuit of wellness." *American Psychologist* 46: 404–8.

Craib, K.J.P., P.M. Spittal, S.H. Patel, W.M. Christian, A. Moniruzzaman, M.E. Pearce, L. Demarais, C. Sherlock, and M. Schechter. 2010. "Prevalence and incidence of hepatitis C virus infection among Aboriginal young people who use drugs: Results from the Cedar Project." *Open Medicine* 3: 220–7.

Crawford, R. 1977. "You are dangerous to your health: The ideology and politics of victim blaming." *International Journal of Health Services* 7: 663–80.

——— 1980. "Healthism and medicalisation of everyday life." *International Journal of Health Services* 10: 365–88.

——— 1986. "Individual responsibility and health politics." In P. Conrad and R. Kern, eds, *The Sociology of Health and Illness: Critical Perspectives*, 369–77. New York: St Martin's Press.

Crooks, C.V., G.R. Goodall, R. Hughes, P.G. Jaffe, and L. Baker. 2007. "Engaging men and boys in preventing violence against women: Applying a cognitive-behavioral model." *Violence against Women* 13: 217–39.

CSHA (Canadian Study of Health and Aging). 1994. "Patterns of caring for people with dementia in Canada." *Canadian Journal on Aging* 13(4): 470–87.

Cullis, P. 2015. *The Personalized Medicine Revolution: How Diagnosing and Treating Disease Are about to Change Forever*. Vancouver: Greystone Books.

Curry-Stevens, A. 2009. "When economic growth doesn't trickle down: The wage dimensions of income polarization." In D. Raphael, ed., *Social Determinants of Health: Canadian Perspectives*, 2nd edn, 41–60. Toronto: Canadian Scholars Press.

Curtis, L.J. 2007. "Health status of on and off-reserve Aboriginal peoples: Analysis of the Aboriginal Peoples Survey." SEDAP Research Paper no. 191. http://socserv.mcmaster.ca/sedap.

Cutler, D., and A. Lleras-Muney. 2010. "Understanding differences in health behaviors by education." *Journal of Health Economics* 29: 1–28.

Dannenberg, A., H. Frumkin, and R. Jackson, eds. 2011. *Making Healthy Places: Designing and Building for Health, Well-Being, and Sustainability*. Washington: Island Press.

D'Arcy, C. 1986. "Unemployment and health: Data and implications." *Canadian Journal of Public Health* 77: S124–31.

——— and C. Siddique. 1985. "Unemployment and health: An analysis of 'Canada Health Survey' data." *International Journal of Health Services* 15: 609–35.

Das-Munshi, J., L. Becares, M.E. Dewey, S.A. Stansfeld, and M.J. Prince. 2010. "Understanding the effect of ethnic density on mental health: Multi-level investigation of survey data from England." *British Medical Journal* 21: 341.

Dean, J.A., and K. Wilson. 2010. "'My health has improved because I always have everything I need here . . .': A qualitative exploration of health improvement and decline among immigrants." *Social Science and Medicine* 70(8): 1219–28.

Dean, K. 1981. "Self-care responses to illness: A selected review." *Social Science and Medicine* 15A: 673–87.

——— 1986. "Lay care in illness." *Social Science and Medicine* 22: 275–84.

de Leeuw, S., and M. Greenwood. 2011. "Beyond borders and boundaries: Addressing Indigenous health inequities in Canada through theories of social determinants of health and intersectionality." In O. Hankivsky, ed., *Health Inequities in Canada: Intersectional Frameworks and Practices*, 53–70. Vancouver: University of British Columbia Press.

De Maio, F. 2010a. *Health and Social Theory*. New York: Palgrave MacMillan.

——— 2010b. "Immigration as pathogenic: A systematic review of the health of immigrants to Canada." *International Journal for Equity in Health* 9(27): 1–20.

——— 2012. "Advancing the income inequality–health hypothesis." *Critical Public Health* 22(1): 39–46.

——— and E. Kemp. 2010. "The deterioration of health status among immigrants to Canada." *Global Public Health* 5: 462–78.

Demakakos, P., J. Nazroo, E. Breeze, and M. Marmot. 2008. "Socioeconomic status and health: The role of subjective social status." *Social Science and Medicine* 67: 330–40.

Denburg, A., and D. Daneman. 2010. "The link between social inequality and child health outcomes." *Healthcare Quarterly* 14: 21–31.

Denton, M., S. Prus, and V. Walters. 2004. "Gender differences in health: A Canadian study of the psychosocial, structural, and behavioural determinants." *Social Science and Medicine* 58: 2585–600.

Denton, M., and V. Walters. 1999. "Gender differences in structural and behavioral determinants of health: An analysis of the social production of health." *Social Science and Medicine* 48: 1221–35.

Desesquelles, A.F., V. Egidi, and M.A. Salvatore. 2009. "Why do Italian people rate their health worse than French people do? An exploration of cross-country differentials of self-rated health." *Social Science and Medicine* 68: 1124–8.

DesMeules, M., D. Manuel, and R. Cho. 2003. "Mortality: Life and health expectancy of Canadian women." In M. DesMeules, D. Stewart, A. Kazanjian, H. Maclean, J. Payne, and B. Vissandjée, eds, *Women's Health Surveillance Report: A Multidimensional Look at the Health of Canadian Women*, 1–18. Ottawa: Canadian Institute for Health Information.

DesMeules, M., L. Turner, and R. Cho. 2003. "Morbidity experiences and disability among Canadian women." In M. DesMeules,

D. Stewart, A. Kazanjian, H. Maclean, J. Payne, and B. Vissandjée, eds, *Women's Health Surveillance Report: A Multidimensional Look at the Health of Canadian Women*, 1–14. Ottawa: Canadian Institute for Health Information.

DesMeules, M., D. Stewart, A. Kazanjian, H. Maclean, J. Payne, and B. Vissandjée, eds. 2003. *Women's Health Surveillance Report: A Multidimensional Look at the Health of Canadian Women*. Ottawa: Canadian Institute for Health Information.

DeSousa, C. 2006. "Urban brownfields redevelopment in Canada: The role of local government." *Canadian Geographer* 50: 392–407.

Dhanoon, R.K., and O. Hankivsky. 2011. "Why the theory and practice of intersectionality matter to health research and policy." In O. Hankivsky, ed., *Health Inequities in Canada: Intersectional Frameworks and Practices*, 16–52. Vancouver: University of British Columbia Press.

d'Houtaud, A., and M. Field. 1984. "The image of health: Variations in perception by social class in a French population." *Sociology of Health and Illness* 6: 30–60.

Dines, A., and A. Cribb, eds. 1993. *Health Promotion Concepts and Practice*. Oxford: Blackwell.

Dingwall, R., C. Heath, M. Reid, and M. Stacey, eds. 1977. *Health Care and Health Knowledge*. London: Croom Helm.

Douglas, V. 2013. *Introduction to Aboriginal Health and Health Care in Canada: Bridging Health and Healing*. New York: Springer.

Dovidio, J.F., and, S.L. Gaertner. 2004. "Aversive racism." *Advances in Experimental Social Psychology* 36: 1–52.

Dowd, J. 2012. "Whiners, deniers, and self-rated health: What are the implications for measuring health inequalities? A commentary on Layes, et al." *Social Science and Medicine* 75: 10–13.

Downey, C., and E. Chang. 2013. "Assessment of everyday beliefs about health: The lay concepts of health inventory, college student version." *Psychology and Health* 28: 818–32.

Dubos, R.J. 1959. *Mirage of Health: Utopias, Progress, and Biological Change*. New York: Harper.

——— 1968. *Man, Medicine and Environment*. New York: Mentor Books.

——— 1969. *So Human and Animal: How We Are Shaped by Our Surroundings and Events*. New Brunswick, NJ: Charles Scribner and Sons.

Ducey, A. 2009. *Never Good Enough: Health Care Workers and the False Promise of Job Training*. Ithaca, NY: Cornell University Press.

Dumas, A., J. Robitaille, and S.L. Jette. 2014. "Lifestyle as a choice of necessity: Young women, health and obesity." *Social Theory and Health* 12(2): 138–58.

Dunn, J.R. 2006. "Speaking theoretically about population health." *Journal of Epidemiology and Community Health* 60: 572–3.

——— and I. Dyck. 2000. "Social determinants of health in Canada's immigrant population: Results from the National Population Health Survey." *Social Science and Medicine* 51: 1573–93.

Dunn, J.R., and M. Hayes. 1999. "Toward a lexicon of population health." *Canadian Journal of Public Health* 90: S7–10.

Duster, T. 2003. "Buried alive: The concept of race in science." In A.H. Goodman, D. Heath, and M.S. Lindee, eds, *Genetic Nature/Culture: Anthropology and Science beyond the Two Culture Divide*, 258–77. Berkeley: University of California Press.

——— 2015. "A post-genomic surprise: The molecular reinscription of race in science, law and medicine." *British Journal of Sociology* 66(1): 1–27.

Eakin, J. 1992. "Leaving it up to the workers: Sociological perspective on the management of health and safety in small workplaces." *International Journal of Health Services* 22: 689–704.

Earle, A., J. Heymann, and J. Lavis. 2006. "Where do we go from here? Translating research to policy." In J. Heymann, C. Hertzman, M. Barer, and R. Evans, eds, *Healthier Societies: From Analysis to Action*, 381–404. New York: Oxford University Press.

Ecob, R., and G. Davey Smith. 1999. "Income and health: What is the nature of the relationship?" *Social Science and Medicine* 48: 693–705.

Edelstein, M. 1988. *Contaminated Communities: The Social and Psychological Impacts of Residential Toxic Exposure*. Boulder, CO: Westview.

Egolf, B., J. Lasker, S. Wolf, and L. Potvin. 1992. "The Roseto effect: A 50-year comparison of mortality rates." *American Journal of Public Health* 82: 1089–92.

Ehrenreich, B., and D. English. 1979. *For Her Own Good: 150 Years of the Experts' Advice to Women*. London: Pluto Press.

Ehrenreich, J., ed. 1978. *The Cultural Crisis of Modern Medicine*. New York: Monthly Review Press.

Eide, E., and M. Showalter. 2011. "Estimating the relation between health and education: What do we know and what do we need to know?" *Economics of Education Review* 30: 778–91.

Eisenberg, D.M., R. Davis, S. Ettner, S. Appel, S. Wilkey, M. Van Rompay, and R. Kessler. 1998. "Trends in alternative medicine use in the United States, 1990–1997: Results of a follow-up national survey." *Journal of the American Medical Association* 280: 1569–75.

Eiser, J., and P. Gentle. 1988. "Health behavior as goal-directed action." *Journal of Behavioral Medicine* 11: 523–35.

Elder, G. 1975. "Age differentiation and the life course." *Annual Review of Sociology* 1: 165–90.

——— 1994. "Time, human agency, and social change: Perspectives on the life course." *Social Psychology Quarterly* 57: 4–15.

Elias, B. 2014. "Moving beyond the historical quagmire of measuring infant mortality for the First Nations population in Canada." *Social Science and Medicine* 123:125–32.

Ellison, C., M. Musick, and A. Henderson. 2008. "Balm in Gilead: Racism, religious involvement, and psychological distress among African-American adults." *Journal for the Scientific Study of Religion* 47(2): 291–309.

Elston, M.A. 1993. "Women doctors in a changing profession: The case of Britain." In E. Riska and K. Wegar, eds, *Gender, Work and Medicine: Women and the Medical Division of Labour*, 27–61. Newbury Park, CA: Sage.

Engels, F. (1845) 1999. *The Condition of the Working Class in England*. Oxford: Oxford University Press.

Epp, J. 1986. *Achieving Health for All: A Framework for Health Promotion*. Ottawa: Health and Welfare Canada.

——— 1987. *The Active Health Report: Perspectives on Canada's Health Promotion Survey*. Ottawa: Health and Welfare Canada.

Erickson, P., A. Kendall, J. Anderson, and R. Kaplan. 1989. "Using composite health status measures to assess the nation's health." *Medical Care* 27: S66–76.

Eriksson, M., and B. Lindstrom. 2005. "Validity of Antonovsky's sense of coherence scale: A systematic review." *Journal of Epidemiology and Community Health* 59: 460–6.

——— 2006. "Antonovsky's sense of coherence scale and the relation with health: A systematic review." *Journal of Epidemiology and Community Health* 60: 376–81.

——— 2007. "Antonovsky's sense of coherence scale and its relation with quality of life: A systematic review." *Journal of Epidemiology and Community Health* 61: 938–44.

——— 2008. "A salutogenic interpretation of the Ottawa Charter." *Health Promotion International* 23: 190–9.

——— 2010. "Bringing it all together: The salutogenic response to some of the most pertinent public health dilemmas." In A. Morgan, M. Davies, and E. Ziglio, eds, *Health Assets in a Global Context: Theory, Methods, Action*, 339–51. New York: Springer.

Esmail, N. 2007. "Complementary and alternative medicine in Canada: Trends in use and public attitudes, 1997–2006." *Public Policy Sources* 87: 3–53. Vancouver: Fraser Institute.

Estey, E.A., A.M. Kmetic, and J. Reading. 2007. "Innovative approaches in public health research: Applying life course epidemiology to Aboriginal health research." *Canadian Journal of Public Health* 98(6): 444–6.

Etches, V., J. Frank, E. Di Ruggiero, and D. Manuel. 2006. "Measuring population health: A review of indicators." *Annual Review of Public Health* 27: 29–55.

Evans, J., L. Butler, J. Etowa, I. Crawley, D. Rayson, and D.G. Bell. 2005. "Gendered and cultured relations: Exploring African Nova Scotians' perceptions and experiences of breast and prostate cancer." *Research and Theory for Nursing Practice* 19(3): 257–73.

Evans, J., B. Frank, J.L. Oliffe, and D. Gregory. 2011. "Health, illness, men and masculinities (HIMM): A theoretical framework for understanding men and their health." *Journal of Men's Health* 8(1): 7–15.

Evans, M., H. Prout, L. Prior, L. Tapper-Jones, and C. Butler. 2007. "A qualitative study of lay beliefs about influenza immunisation in older people." *British Journal of General Practice* 57: 352–8.

Evans, R. 1994. Introduction. In R. Evans, M. Barer, and T. Marmor, eds, *Why Are Some People Healthy and Others Not?* 3–26. New York: Aldine de Gruyter.

——— M. Barer, and T. Marmor, eds. 1994. *Why Are Some People Healthy and Others Not?* New York: Aldine de Gruyter.

Evans, R., K. Cardiff, and S. Sheps. 2006. "High reliability versus high autonomy: Dryden, Murphy and patient safety." *Health Care Policy* 1: 12–20.

Evans, R., and G. Stoddart. 1990. "Producing health, consuming health care." *Social Science and Medicine* 31: 1347–63.

——— 2003. "Consuming research, producing policy?" *American Journal of Public Health* 93: 371–9.

Ewing, R., G. Meakins, S. Hamidi, and A. Nelson. 2014. "Relationship between urban sprawl and physical activity, obesity, and morbidity—Update and refinement." *Health and Place* 26:118–26.

Eyles, J., M. Brimacombe, P. Chaulk, G. Stoddart, T. Pranger, and O. Moase. 2001. "What determines health? To where should we shift resources? Attitudes toward the determinants of health among multiple stakeholder groups in PEI, Canada." *Social Science and Medicine* 53: 1611–19.

Fausto-Sterling, A. 1993. "The five sexes." *The Sciences* 33: 20–4.

——— 2000. "The five sexes, revisited." *The Sciences* 40: 18–23.

Feldt, T., E. Leskinen, M. Koskenvuo, S. Suominen, J. Vehtera, and M. Kivimaki. 2011. "Development of sense of coherence in adulthood: A person-centered approach: The Population-Based HeSSup Cohort Study." *Quality of Life Research* 20: 69–79.

Findlay, D.A., and L.J. Miller. 2002. "Through medical eyes: The medicalization of women's bodies and women's lives." In B.S. Bolaria and H.D. Dickinson, eds, *Health, Illness, and Health Care in Canada*, 185–210. Toronto: Nelson Thompson Learning.

Fiori, K., and J. Jager. 2011. "The impact of social support networks on mental and physical health in the transition to older adulthood: A longitudinal, pattern-centered approach." *International Journal of Behavioral Development* 36: 117–29.

First Nations Information Governance Centre (FNIGC). 2012. *First Nations Regional Health Survey (RHS) 2008/10: National Report on Adults, Youth and Children Living in First Nations Communities*. Ottawa: FNIGC.

Fisher, C., L. Hunt, R. Adamsam, and W. Thurston. 2007. "'Health's a difficult beast': The interrelationships between domestic violence, women's health and the health sector: An Australian case study." *Social Science and Medicine* 65: 1742–50.

Fitzcharles, M.-A., P. Ste-Marie, and J. Pereira. 2013. "Fibromyalgia: Evolving concepts over the past 2 decades." *Canadian Medical Association Journal* 185: E645–51.

Fontanarosa, P., and G. Lundberg. 1998. "Alternative medicine meets science." *Journal of the American Medical Association* 280: 1618–19.

Ford, E., M. Bergmann, H. Boeing, C. Li, and S. Capewell. 2012. "Healthy lifestyle behaviors and all-cause mortality among adults in the United States." *Preventive Medicine* 55: 23–7.

Forde, O.H. 1998. "Is imposing risk awareness cultural imperialism?" *Social Science and Medicine* 47: 1155–9.

Forget, E. 2011. "The town with no poverty: The health effects of a Canadian guaranteed annual income field experiment." *Canadian Public Policy* 37: 283–305.

Fortin, N., D.A. Green, T. Lemieux, K. Milligan, and W.C. Riddell. 2012. "Canadian inequality: Recent developments and policy options. *Canadian Public Policy* 38(2): 121–45.

Foucault, M. 1973. *The Birth of the Clinic: An Archaeology of Medical Perception*. New York: Vintage.

—— 1977. *Discipline and Punish: The Birth of the Prison*. New York: Vintage.

—— 1978. *The History of Sexuality: Volume 1: An Introduction*. New York: Vintage.

—— 1980. "Two lectures." In C. Gordon, ed., *Michel Foucault: Power/Knowledge: Selected Interviews and Other Writings, 1972–1977*, 78–108. New York: Vintage.

—— 2000. "The risks of security." In J. Faubion, ed., *Power*, 365–81. New York: New Press.

—— 2004. "The crisis of medicine or the crisis of antimedicine?" *Foucault Studies* 1: 5–19.

Fox, N.J. 1994. *Postmodernism, Sociology and Health*. Toronto: University of Toronto Press.

Frank, A. 1990. "Bring bodies back in: A decade review." *Theory, Culture and Society* 7(1): 131–62.

—— 1991a. *At the Will of the Body*. New York: Houghton Mifflin.

—— 1991b. "For a sociology of the body: An analytical review." In M. Featherstone, M. Hepworth, and B. Turner, eds, *The Body: Social Processes and Cultural Theory*, 36–102. London: Sage.

—— 1991c. "From sick role to health role: Deconstructing Parsons." In R. Robertson and B. Turner, eds, *Parsons: Theorist of Modernity*, 205–16. London: Sage.

—— 1995. *The Wounded Storyteller: Body, Illness, and Ethics*. Chicago: University of Chicago Press.

—— 2004. *The Renewal of Generosity: Illness, Medicine, and How to Live*. Chicago: University of Chicago Press.

Frank, L., B. Saelens, K. Powell, and J. Chapman. 2007. "Stepping towards causation: Do built environments or individual preferences explain walking, driving, and obesity?" *Social Science and Medicine* 65: 1898–914.

Frank, R., and G. Stollberg. 2004. "Medical acupuncture in Germany: Patterns of consumerism among physicians and patients." *Sociology of Health and Illness* 26: 351–72.

Frankel, S. 1991. "Health needs, health-care requirements, and the myth of infinite demand." *The Lancet* 337: 1588–90.

Frankish, C., C. Milligan, and C. Reid. 1998. "A review of relationships between active living and determinants of health." *Social Science and Medicine* 47: 287–301.

Frankish, J., G. Veenstra, and G. Moulton. 1999. "Population health in Canada: Issues and challenges for policy, practice and research." *Canadian Journal of Public Health* 90: S71–5.

Frappier, J., M. Kaufman, F. Baltzer, A. Elliott, M. Lane, J. Pinzon, and P. McDuff. 2008. "Sex and sexual health: A survey of Canadian youth and mothers." *Paediatrics and Child Health* 13: 25–30.

Freer, A. 1980. "Self-care: A health diary study." *Medical Care* 18: 853–61.

Freidson, E. 1970a. *Professional Dominance: The Social Structure of Medical Care*. New York: Atherton.

—— 1970b. *Profession of Medicine: A Study of the Sociology of Applied Knowledge*. New York: Harper and Row.

Freund, P.E.S., M. McGuire, and S. Podhurst. 2003. *Health, Illness and the Social Body*. London: Prentice-Hall.

Frideres, J.S. 1999. "Managing immigrant social transformations." In S. Halli and L. Driedger, eds, *Immigrant Canada: Demographic, Economic, and Social Challenges*, 70–90. Toronto: University of Toronto Press.

—— 2011. *First Nations in the Twenty-First Century*. Don Mills, ON: Oxford University Press.

Friedman, H.S., and M.R. DiMatteo. 1979. "Health care as an interpersonal process." *Journal of Social Issues* 35: 1–11.

Friel, S., R. Bell, T. Houweling, and M. Marmot. 2009. "Calling all Don Quixotes and Sancho Panzas: Achieving the dream of global health equity through practical action on the social determinants of health." *Global Health Promotion* 1 (Supplement): 9–13.

Friel, S., and M. Marmot. 2011. "Action on the social determinants of health and health equities goes global." *Annual Review of Public Health* 32: 225–36.

Fries, C.J. 2005. "Ethnocultural space and the symbolic negotiation of alternative as 'cure.'" *Canadian Ethnic Studies* 37(1): 87–100.

—— 2006. "Pursuing health, negotiating 'cure': A reflexive sociology of alternative medical practices." (Unpublished PhD dissertation, University of Calgary).

—— 2008. "Governing the health of the hybrid self: Integrative medicine, neoliberalism, and the shifting biopolitics of subjectivity." *Health Sociology Review* 17: 353–67.

——— 2009. "Bourdieu's reflexive sociology as a theoretical basis for mixed methods research: An application to complementary and alternative medicine." *Journal of Mixed Methods Research* 3: 326–48.

——— 2012. "Ethnicity and the use of 'accepted' and 'rejected' complementary/alternative medical therapies in Canada: Evidence from the Canadian Community Health Survey." In J. Kronenfeld, ed., *Issues in Health and Health Care Related to Race/Ethnicity, Immigration, SES and Gender* (Research in the Sociology of Health Care, vol. 30). Emerald Group Publishing Limited.

——— 2013. "Self-care and complementary and alternative medicine as care for the self: An embodied basis for distinction." *Health Sociology Review* 22(1): 37–51.

——— 2014. "Older adults' use of complementary and alternative medical therapies to resist biomedicalization of aging." *Journal of Aging Studies* 28: 1–10.

Fries, C.J., and K. Menzies. 2000. "Gullible fools or desperate pragmatists? A profile of people who use rejected alternative health care providers." *Canadian Journal of Public Health* 91: 217–19.

Fries, J.F. 1980. "Aging, natural death, and the compression of morbidity." *New England Journal of Medicine* 303: 130–5.

Frohlich, K., and T. Abel. 2014. "Environmental justice and health practices: Understanding how health inequities arise at the local level." *Sociology of Health and Health and Illness* 36: 199–212.

Frohlich, K., E. Corin, and L. Potvin. 2001. "A theoretical proposal for the relationship between context and disease." *Sociology of Health and Illness* 23: 776–97.

Frohlich, K., and L. Potvin. 1999. "Health promotion through the lens of population health: Toward a salutogenic setting." *Critical Public Health* 9: 211–22.

Frumkin, H. 2002. "Urban sprawl and public health." *Public Health Reports* 117: 201–17.

———, L. Frank, and R. Jackson. 2004. *Urban Sprawl and Public Health: Designing, Planning and Building for Healthy Communities*. Washington: Island Press.

Fuller-Thomson, E., A.M., Noack, and U. George. 2011. "Health decline among recent immigrants to Canada: Findings from a nationally-representative longitudinal survey." *Canadian Journal of Public Health* 102(4): 273–80.

Funk, L. 2010. "The interpretive dynamics of filial and collective responsibility for elderly people." *Canadian Review of Sociology* 47: 71–92.

Furedi, F. 2004. *Therapy Culture: Cultivating Vulnerability in an Uncertain Age*. London: Routledge.

——— 2008. "Medicalisation in a therapy culture." In D. Wainright, ed., *A Sociology of Health*, 97–114. London: Sage.

Furlong, W., D. Feeny, G. Torrance, and R. Barr. 2001. "The Health Utilities Index (HUI) system for assessing health-related quality of life in clinical studies." *Annals of Medicine* 33: 375–84.

Furnham, A. 1988. *Lay Theories: Everyday Understanding of Problems in the Social Sciences*. Oxford: Pergamon Press.

——— and J. Forey. 1994. "The attitudes, behaviours, and beliefs of patients of conventional vs. complementary (alternative) medicine." *Journal of Clinical Psychology* 50: 458–69.

Fylkesnes, K., and O. Forde. 1992. "Determinants and dimensions involved in self-evaluation of health." *Social Science and Medicine* 35: 271–9.

Gabe, J., M. Bury, and M. Elston. 2004. *Key Concepts in Medical Sociology*. London: Sage.

Gaboury, I., M. Bujold, H. Boon, and D. Moher. 2009. "Interprofessional collaboration within Canadian integrative healthcare clinics: Key components." *Social Science and Medicine* 69: 707–15.

Gadalla, T. 2009. "Sense of mastery, social support, and health in elderly Canadians." *Journal of Aging and Health* 21: 581–95.

Galabuzi, G. 2012. "Social exclusion as a determinant of health." In E. McGibbon, ed., *Oppression: A Social Determinant of Health*, 97–112. Halifax: Fernwood.

Gale, N. 2014. "The sociology of traditional, complementary and alternative medicine." *Sociology Compass* 8(6): 805–22.

Galea, S., N. Freudenberg, and D. Vlahov. 2005. "Cities and population health." *Social Science and Medicine* 60: 1017–33.

Gallant, M. 2003. "The influence of social support on chronic illness self-management: A review and directions for research." *Health Education and Behavior* 30: 170–95.

Gandhi, T.K., H.R. Burstin, F. Cook, A.L. Puopolo, J.S. Haas, T.A. Brennan, and D. Bates. 2000. "Drug complications in outpatients." *Journal of General Internal Medicine* 15: 149–54.

Garbarski, D. 2010. "Perceived social position and health: Is there a reciprocal relationship?" *Social Science and Medicine* 70: 692–9.

Gardam, M.A., C. Lemieux, P. Reason, M. van Dijk, and V. Goel. 2009. "Healthcare-associated infections as patient safety indicators." *Healthcare Papers* 9: 8–24.

Garden, R. 2010, "Telling stories about illness and disability." *Perspectives in Biology and Medicine* 53: 121–35.

Garfinkel, H. 1967. *Studies in Ethnomethodology*. Englewood Cliffs, NJ: Prentice-Hall.

Gatrell, A., J. Popay, and C. Thomas. 2004. "Mapping the determinants of health inequalities in social space: Can Bourdieu help us?" *Health and Place* 10: 245–57.

Gee, E., K. Kobayashi, and S. Prus. 2004. "Examining the healthy immigrant effect in mid to later life Canadians: Findings from the Canadian Community Health Survey." *Canadian Journal on Aging* 23: S61–9.

—— 2007. "Ethnic inequality in Canada: Economic and health dimensions." SEDAP Research Paper no. 182. http://socserv.mcmaster.ca/sedap.

Gee, G.C., K.M. Walsemann, and E. Brondolo. 2012. "A life course perspective on how racism may be related to health inequities." *American Journal of Public Health* 102(5): 967–74.

Genné-Bacon, E.A. 2014. "Thinking evolutionarily about obesity." *Yale Journal of Biology and Medicine* 87: 99–112.

George, L.K., C.G. Ellison, and D.B. Larson. 2002. "Explaining the relationships between religious involvement and health." *Psychological Inquiry: An International Journal for the Advancement of Psychological Theory* 13(3): 190–200.

Gerhardt, U. 1989. *Ideas about Illness: An Intellectual and Political History of Medical Sociology*. London: Macmillan.

—— 1990. "Qualitative research on chronic illness: The issue and the story." *Social Science and Medicine* 30: 1149–59.

Gibson, B., and O. Boiko. 2012. "The experience of health and illness: Polycontextual meaning and accounts of illness." *Social Theory and Health* 10: 156–87.

Giddens, A. 1991. *Modernity and Self Identity: Self and Society in Late Modern Age*. Cambridge: Polity Press.

Gijsbers van Wijk, C., H. Huisman, and A. Kolk. 1999. "Gender differences in physical symptoms and illness behavior: A health diary study." *Social Science and Medicine* 49: 1061–74.

Gillet, G. 1994. "Beyond the orthodox: Heresy in medicine and social science." *Social Science and Medicine* 39: 1125–31.

Gillham, O. 2002. *The Limitless City: A Primer on the Urban Sprawl Debate*. Washington: Island Press.

Gilmour, H. 2007. "Physically active Canadians." *Health Reports* 18: 45–65. Ottawa: Statistics Canada.

Giltay, E., A. Vollaard, and D. Kromhout. 2012. "Self-rated health and physician-rated health as independent predictors of mortality in elderly men." *Age and Ageing* 41: 165–71.

Ginsberg, J., M.H. Mohebbi, R.S. Patel, L. Brammer, M.S. Smolinski, and L. Brilliant. 2009. "Detecting influenza epidemics using search engine query data." *Nature* 457: 1012–14.

Giordano, G., and M. Lindstrom. 2010. "The impact of changes in different aspects of social capital and material conditions on self-rated health over time: A longitudinal cohort study." *Social Science and Medicine* 70: 700–10.

Glaser, R., J.K. Kiecolt-Glaser, R. Bonneau, W. Malarkey, and J. Hughes. 1992. "Stress-induced modulation of the immune response to recombinant hepatitis B vaccine." *Psychosomatic Medicine* 54: 22–9.

Glouberman, S., and J. Millar. 2003. "Evolution of the determinants of health, health policy, and health information systems in Canada." *American Journal of Public Health* 93: 388–92.

Goffman, E. 1961. *Asylums: Essays on the Social Situation of Mental Patients and Other Inmates*. Garden City, NY: Anchor.

—— 1963. *Stigma: Notes on the Management of Spoiled Identity*. Englewood Cliffs, NJ: Prentice-Hall.

Gold, M. 1977. "A crisis of identity: The case of medical sociology." *Journal of Health and Social Behavior* 18: 160–8.

Gold, M., P. Franks, and P. Erickson. 1996. "Assessing the health of the nation: The predictive validity of a preference-based measure and self-rated health." *Medical Care* 34: 163–77.

Goldman, D., and J. Smith. 2011. "The increasing value of education to health." *Social Science and Medicine* 72: 1728–37.

Goldman, N., C. Turra, L. Roserio-Bixby, D. Weir, and E. Crimmins. 2011. "Do biological measures mediate the relationship between education and health: A comparative study." *Social Science and Medicine* 72: 307–15.

Good, M.-J., P. Brodwin, B. Good, and A. Kleinman, eds. 1992. *Pain as Human Experience*. Berkeley: University of California Press.

Gordon, C., ed. 1980. *Michel Foucault: Power/Knowledge: Selected Interviews and Other Writings 1972-1977*. New York: Pantheon.

Gould, S. 1990. "Health consciousness and health behavior: The application of a new health consciousness scale." *American Journal of Preventive Medicine* 6: 228–37.

Grabb, E. 2009. "Conceptual issues in the study of social inequality." In E. Grabb and N. Guppy, eds, *Social Inequality in Canada: Patterns, Problems and Policies*, 5th edn, 1–16. Toronto: Pearson Education Canada.

Graham, H. 2002. "Building an inter-disciplinary science of health inequalities: The example of life-course research." *Social Science and Medicine* 55: 2005–16.

Graham, H., and L. Leeseberg Stamler. 2010. "Contemporary perceptions of health from an Indigenous (Plains Cree) perspective." *Journal of Aboriginal Health* 6–17.

Grandinetti, D.A. 2000. "Doctors and the Web: Help your patients surf the net safely." *Medical Economics* 63(8): 28–34.

Greaves, L., and N. Jategaonkar. 2006. "Tobacco policies and vulnerable girls and women: Toward a framework for gender sensitive policy development." *Journal of Epidemiology and Community Health* 60 (Supplement 2): ii57–65.

Green, K. 1985. "Identification of the facets of self-health management." *Evaluation and the Health Professions* 8: 323–38.

Griffith, D.M. 2012. "An intersectional approach to men's health." *Journal of Men's Health* 9(2): 106–12.

Gunning-Scheppers, L., and J. Hagen. 1987. "Avoidable burden of illness: How much can prevention contribute to health?" *Social Science and Medicine* 24: 945–51.

Guralnik, J. 1991. "Prospects for the compression of morbidity." *Journal of Aging and Health* 3: 138–54.

Gurin, D. 2003. *Understanding Sprawl: A Citizen's Guide*. Vancouver: David Suzuki Foundation.

Haas, J., and W. Shaffir. 1992. "Taking on the role of doctor." In D. Coburn, D.C. D'Arcy, G.M. Torrance, and P. New, eds, *Health and Canadian Society: Sociological Perspectives*, 399–421. Richmond Hill, ON: Fitzhenry and Whiteside.

Hadler, N.M. 2004. *The Last Well Person: How to Stay Well despite the Health-Care System*. Montreal: McGill-Queen's University Press.

Hajjaj, F., M. Salek, M. Basra, and A.Y. Finlay. 2010. "Non-clinical influences on clinical decision-making: A major challenge to evidence-based practice." *Journal of the Royal Society of Medicine* 103(5): 178–87.

Halfmann, D. 2011. "Recognizing medicalization and demedicalization: Discourses, practices, and identities." *Health* 16: 186–207.

Halfon, N. 2012. "Addressing health inequalities in the US: A life course health development approach." *Social Science and Medicine* 74: 671–3.

——— and M. Hochstein. 2002. "Life course health development: An integrated framework for developing health, policy, and research." *Milbank Quarterly* 80: 433–79.

Hall, J.E. 2010. *Guyton and Hall Textbook of Medical Physiology*. 12th edn. Philadelphia: Elsevier Saunders.

Hallin, D., M. Brandt, and C. Briggs. 2013. "Biomedicalization and the public sphere: Newspaper coverage of health and medicine, 1960s–2000s." *Social Science and Medicine* 96: 121–8.

Halter, M. 2000. *Shopping for Identity: The Marketing of Ethnicity*. New York: Pantheon Books.

Hancock, T. 1986. "Lalonde and beyond: Looking back at 'A New Perspective on the Health of Canadians.'" *Health Promotion* 1: 93–100.

———, R. Labonte, and R. Edwards. 1999. "Indicators that count! Measuring population health at the community level." *Canadian Journal of Public Health* 90: S22–6.

Hankin, J., and E. Wright. 2010. "Reflections on fifty years of medical sociology." *Journal of Health and Social Behavior* 51(S): S10–14.

Hankivsky, O., ed. 2012a. *An Intersectionality-Based Policy Analysis Framework*. Vancouver: Institute for Intersectionality Research and Policy, Simon Fraser University.

——— 2012b. "The lexicon of mainstreaming equality: Gender based analysis (GBA), gender and diversity analysis (GDA) and intersectionality based analysis (IBA)." *Canadian Political Science Review* 6(2–3): 171–83.

——— 2012c. "Women's health, men's health, and gender and health: Implications of intersectionality." *Social Science and Medicine* 74: 1712–20.

——— 2014. *Intersectionality 101*. Vancouver: Institute for Intersectionality Research and Policy.

——— and A. Christoffersen. 2008. "Intersectionality and the determinants of health: A Canadian perspective." *Critical Public Health* 18(3): 271–83.

Hankivsky, O., and R. Cormier. 2009. *Intersectionality: Moving Women's Health Research and Policy Forward*. Vancouver: Women's Health Research Network.

——— 2011. "Intersectionality and public policy: Some lessons from existing models." *Political Research Quarterly* 64: 217–29.

Hanlon, P., and S. Carlisle. 2009. "Is 'modern culture' bad for our health and well-being?" *Global Health Promotion* 16: 27–34.

Hansen, E., and G. Easthope. 2007. *Lifestyle in Medicine*. New York: Routledge.

Hanson, D., J. Hanson, P. Vardon, K. McFarlane, J. Lloyd, R. Muller, and D. Durrheim. 2005. "The injury iceberg: An ecological approach to planning sustainable community safety interventions." *Health Promotion Journal of Australia* 16: 5–10.

Harcourt, J. 2006. "Current issues in lesbian, gay, bisexual, and transgender (LGBT) health: Introduction." *Journal of Homosexuality* 51: 1–11.

Hardey, M. 1999. "Doctor in the house: The Internet as a source of lay health knowledge and the challenge to expertise." *Sociology of Health and Illness* 21(6): 820–35.

Harris, D., and S. Guten. 1979. "Health protective behavior: An exploratory study." *Journal of Health and Social Behavior* 20: 17–29.

Harvey, I., and K. Alexander. 2012. "Perceived social support and preventive health behavioral outcomes among older women." *Journal of Cross Cultural Gerontology* 27: 275–90.

Harwood, A. 1981. *Ethnicity and Medical Care*. Cambridge, MA: Harvard University Press.

Hasty, R.T., R.C. Garbalosa, V.A. Barbato, P.J. Valdes, jr, D.W. Powers, E. Hernandez, J.S. John, et al. 2014. "Wikipedia vs peer-reviewed medical literature for information about the 10 most costly medical conditions." *Journal of the American Osteopathic Association* 114: 368–73.

Health Canada. 1994. *Strategies for Population Health: Investing in the Health of Canadians*. Ottawa: Minister of Supply and Services Canada.

——— 2003. "Closing the gaps in Aboriginal health." Health Policy Research Bulletin 5. Ottawa: Health Canada.

——— 2004. *Public Opinion Survey on Key Issues Pertaining to Post-Market Surveillance of Marketed Health Products in Canada*. Ottawa: Health Canada.

——— 2005. *The Integrated Pan-Canadian Healthy Living Strategy*. Catalogue no. HP-10-1/2005. Ottawa: Minister of Health. www.phac-aspc.gc.ca/hl-vs-strat/pdf/hls_e.pdf.

——— 2009. *A Statistical Profile on the Health of First Nations in Canada: Determinants of Health, 1999–2003*. Ottawa: Health Canada.

——— 2014a. *A Statistical Profile on the Health of First Nations in Canada: Determinants of Health, 2006–2010.* Ottawa: Health Canada.

——— 2014b. *A Statistical Profile on the Health of First Nations in Canada: Vital Statistics for Atlantic and Western Canada, 2003–2007.* Ottawa: Health Canada.

Health Council of Canada. 2013. *Better Health, Better Care, Better Value for All: Refocusing Health Care Reform in Canada.* Toronto: Health Council of Canada.

Hedwig, T. 2007. "Living communities, health disparities and the everyday health experiences of Inupiaq migrants to Anchorage, Alaska." Copenhagen: Proceedings of the Fifth IPSSAS Seminar on Living Communities, New Perspectives on Inuit Urban Life, May.

Hejazi, S., V.S. Dahinten, S. Marshall, and P. Ratner. 2009. "Developmental pathways leading to obesity in childhood." *Health Reports* 20: 1–7. Catalogue no. 82-003-XPE. Ottawa: Statistics Canada.

Henderson, S., and A. Peterson, eds. 2002. *Consuming Health: The Commodification of Health Care.* London: Routledge.

Henly, S., J. Wyman, and M. Findorff. 2011. "Health and illness over time: The trajectory perspective in nursing science." *Nursing Research* 60: S5–14.

Hertzman, C., and T. Boyce. 2010. "How experience gets under the skin to create gradients in developmental health." *Annual Review of Public Health* 31: 329–47.

Hertzman, C., and C. Power. 2003. "Health and human development: Understandings from life-course research." *Developmental Neuropsychology* 24: 719–44.

——— 2006. "A life course approach to health and human development." In J. Heymann, C. Hertzman, M. Barer, and R. Evans, eds, *Healthier Societies: From Analysis to Action*, 83–106. New York: Oxford University Press.

Herzlich, C. 1973. *Health and Illness: A Social Psychological Analysis.* London: Academic Press.

Hibbard, J.H., and C.R. Pope. 1986. "Another look at sex differences in the use of medical care: Illness orientation and the types of morbidities for which services are used." *Women and Health* 11: 21–36.

Hickey, R., H. Akiyama, and W. Rakowski. 1991. "Daily illness characteristics and health care decisions of older people." *Journal of Applied Gerontology* 10: 169–84.

Higgs, P., M. Leontowitsch, F. Stevenson, and I. Jones. 2009. "Not just old and sick—The 'will to health' in later life." *Ageing and Society* 29: 687–707.

Hills, M., and D. McQueen. 2007. "At issue: Two decades of the Ottawa Charter." *Promotion and Education* 5 (Supplement).

Hiscock, R., L. Bauld, A. Amos, J.A. Fidler, and M. Munafo. 2012. "Socioeconomic status and smoking: A review." *Annals of the New York Academy of Sciences* 1248(1): 107–23.

Hislop, T.G., C.Z. The, A. Lai, T. Labo, and V. Taylor. 2000. "Cervical cancer screening in BC Chinese women." *British Columbia Medical Journal* 42: 456–60.

Hoffer, J.L. 2003. "Complementary or alternative medicine: The need for plausibility." *Canadian Medical Association Journal* 168: 180–1.

Hoffman, S.J., and C. Tan. 2013. "Following celebrities' medical advice: Meta-narrative analysis." *British Medical Journal* 347: f7151.

Hoffman-Goetz, L., L. Donelle, and R. Ahmed. 2014. *Health Literacy in Canada.* Toronto: Canadian Scholars Press.

Hofrichter, R., ed. 2000. *Reclaiming the Environmental Debate: The Politics of Health in a Toxic Culture.* Cambridge, MA: MIT Press.

Hole, R., M. Evans, L.D. Berg, J.L. Bottorff, C. Dingwall, C. Alexis, J. Nyberg, and M.L. Smith. 2015. "Visibility and voice: Aboriginal people experience culturally safe and unsafe health care." *Qualitative Health Research* 25(12): 1662–74.

Holland, P., L. Berney, D. Blane, G. Davey-Smith, D. Gunnell, and S. Montgomery. 2000. "Life course accumulation of disadvantage: Childhood health and hazard exposure during adulthood." *Social Science and Medicine* 50: 1285–95.

Hollenberg, D. 2006. "Uncharted ground: Patterns of professional interaction among complementary/alternative and biomedical practitioners in integrative health care settings." *Social Science and Medicine* 62: 731–44.

——— 2007. "How do private CAM therapies affect integrative health care settings in a publicly funded health care system?" *Journal of Complementary and Integrative Medicine* 4: Article 5.

Holmefur, M., K. Sunberg, L. Wettergren, and A. Langius-Eklof. 2014. "Measurement properties of the 13-item sense of coherence scale using Rasch analysis." *Quality of Life Research*, doi: 10.1007/s11136-014-0866-6.

Holmes, T., and R. Rahe. 1967. "The social readjustment rating scale." *Journal of Psychosomatic Research* 11: 213–18.

Hou, F., and J. Myles. 2005. "Neighbourhood inequality, neighbourhood affluence and population health." *Social Science and Medicine* 60: 1557–69.

House, J. 2001. "Understanding social factors and inequalities in health: 20th century progress and 21st century prospects." *Journal of Health and Social Behavior* 43: 125–42.

Howson, Alexandra. 2013. *The Body in Society: An Introduction.* 2nd edn. Cambridge: Polity Press.

Hsieh, A.Y., D.A. Tripp, L.J. Ji, and M.J. Sullivan. 2010. "Comparisons of catastrophizing, pain attitudes, and cold-pressor pain experience between Chinese and European Canadian young adults." *Journal of Pain* 11(11): 1187–94.

Hughner, R., and S. Kleine. 2004. "Views of health in the lay sector:

A compilation and review of how individuals think about health." *Health: An Interdisciplinary Journal for the Social Study of Health, Illness, and Medicine* 8: 395–422.

——— 2008. "Variations in lay health theories: Implications for consumer health care decision making." *Qualitative Health Research* 18: 1687–703.

Huisman, H., A. Kunst, O. Andersen, M. Bopp, J. Borgan, C. Borell, G. Costa, et al. 2004. "Socioeconomic inequalities in mortality among elderly people in 11 European populations." *Journal of Epidemiology and Community Health* 58: 468–75.

Humphries, K., and E. van Doorslaer. 2000. "Income-related health inequality in Canada." *Social Science and Medicine* 50: 663–71.

Hunter, D.J., J. Popay, C. Tannahill, M. Whitehead, and T. Elson. 2009. "Learning lessons from the past: Shaping a different future." Marmot Review Working Committee 3.

Hurst, M. 2009. "Who participates in active leisure?" *Canadian Social Trends*. Catalogue no. 11-008. Ottawa: Statistics Canada.

Hurwitz, B., T. Greenhalgh, and V. Skultans, eds. 2004. *Narrative Research in Health and Illness*. Oxford: Blackwell Publishing.

Idler, E. 1979. "Definitions of health and illness and medical sociology." *Social Science and Medicine* 13A: 723–31.

——— 1987. "Religious involvement and the health of the elderly: Some hypotheses and an initial test." *Social Forces* 66: 226–38.

——— and Y. Benyamini. 1997. "Self-rated health and mortality: A review of twenty-seven community studies." *Journal of Health and Social Behavior* 38: 21–37.

Idler, E., S. Hudson, and H. Leventhal. 1999. "The meanings of self-ratings of health." *Research on Aging* 21: 458–76.

Idler, E., and S. Kasl. 1991. "Health perceptions and survival: Do global evaluations of health status really predict mortality?" *Journal of Gerontology: Social Sciences* 46: S55–65.

Iedema, R., and I. Veljanova. 2013. "Editorial: Lifestyle science: Self-healing, co-production and DIY." *Health Sociology Review* 22: 2–7.

Illich, I. 1976. *Medical Nemesis: The Expropriation of Health*. New York: Pantheon Books.

Institute of Medicine. 2000. *To Err Is Human: Building a Safer Health System*. Washington: National Academies Press.

——— 2005. *Complementary and Alternative Medicine in the United States*. Washington: National Academies Press.

Irvine, K. 2009. *Supporting Aboriginal Parents: Teachings for the Future*. Prince George, BC: National Collaborating Centre for Aboriginal Health.

Isajiw, W. 1993. "Definitions and dimensions of ethnicity: A theoretical framework." In Statistics Canada and US Bureau of the Census, eds, *Challenges of Measuring an Ethnic World: Science, Politics and Reality: Proceedings of the Joint Canada–United States Conference on the Measurement of Ethnicity, April 1–3, 1992*, 407–27. Washington: US Government Printing Office.

Jackson, A. 2009. "The unhealthy Canadian workplace." In D. Raphael, ed., *Social Determinants of Health: Canadian Perspectives*, 2nd edn, 99–113. Toronto: Canadian Scholars Press.

James, W. 2008. "The epidemiology of obesity: The size of the problem." *Journal of Internal Medicine* 263: 336–52.

Janssen, I. 2012. "Health care costs of physical inactivity in Canadian adults." *Applied Physiology, Nutrition, and Metabolism* 37: 803–6.

——— 2013. "The public health burden of obesity in Canada." *Canadian Journal of Diabetes* 37: 90–6.

Janzen, B.L., and N. Muhajarine. 2003. "Social role occupancy, gender, income adequacy, life stage and health: A longitudinal study of employed Canadian men and women." *Social Science and Medicine* 57: 1491–503.

Jerrett, M., P. Kanaroglou, J. Eyles, N. Finkelstein, and C. Giovis. 2001. "A GIS-environmental justice analysis of particulate air pollution in Hamilton, Canada." *Environmental Planning* 33: 1–19.

Jewson, N.D. 1976. "The disappearance of the sick-man from medical cosmology, 1770–1870." *Sociology* 10: 225–43.

Johnson, M. 1975. "Medical sociology and sociological theory." *Social Science and Medicine* 9: 227–32.

Johnson, R., and R. Schoeni. 2011. "Early-life origins of adult disease: National longitudinal population-based study of the United States." *American Journal of Public Health* 101: 2317–24.

——— and J. Rogowski. 2012. "Health disparities in mid-to-late life: The role of earlier life family and neighborhood socioeconomic conditions." *Social Science and Medicine* 74: 625–36.

Jonas, W.B. 2002. "Policy, the public, and priorities in alternative medicine research." *Annals of the American Academy of Political and Social Sciences* 583: 29–43.

Jones, R. 2000. "Self care." *British Medical Journal* 320: 596.

Josewski, V. 2012. "Analysing 'cultural safety' in mental health policy reform: Lessons from British Columbia, Canada." *Critical Public Health* 22(2): 223–34.

Judge, K., J. Mulligan, and M. Benzeval. 1998. "Income inequality and population health." *Social Science and Medicine* 46: 567–79.

Jurcik, T., R. Ahmed, E. Yakobov, and L. Solopieieva-Jurcikova. 2013. "Understanding the role of the ethnic density effect: Issues of acculturation, discrimination and social support." *Journal of Community Psychology* 41(6): 662–78.

Jyhla, M. 1994. "Self-rated health revisited: Exploring survey interview episodes with elderly respondents."

Social Science and Medicine 39: 983–90.

——— 2009. "What is self-rated health and why does it predict mortality? Towards a unified conceptual model." *Social Science and Medicine* 69: 307–16.

Kandrack, M.-A., K. Grant, and A. Segall. 1991. "Gender differences in health related behaviour: Some unanswered questions." *Social Science and Medicine* 32: 579–90.

Kangas, I. 2002. "'Lay' and 'expert': Illness knowledge construction in the sociology of health and illness." *Health: An Interdisciplinary Journal for the Social Study of Health, Illness, and Medicine* 6: 301–4.

Kaplan, G. 1991. "Epidemiologic observations on the compression of morbidity." *Journal of Aging and Health* 3: 155–71.

———V. Barell, and A. Lusky. 1988. "Subjective state of health and survival in elderly adults." *Journal of Gerontology: Social Sciences* 43: S114–20.

Kaplan, G., and O. Baron-Epel. 2003. "What lies behind the subjective evaluation of health status?" *Social Science and Medicine* 56: 1669–76.

Kark, R.L., S. Carmel, R. Sinnreich, N. Goldberger, and Y. Friedlander. 1996. "Psychosocial factors among members of religious and secular kibbutzim." *Israeli Journal of Medical Science* 32: 185–94.

Kark, R.L., G. Shermi, Y. Friedlander, O. Martin, O. Manor, and S. H. Bondheim. 1996. "Does religious observance promote health? Mortality in secular vs. religious kibbutzim in Israel." *American Journal of Public Health* 86: 341–6.

Karlsson, M., T. Nilsson, C. Lyttkens, and G. Leeson. 2010. "Income inequality and health: Importance of a cross-country perspective." *Social Science and Medicine* 70: 875–85.

Kaskutas, L., and T. Greenfield. 1997. "The role of health consciousness in predicting attention to health warning messages." *American Journal of Health Promotion* 11: 186–93.

Katz, S.H. 1995. *Is Race a Legitimate Concept for Science? The AAPA Revised Statement on Race: A Brief Analysis and Commentary*. Philadelphia: University of Pennsylvania Press.

Kawachi, I., N. Adler, and W. Dow. 2010. "Money, schooling, and health: Mechanisms and causal evidence." *Annals of the New York Academy of Sciences* 1186: 56–68.

Kawachi, I., and S.V. Subramanian. 2014. "Income inequality." In L. Berkman, I Kawachi, and M. Glymour, eds, *Social Epidemiology*, 2nd edn, 126–51. New York: Oxford University Press.

Kazanjian, A., D. Morettin, and R. Cho. 2003. "Health care utilization by Canadian women." In M. DesMeules, D. Stewart, A. Kazanjian, H. Maclean, J. Payne, and B. Vissandjée, eds, *Women's Health Surveillance Report: A Multidimensional Look at the Health of Canadian Women*, 5–6. Ottawa: Canadian Institute for Health Information.

Kehoe, A. 1990. "Primal gaia: Primitivists and plastic medicine men." In J. Clifton, ed., *The Invented Indian: Cultural Fictions and Government Policies*, 193–209. New York: Transaction Publishers.

Kelner, M., and P. New, eds. 1984. "Social science and health in Canada." *Social Science and Medicine* (Special Issue) 18: 3.

Kelner, M., and B. Wellman. 1997. "Health care and consumer choice: Medical and alternative therapies." *Social Science and Medicine* 45: 203–12.

——— 2000. *Complementary Alternative Medicine: Challenge and Change*. New York: Harwood Academic Publishers.

Kendall, O., T. Lipskie, and S. MacEachern. 1997. "Canadian health surveys, 1950–1997." *Chronic Diseases in Canada* 18: 70–90.

Keon, W., and L. Pepin. 2009. *A Healthy, Productive Canada: A Determinant of Health Approach*. Final Report of the Senate Subcommittee on Population Health. Ottawa: Standing Senate Committee on Social Affairs, Science and Technology. http://senate-senat.ca/health-e.asp.

Kickbusch, I. 1986. "Life-styles and health." *Social Science and Medicine* 22: 117–24.

——— 1989. "Self-care in health promotion." *Social Science and Medicine* 29: 125–30.

——— 2001. "Health literacy: Addressing the health and education divide." *Health Promotion International* 16: 289–97.

——— 2007. "Health governance: The health society." In D. McQueen, I. Potvin, J. Pelikan, L. Balbo, and T. Abel, eds, *Health and Modernity: The Role of Theory in Health Promotion*, 144–61. New York: Springer.

Kielmann, T., G. Huby, A. Powell, A. Sheikh, D. Price, S. Williams, and H. Pinnock. 2010. "From support to boundary: A qualitative study of the border between self-care and professional care." *Patient Education and Counseling* 79: 55–61.

Kim, I.H., C. Carrasco, C. Muntaner, K. McKenzie, and S. Noh. 2013. "Ethnicity and postmigration health trajectory in new immigrants to Canada." *American Journal of Public Health* 103(4): e96–104.

Kindig, D. 2007. "Understanding population health terminology." *Milbank Quarterly* 85: 139–61.

———and G. Stoddart. 2003. "What is population health?" *American Journal of Public Health* 93: 380–3.

King, S. 1962. *Perceptions of Illness and Medical Practice*. New York: Russell Sage Foundation.

Kirkland, A. 2014a. "Critical perspectives on wellness." *Journal of Health Politics, Policy and Law* 39: 971–88.

——— 2014b. "What is wellness now?" *Journal of Health Politics, Policy and Law* 39: 957–70.

Kirkpatrick, S., and L. McIntyre. 2009. "The chief public health officer's report on health inequalities: What are the implications for public health practitioners and researchers?" *Canadian Journal of Public Health* 100: 93–5.

Kirmayer, L.J. 2011. "Multicultural medicine and the politics of recognition." *Journal of Medicine and Philosophy* 36(4): 410–23.

Kleinman, A. 1988. *The Illness Narratives: Suffering, Healing and the Human Condition*. New York: Basic Books.

Klumb, P.L., and T. Lampert. 2004. "Women, work, and well-being 1950–2000: A review and methodological critique." *Social Science and Medicine* 58: 1007–24.

Knowles, J. 1977. "The responsibility of the individual." In J. Knowles, ed., *Doing Better and Feeling Worse*, 57–80. New York: W.W. Norton

Kobayashi, K. 2003. "Do intersections of diversity matter? An exploration of the relationship between identity markers and health for mid- to later-life Canadians." *Canadian Ethnic Studies* 35: 85–98.

—— and S. Prus. 2005. "Explaining the health gap between Canadian- and foreign-born older adults: Findings from the 2000/2001 Canadian Community Health Survey." *Recent Advances and Research Updates: Journal of the International Research Promotion Council* 6: 269–73.

Kobayashi, L., J. Wardle, and C. von Wagner. 2014. "Internet use, social engagement and health literacy decline during ageing in a longitudinal cohort of older English adults." *Journal of Epidemiology and Community Health* 0: 1–6.

Koh, H., J. Piotrowski, S. Kumanyika, and J. Fielding. 2011. "Healthy people: A 2020 vision for the social determinants approach." *Health Education and Behavior* 38: 551–7.

Köhler, N., and B. Righton. 2006. "Overeaters, smokers, and drinkers: The doctor won't see you now." *Maclean's* 119 (24 April): 34–40.

Kompier, M., and V. Di Martino. 1995. "Review of bus drivers' occupational stress and stress prevention." *Stress Medicine* 11: 253–62.

Kondo, N., R.M. van Dam, G. Sembajwe, S.V. Subramanian, I. Kawachi, and Z. Yamagata. 2011. "Income inequality and health: The role of population size, inequality threshold, period effects and lag effects." *Journal of Epidemiology and Community Health* 66(6): e11–11, doi: 10.1136/jech-2011-200321.

Kooiker, S. 1995. "Exploring the iceberg of morbidity: A comparison of different survey methods for assessing the occurrence of everyday illness." *Social Science and Medicine* 41: 317–32.

Kopec, J.A., J.I. Williams, T. To, and P.C. Austin. 2001. "Cross-cultural comparisons of health status in Canada using the Health Utilities Index." *Ethnicity and Health* 61: 41–50.

Kornelson, J., C. Atkins, K. Brownell, and R. Woollard. 2015. "The meaning of patient experiences of medically unexplained physical symptoms." *Qualitative Health Research*, doi:10.1177/1049732314566326.

Korp, P. 2008. "The symbolic power of 'healthy lifestyles.'" *Health Sociology Review* 17: 18–26.

—— 2010. "Problems of the healthy lifestyle discourse." *Sociology Compass* 4(9): 800–10.

Kosteniuk, J., and H. Dickinson. 2003. "Tracing the social gradient in the health of Canadians: Primary and secondary determinants." *Social Science and Medicine* 57: 263–76.

Krause, N. 1987. "Understanding the stress process: Linking social support with locus of control beliefs." *Journal of Gerontology* 42: 589–93.

—— A.R. Herzog, and E. Baker. 1992. "Providing support to others and well-being in late life." *Journal of Gerontology: Psychological Sciences* 47: P300–11.

Krause, N., and G. Jay. 1994. "What do global self-rated health items measure?" *Medical Care* 32: 930–42.

Kreindler, S. 2008. "Lifting the burden of chronic disease: What's worked, what hasn't, what's next." Winnipeg: Winnipeg Regional Health Authority. www.longwoods.com/articles/images/ChronicDiseaseReport.pdf.

Krick, J., and J. Sobal. 1990. "Relationships between health protective behaviors." *Journal of Community Health* 15: 19–34.

Krieger, N. 2003. "Does racism harm health? Did child abuse exist before 1962? On explicit questions, critical science, and current controversies: An ecosocial perspective." *American Journal of Public Health* 93: 194–9.

Kronenfeld, J., N. Goodyear, R. Pate, A. Blair, H. Howe, G. Parker, and S. Blair. 1988. "The interrelationship among preventive health habits." *Health Education Research* 3: 317–23.

Labonte, R. 2012. "Global action on social determinants of health." *Journal of Public Health Policy* 33: 139–47.

Lai, D. 2004. "Health status of older Chinese in Canada: Findings from the SF-36 health survey." *Canadian Journal of Public Health* 95: 193–200.

Laing, R.D. 1961. *The Divided Self: An Existential Study in Sanity and Madness*. London: Tavistock.

Lalonde, M. 1974. *A New Perspective on the Health of Canadians*. Ottawa: Health and Welfare Canada.

Lambert, C. 2002. "The new ancient trend in medicine: Scientific scrutiny of 'alternative' therapies." *Harvard Magazine* 104: 46–9, 99–101.

La Rue, A., L. Bank, L. Jarvik, and M. Hetland. 1979. "Health in old age: How do physicians' ratings and self-ratings compare?" *Journal of Gerontology* 34: 687–91.

Lasser, K., D. Himmelstein, and S. Woolhandler. 2006. "Access to care, health status, and health disparities in the United States and Canada: Results of a cross-national population-based survey." *American Journal of Public Health* 96: 1300–7.

Last, J., and M. Adelaide. 2013. "The iceberg: Completing the clinical picture in general practice." *International Journal of Epidemiology* 42: 1608–13.

Lau, R. 1997. "Cognitive representations of health and illness." In D. Gochman, ed., *Handbook of Health Behavior Research I: Personal and Social Determinants*, 51–69. New York: Plenum Press.
——— and K. Hartman. 1983. "Common sense representations of common illnesses." *Health Psychology* 2: 167–85.
——— and J. Ware. 1986. "Health as a value: Methodological and theoretical considerations." *Health Psychology* 5: 25–43.
Launsø, L. 1989. "Integrated medicine—A challenge to the health care system." *Acta Sociologica* 32: 237–51.
Layes, A., Y. Asada, and G. Kephart. 2012. "Whiners and deniers—What does self-rated health measure?" *Social Science and Medicine* 75: 1–9.
Leading Edge. 2009. "Beauty and the beast." *The Lancet Oncology* 10: 835.
Leduc, N., and M. Proulx. 2004. "Patterns of health services utilization by recent immigrants." *Journal of Immigrant Health* 6: 15–27.
Lee, J., C. Dallaire, M.-P. Markon, L. Lemrye, D. Kewski, and M. Turner. 2014. "I can choose: The reflected prominence of personal control in representations of health risk in Canada." *Health, Risk and Society* 16: 117–35.
Lee, K. 2010. "How do we move forward on the social determinants of health: The global governance challenges." *Critical Public Health* 20: 5–14.
Lee, T.C., C. Moore, J.M. Raboud, M.P. Muller, K. Green, A. Tong, J. Dhaliwal, and A. McGeer. 2009. "Impact of a mandatory infection control education program on nosocomial acquisition of methicillin-resistant staphylococcus aureus." *Infection Control and Hospital Epidemiology* 30: 249–56.
Leichter, H. 1997. "Lifestyle correctness and the new secular morality." In A. Brandt and P. Rozin, eds, *Morality and Health*, 359–78. New York: Routledge.

Leinonen, R., E. Heikkinen, and M. Jylha. 1998. "Self-rated health and self-assessed change in health in elderly men and women: A five-year longitudinal study." *Social Science and Medicine* 46: 591–7.
Lemchuk-Favel, L., and R. Jock. 2004. "Aboriginal health systems in Canada: Nine case studies." *International Journal of Indigenous Health* 1(1): 28–51.
Leon, D.A., G. Walt, and L. Gilson. 2001. "International perspectives on health inequalities and policy." *British Medical Journal* 322: 591–4.
Le Petit, C., and J.-M. Berthelot. 2006. "Obesity: A growing issue." *Health Reports* 17: 43–50. Catalogue no. 82-003. Ottawa: Statistics Canada.
Levesque, A., and H. Li. 2014. "The relationship between culture, health conceptions, and health practices: A qualitative-quantitative approach." *Journal of Cross-Cultural Psychology* 45: 628–45.
——— and M. Bohemier. 2013. "Cultural variations in health conceptions: A qualitative approach." *Pimatisiwin: A Journal of Aboriginal and Indigenous Community Health* 2: 215–29.
Levin, L. 1976. "The layperson as the primary health care practitioner." *Public Health Reports* 91: 206–10.
——— and E. Idler. 1981. *The Hidden Health Care System: Mediating Structures and Medicine*. Cambridge, MA: Ballinger.
———. 1983. "Self-care in health." *Annual Review of Public Health* 4: 181–201.
Levin, L., A. Katz, and E. Holst. 1976. *Self-Care: Lay Initiatives in Health*. New York: Prodist.
Levine, S., and M. Kozloff. 1978. "The sick role: Assessment and overview." *Annual Review of Sociology* 4: 317–43.
Lewis, S. 2010. "Neoliberalism, conflict of interest, and the governance of health research in Canada." *Open Medicine* 1: 28–30.
Lewontin, R.C. 1991. *Biology as Ideology: The Doctrine of DNA*. Toronto: House of Anansi Press.

——— and R. Levins. 2007. *Biology under the Influence: Dialectical Essays on Ecology, Agriculture, and Health*. New York: Monthly Review Press.
Lexchin, J., L.A. Bero, B. Djulbegovic, and O. Clark. 2003. "Pharmaceutical industry sponsorship and research outcome and quality: Systematic review." *British Medical Journal* 326: 1167–70.
Li, P.S. 1999. "The multiculturalism debate." In P.S. Li, ed., *Race and Ethnic Relations in Canada*, 2nd edn, 148–77. Don Mills, ON: Oxford University Press.
Lindbladh, E., and C. Lyttkens. 2002. "Habit versus choice: The process of decision-making in health-related behaviour." *Social Science and Medicine* 55: 451–65.
Lindmark, U., U. Stenstrom, E. Gerdin, and A. Hugoson. 2010. "The distribution of 'sense of coherence' among Swedish adults: A quantitative cross-sectional population study." *Scandinavian Journal of Public Health* 38: 1–8.
Lindsay, S. 2009. "Prioritizing illness: Lessons in self-managing multiple chronic diseases." *Canadian Journal of Sociology* 34: 983–1002.
Lindstrom, B., and M. Eriksson. 2005. "Salutogenesis." *Journal of Epidemiology and Community Health* 59: 440–2.
———. 2006. "Contextualizing salutogenesis and Antonovsky in public health development." *Health Promotion International* 21: 238–44.
———. 2009. "The salutogenic approach to the making of HiAP/healthy public policy: Illustrated by a case study." *Global Health Promotion* 16: 17–28.
———. 2010. *The Hitchhiker's Guide to Salutogenesis*. Helsinki: Folkhalsan Health Promotion Research Report. www.salutogenesis.fi.
Link, B.G., R. Carpiano, and M. Weden. 2013. "Can honorific awards give us clues about the connection between socioeconomic status and mortality?" *American Sociological Review* 78: 192–212.

Link, B.G., and J. Phelan. 1995. "Social conditions as fundamental causes of disease." *Journal of Health and Social Behaviour* 35: 80–94.

Lipton, J.A., and J.J. Marbach. 1984. "Ethnicity and the pain experience." *Social Science and Medicine* 19: 1279–98.

Litva, A., and J. Eyles. 1994. "Health or healthy: Why people are not sick in a southern Ontarian town." *Social Science and Medicine* 39: 1083–91.

Liu, S., R. Jones, and M. Glymour. 2010. "Implications of lifecourse epidemiology for research on determinants of adult disease." *Public Health Reviews* 32: 489–511.

Loader, B.D., S. Muncer, R. Burrows, N. Pleace, and S. Nettleton. 2002. "Medicine on the line? Computer-mediated social support and advice for people with diabetes." *International Journal of Social Welfare* 11(1): 53–65.

Lobmayer, P., and R. Wilkinson. 2000. "Income, inequality and mortality in 14 developed countries." *Sociology of Health and Illness* 22: 401–14.

Locust, C. 1999. "Overview of health programs for Canadian Aboriginal peoples." In J. Galloway, B. Goldberg, and J. Alpert, eds, *Primary Care of Native American Patients*, 17–21. Woburn, MA: Butterworth.

Long, K.A. 1993. "The concept of health: Rural perspectives." *Nursing Clinics of North America* 2: 123–30.

Loppie, S., C. Reading, and S. de Leeuw. 2014. *Aboriginal Experiences with Racism and its Impacts*. Prince George, BC: National Collaborating Centre for Aboriginal Health.

Low, J. 2004. *Using Alternative Therapies: A Qualitative Analysis*. Toronto: Canadian Scholars Press.

Lowenberg, J.S., and F. Davis. 1994. "Beyond medicalisation—Demedicalisation: The case of holistic health." *Sociology of Health and Illness* 16: 579–99.

Luchenski, S., A. Quesnel-Vallée, and J. Lynch. 2007. "Differences between women's and men's socioeconomic inequalities in health: Longitudinal analysis of the Canadian population, 1994-2003." *Journal of Epidemiology and Community Health* 62: 1036–44.

Lundell, H., J. Niederdeppe, and C. Clarke. 2013. "Public views about health causation, attributions of responsibility, and inequality." *Journal of Health Communication* 18: 1116–30.

Lupton, D. 1995. *The Imperative of Health: Public Health and the Regulated Body*. London: Sage.

——— 1996. "Your life in their hands: Trust in the medical encounter." In J. Gabe and V. James, eds, *Health and the Sociology of Emotion*, 158–72. Sociology of Health and Illness Monograph Series. Oxford: Blackwell.

——— 1997a. "Consumerism, reflexivity and the medical encounter." *Social Science and Medicine* 45: 373–81.

——— 1997b. "Foucault and the medicalisation critique." In R. Bunton, ed., *Foucault, Health and Medicine*, 94–110. Florence, KY: Routledge.

——— 2012a. *Medicine as Culture: Illness, Disease and the Body in Western Societies*. 3rd edn. London: Sage.

——— 2012b. "M-health and health promotion: The digital cyborg and surveillance society." *Social Theory and Health* 10: 229–44.

——— 2013. "The digitally engaged patient: Self-monitoring and self-care in the digital health era." *Social Theory and Health* 11: 256–70.

——— 2014. "Critical perspectives on digital health technologies." *Sociology Compass* 8: 1344–59.

Lynam, M., and S. Cowley. 2007. "Understanding marginalization as a social determinant of health." *Critical Public Health* 17: 137–49.

Lynch, J. 2000. "Income inequality and health: Expanding the debate." *Social Science and Medicine* 51: 1001–5.

Lynn, T.N., R. Duncan, J. Naughton, E.N. Brandt, J. Wulff, and S. Wolf. 1967. "Prevalence of evidence of prior myocardial infarction, hypertension, diabetes and obesity in three neighboring communities in Pennsylvania." *American Journal of Medical Science* 254: 385–91.

Lyotard, J. 1979. *The Postmodern Condition: A Report on Knowledge*. Manchester: Manchester University Press.

McAteer, A., A. Elliott, and P. Hannaford. 2011. "Ascertaining the size of the symptom iceberg in a UK-wide community-based survey." *British Journal of General Practice* 61: e1–11.

McCarthy, D., and D. Blumenthal. 2006. "Stories from the sharp end: Case studies in safety improvement." *Milbank Quarterly* 84: 165–200.

McDaniel, S. 2013. "Understanding health sociologically." *Current Sociology Review* 0: 1–16.

——— and P. Bernard. 2011. "Life course as a policy lens: Challenges and opportunities." *Canadian Public Policy* 37 (Supplement): S1–13.

Macdonald, D. 2014. *Outrageous Fortune: Documenting Canada's Wealth Gap*. Ottawa: Canadian Centre for Policy Alternatives.

McDonald, J. 2006. "The health behaviours of immigrants and native-born people in Canada." Working Paper no. 01-06. Halifax: Atlantic Metropolis Centre.

——— and S. Kennedy. 2004. "Insights into the 'healthy immigrant effect': Health status and health service use of immigrants to Canada." *Social Science and Medicine* 59: 1613–27.

Macdonald, J., D. Raphael, R. Labonte, R. Colman, R. Torgerson, and K. Hayward. 2009. "Income and health in Canada: Canadian researchers' conceptualizations make policy change unlikely." *International Journal of Health Services* 39: 525–43.

McDonald, L. 2004. *The Women Founders of the Social Sciences*. Montreal: McGill-Queen's University Press.

McDonnell, O., M. Lohan, A. Hyde, and S. Porter, 2009. *Social Theory, Health and Healthcare*. New York: Palgrave Macmillan.

McDonough, P. 2001. "Work and health in the global economy." In P. Armstrong, H. Armstrong, and D. Coburn, eds, *Unhealthy Times: Political Economy Perspectives on Health and Health Care*, 195–222. Toronto: Oxford University Press.

——— and B. Amick. 2001. "The social context of health selection: A longitudinal study of health and employment." *Social Science and Medicine* 53: 135–45.

McDonough, P., and V. Walters. 2001. "Gender and health: Reassessing patterns and explanations." *Social Science and Medicine* 52: 547–59.

McDonough, P., D. Williams, J. House, and G. Duncan. 1999. "Gender and the socioeconomic gradient in mortality." *Journal of Health and Social Behavior* 40: 17–31.

McDowell, I., R. Spasoff, and B. Kristjansson. 2004. "On the classification of population health measurements." *American Journal of Public Health* 94: 388–93.

McGibbon, E., and C. McPherson. 2011. "Applying intersectionality & complexity theory to address the social determinants of women's health." *Women's Health and Urban Life* 10: 59–86.

McGibbon, E., and M. Shebib. 2012. "Health as human right: Challenges and supports for accountability." In E. McGibbon, ed., *Oppression: A Social Determinant of Health*, 186–203. Halifax: Fernwood.

McHorney, C. 2000. "Concepts and measurement of health status and health-related quality of life." In G. Albrecht, R. Fitzpatrick, and S. Scrimshaw, eds, *The Handbook of Social Studies in Health and Medicine*, 339–58. London: Sage.

Macintyre, S., G. Ford, and K. Hunt. 1999. "Do women 'over-report' morbidity? Men's and women's responses to structured prompting on a standard question on long standing illness." *Social Science and Medicine* 48: 89–98.

Macintyre, S., K. Hunt, and H. Sweeting. 1996. "Gender differences in health: Are things really as simple as they seem?" *Social Science and Medicine* 42: 617–24.

Macintyre, S., L. McKay, and A. Ellaway. 2005. "Are rich people or poor people more likely to be ill? Lay perceptions, by social class and neighbourhood, of inequalities in health." *Social Science and Medicine* 60: 313–17.

McKay, A. 2004. "Sexual health education in the schools: Questions and answers." *Canadian Journal of Human Sexuality* 13: 129–41.

McKee, J. 1988. "Holistic health and the critique of Western medicine." *Social Sciences and Medicine* 26: 775–84.

Mackenbach, J., J. Van Den Bos, I. Joung, H. Van De Mheen, and K. Stronks. 1994. "The determinants of excellent health: Different from the determinants of ill-health?" *International Journal of Epidemiology* 23: 1273–81.

McKeown, T. 1976. *The Modern Rise of Population*. London: Edward Arnold.

——— 1979. *The Role of Medicine: Dream, Mirage or Nemesis?* Princeton, NJ: Princeton University Press.

——— R.G. Record, and R.D. Turner. 1975. "An interpretation of the decline of mortality in England and Wales during the twentieth century." *Population Studies* 29: 391–422.

McKinlay, J.B. 1979. "A case for refocusing upstream: The political economy of illness." In E.G. Jaco, ed., *Patients, Physicians, and Illness*, 3rd edn, 9–25. New York: Free Press.

——— 1996. "Some contributions from the social system to gender inequalities in heart disease." *Journal of Health and Social Behavior* 37: 1–26.

——— and S.M. McKinlay. 1977. "The questionable contribution of medical measures to the decline of mortality in the United States in the twentieth century." *Milbank Memorial Fund Quarterly. Health and Society* 55: 405–28.

Maclean, H., K. Glynn, and D. Ansara. 2003. "Multiple roles and women's mental health in Canada." In M. DesMeules, D. Stewart, A. Kazanjian, H. Maclean, J. Payne, and B. Vissandjée, eds, *Women's Health Surveillance Report: A Multi-dimensional Look at the Health of Canadian Women*, 1–15. Ottawa: Canadian Institute for Health Information.

McLeod, C., J. Lavis, C. Mustard, and G. Stoddart. 2003. "Income inequality, household income, and health status in Canada: A prospective cohort study." *American Journal of Public Health* 93: 287–93.

McMullin, J. 2004. *Understanding Social Inequality: Intersections of Class, Age, Gender, Ethnicity, and Race in Canada*. Don Mills, ON: Oxford University Press.

——— 2010. *Understanding Social Inequality: Intersections of Class, Age, Gender, Ethnicity, and Race in Canada*. 2nd edn. Don Mills, ON: Oxford University Press.

McMunn, A., E. Breeze, A. Goodman, J. Nazroo, and Z. Oldfield. 2006. "Social determinants of health in older age." In M. Marmot and R. Wilkinson, eds, *Social Determinants of Health*, 2nd edn, 265–96. New York: Oxford University Press.

McPherson, C. 2012. "A rights-based approach to primary health care: Increasing accountability for health inequities within health systems strengthening." In E. McGibbon, ed., *Oppression: A Social Determinant of Health*, 150–66. Halifax: Fernwood.

Madden, S., and J. Sim. 2006. "Creating meaning in fibromyalgia syndrome." *Social Science and Medicine* 63: 2962–73.

Mahamoud, A., B. Roche, and J. Homer. 2013. "Modelling the social determinants of health and simulating short-term and long-term intervention impacts for the City of Toronto, Canada." *Social Science and Medicine* 93: 247–55.

Malacrida, C. 2005. "Discipline and dehumanization in a total institution: Institutional survivors' descriptions of time-out rooms." *Disability and Society* 20(5): 523–37.

—— 2015. "Always, already-medicalized: Women's prenatal knowledge and choice in two Canadian contexts." *Current Sociology* 63(5): 636–51.

Maller, C.J. 2015. "Understanding health through social practices: Performance and materiality in everyday life." *Sociology of Health and Illness* 37(1): 52–66.

Mandich, S., and R. Margolis. 2014. "Changes in disability-free life expectancy in Canada between 1994 and 2007." *Canadian Studies in Population* 41(1–2): 192–208.

Mansour, A. 1994. "The conceptualisation of health among residents of Saskatoon." *Journal of Community Health* 19: 165–79.

Manton, K., and E. Stallard. 1991. "Cross-sectional estimates of active life expectancy for the US elderly and oldest-old populations." *Journal of Gerontology: Social Sciences* 46: S170–82.

Manuel, D., A. Schultz, and J. Kopec. 2002. "Measuring the health burden of chronic disease and injury using health adjusted life expectancy and the Health Utilities Index." *Journal of Epidemiology and Community Health* 56: 843–50.

Marcus, B.H., N. Owen, L.H. Forsyth, N.A. Cavill, and F. Fridinger. 1998. "Physical activity interventions using mass media, print media, and information technology." *American Journal of Preventative Medicine* 15: 362–78.

Marmot, M. 2004a. "Social determinants of health: A panoramic view." http://balzan.com/en/Prizewinners/MichaelMarmot/Socialdeterminantsofhealthapanoramicview.aspx.

—— 2004b. *The Status Syndrome: How Social Standing Affects Our Health and Longevity*. New York: Times Books.

—— 2005. "Social determinants of health inequalities." *The Lancet* 365: 1099–104.

—— 2006. Introduction. In M. Marmot and R. Wilkinson, eds, *Social Determinants of Health*, 2nd edn, 1–5. Oxford: Oxford University Press.

Marmot, M., J. Allen, and P. Goldblatt. 2010. "A social movement, based on evidence, to reduce inequalities in health." *Social Science and Medicine* 71: 1254–8.

Marmot, M., and R. Bell. 2012. "Fair society, healthy lives." *Public Health* 126: S4–10.

—— and P. Goldblatt. 2013. "Action on the social determinants of health." *Revue d'Épidemiologie et de santé publique* 61S: S127–32.

Marmot, M., C. Ryff, L. Bumpass, M. Shipley, and N. Marks. 1997. "Social inequalities in health: Next questions and converging evidence." *Social Science and Medicine* 44: 901–10.

Marmot, M., and R. Wilkinson, eds. 2006. *Social Determinants of Health*. 2nd edn. Oxford: Oxford University Press.

Marshall, B. 2000. *Configuring Gender: Explorations in Theory and Politics*. Peterborough, ON: Broadview Press.

Martel, L., and A. Bélanger. 2000. "Dependence-free life expectancy in Canada." *Canadian Social Trends* 58: 26–9. Catalogue no. 11-008. Ottawa: Statistics Canada.

—— J.-M. Berthelot, and Y. Carriere. 2005. *Healthy Aging*. Ottawa: Statistics Canada.

Matthews, S., O. Manor, and C. Power. 1999. "Social inequalities in health: Are there gender differences?" *Social Science and Medicine* 48: 49–60.

Mavaddat, N., A. Kinmonth, S. Sanderson, P. Surtees, S. Bingham, and K. Khaw. 2011. "What determines self-rated health (SRH)? A cross-sectional study of SF-36 health domains in the EPIC-Norfolk cohort." *Journal of Epidemiology and Community Health* 65: 800–6.

Mechanic, D. "Religion, religiosity, and illness behavior." 1963. *Human Organization* 22: 202–8.

—— and P. Cleary. 1980. "Factors associated with the maintenance of positive health behavior." *Preventive Medicine* 9: 805–14.

Medved, M.I., and J. Brockmeier. 2008. "Continuity amidst chaos: Neurotrauma, loss of memory and sense of self." *Qualitative Health Research* 18: 469–79.

Meili, R. 2012. *A Healthy Society: How a Focus on Health Can Revive Canadian Democracy*. Saskatoon: Purich Publishing.

Mikkonen, J., and D. Raphael. 2010. *Social Determinants of Health: The Canadian Facts*. Toronto: York University School of Health Policy and Management.

Millar, J., and C. Hull. 1997. "Measuring human wellness." *Social Indicators Research* 40: 147–58.

Miller, G., and L. Foster. 2010. *Critical Synthesis of Wellness Literature*. Victoria, BC: University of Victoria, Faculty of Human and Social Development and Department of Geography.

Milligan, C., A. Bingley, and A. Gatrell. 2005. "Digging deep: Using diary techniques to explore the place of health and well-being amongst older people." *Social Science and Medicine* 61: 1882–92.

Mills, C.W. 1959. *The Sociological Imagination*. New York: Oxford University Press.

Minassian, V., X. Yan, M. Lichtenfeld, H. Sun, and W. Stewart. 2012. "The iceberg of health care utilization in women with urinary incontinence." *International Urogynecology Journal* 23: 1087–93.

Mishra, G., K. Ball, A. Dobson, and J. Byles. 2004. "Do socioeconomic gradients in women's health widen over time and with age?" *Social Science and Medicine* 58:1585–95.

Mittelmark, M., and T. Bull. 2013. "The salutogenic model of health in health promotion research." *Global Health Promotion* 20: 30–8.

Mizrahi, T. 1984. "Managing medical mistakes: Ideology, insularity and accountability amongst internists-in-training." *Social Science and Medicine* 19: 135–46.

Mokdad, A., J. Marks, D. Stroup, and J. Gerberding. 2004. "Actual causes of death in the United States, 2000." *Journal of the American Medical Association* 291: 1238–45.

——— 2005. "Correction: Actual causes of death in the United States, 2000." *Journal of the American Medical Association* 293: 293–4.

Monette, L.E., S.B. Rourke, K. Gibson, T.M. Bekele, R. Tucker, S. Greene, and S. Bhuiyan. 2011. "Inequalities in determinants of health among Aboriginal and Caucasian persons living with HIV/AIDS in Ontario: Results from the Positive Spaces, Healthy Places Study. *Canadian Journal of Public Health* 102(3): 215–19.

Morgan, A., and E. Ziglio. 2007. "Revitalising the evidence base for public health: An assets model." *Global Health Promotion* 2 (Supplement): 17–22.

Morissette, R., G. Picot, and Y. Lu. 2013. "The evolution of Canadian wages over the last three decades." 11F0019M, no. 347. Ottawa: Statistics Canada.

Mortimer, J., and M. Shanahan. 2002. *Handbook of the Life Course*. New York: Kluwer Academic Publishers.

Moss, N. 2002. "Gender equity and socioeconomic inequality: A framework for the patterning of women's health." *Social Science and Medicine* 54: 649–66.

Mossakowski, K.N. 2003. "Coping with perceived discrimination: Does ethnic identity protect mental health?" *Journal of Health and Social Behavior* 44(3): 318–31.

Mossey, J., and E. Shapiro. 1982. "Self-rated health: A predictor of mortality among the elderly." *American Journal of Public Health* 72: 800–8.

Moynihan, R., and A. Cassels. 2005. *Selling Sickness: How the World's Biggest Pharmaceutical Companies Are Turning Us All into Patients*. Toronto: Greystone Press.

Moynihan, R., I. Heath, and D. Henry. 2002. "Selling sickness: The pharmaceutical industry and disease mongering." *British Medical Journal* 324: 886–91.

Mulé, N., and M. Smith. 2014. "Invisible populations: LGBTQ people and federal health policy in Canada." *Canadian Public Administration* 57: 234–55.

Munch, S. 2004. "Gender-biased diagnosing of women's medical complaints: Contributions of feminist thought, 1970–1995." *Women and Health* 40: 101–21.

Muntaner, C., C. Borrell, A. Kunst, H. Chung, J. Benach, and S. Ibrahim. 2006. "Social class inequalities in health." In D. Raphael, T. Bryant, and M. Rioux, eds, *Staying Alive: Critical Perspectives on Health, Illness, and Health Care*, 139–58. Toronto: Canadian Scholars Press.

Muntaner, C., C. Borrell, E. Ng, H. Chung, A. Espelt, M. Rodriguez-Sanz, J. Benach, and P. O'Campo. 2011. "Review article: Politics, welfare regimes, and population health: Controversies and evidence." *Sociology of Health and Illness* 33: 946–64.

Muntaner, C., C. Borrell, C. Vanroelen, H. Chung, J. Benach, I. Kim, and E. Ng. 2010. "Employment relations, social class and health: A review and analysis of conceptual and measurement alternatives." *Social Science and Medicine* 71: 2130–40.

Murray, C., and A. Lopez. 2013. "Measuring the global burden of disease." *New England Journal of Medicine* 369: 448–57.

Murray, M. 1990. "Lay representations of illness." In P. Bennett, J. Weinman, and P. Spurgeon, eds, *Current Developments in Health Psychology*, 63–92. London: Harwood Academic.

Murray, S., J. Brophy, and A. Palepu. 2010. "Open medicine's ghost and guest authorship policy." *Open Medicine* 4: 1–2.

Mustard, C., J. Lavis, and A. Ostry. 2006. "Work and health: New evidence and enhanced understandings." In J. Heymann, C. Hertzman, M. Barer, and R. Evans, eds, *Healthier Societies: From Analysis to Action*, 173–201. New York: Oxford University Press.

Mustard, C., M. Vermeulen, and J. Lavis. 2003. "Is position in the occupational hierarchy a determinant of decline in perceived health status?" *Social Science and Medicine* 57: 2291–303.

Nakhaie, A., L. Smylie, and R. Arnold. 2007. "Social inequalities, social capital, and health of Canadians." *Review of Radical Political Economics* 39: 562–85.

Nandi, A., M.M. Glymour, and S.V. Subramanian. 2014. "Association among socioeconomic status, health behaviors, and all-cause mortality in the United States." *Epidemiology* 25(2): 170–7.

National Center for Complementary and Alternative Medicine (NCCAM). 2007. "Selecting a practitioner; CAM basics." http://nccam.nih.gov/health/decisions/D346.pdf.

National Collaborating Centre for Aboriginal Health (NCCAH). 2012. *State of Knowledge of Aboriginal Health: A Review of Aboriginal Public Health in Canada*. Prince George, BC: NCCAH.

——— 2013. *An Overview of Aboriginal Health in Canada*. Prince George, BC: NCCAH.

National Collaborating Centre for Healthy Public Policy. 2010. *Thirteen Public Interventions in Canada That Have Contributed to a Reduction in Health Inequalities*. www.ncchpp.ca.

National Forum on Health. 1996. *What Determines Health?* Ottawa: National Forum on Health.

——— 1997. *Canada Health Action: Building on the Legacy*. Vol. 1, *The Final Report*. Ottawa: National Forum on Health.

Navarro, V. 1976. *Medicine under Capitalism*. New York: Prodist.

——— 1998. "Book review of *Private Medicine and Public Health: Profits, Politics and Prejudice in the American Health Care Enterprise* by Lawrence D. Weiss." *Contemporary Sociology* 27: 419–20.

—— and L. Shi. 2001. "The political context of social inequalities and health." *Social Science and Medicine* 52: 481–91.

Neel, J.V. 1962. "Diabetes mellitus: A 'thrifty' genotype rendered detrimental by progress?" *American Journal of Human Genetics* 14: 353–62.

Nelson, E., and B. Robinson. 1999. *Gender in Canada*. Scarborough, ON: Prentice Hall Allyn and Bacon Canada.

Nettleton, S. 2004. "The emergence of E-scaped Medicine?" *Sociology* 38(4): 661–79.

—— 2009. "The appearance of new medical cosmologies and the re-appearance of sick and healthy men and women: A comment on the merits of social theorizing." *International Journal of Epidemiology* 38: 633–6.

—— 2013. *Sociology of Health and Illness*. 3rd edn. Cambridge: Polity Press.

—— R. Burrows, and L. O'Malley. 2005. "The mundane realities of the everyday lay use of the Internet for health, and their consequences for media convergence." *Sociology of Health and Illness* 27: 972–92.

New, P. 1977. "Traditional and modern health care: An appraisal of complementarity." *International Social Science Journal* 29: 483–95.

Newbold, K. 2005. "Self-rated health within the Canadian immigrant population: Risk and the healthy immigrant effect." *Social Science and Medicine* 60: 1359–70.

—— 2009. "Health care use and the Canadian immigrant population." *International Journal of Health Services* 39: 545–65.

—— and J. Danforth. 2003. "Health status and Canada's immigrant population." *Social Science and Medicine* 51: 1981–95.

Newsom, J., T. McFarland, M. Kaplan, N. Huguet, and B. Zani. 2005. "The health consciousness myth: Implications of the near independence of major health behaviors in the North American population." *Social Science and Medicine* 60: 433–7.

Ng, E., K. Pottie, and D.L. Spitzer. 2011. *Official Language Proficiency and Self-Reported Health among Immigrants to Canada*. Catalogue no. 82-003-X. Ottawa: Statistics Canada.

Nicholas, A.B. 2008. "The assault on Aboriginal oral traditions: Past and present." In E. Renate and R. Hulan, eds, *Aboriginal Oral Traditions: Theory, Practice, Ethics*, 13–43. Halifax: Fernwood.

Nicolau, B., and W. Marcenes. 2012. "How will a life course framework be used to tackle wider social determinants of health?" *Community Dentistry and Oral Epidemiology* 40: 33–8.

Nielsen//NetRatings. 2008. http://www.nielsen-netratings.com/pr/pr_020213.pdf.

Nilsson, K., J. Leppert, B. Simonsson, and B. Starrin. 2010. "Sense of coherence and psychological well-being." *Journal of Epidemiology and Community Health* 64: 347–52.

Nolte, E., and C. McKee. 2008. "Measuring the health of nations: Updating an earlier analysis." *Health Affairs* 27: 58–71.

Norman, R. 1985. "Studies of the interrelationships amongst health behaviours." *Canadian Journal of Public Health* 76: 407–10.

Northcott, H., L. Vanderheyden, J. Northcott, C. Adair, C. McBrien-Morrison, P. Norton, and J. Cowell. 2007. "Perceptions of preventable medical errors in Alberta, Canada." *International Journal for Quality in Health Care* 20: 115–22.

Nowatzki, N. 2011. "Income inequality and health: A theoretical quagmire." In T. McIntosh, B. Jeffery, and N. Muharine, eds, *Redistributing Health: New Directions in Population Health Research in Canada*, 35–53. Regina: CPRC Press.

Nutbeam, D. 2008. "The evolving concept of health literacy." *Social Science and Medicine* 67: 2072–8.

Nye, R.A. 2003. "The evolution of the concept of medicalization in the late twentieth century." *Journal of History of the Behavioral Sciences* 39: 115–29.

Oakley, A. 1980. *Women Confined: Towards Sociology of Childbirth*. Oxford: Martin Robertson.

—— 1981. *Becoming a Mother*. Harmondsworth, UK: Penguin.

—— 1984. *The Captured Womb: A History of the Medical Care of Pregnant Women*. Oxford: Basil Blackwell.

—— 1994. "Who cares for health? Social relations, gender and the public health." *Journal of Epidemiology and Community Health* 48: 427–34.

—— 2005. *The Ann Oakley Reader: Gender, Women and Social Science*. Bristol, UK: Policy Press.

O'Brien, M. 1981. *The Politics of Reproduction*. Boston: Routledge and Kegan Paul.

O'Campo, P., and J.R. Dunn. 2012. *Rethinking Social Epidemiology: Towards a Science of Change*. New York: Springer.

O'Connor, B. 1995. *Healing Traditions: Alternative Medicine and the Health Professions*. Philadelphia: University of Pennsylvania Press.

OECD (Organisation for Economic Co-operation and Development). 2013. "Health at a glance 2013: OECD indicators." http://dx.doi.org/10.1787/health_glance-2013-en.

Ojala, T., A. Hakkinen, J. Karppinen, K. Sipila, T. Suutama, and A. Piiranen. 2015. "Chronic pain affects the whole person—A phenomenological study. *Disability and Rehabilitation* 37: 363–71.

Oldani, M.J. 2004. "Thick prescriptions: Towards an interpretation of pharmaceutical sales practices." *Medical Anthropology Quarterly* 18: 325–56.

Oliver, J.E. 2005. *Fat Politics: The Real Story behind America's Obesity Epidemic*. New York: Oxford University Press.

Olshansky, A., M. Rudberg, B. Carnes, C. Cassel, and J. Brody. 1991. "Trading off longer life for worsening health: The expansion of morbidity hypothesis." *Journal of Aging and Health* 3: 194–216.

Omariba, D.W.R. 2015. "Immigration, ethnicity, and avoidable mortality in Canada, 1991–2006." *Ethnicity and Health*, doi: 10.1080/13557858.2014.995155.

O'Neill, J. 1985. *Five Bodies: The Human Shape of Modern Society*. Ithaca, NY: Cornell University Press.

O'Neill, M.S., M. Jerrett, I. Kawachi, J.I. Levy, A.J. Cohen, N. Gouveia, P. Wilkinson, T. Fletcher, L. Cifuentes, and J. Schwartz. 2003. "Health, wealth, and air pollution: Advancing theory and methods." *Environmental Health Perspectives* 111(16): 1861–70.

Orpana, H., and L. Lemrye. 2004. "Explaining the social gradient in health in Canada: Using the National Population Health Survey to examine the role of stressors." *International Journal of Behavioural Medicine* 11: 143–51.

Osborn, C., M. Paasche-Orlow, S. Bailey, and M. Wolf. 2011. "The mechanisms linking health literacy to behavior and health status." *American Journal of Health Behavior* 35: 118–28.

Osler, W. 1906. *Aequanimitas*. New York: McGraw Hill.

Ostberg, V., and C. Lennartsson. 2007. "Getting by with a little help: The importance of various types of social support for health problems." *Scandinavian Journal of Public Health* 35: 197–204.

O'Sullivan, S., and A. Stakelum. 2004. "Lay understandings of health: A qualitative study." In I. Shaw and K. Kauppinen, eds, *Constructions of Health and Illness: European Perspectives*, 26–43. Aldershot, UK: Ashgate.

Oxman-Martinez, J., and J. Hanley. 2005. *Health and Social Services for Canada's Multicultural Population: Challenges for Equity*. Ottawa: Heritage Canada.

Paasche-Orlow, M., and M. Wolf. 2007. "The causal pathways linking health literacy to health outcomes." *American Journal of Health Behavior* 31 (Supplement): S19–26.

Padamsee, T. 2011. "The pharmaceutical corporation and the 'good work' of managing women's bodies." *Social Science and Medicine* 72: 1342–50.

Park, J. 2005. "Use of alternative health care." *Health Reports* 16: 39–42. Catalogue no. 82-003-XIE. Ottawa: Statistics Canada.

—— and S. Knudson. 2007. "Medically unexplained physical symptoms." *Health Reports* 18: 43–7. Ottawa: Statistics Canada.

Parliament of Canada. 2013. *Income Inequality in Canada: An Overview*. Report of the Standing Committee on Finance. Ottawa: House of Commons Canada.

Parsons, T. 1951. *The Social System*. New York: Free Press.

Pavalko, E., and J. Caputo. 2013. "Social inequality and health across the life course." *American Behavioral Scientist* 57: 1040–56.

Pavalko, E., and A. Willson. 2011. "Life course approaches to health, illness and healing." In B.A. Pescosolido, J.K. Martin, J.D. McLeod, and A. Rogers, eds, *Handbook of the Sociology of Health, Illness, and Healing: A Blueprint for the 21st Century*, 449–64. New York: Springer.

Payne, J., I. Neutel, R. Cho, and M. DesMeules. 2003. "Factors associated with women's medication use." In M. DesMeules, D. Stewart, A. Kazanjian, H. Maclean, J. Payne, and B. Vissandjée, eds, *Women's Health Surveillance Report: A Multidimensional Look at the Health of Canadian Women*, 1–16. Ottawa: Canadian Institute for Health Information.

Pederson, A. 2013. "To be welcome: A call for narrative interviewing methods in illness contexts." *Qualitative Inquiry* 19: 411–18.

—— M.J. Haworth-Brockman, B. Clow, H. Isfeld, and A. Liwander, eds. 2013. *Rethinking Women and Healthy Living in Canada*. Vancouver: British Columbia Centre of Excellence for Women's Health.

Peerson, A., and M. Saunders. 2009. "Health literacy revisited: What do we mean and why does it matter?" *Health Promotion International* 24: 285–96.

Pendakur, K., and R. Pendakur. 2011. "Color by numbers: Minority earnings in Canada 1995–2005." *International Migration and Integration* 12: 305–29.

Perez, C.E. 2002. "Health status and health behaviour among immigrants." *Health Reports* 13 (Supplement): 1–13. Catalogue no. 82-0032002. Ottawa: Statistics Canada.

Pescosolido, B., J. McLeod, and M. Alegría. 2000. "Confronting the second social contract: The place of medical sociology in research and policy for the twenty-first century." In C. Bird, P. Conrad, and A. Fremont, eds, *Handbook of Medical Sociology*, 5th edn, 411–26. Upper Saddle River, NJ: Prentice-Hall.

Petersen, A. 2012. "Foucault, health and healthcare." In G. Scambler, ed., *Contemporary Theorists for Medical Sociology*, 7–19. New York: Routledge.

—— and D. Lupton. 1996. *The New Public Health: Health and Self in the Age of Risk*. London: Sage.

Peterson, C., and A. Stunkard. 1989. "Personal control and health promotion." *Social Science and Medicine* 28: 819–28.

Pfifferling, J. 1975. "Some issues in the consideration of non-Western and Western folk practices as epidemiologic data." *Social Science and Medicine* 9: 655–8.

Pflanz, M. 1974. "A critique of Anglo-American medical sociology." *International Journal of Health Services* 4: 565–74.

—— 1975. "Relations between social scientists, physicians and medical organizations in health research." *Social Science and Medicine* 9: 7–13.

Pham-Kanter, G. 2009. "Social comparisons and health: Can having richer friends and neighbors make you sick?" *Social Science and Medicine* 69: 335–44.

Philips, R., C. Benoit, H. Hallgrimsdottir, and K. Vallance, 2012. "Courtesy stigma: A hidden health concern among front-line service providers to sex workers." *Sociology of Health and Illness* 34(5): 681–96.

Picard, A. 2009. "The man from Pfizer: Should big pharma help steer health research?" *Globe and Mail*. www.theglobeandmail.com/life/health/the-man-from-pfizer-should-big-pharma-help-steer-health-research/article1386213.

Picard, M., R.-P. Juster, and C. Sabiston. 2013. "Is the whole greater than the sum of the parts? Self-rated health and transdisciplinarity." *Health* 5: 24–30.

Pickard, S., and A. Rogers. 2012. "Knowing as practice: Self-care in the case of chronic multi-morbidities." *Social Theory and Health* 10: 101–20.

Pickett, K.E., and R.G. Wilkinson. 2008. "People like us: Ethnic group density effects on health." *Ethnicity and Health* 13(4): 321–34.

——— 2014. "Income inequality and health: A causal review." *Social Science and Medicine* 128: 316–26.

Pickstone, J.V. 2009. "From history of medicine to a general history of 'working knowledges.'" *International Journal of Epidemiology* 38: 646–9.

Pill, R., and N. Stott. 1982. "Concepts of illness causation and responsibility: Some preliminary data from a sample of working class mothers." *Social Science and Medicine* 16: 43–52.

——— 1985. "Choice or chance: Further evidence on ideas of illness and responsibility for health." *Social Science and Medicine* 20: 981–91.

Pilnick, A., and R. Dingwall. 2011. "On the remarkable persistence of asymmetry in doctor/patient interaction: A critical review." *Social Science and Medicine* 72: 1374–82.

Pilote, L., K. Dasgupta, V. Guru, K. Humphries, J. McGrath, C. Norris, and V. Tagalakis. 2007. "A comprehensive view of sex-specific issues related to cardiovascular disease."

Canadian Medical Association Journal 176(6): S1–44.

Pinxten, W., and J. Lievens. 2014. "The importance of economic, social and cultural capital in understanding health inequalities: Using a Bourdieu-based approach in research on physical and mental health perceptions." *Sociology of Health and Illness* 36(7): 1095–110.

Pluijm, S., M. Visser, M. Puts, M. Dik, B. Schalk, N. van Schoor, L. Schaap, R. Bosscher, and D. Deeg. 2007. "Unhealthy lifestyles during the lifecourse: Association with physical decline in late life." *Aging Clinical and Experimental Research* 19: 75–83.

Poland, B., D. Coburn, A. Robertson, and J. Eakin. 1998. "Wealth, equity and health care: A critique of a 'population health' perspective on the determinants of health." *Social Science and Medicine* 46: 785–98.

Poland, B., K. Frohlich, R. Haines, E. Mykhalovskiy, M. Rock, and R. Sparks. 2006. "The social context of smoking: The next frontier in tobacco control?" *Tobacco Control* 15: 59–63.

Poortinga, W. 2006. "Social relations or social capital? Individual and community health effects of bonding social capital." *Social Science and Medicine* 63: 255–70.

Pop, I., E. van Ingen, and W. van Oorschot. 2013. "Inequality, wealth and health: Is decreasing income inequality the key to create healthier societies?" *Social Indicators Research* 113: 1025–43.

Popay, J., G. Williams, C. Thomas, and T. Gatrell. 1998. "Theorising inequalities in health: The place of lay knowledge." *Sociology of Health and Illness* 20: 619–44.

Porter, C. 2007. "Ottawa to Bangkok: Changing health promotion discourse." *Health Promotion International* 22: 72–9.

Porter, J. 1965. *The Vertical Mosaic*. Toronto: University of Toronto Press.

Porter, R. 1997. *The Greatest Benefit to Mankind: A Medical History*

of Humanity from Antiquity to Present. New York: W.W. Norton.

Poudrier, J. 2007. "The geneticization of Aboriginal diabetes and obesity: Adding another scene to the story of the thrifty gene." *Canadian Review of Sociology* 44(2): 237–61.

——— and J. Kennedy. 2007. "Embodiment and the meaning of the 'healthy body': An exploration of Aboriginal women's perspectives of healthy body weight and body image." *Journal of Aboriginal Health* 4: 15–24.

Power, C., and D. Kuh. 2006. "Life course development of unequal health." In J. Siegrist and M. Marmot, eds, *Social Inequalities in Health: New Evidence and Policy Implications*, 27–52. New York: Oxford University Press.

Press, I. 1980. "Problems in the definition and classification of medical systems." *Social Science and Medicine* 14B: 45–57.

Prior, L. 2003. "Belief, knowledge and expertise: The emergence of the lay expert in medical sociology." *Sociology of Health and Illness* 25: 41–57.

——— 2009. "From sick men and women, to patients, and thence to clients and consumers—The structuring of the 'patient' in the modern world." *International Journal of Epidemiology* 38: 637–9.

——— M. Evans, and H. Prout. 2011. "Talking about colds and flu: The lay diagnosis of two common illnesses among older British people." *Social Science and Medicine* 73: 922–8.

Prus, S. 2007. "Age, SES, and health: A population level analysis of health inequalities over the lifecourse." *Sociology of Health and Illness* 29: 275–96.

——— 2011. "Comparing social determinants of self-rated health across the United States and Canada." *Social Science and Medicine* 73: 50–9.

——— and Z. Lin. 2005. "Ethnicity and health: An analysis of physical health differences across twenty-one ethnocultural groups in Canada." SEDAP Research Paper

no. 143. http://socserv.mcmaster.ca/sedap.
Public Health Agency of Canada. 1999. *Toward a Healthy Future: Second Report on the Health of Canadians.* www.phac-aspc.gc.ca/ph-sp/determinants/determinants.html.
—— 2004. "The social determinants of health: Income inequality as a determinant of health." www.phac-aspc.gc.ca/ph-sp/oi-ar/02_income-eng.
—— 2011. *Diabetes in Canada: Facts and Figures from a Public Health Perspective.* Ottawa: Public Health Agency of Canada.
—— 2012. "Health-adjusted life expectancy in Canada." Ottawa: Public Health Agency of Canada.
—— 2013. "What makes Canadians healthy or unhealthy?" http://www.phac-aspc.gc.ca/ph-sp/determinants/determinants-eng.php.
—— 2014. *HIV and AIDS in Canada: Surveillance Report to December 31, 2013.* Ottawa: Minister of Public Works and Government Services Canada.
—— 2015. *Report on Sexually Transmitted Infections in Canada: 2012.* Catalogue no. HP37-10/2012E-PDF. Ottawa: Centre for Communicable Diseases and Infection Control, Infectious Disease Prevention and Control Branch.
Puig-Barranchina, V., D. Malmusi, J. Martinez, and J. Benach. 2011. "Monitoring social determinants of health inequalities: The impact of unemployment among vulnerable groups." *International Journal of Health Services* 41: 459–82.
Quah, S.R. 2008. "In pursuit of health: Pragmatic acculturation in everyday life." *Health Sociology Review* 17: 419–22.
Rabinow, P. 1996. *Artificiality and Enlightenment: From Sociobiology to Biosociality. Essays on the Anthropology of Reason.* Princeton, NJ: Princeton University Press.
Rachlis, M. "Health care and health." 2004. In D. Raphael, ed., *Social Determinants of Health: Canadian Perspectives,* 297–310. Toronto: Canadian Scholars Press.
Radley, A., and M. Billig. 1996. "Accounts of health and illness: Dilemmas and representations." *Sociology of Health and Illness* 18: 220–40.
Raffle, A.E., and J.A.M. Gray. 2007. *Screening: Evidence and Practice.* Cambridge: Oxford University Press.
Rakowski, W., J. Fleishman, V. Mor, and S. Bryant. 1993. "Self-assessments of health and mortality among older persons." *Research on Aging* 15: 92–116.
Raphael, D. 2001. "From increasing poverty to societal disintegration: How economic inequality affects the health of individuals and communities." In H. Armstrong, P. Armstrong, and D. Coburn, eds, *Unhealthy Times: The Political Economy of Health and Care in Canada,* 223–46. Toronto: Oxford University Press.
—— 2003a. "Addressing the social determinants of health in Canada: Bridging the gap between research findings and public policy." *Policy Options* 24: 35–40.
—— 2003b. "Barriers to addressing the societal determinants of health: Public health units and poverty in Ontario, Canada." *Health Promotion International* 18: 397–405.
—— 2006. "Social determinants of health: An overview of concepts and issues." In D. Raphael, T. Bryant, and M. Rioux, eds, *Staying Alive: Critical Perspectives on Health, Illness, and Health Care,* 115–38. Toronto: Canadian Scholars Press.
—— 2008. "Getting serious about the social determinants of health: New directions for public health workers." *Promotion and Education* 15: 15–20.
—— 2009. "Social determinants of health: An overview of key issues and themes." In D. Raphael, ed., *Social Determinants of Health: Canadian Perspectives,* 2nd edn, 2–19. Toronto: Canadian Scholars Press.
—— 2010. "Social determinants of health: An overview of concepts and issues." In D. Raphael, T. Bryant, and M. Rioux, eds, *Staying Alive: Critical Perspectives on Health, Illness, and Health Care,* 2nd edn, 145–80. Toronto: Canadian Scholars Press.
—— 2011. "A discourse analysis of the social determinants of health." *Critical Public Health* 21: 221–36.
—— and T. Bryant. 2002. "The limitations of population health as a model for a new public health." *Health Promotion International* 17: 189–99.
Raphael, D., R. Labonte, R. Colman, K. Hayward, R. Torgerson, and J. Macdonald. 2006. "Income and health in Canada: Research gaps and future opportunities." *Canadian Journal of Public Health* 97: S16–23.
Raphael, D., J. Macdonald, R. Colman, R. Labonte, K. Hayward, and R. Torgerson. 2005. "Researching income and income distribution as determinants of health in Canada: Gaps between theoretical knowledge, research practice, and policy implementation." *Health Policy* 72: 217–32.
Ravelli, B., and M. Webber. 2016. *Exploring Sociology: A Canadian Perspective.* 3rd edn. Toronto: Pearson.
Ray, P.H. 1997. "The emerging culture." *American Demographics* 19: 29–56.
—— and S.R. Anderson. 2000. *The Cultural Creatives: How 50 Million People Are Changing the World.* New York: Harmony Books.
Read, J.N.G., and B.K. Gorman. 2011. "Gender and health revisited." In B.A. Pescosolido, J.K. Martin, J.D. McLeod, and A. Rogers, eds, *Handbook of the Sociology of Health, Illness, and Healing,* 411–29. New York: Springer.
Reading, C. 2013. *Understanding Racism.* Prince George, BC: National Collaborating Centre for Aboriginal Health.
Reading, J. 2009. "A life course approach to the social determinants of health for Aboriginal peoples."

For the Senate Subcommittee on Population Health. Appendix A. http://senate-senat.ca/health-e.asp.

Reason, J. 2000. "Human error: Models and management." *British Medical Journal* 320: 768–70.

Redelmeier, D., and S. Singh. 2001. "Survival in Academy Award-winning actors and actresses." *Annals of Internal Medicine* 134: 955–62.

Rehm, J., S. Geisbrecht, S. Popova, J. Patra, E. Adlaf, and R. Mann. 2006. *Overview of Positive and Negative Effects of Alcohol Consumption: Implications for Preventative Policies in Canada*. Toronto: Centre for Addiction and Mental Health.

Rehm, J., J. Patra, and S. Popova. 2006. "Alcohol-attributable mortality and potential years of life lost in Canada 2001: Implications for prevention and policy." *Addiction* 101: 373–84.

Relman, A. 1980. "The new medical-industrial complex." *New England Journal of Medicine* 303: 963–70.

—— and A. Weil. 1999. "Is integrative medicine the medicine of the future? A debate between Arnold S. Relman, MD, and Andrew Weil, MD." *Archives of Internal Medicine* 159: 2122–6.

Remennick, L. 1998. "Race, class, and occupation as determinants of cancer risk and survival: Trend report. The cancer problem in the context of modernity: Sociology, demography, and politics." *Current Sociology* 46: 25–39.

Renaud, M., D. Good, L. Nadeau, J. Ritchie, R. Way-Clark, and C. Connolly. 1996. *Determinants of Health Working Group Synthesis Report*. Vol. 2, *Canada Health Action: Building on the Legacy: Synthesis Reports and Issues Papers*. Ottawa: National Forum on Health.

Ricciuto, L.E., and V.S. Tarasuk. 2007. "An examination of income-related disparities in the nutritional quality of food selections among Canadian households from 1986–2001. *Social Science and Medicine* 64: 186–98.

Richman, J., L. Jason, R. Taylor, and S. Jahn. 2000. "Feminist perspectives on the social construction of chronic fatigue syndrome." *Health Care for Women International* 21: 173–85.

Richmond, C., N. Ross, and G. Egeland. 2007. "Social support and thriving health: A new approach to understanding the health of Indigenous Canadians." *American Journal of Public Health* 97: 1827–33.

Ridde, V., A. Guichard, and D. Houeto. 2007. "Social inequalities in health from Ottawa to Vancouver: Action for fair equality of opportunity." *Promotion and Education* 14 (Supplement): 12–16.

Reid, J.L, D. Hammond, V.L. Rynard, and R. Burkhalter. 2015. *Tobacco Use in Canada: Patterns and Trends, 2015 Edition*. Waterloo, ON: Propel Centre for Population Health Impact, University of Waterloo.

Rieker, P., and C. Bird. 2000. "Sociological explanations of gender differences in mental and physical health." In C. Bird, P. Conrad, and A. Fremont, eds, *Handbook of Medical Sociology*, 5th edn, 98–113. Upper Saddle River, NJ: Prentice-Hall.

—— M. Lang. 2010. "Understanding gender and health: Old patterns, new trends, and future directions." In C. Bird, P. Conrad, A. Fremont, and S. Timmermans, eds, *Handbook of Medical Sociology*, 6th edn, 53–74. Nashville: Vanderbilt University Press.

Rinzler, C. 1981. *The Dictionary of Medical Folklore*. New York: Ballantine Books.

Riska, E., and K. Wegar. 1993. "Women physicians: A new force in medicine?" In E. Riska and K. Wegar, eds, *Gender, Work and Medicine: Women and the Medical Division of Labour*, 27–60. Newbury Park, CA: Sage.

Ritzer, G. 1992. *Sociological Theory*. 3rd edn. New York: McGraw-Hill.

Robles, T., F. Reynolds, R. Repetti, and P. Chung. 2013. "Using daily diaries to study family settings, emotions, and health in everyday life." *Journal of Social and Personal Relationships* 30: 179–88.

Roizen, M.F., and M. Oz. 2005. *YOU: The Owner's Manual— An Insider's Guide to the Body That Will Make You Healthier and Younger*. New York: HarperCollins.

Rollman, G.B. 2004. "Ethnocultural variations in the experience of pain." In T. Hadjistavropoulos and K.D. Craig, eds, *Pain: Psychological Perspectives*, 155–78. Mahwah, NJ: Lawrence Erlbaum.

—— 2005. "The need for ecological validity in studies of pain and ethnicity." *Pain* 113(1–2): 3–4.

Romanow, R. 2002. "Building on values: The future of health care in Canada." www.hc-sc.gc.ca/hcs-sss/com/fed/romanow/index-eng.php.

—— 2006. "Canada's medicare: At the crossroads?" *Canadian Psychology* 47: 1–8.

Rootman, I., and D. Gordon-El-Bihbety. 2008. "A vision for a health literate Canada." Ottawa: Canadian Public Health Association. www.cpha.ca.

Rootman, I., and B. Ronson. 2005. "Literacy and health research in Canada." *Canadian Journal of Public Health* 96: S62–77.

Rosch, P.J., and H.M. Kearney. 1985. "Holistic medicine and technology: A modern dialectic." *Social Sciences and Medicine* 21: 1405–9.

Rose, N. 1999. *Powers of Freedom: Reframing Political Thought*. Cambridge: Cambridge University Press.

—— 2003. "Neurochemical selves." *Society* 41: 46–59.

—— 2007. *The Politics of Life Itself: Biomedicine, Power, and Subjectivity in the Twenty-First Century*. Princeton, NJ: Princeton University Press.

—— 2013. "Personalized medicine: Promises, problems and perils of a new paradigm for healthcare." *Procedia—Social and Behavioral Sciences* 77: 34–52.

Rose, S., R.C. Lewontin, and L.J. Kamin. 1984. *Not in Our Genes:*

Biology, Ideology, and Human Nature. New York: Penguin.

Rosenberg, E., L.J. Kirmayer, S. Xenocostas, M. Dao, and C. Loignon. 2007. "GPs' strategies in intercultural clinical encounters." *Family Practice* 24(2): 145–51.

Rosenthal, L., A. Carroll-Scott, V. Earnshaw, A. Santilli, and J. Ickovics. 2012. "The importance of full-time work for urban adults' mental and physical health." *Social Science and Medicine* 75: 1692–6.

Rosenthal, M. 1995. *The Incompetent Doctor*. Buckingham, UK: Open University Press.

Rosich, K., and J. Hankin. 2010. "Executive summary: What do we know? Key findings from 50 years of medical sociology." *Journal of Health and Social Behavior* 51(S): S1–9.

Ross, C., and J. Mirowsky. 2011. "The interaction of personal and parental education on health." *Social Science and Medicine* 72: 591–9.

Ross, N., D. Dorling, J. Dunn, G. Henriksson, J. Glover, J. Lynch, and G. Weitoft. 2005. "Metropolitan income inequality and working-age mortality: A cross-sectional analysis using comparable data from five countries." *Journal of Urban Health* 82: 101–10.

Ross, N., M. Wolfson, J. Dunn, J.-M. Berthelot, G. Kaplan, and J. Lynch, 2000. "Relation between income inequality and mortality in Canada and the United States: Cross sectional assessment using census data and vital statistics." *British Medical Journal* 320: 898–902.

Rottermann, M. 2012. "Sexual behaviour and condom use of 15- to 24-year-olds in 2003 and 2009/2010." *Health Reports* 23(1). Catalogue no. 82-003-XPE. Ottawa: Statistics Canada.

Roy, R. 1992. *The Social Context of the Chronic Pain Sufferer*. Toronto: University of Toronto Press.

Ruggie, M. 2004. *Marginal to Mainstream: Alternative Medicine in America*. New York: Cambridge University Press.

Rütten, A., and P. Gelius, 2011. "The interplay of structure and agency in health promotion: Integrating a concept of structural change and the policy dimension into a multi-level model and applying it to health promotion principles and practice." *Social Science and Medicine* 73(7): 953–9.

Sahai, V., M. Ward, T. Zmijowskyj, and B. Rowe. 2005. "Quantifying the iceberg effect for injury." *Canadian Journal of Public Health* 96: 328–32.

Salmon, J.W. 1984. *Alternative Medicines: Popular and Policy Perspectives*. New York: Tavistock.

Saltonstall, R. 1993. "Healthy bodies, social bodies: Men's and women's concepts and practices of health in everyday life." *Social Science and Medicine* 36: 7–14.

Sargent-Cox, K., N. Cherbuin, L. Morris, P. Butterworth, and K. Anstey. 2014. "The effect of health behaviour change on self-rated health across the adult life course: A longitudinal cohort study." *Preventive Medicine* 58: 75–80.

Sarma, S., G.S. Zaric, M.K. Campbell, and J. Gilliland. 2014. "The effect of physical activity on adult obesity: Evidence from the Canadian NPHS panel." *Economics and Human Biology* 14: 1–21.

Savitch, H. 2003. "How suburban sprawl shapes human well-being." *Journal of Urban Health* 80: 590–601.

Scambler, G., ed. 2012. *Contemporary Theorists for Medical Sociology*. New York: Routledge.

Schofield, T. 2007. "Health inequity and its social determinants: A sociological commentary." *Health Sociology Review* 16: 105–14.

Schultz, S., and J. Kopec. 2003. "Impact of chronic conditions." *Health Reports* 14: 41–53. Ottawa: Statistics Canada.

Schutz, A. 1967. *Collected Papers: The Problem of Social Reality*. The Hague: Martinus Nijhoff.

Schwartz, R.S. 2001. "Racial profiling in medical research." *New England Journal of Medicine* 344: 1392–3.

Seabrook, J., and W. Avison. 2012. "Socioeconomic status and cumulative disadvantage processes across the life course: Implications for health outcomes." *Canadian Review of Sociology* 49: 50–68.

Seale, C. 2003. "Health and media: An overview." *Sociology of Health and Illness* 25(6): 513–31.

Searight, H.R. 1994. "Psychosocial knowledge and allopathic medicine: Points of consequence and departure." *Journal of Medical Humanities* 15: 221–32.

Seeman, M., and T. Seeman. 1983. "Health behavior and personal autonomy: A longitudinal study of the sense of control in illness." *Journal of Health and Social Behavior* 24: 144–60.

Segall, A. 1976a. "Sociocultural variation in sick role behavioural expectations." *Social Science and Medicine* 10: 47–51.

———. 1976b. "The sick role concept: Understanding illness behavior." *Journal of Health and Social Behavior* 17: 163–70.

——— 1988. "Cultural factors in sick-role expectations." In D. Gochman, ed., *Health Behavior: Emerging Research Perspectives*, 249–60. New York: Plenum Press.

——— 1997. "Sick role concepts and health behavior." In D. Gochman, ed., *Handbook of Health Behavior Research I: Personal and Social Determinants*, 289–301. New York: Plenum Press.

Segall, A., and N. Chappell. 1991. "Making sense out of sickness: Lay explanations of chronic illness among older adults." *Advances in Medical Sociology* 2: 115–33.

——— 2000. *Health and Health Care in Canada*. Toronto: Pearson Education.

Segall, A., and J. Goldstein. 1989. "Exploring the correlates of self-provided health care behaviour." *Social Science and Medicine* 29: 153–61.

Segrin, C., and T. Domschke. 2011. "Social support, loneliness, recuperative processes, and their direct and indirect effects on health." *Health Communication* 26: 221–32.

Seliske, L., W. Pickett, and I. Janssen. 2012. "Urban sprawl and its relationship with active transportation, physical activity and obesity in Canadian youth." *Health Reports* 23:17–25. Catalogue no. 82-003-XPE. Ottawa: Statistics Canada.

Senate of Canada. 2007. *Safe Drinking Water for First Nations*. Final Report of the Standing Senate Committee on Aboriginal Peoples. www.parl.gc.ca/39/1/parlbus/commbus/sentate/Com-e/abor-e/rep08jun07-e.pdf.

Setia, M.S., J. Lynch, M. Abrahamowicz, P. Tousignant, and A. Quesnel-Vallée. 2011a. "Self-rated health in Canadian immigrants: Analysis of the longitudinal survey of immigrants to Canada." *Health and Place* 17(2): 658–70.

Setia, M.S., A. Quesnel-Vallée, M. Abrahamowicz, P. Tousignant, and J. Lynch. 2011b. "Access to health-care in Canadian immigrants: A longitudinal study of the National Population Health Survey." *Health and Social Care in the Community* 19(1): 70–9.

Shah, C. 2004. "The health of Aboriginal Peoples." In D. Raphael, ed., *Social Determinants of Health: Canadian Perspectives*, 1–18. Toronto: Canadian Scholars Press.

Shavers, V., A. Bakos, and V. Sheppard. 2010. "Race, ethnicity, and pain among the U.S. adult population." *Journal of Health Care for the Poor and Underserved* 21(1) 177–220.

Shaw, G.B. 1913. *Pygmalion*. New York: Simon and Schuster.

Shaw, I. 2002. "How lay are lay beliefs?" *Health: An Interdisciplinary Journal for the Social Study of Health, Illness and Medicine* 6: 287–99.

Shealy, C.N. 1999. *The Complete Illustrated Encyclopedia of Alternative Healing Therapies*. Boston: Element.

Sheps, S., and K. Cardiff. 2005. *Governing for Patient Safety: Lessons from Non-Health Risk-Critical High-Reliability Industries*. Ottawa: Health Canada.

Shield, K., B. Taylor, T. Kehoe, J. Patra, and J. Rehm. 2012. "Mortality and potential years of life lost attributable to alcohol consumption in Canada in 2005." *BMC Public Health* 12 (91).

Shields, M. 2008. "Community belonging and self-perceived health." *Health Reports* 19: 1–10. Ottawa: Statistics Canada.

Shilling, C. 2002. "Culture, the sick role and the consumption of health." *British Journal of Sociology* 53: 621–38.

—— 2003. *The Body and Social Theory*. London: Sage.

—— 2012. *The Body and Social Theory*. 3rd edn. London: Sage.

Shooshtari, S., V. Menec, and R. Tate. 2007. "Comparing predictors of positive and negative self-rated health between younger (25–54) and older (55+) Canadian adults." *Research on Aging* 29: 512–54.

Siahpush, M., A. McNeill, D. Hammond, and G.T. Fong. 2006. "Socioeconomic and country variations in knowledge of health risks of tobacco smoking and toxic constituents of smoke: Results from the 2002 International Tobacco Control (ITC) four country survey." *Tobacco Control* 15: 65–70.

Siegrist, J., and M. Marmot. 2006. Introduction. In J. Siegrist and M. Marmot, eds, *Social Inequalities in Health: New Evidence and Policy Implications*, 1–25. New York: Oxford University Press.

Siegrist, J., and T. Theorell. 2006. "Socio-economic position and health: The role of work and employment." In J. Siegrist and M. Marmot, eds, *Social Inequalities in Health: New Evidence and Policy Implications*, 73–100. New York: Oxford University Press.

Sim, J., and S. Madden. 2008. "Illness experience in fibromyalgia syndrome: A metasynthesis of qualitative studies." *Social Science and Medicine* 67: 57–67.

Sinding, C. 2004. "Informal care—Two-tiered care? The work of family members and friends in hospitals and cancer centres."

Journal of Sociology and Social Welfare 31: 69–86.

Singer, N. 2009. "Medical papers by ghostwriters pushed therapy." *New York Times* 5 August.

Singh-Manoux, A., and M. Marmot. 2005. "Role of socialization in explaining social inequalities in health." *Social Science and Medicine* 60: 2129–33.

Sinha, M., and A. Bleakney. 2014. *Receiving Care at Home*. Catalogue no. 89-652-X, no. 002. Ottawa: Statistics Canada.

Sismondo, S. 2015. "Pushing knowledge in the drug industry: Ghost managed science." In S. Sismondo and J. Greene, eds, *The Pharmaceutical Studies Reader*, 150–64. London: Wiley-Blackwell.

Skolbekken, J. 1995. "The risk of epidemic in medical journals." *Social Science and Medicine* 40: 291–305.

Smaje, C. 2000. "Race, ethnicity and health." In C. Bird, P. Conrad, and A. Freemont, eds, *Handbook of Medical Sociology*, 5th edn, 114–28. Upper Saddle River, NJ: Prentice-Hall.

Smith, B., P. Smith, S. Harper, D. Manuel, and C. Mustard. 2014. "Reducing social inequalities in health: The role of simulation modelling in chronic disease epidemiology to evaluate the impact of population health interventions." *Journal of Epidemiology and Community Health* 68: 384–9.

Smith, D. 1990. *The Conceptual Practices of Power*. Toronto: University of Toronto Press.

Smith, K., and N. Christakis. 2008. "Social networks and health." *Annual Review of Sociology* 34: 405–29.

Smith, P., R. Glazier, and L. Sibley. 2010. "The predictors of self-rated health and the relationship between self-rated health and health service needs are similar across socioeconomic groups in Canada." *Journal of Clinical Epidemiology* 63: 412–21.

Smylie, J. 2009. "The health of Aboriginal peoples." In D. Raphael, ed., *Social Determinants of Health:*

Canadian Perspectives, 280–304. Toronto: Canadian Scholars Press.

Snyderman, R., and A.T. Weil. 2002. "Integrative medicine: Bringing medicine back to its roots." *Archives of Internal Medicine* 162: 395–7.

Sointu, E. 2005. "The rise of an ideal: Tracing changing discourses of wellbeing." *Sociological Review* 53(2): 255–74.

Speakman, J.R. 2013. "Evolutionary perspectives on the obesity epidemic: Adaptive, maladaptive, and neutral viewpoints." *Annual Review of Nutrition* 33: 289–317.

Spitzer, D. 2005. "Engendering health disparities." *Canadian Journal of Public Health* 96: S78–96.

——— 2012. "Oppression and im/migrant health in Canada." In E. McGibbon, ed., *Oppression: A Social Determinant of Health*, 113–122. Halifax: Fernwood.

Stafford, M., B.K. Newbold, and N.A. Ross. 2010. "Psychological distress among immigrants and visible minorities in Canada: A contextual analysis." *International Journal of Social Psychiatry* 57(4): 428–41.

Stansfeld, A. 2006. "Social support and social cohesion." In M. Marmot and R. Wilkinson, eds, *Social Determinants of Health*, 2nd edn, 148–71. New York: Oxford University Press.

Starky, S. 2005. *The Obesity Epidemic in Canada*. Ottawa: Library of Parliament. www.parl.gc.ca/information/library/prbpubs/prb0511-e.htm.

Statistics Canada. 1994. *Profile of Canada's Seniors*. Catalogue no. 96-312E. Ottawa: Minister of Industry, Science and Technology.

——— 1999. "Personal health practices: Smoking, drinking, physical activity and weight." *Health Reports* 11: 83–90. Catalogue no. 82-003. Ottawa: Statistics Canada.

——— 2001. "Health care/self-care." *Health Reports* 12: 33–9. Dept. IST, Catalogue no. 96-312-XPE1991000. Ottawa: Statistics Canada.

——— 2003. *Ethnic Diversity Survey: Portrait of a Multicultural Society*. Catalogue no. 89-593-XIE. Ottawa: Ministry of Industry.

——— 2008a. *Aboriginal Peoples in Canada in 2006: Inuit, Métis, and First Nations, 2006 Census*. Catalogue no. 7-558-XIE. Ottawa: Ministry of Industry.

——— 2008b. *Canada's Ethnocultural Mosaic, 2006 Census*. Catalogue no. 97-562-X2008. Ottawa: Ministry of Industry.

——— 2009. "Life expectancy at birth and at age 65, by sex, Canada, provinces and territories." CANSIM Table 102-0512. Ottawa: Statistics Canada.

——— 2011a. *Disparities in Life Expectancy at Birth*. Catalogue no. 82-624-X. Ottawa: Ministry of Industry.

——— 2011b. "The 10 leading causes of death, 2011." CANSIM Table 102-0561. Ottawa: Statistics Canada.

——— 2012a. *Annual Demographic Estimates: Canada, Provinces and Territories*. Catalogue no. 91-215-X. Ottawa: Minister of Industry.

——— 2012b. "Deaths and mortality rates, by age group and sex, Canada, provinces and territories." CANSIM Table 102-0504. Ottawa: Statistics Canada.

——— 2012c. *Linguistic Characteristics of Canadians: Language, 2011 Census of Population*. Catalogue no. 98-314-X2011001. Ottawa: Minister of Industry.

——— 2012d. *The Canadian Population in 2011: Age and Sex*. Catalogue no. 98-311-X2011001. Ottawa: Minister of Industry.

——— 2013a. *Aboriginal Peoples in Canada: First Nations People, Métis and Inuit: National Household Survey, 2011*. Catalogue no. 99-011-X2011001. Ottawa: Statistics Canada.

——— 2013b. "Cause-specific mortality by income adequacy in Canada: A 16-year follow-up study." *Health Reports* 24: 14–22. Catalogue no. 82-003-X. Ottawa: Statistics Canada.

——— 2013c. "High-income trends among Canadian taxfilers, 1982 to 2010." *The Daily* 28 January. Catalogue no. 11-001-X 3. Ottawa: Statistics Canada.

——— 2013d. *Immigration and Ethnocultural Diversity in Canada: National Household Survey, 2011*. Catalogue no. 99-010-X2011001. Ottawa: Statistics Canada.

——— 2014a. "High-income trends among Canadian taxfilers, 1982 to 2012. *The Daily* 18 November. Catalogue no. 11-001-X. Ottawa: Statistics Canada.

——— 2014b. *Smoking, 2014*. Catalogue no. 82-625X. Ottawa: Statistics Canada.

Steele, J., and W. McBroom. 1972. "Conceptual and empirical dimensions of health behavior." *Journal of Health and Social Behavior* 13: 382–92.

Steingraber, S. 1997. *Living Downstream: A Scientist's Personal Investigation of Cancer and the Environment*. New York: Vintage Books.

Stephens, C., F. Alpass, A. Towers, and B. Stevenson. 2011. "The effects of types of social networks, perceived social support, and loneliness on the health of older people: Accounting for the social context." *Journal of Aging and Health* 23: 887–911.

Stephens, T. 1986. "Health practices and health status: Evidence from the Canada Health Survey." *American Journal of Preventive Medicine* 2: 209–15.

Stewart, M., L. Reutter, E. Makwarimba, G. Veenstra, R. Love, and D. Raphael. 2008. "Left out: Perspectives on social exclusion and inclusion across income groups." *Health Sociology Review* 17: 78–94.

Stoddart, G., J. Eyles, J. Lavis, and P. Chaulk. 2006. "Reallocating resources across public sectors to improve population health." In J. Heymann, C. Hertzman, M. Barer, and R. Evans, eds, *Healthier Societies: From Analysis to Action*, 327–47. New York: Oxford University Press.

Stoller, E. 1993. "Interpretations of symptoms by older people." *Journal of Aging and Health* 5: 58–81.

——— L. Forster, and S. Portugal. 1993. "Self-care responses to symptoms by older people." *Medical Care* 31: 24–42.

Stout, C., J. Morrow, E.N. Brandt, and S. Wolf. 1964. "Unusually low incidence of death from myocardial infarction: Study of an Italian American community in Pennsylvania. *Journal of the American Medical Association* 188(10): 845–9.

Straus, R. 1957. "The nature and status of medical sociology." *American Sociological Review* 22: 200–4.

——— 1999. "Medical sociology: A personal fifty year perspective." *Journal of Health and Social Behavior* 40(2): 103–10.

Streiner, D.L. 1997. Book review: I. McDowell and C. Newell, *Measuring Health: A Guide to Rating Scales and Questionnaires*. *Chronic Diseases in Canada* 17: 124–5.

Subramanian, S., and I. Kawachi. 2004. "Income inequality and health: What have we learned so far?" *Epidemiologic Reviews* 26: 78–91.

Suchman, E. 1964. "Sociomedical variations among ethnic groups." *American Journal of Sociology* 70: 319–31.

Sulik, G. 2011. "Our diagnoses, our selves: The rise of the technoscientific illness identity." *Sociology Compass* 5/6: 463–77.

Sullivan, M. 1986. "In what sense is contemporary medicine dualistic?" *Culture, Medicine, and Psychiatry* 10: 331–50.

Switankowsky, I. 2000. "Dualism and its importance for medicine." *Theoretical Medicine* 21: 567–80.

Sylvestre, M.-P., B. Huszti, and J. Hanley. 2006. "Do Oscar winners live longer than less successful peers? A reanalysis of the evidence." *Annals of Internal Medicine* 145: 361–3.

Syme, S.L. 1994. "The social environment and health." *DAEDALUS, Journal of the American Academy of Arts and Sciences* 123: 79–86.

Szasz, T. 1971. *The Manufacture of Madness: A Comparative Study of the Inquisition and the Mental Health Movement*. London: Routledge.

Tambay, J., and G. Catlin. 1995. "Sample design of the National Population Health Survey." *Health Reports* 7: 1–11. Ottawa: Statistics Canada.

Tarlov, A. 1996. "Social determinants of health: The sociobiological translation." In D. Blane, E. Brunner, and R. Wilkinson, eds, *Health and Social Organisation*, 71–93. London: Routledge.

Taylor, M. 2011. "The causal pathway from socioeconomic status to disability trajectories in later life: The importance of mediating mechanisms for onset and accumulation." *Research on Aging* 33: 84–108.

——— 2010. "Capturing transitions and trajectories: The role of socioeconomic status in later life disability." *Journal of Gerontology: Social Sciences* 65: 733–43.

Taylor, R., and A. Rieger. 1984. "Rudolf Virchow on the typhus epidemic in Upper Silesia: An introduction and translation." *Sociology of Health and Illness* 6: 201–17.

Taylor, R.C.R. 1984. "Alternative medicine and the medical encounter in Britain and the United States." In J.W. Salmon, ed., *Alternative Medicines, Popular and Policy Perspectives*, 191–228. New York: Tavistock.

Teelucksingh, C. 2007. "Environmental racialization: Linking racialization to the environment in Canada." *Local Environment* 12: 645–61.

Thoits, P. 1995. "Stress, coping and social support processes: Where are we? What's next?" *Journal of Health and Social Behavior* (Extra issue): 53–79.

——— 2011. "Mechanisms linking social ties and support to physical and mental health." *Journal of Health and Social Behavior* 52: 145–61.

Thorslund, M., and T. Norstrom. 1993. "The relationship between different survey measures of health in an elderly population." *Journal of Applied Gerontology* 12: 61–70.

Timmermans, S. 2013. "Seven warrants for qualitative health sociology." *Social Science and Medicine* 77: 1–8.

Tjepkema, M. 2005. *Measured Obesity, Adult Obesity in Canada: Measured Height and Weight from Nutrition*. Findings from the Canadian Community Health Survey. Catalogue no. 82-620-MWE2005001. Ottawa: Statistics Canada.

——— and R. Wilkins. 2011. "Remaining life expectancy at age 25 and probability of survival to age 75, by socioeconomic status and Aboriginal ancestry." *Health Reports* 22: 1–5. Catalogue No. 82-003-XPE. Ottawa: Statistics Canada.

——— and A. Long. 2013. "Cause-specific mortality by income adequacy in Canada: A 16-year follow-up study." *Health Reports* 24: 14–22. Catalogue no. 82-003-X. Ottawa: Statistics Canada.

Tremblay, M., M. Wolfson, and S. Gorber. 2007. "Canadian Health Measures Survey. Rationale, background and overview." *Health Reports* 18 (Supplement): 7–20.

Tuana, N. 2006. "The speculum of ignorance: The women's health movement and epistemologies of ignorance." *Hypatia* 21: 1–19.

Turcotte, M. 2011. *Women in Canada: A Gender-Based Statistical Report*. Catalogue no. 89-503-X. Ottawa: Statistics Canada.

——— 2013. *Family Caregiving: What Are the Consequences?* Catalogue no. 75-006-X. Ottawa: Statistics Canada.

——— and G. Schellenberg. 2007. *A Portrait of Seniors in Canada*. Catalogue no. 89-519-XIE. Ottawa: Statistics Canada.

Turk, D., T. Rudy, and P. Salovey. 1986. "Implicit models of illness." *Journal of Behavioral Medicine* 9: 453–74.

Turner, B.S. 1992. *Regulating Bodies: Essays in Medical Sociology*. London: Routledge.

——— 1995. *Medical Power and Social Knowledge*. London: Sage.

Turner, R.J., and S. Noh. 1988. "Physical disability and depression:

A longitudinal analysis." *Journal of Health and Social Behavior* 29: 23–37.

Tutton, R. 2012. "Personalizing medicine: Futures present and past." *Social Science and Medicine* 75: 1721–8.

Twaddle, A. 1974. "The concept of health status." *Social Science and Medicine* 8: 29–38.

——— 1982. "From medical sociology to the sociology of health: Some changing concerns in the sociological study of sickness and treatment." In T. Bottomore, M. Sokolowska, and S. Novak, eds, *Sociology: The State of the Art*, 323–58. Beverley Hills, CA: Sage.

Twells, L.K., D.M. Gregory, J. Reddigan, and W.K. Midodzi. 2014. "Current and predicted prevalence of obesity in Canada: A trend analysis." *Canadian Medical Association Open* 2(1): 18–26.

Uchino, B. 2009. "What a lifespan approach might tell us about why distinct measures of social support have differential links to physical health." *Journal of Social and Personal Relationships* 26: 53–62.

——— K. Bowen, M. Carlisle, and W. Birmingham. 2012. "Psychological pathways linking social support to health outcomes: A visit with the 'ghosts' of research past, present, and future." *Social Science and Medicine* 74: 949–57.

Umberson, D., R. Crosnoe, and C. Reczek. 2010. "Social relationships and health behavior across the life course." *Annual Review of Sociology* 36: 139–57.

Underhill, C., and L. McKeown. 2008. "Getting a second opinion: Health information and the Internet." *Health Reports* 19: 1–5. Catalogue no. 82-003. Ottawa: Statistics Canada.

US President's Cancer Panel. 2007. *Promoting Healthy Lifestyles: Policy, Program, and Personal Recommendations for Reducing Cancer Risk*. Washington: US Department of Health and Human Services, National Institutes of Health, National Cancer Institute.

Vafaei, A., M.W. Rosenberg, and W. Pickett. 2010. "Relationships between income inequality and health: A study on rural and urban regions of Canada." *Rural and Remote Health* 10(2): 1430.

van Dalen, H., A. Williams, and C. Gudex. 1994. "Lay people's evaluations of health: Are there variations between different subgroups?" *Journal of Epidemiology and Community Health* 48: 248–53.

van de Mheen, H., S. Stronks, and J. Mackenbach. 1998. "A life course perspective on socio-economic inequalities in health: The influence of childhood socio-economic conditions and selection processes." *Sociology of Health and Illness* 20: 754–77.

Vang, Z., J. Sigouin, A. Flenon, and A. Gagnon. 2015. "The healthy immigrant effect in Canada: A systematic review." *Population Change and Lifecourse Strategic Knowledge Cluster Discussion Paper Series* 3(1): 1–40.

Vannini, P., and A. McCright. 2004. "To die for: The semiotic seductive power of the tanned body." *Symbolic Interaction* 27: 309–32.

van Oostrom, S., H.A. Smit, G.C.W. Wendel-Vos, M. Visser, W.M.M. Verschuren, and S.J. Picavet. 2012. "Adopting an active lifestyle during adulthood and health-related quality of life: The Doetinchem Cohort Study." *American Journal of Public Health* 102(11): 62–8.

Varcoe, C., O. Hankivsky, M. Ford-Gilboe, J. Wuest, P. Wilk, J. Hammerton, and J.Campbell. 2011. "Attributing selected costs to intimate partner violence in a sample of women who have left abusive partners: A social determinants of health approach." *Canadian Public Policy* 37(3): 359–80.

Veenstra, G. 2002a. "Income inequality and health." *Canadian Journal of Public Health* 93: 374–9.

——— 2002b. "Social capital and health (plus wealth, income inequality and regional health governance)." *Social Science and Medicine* 54: 849–68.

——— 2007. "Social space, social class and Bourdieu: Health inequalities in British Columbia, Canada." *Health and Place* 13: 14–31.

——— 2009. "Racialized identity and health in Canada: Results from a nationally representative survey." *Social Science and Medicine* 69: 538–42.

——— 2011a. "Mismatched racial identities, colourism, and health in Toronto and Vancouver." *Social Science and Medicine* 73(8): 1152–62.

——— 2011b. "Race, gender, class, and sexual orientation: Intersecting axes of inequality and self-rated health in Canada." *International Journal for Equity in Health* 10(3): 1–11.

——— 2012. "Expressed racial identity and hypertension in a telephone survey sample from Toronto and Vancouver, Canada: Do socio-economic status, perceived discrimination and psychosocial stress explain the relatively high risk of hypertension for black Canadians?" *International Journal for Equity in Health* 11(58): 1–10.

——— 2013. "Race, gender, class, sexuality (RGCS) and hypertension." *Social Science and Medicine* 89: 16–24.

Veenstra, G., and P.J. Burnett. 2014. "A relational approach to health practices: Towards transcending the agency-structure divide." *Sociology of Health and Illness* 36(2): 187–98.

Veenstra, G., and A. Patterson. 2012. "Capital relations and health: Mediating and moderating effects of cultural, economic, and social capitals on mortality in Alameda County, California." *International Journal of Health Services* 42: 277–91.

Verbrugge, L.M. 1980. "Health diaries." *Medical Care* 18: 73–95.

——— 1986. "From sneezes to adieux: Stages of health for American men and women." *Social Science and Medicine* 22: 1195–212.

——— 1990. "The iceberg of disability." In S. Stahl, ed., *The Legacy of*

Longevity: Health and Health Care in Later Life, 55–75. Thousand Oaks, CA: Sage.

—— and F. Ascione. 1987. "Exploring the iceberg: Common symptoms and how people care for them." *Medical Care* 25: 539–69.

Verbrugge, L.M., and R.P. Steiner. 1981. "Physician treatment of men and women patients: Sex bias or appropriate care?" *Medical Care* 19: 609–32.

Vissandjée, B., M. DesMeules, Z. Cao, S. Abdool, and A. Kazanjian. 2003. "Integrating ethnicity and immigration as determinants of Canadian women's health." In M. DesMeules, D. Stewart, A. Kazanjian, H. Maclean, J. Payne, and B. Vissandjée, eds., *Women's Health Surveillance Report: A Multidimensional Look at the Health of Canadian Women*, 1–3. Ottawa: Canadian Institute for Health Information.

Vlahov, D., S. Galea, and N. Freudenberg. 2005. "The urban health 'advantage.'" *Journal of Urban Health* 82: 1–4.

Wadsworth, M. 1997. "Health inequalities in the life course perspective." *Social Science and Medicine* 44: 859–69.

Waitzkin, H. 2000. *The Second Sickness: Contradictions of Capitalist Health Care*. 2nd edn. Lanham, MD: Rowman and Littlefield.

Waldram, J.B., A. Herring, and T.K. Young. 2006. *Aboriginal Health in Canada: Historical, Cultural, and Epidemiological Perspectives*. Toronto: University of Toronto Press.

Waldron, I. 1997. "Changing gender roles and gender differences in health behavior." In D. Gochman, ed., *Handbook of Health Behavior Research I: Personal and Social Determinants*, 303–28. New York: Plenum Press.

—— C. Weiss, and M. Hughes. 1998. "Interacting effects of multiple roles on women's health." *Journal of Health and Social Behavior* 39: 216–36.

Wallace, J.E., J.B. Lemaire, and W.A. Ghali. 2009. "Physician wellness: A missing quality indicator." *The Lancet* 374: 1714–21.

Wallace, L., R. Wexler, L. McDougle, W. Miser, and J. Haddox. 2014. "Voices that may not otherwise be heard: A qualitative exploration into the perspectives of primary care patients living with chronic pain." *Journal of Pain Research* 7: 291–9.

Wallace, R. 1994. "Assessing the health of individuals and populations in surveys of the elderly: Some concepts and approaches." *The Gerontologist* 34: 449–53.

Walters, V. 1992. "Women's views of their main health problem." *Canadian Journal of Public Health* 83: 371–4.

—— 2003. "The social context of women's health." In M. DesMeules, D. Stewart, A. Kazanjian, H. Maclean, J. Payne, and B. Vissandjée, eds, *Women's Health Surveillance Report: A Multidimensional Look at the Health of Canadian Women*, 1–9. Ottawa: Canadian Institute for Health Information.

—— P. McDonough, and L. Strohschein. 2002. "The influence of work, household structure, and social, personal and material resources on gender differences in health: An analysis of the 1994 Canadian National Population Health Survey." *Social Science and Medicine* 54: 677–92.

Wang, L. 2014. "Immigrant health, socioeconomic factors and residential neighbourhood characteristics: A comparison of multiple ethnic groups in Canada." *Applied Geography* 51: 90–8.

Waring, J. 2005. "Beyond blame: Cultural barriers to medical incident reporting." *Social Science and Medicine* 60: 1927–35.

—— 2007. "Doctors' thinking about 'the system' as a threat to patient safety." *Health: An Interdisciplinary Journal for the Social Study of Health, Illness and Medicine* 11: 29–46.

Warren, J., P. Hoonakker, P. Carayon, and J. Brand. 2004. "Job characteristics as mediators in SES-health relationships." *Social Science and Medicine* 59: 1367–78.

Weber, M. 1922. *Wirtsckfi und Gesellschaft* [Economy and Society]. Tübingen, Germany: Mohr.

—— 1947. *The Theory of Social and Economic Organization*. New York: Free Press.

—— 1958. *The Protestant Ethic and the Spirit of Capitalism*. New York: Charles Scribner's Sons.

Welch, G. 2004. *Should I Be Tested for Cancer? Maybe Not and Here's Why*. Berkeley: University of California Press.

West, C., and D.H. Zimmerman. 1987. "Doing gender." *Gender and Society* 1(2): 125–51.

West, C., K. Usher, K. Foster, and L. Stewart. 2012. "Chronic pain and the family: The experience of the partners of people living with chronic pain." *Journal of Clinical Nursing* 21: 3352–60.

Whelan, E. 2003. "Putting pain to paper: Endometriosis and the documentation of suffering." *Health: An Interdisciplinary Journal for the Social Study of Health, Illness and Medicine* 7: 463–82.

White, K., and R. Wilkins. 2006. "Socioeconomic status and birth outcomes in Quebec." *Newsletter of the Health Analysis and Measurement Group*. September. Catalogue no. 82-005-XIE2006002. Ottawa: Statistics Canada. www.statcan.gc.ca/bsolc/olc-cel/olc-cel?cat-no=82-005-XIE&lang=eng#-formatdisp.

White, K. 2002. *An Introduction to the Sociology of Health and Illness*. London: Sage.

Whitehead, M., and J. Popay. 2010. "Swimming upstream? Taking action on the social determinants of health inequalities." *Social Science and Medicine* 71: 1234–6.

Whorton, J.C. 1985. "The first holistic revolution: Alternative medicine in the nineteenth century." In D. Stalker and C. Glymour, eds, *Examining Holistic Medicine*, 29–48. New York: Prometheus Books.

Wickrama, K., J. Mancini, K. Kwag, and J. Kwon. 2013. "Heterogeneity

in multidimensional health trajectories of late old years and socioeconomic stratification: A latent trajectory class analysis." *Journals of Gerontology Series B: Psychological Sciences and Social Sciences* 68: 290–7.
Wiesmann, U., and H.-J. Hannich. 2010. "A salutogenic analysis of healthy aging in active elderly persons." *Research on Aging* 32: 349–71.
Wilkins, K. 2005. "Predictors of death in seniors." *Health Reports* 16 (Supplement): 57–67. Ottawa: Statistics Canada.
—— N. Campbell, M. Joffres, F. McAlister, M. Nichol, S. Quach, H. Johansen, and M. Tremblay. 2010. "Blood pressure in Canadian adults." *Health Reports* 21: 1–10. Ottawa: Statistics Canada.
Wilkins, R., J.-M. Berthelot, and E. Ng. 2002. "Trends in mortality by neighbourhood income in urban Canada from 1971 to 1996." *Health Reports* 13 (Supplement): 1–28. Catalogue No. 82-003. Ottawa: Statistics Canada.
Wilkinson, R. 1992. "Income distribution and life expectancy." *British Medical Journal* 304: 165–8.
—— 1996. *Unhealthy Societies: The Afflictions of Inequality*. New York: Routledge.
—— and M. Marmot, eds. 2003. *Social Determinants of Health: The Solid Facts*. 2nd edn. Copenhagen: World Health Organization.
Wilkinson, R., and K. Pickett. 2006. "Income inequality and population health: A review and explanation of the evidence." *Social Science and Medicine* 62: 1768–84.
—— 2010. *The Spirit Level: Why Equality Is Better for Everyone*. New York: Bloomsbury Press.
Williams, D.R., and S.A. Mohammed. 2013a. "Racism and health I: Pathways and scientific evidence." *American Behavioral Scientist* 57(8): 1152–73.
—— 2013b. "Racism and health II: A needed research agenda for effective interventions." *American Behavioral Scientist* 57(8) 1200–26.

—— and M. Sternthal. 2010. "Understanding racial-ethnic disparities in health: Sociological contributions." *Journal of Health and Social Behavior* 51(S): S15–27.
Williams, G. 1984. "The genesis of chronic illness: Narrative reconstruction." *Sociology of Health and Illness* 6: 175–200.
—— 2003. "The determinants of health: Structure, context and agency." *Sociology of Health and Illness* 25: 131–54.
Williams, R. 1983. "Concepts of health: An analysis of lay logic." *Sociology* 17: 185–205.
Williams, S. 1995. "Theorising class, health and lifestyles: Can Bourdieu help us?" *Sociology of Health and Illness* 17: 577–604.
—— 2000. "Chronic illness as biographical disruption or biographical disruption as chronic illness? Reflections on a core concept." *Sociology of Health and Illness* 22: 40–67.
—— 2005. "Parsons revisited: From the sick role to . . . ? *Health: An Interdisciplinary Journal for the Social Study of Health, Illness and Medicine* 9: 123–44.
—— L. Birke, and G.A. Bendelow. 2003. *Debating Biology: Sociological Reflections on Health, Medicine and Society*. London: Routledge.
Williamson, J., and K. Danaher. 1978. *Self-Care in Health*. London: Croom Helm.
Willson, A. 2009. "'Fundamental causes' of health disparities: A comparative analysis of Canada and the United States." *International Sociology* 24: 93–113.
Winkleby, M., D. Ragland, J. Fisher, and L. Syme. 1988. "Excess risk of sickness and disease in bus drivers: A review and synthesis of epidemiological studies." *International Journal of Epidemiology* 17: 255–62.
Winnipeg Regional Health Authority. 2013. *Health for All: Building Winnipeg's Health Equity Action Plan*. Winnipeg: Winnipeg Regional Health Authority.
Wolf, M., J. Feinglass, J. Thompson, and D. Baker. 2010. "In search

of 'low health literacy': Threshold vs. gradient effect of literacy on health status and mortality." *Social Science and Medicine* 70: 1335–41.
Wolf, M., J. Gazmararian, and D. Baker. 2005. "Health literacy and functional health status among older adults." *Archives of Internal Medicine* 165: 1946–52.
Wolpe, P.R. 1987. "Shamans of the metropolis: Holistic physicians and cultural movements in modern medicine." (PhD dissertation, Yale University).
Woolf, S., and P. Braveman. 2011. "Where health disparities begin: The role of social and economic determinants—and why current policies may make matters worse." *Health Affairs* 30: 1852–9.
World Health Organization. 1948. *Official Records of the World Health Organization*. No. 2. Geneva: United Nations, WHO Interim Commission.
—— 1986. *Ottawa Charter for Health Promotion*. Geneva: World Health Organization.
—— 2001. *Legal Status of Traditional Medicine and Complementary/Alternative Medicine: A Worldwide Review*. Geneva: World Health Organization.
—— 2008. *Closing the Gap in a Generation: Health Equity through Action on the Social Determinants of Health*. Final Report of the Commission on Social Determinants of Health. Geneva: World Health Organization. www.who.int/social_determinants/thecommission/finalreport/en/index.html.
—— 2011a. *Closing the Gap: Policy into Practice on Social Determinants of Health*. Geneva: World Health Organization.
—— 2011b. *Global Health and Aging*. NIH Publication no. 11-7737. Washington: National Institute on Aging and National Institutes of Health.
—— 2014a. *Global Status Report on Noncommunicable Diseases 2014*. Geneva, Switzerland: World Health Organization.

——— 2014b. "Social determinants of health." Geneva: World Health Organization. www.who.int/topics/social_determinants/en.

——— 2014c. "World health statistics 2014." Geneva: World Health Organization. http://www.who.int/mediacentre/news/releases/2014/world-health-statistics-2014/en.

Wright, C.J. 2009. "Too much health care." *Literary Review of Canada* 17: 3–5.

Wright, P. 2003. "Ivan Illich." *The Lancet* 361: 185.

Wu, Z., S. Noh, V. Kaspar, and C. Schimmele. 2003. "Race, ethnicity, and depression in Canadian society." *Journal of Health and Social Behavior* 44: 426–41.

Wu, Z., and C. Schimmele. 2005. "Racial/ethnic variation in functional and self-reported health." *American Journal of Public Health* 95: 710–16.

Xiong, H., M. Murphy, M. Mathews, V. Gadag, and P. Wang. 2010. "Cervical cancer screening among Asian Canadian immigrant and non-immigrant women." *American Journal of Health Behavior* 34(2): 131–43.

Yang, A.I., K.M. Fong, P.V. Zimmerman, S.T. Holgate, and J.W. Holloway. 2008. "Genetic susceptibility to the respiratory effects of air pollution." *Thorax* 63: 555–63.

Zborowski, M. 1969. *People in Pain*. San Francisco: Jossey-Bass.

Zhao, Z., and R. Kaestner. 2010. "Effects of urban sprawl on obesity." *Journal of Health Economics* 29:779–87.

Zheng, H. 2012. "Do people die from income inequality of a decade ago?" *Social Science and Medicine* 75(1): 36–45.

Ziebland, S., and S. Wyke. 2012. "Health and illness in a connected world: How might sharing experiences on the Internet affect people's health?" *Milbank Quarterly* 90: 219–49.

Ziguras, C. 2004. *Self-Care: Embodiment, Personal Autonomy and the Shaping of Health Consciousness*. New York: Routledge.

Zimbardo, P. 2001. "Sex and gender." Episode 17 in "Discovering psychology today" series. Produced by WGBH Boston with the American Psychological Association.

Zola, I. 1964. "Culture and symptoms: An analysis of patients' presenting complaints." *American Sociological Review* 31: 615–30.

——— 1972a. "The concept of trouble and sources of medical assistance: To whom one can turn, with what and why." *Social Science and Medicine* 6: 673–9.

——— 1972b. "Medicine as an institution of social control." *Sociological Review* 20: 487–504.

Index

Aboriginal peoples: disparities in health, 199–200, 204; diversity in, 196; health outcomes, 198–201; hepatitis C, 323–4; income and poverty, 196; intergenerational trauma and residential schools, 199; living conditions, 196–8; medicalization, 200–1; medical profession and health-care system, 201–4; medicine wheel, 204, 205; social exclusion and racism, 196–7, 201–3; view of health and wellbeing, 204–6
Achieving Health for All: A Framework for Health Promotion, 389–90
age and aging: causality of illness, 277–8; demographic transition, 365–6; determinants of health, 115–16; gender differences, 190; and health, 88; percentages and projections, 115–16; population aging, 115–16, 118, 365–6; pyramid in Canada, 117
agency, in structure–agency issue, 249, 256
age stratification, 116–18
age structure, in Canada, 116–18
alcohol use, as unhealthy behaviour, 230
allopathy, 363
alternative medicine: *vs.* biomedical model, 359–63; and CAM, 363; in Canada, 360–1, 365; definition, 362, 363; interest in, 355; labelling of, 362–3; marketing of, 370–1; persistence of, 358; stereotypes of marginality, 361–2; streams of, 363–4; *see also* pluralism
alternative models of health care, 288–91
American Sociological Association, 23
Antonovsky, Aaron: dimensions of health, 72; and good health, 2; mystery of health, 260–1; salutogenic model, 3, 66–7, 85–6, 102–3, 127, 393; sense of coherence, 85–7, 91, 221
assets model of health, 84–5
attention deficit hyperactivity disorder (ADHD), 331–2
automobiles, impact on health, 112–13

Bedside Medicine, 315–17
behaviour. *see* health behaviour; health lifestyle; lifestyle behaviour
beliefs. *see* health belief systems; lay beliefs
Big Pharma. *see* pharmaceutical industry
biographical disruption, 308
biological determinism, 6, 49, 216–18
biology, 106–7, 258, 259
biomedicalization, 350
biomedical model: *vs.* alternative medicine, 359–63; basic ideas of, 320–8, 352; and CAM therapies, 373–4; contribution to humanity, 328–9; definition, 320; and diagnosis, 68; and disease origins, 103; dominance in health care, 328–31, 358, 374; and feminism, 46–7; health and illness/disease, 5–6; as health belief, 358; knowledge development, 315, 316; medical-industrial complex, 348–9; and medicalization, 350; origins and development, 315–20, 352, 358; and population health, 328–9; *vs.* TCM, 43
biomedicine, dissatisfaction with, 355, 366
biopower, 52, 53, 351
biosocial reality, 258–60, 262
birth, outcomes by income, 135, 136; *see also* childbirth
Blaxter, Mildred: on beliefs and inequalities, 152, 271; causality in illness, 273, 276–7; lifestyle practices, 125, 257
BMI, and obesity, 231–2
body: Bourdieu's view, 53–4; Foucault's views, 50–1; in sociology, 48–50, 55; *see also* sociology of the body paradigm
Bourdieu, Pierre: and "health lifestyle theory," 254–6; relational theory, 250–4, 256–7, 258, 263; role of, 250; social exclusion, 239; sociology of the body and habitus, 52–4, 149, 150, 251
Britain, universal health insurance, 398
brownfields, 113
Building on Values: The Future of Health Care in Canada, 391–2

built environment, health problems, 110–13
CAM (complementary/alternative medicine): in biomedical model, 373–4; and consumerism, 367–8; definition, 363; marketing, 371; popularity, 365–8; streams of, 363–4; *see also* alternative medicine
Canada Health Survey, 90, 232
Canadian Adverse Events Study, 337
Canadian Community Health Survey (CCHS): alternative medicine and CAM, 360–1, 365; description and goal, 77, 91–2; gender, 178; immigrant health, 207, 213; income inequality, 158; lifestyle behaviour, 229; self-rated health, 79; social support, 300; unsafe sex, 234
Canadian Health Measures Survey (CHMS), 92
Canadian Index of Wellbeing (CIW), 87
Canadian Institute for Health Information (CIHI), 82, 177, 337, 338–9
Canadian Institutes of Health Research (CIHR), 347–9
Canadian Longitudinal Study of Aging (CLSA), 92–3
Canadian Medical Association, 112
Canadian Sickness Survey, 90
capitalism, 36, 37–8, 40–1, 335–6
cardiovascular disease, and gender, 169–70
caregiving, 189, 296
cars, impact on health, 112–13
causality (origins of disease), 276–8, 279
cellular pathology, 319, 321
childbirth, 39, 46–7, 284, 332
children, 164–6, 233; infant mortality, 135, 136, 148
chronic disease, 81–2, 276, 311
chronic illness work, 308–9
chronic pain. *see* pain
chronic stressors, 260
class. *see* social class
clinical iatrogenesis, 336–9, 340
Closing the Gap: Policy into Practice on Social Determinants of Health, 394
Cockerham, W.C., "health lifestyle theory," 254–6
coherence, sense of, 85–7

cold/common cold, 58, 59
colonization, 200–1
Commission on Social Determinants of Health (WHO), 160, 394
co-morbidity, 82
complementary/alternative medicine (CAM). *see* CAM
complementary medicine, definition, 363
conflict paradigm, 36–41, 56, 335, 378
Conrad, Peter: on medicalization, 314–15, 331–3, 336, 342, 343, 346, 349–50; on pluralism, 358; values and morals in wellness, 7, 404
consumers and consumerism: and CAM, 367–8; consumer culture, 11–12; ethnicity and pluralism, 367–72; health lifestyle, 236, 237, 255; and identity, 369–70; and individualization, 367–8; and integrative medicine, 373; pharmaceutical industry, 344; *vs.* producing health care, 7–12, 406–7; and wellness, 12, 403
control and regimen, 326–8
controllability of illness, 278–9
critical sociological perspective, 166
cultural behaviour, 148–50, 218–19, 253–4
cultural capital, 150, 253
cultural competency, 203
cultural iatrogenesis, 341
cultural safety, 203
cultural sensitivity, 203
culture: as concept, 194; crossing of, 368–9; and ethnicity, 194; and healing, 356–8; health and illness, 4–5, 30; and pursuit of health, 368

Dauphin, Manitoba, 162
death: causes, 108–9, 200, 201; and gender, 176–7; rates, 82, 83; *see also* mortality
deficit model of health, 84
delivery of health services, 16–17
demand–control model, 138
demedicalization, 333
demographic transition, 365–6
Descartes, René, 322
determinants of health: in Canada, 106; as categories, 227; causal relationship with health, 129; cumulative effects, 123–4; disparities in health, 227–8, 382–3; gender and sex, 172; good and ill health, 125–8, 382; health benefits of, 124–5;

horizontal and vertical structures, 122; inputs *vs.* outcomes, 75–6; intersectionality, 128; key factors, 106–19, 382; lifestyle behaviour as, 107–9, 124; personal determinants, 104–6, 382; and population health, 106–19; primary and secondary, 121–3; and risk factors, 126; structural determinants, 104–6, 181–2, 382; upstream and downstream, 120–3; *see also* social determinants of health
diaries, 93–5, 178, 381
differential exposure hypothesis, 148, 149
differential vulnerability hypothesis, 148–9
digital technologies, 141, 294–5, 350–1
dimensions of health, mixed-methods for, 380–1
disability, as indicator, 82
disease: absence of, 272–3; biomedical model, 5–6; in life course perspective, 74; meaning and measurement, 68–9; morbidity patterns, 14; origins of, 103, 276–8, 279; prevalence and incidence rates, 81; specific etiology, 323; *see also* illness; sickness
disparities in health: Aboriginal peoples, 199–200, 204; and determinants of health, 227–8, 382–3; gap in, 394; and gender, 169–71, 382–3; and health lifestyle, 248; and inequality, 132; intersectionality in, 226–9, 247, 382–3; and life course perspective, 163–5; and medicare, 397–9; reduction, 159–61; and socioeconomic status, 133, 134, 159–61, 382–3; *see also* inequalities in health
doctors. *see* physicians
dominance: and biomedical model, 328–31, 358, 374; and conflict paradigm, 36–7, 39–40; and medicalization, 331–6

education, 114, 139–42, 318
effort–reward imbalance model, 138
e-health, 9–10
Elder, Glen H., Jr., 58, 60
embodiment, 49
emotional support, 295
employment: models of health effects, 138; and social determinants of

health, 25, 136–9, 141–2; and social gradient, 143, 147; stress and illness, 137–8; unemployment, 114, 136–7, 142, 147
environment, as determinant of health, 107, 109–19
environmental pollution, 38, 110, 112
"E-scaped Medicine", 350–1
ethics, and conflict paradigm, 39–40
ethnic ancestry and origin, 194–5
ethnic density effect, 219–20
ethnic identity, 194, 195
ethnicity: Aboriginal peoples, 196–206; biological differences, 216–17; in Canada, 193–4; as concept, 194; consumerism and pluralism, 367–72; and culture, 194; differences in health, 195–216, 223–4; differences in health, explanations, 216–22; disparities in health, 382–3; and formal health care, 185, 212–13; and gender, 185, 209; and health-care behaviour, 212–13; health promotion, 214; healthy immigrant effect, 206–10; intercultural care, 203; intersectionality in, 210, 215–16, 222–3; life course perspective, 222–3; marketing, 368–72; measurement, 194–5; and mental health, 215; and pain, 211–12; and racism, 219; and religion, 220–2; social determinants of health, 213–16, 222; and socioeconomic status, 219–20; and symptoms, 210–12; *see also* immigrants
ethnic stratification, 213–14
ethnoculture, 194
evidence-based in CAM, 373

family upbringing, 149–50
Federal, Provincial and Territorial Advisory Committee on Population Health, 391
feeling-state orientation of good health, 272
feminist paradigm, 44–8, 57, 169, 171, 228–9
fibromyalgia and pain, 302–7
First International Conference on Health Promotion, 389
First Nations, 55, 197, 200, 201, 211–12; *see also* Aboriginal peoples
fitness, 71, 273–4
Flexner Report, 318, 358
formal care: and ethnicity, 185, 212–13; iceberg metaphor, 267–8, 269; responsibility, 386; sustainability,

Index

391–2; system in Canada, 288–9, 290; *see also* health-care system and services
Foucault, Michel: and cultural influences, 357; development of medicine, 319; knowledge and power, 61, 342, 351; and medical gaze, 324, 342, 351; and medicalization, 342, 346; sociology of the body, 50–2
Freidson, Eliot, 37, 330
functional ability, health as, 274
funding, and conflict paradigm, 39–40

gender: and age, 117, 190; in Canada, 77, 117, 171; causes of death, 176–7; as determinant of health, 172; differences in health, 173–82, 189–91; differences in health, explanations, 182–8, 190; disparities in health, 169–71, 382–3; ethnicity and immigrants, 185, 209; and formal health care, 178–80, 185, 189; health diaries, 178; in health research, 171–3; heart attacks, 169–70; hospitalization, 178, 179; illness, 177–8; inequalities in health, 45–8, 171, 191; intersectionality in, 47–8, 189–91; intimate partner violence, 187–8; life course perspective, 189–91; life expectancy, 174–7; and medicalization, 180; and mental health, 177; and physicians, 178–80; and risk-taking, 186–7, 188; and roles, 183–4; self-rated health in Canada, 77; *vs.* sex, 171–2; smoking, 229–30; social determinants of health, 48, 180–2; social support, 185; structural determinants of health, 181–2
general determinants of health. *see* determinants of health
genes and heredity, 107, 217
ghostwriting, 347
Gini coefficient, 154
Goffman, Erving, 42–3, 44
good health: components and continuum, 71, 72–3; crossing of cultures, 368–9; definition and meaning, 4, 63, 70, 96; determinants of health, 125–8, 382; *vs.* illness, 72–5; indicators, 84–9; and lay beliefs, 272–5; mystery of, 2–3, 377–8; orientations of, 272; and salutogenic model, 66–7, 103, 377–8; thematic conceptions, 272–5; as value, 403–5; *see also* wellness
governance of health, 386–8

guaranteed annual income, 161–2

habitus, 53–4, 149; in lifestyle and behaviour, 251–2, 253, 256–7, 258–60
Hall Royal Commission on Health Services, 387
Handbook of Medical Sociology, 23
hand washing, 53
healing, and culture, 356–8
health: biomedical view, 5–6; as concept, 4, 5; as continuum, 72–3; dimensions of, 72–5, 380–1; inputs *vs.* outcomes, 75–6; meaning, 63–4, 68; multi-dimensional aspect, 63–4, 78, 96, 150, 272, 373, 380; and society, 4–5, 30; sociological view, 6; value of, 7; vision *vs.* reform, 393–6; *vs.* wellness, 3–4; *see also* good health; illness; sickness; wellness
health assets, 85
health behaviour: definition, 25; and health sociology, 25; intersectionality in, 253; lay beliefs, 271; patterns in, 245, 246, 249, 252–3; relational theory and habitus, 251–3; relationships in, 243–5, 262–3; and self-care, 291–2; and value of health, 403–4; *see also* health lifestyle
health belief systems: definition, 282, 356; in hidden health-care system, 281–5; in pluralism, 282, 356, 361–2
health-care system and services: cultural influence ideas, 320–8; delivery of services, 16–17; as determinant of health, 119; discrimination towards patients, 238; expenditure in, 313–14, 327, 328; as formal system, 288–9, 290; and health sociology, 25–6; hidden components (*see* hidden health-care system); human-rights based approach, 387; as iceberg, 267–70; and immigrants, 209–10; and lifestyle behaviour, 108–9; limits of, 119; medical dominance of, 328–31; and medical harm, 336–9, 340; and medicalization, 314–15; morbidity patterns, 14–15; *vs.* popular belief system, 281–5; regulation, 339–40, 386–7; safety culture, 338–40; sustainability in Canada, 391–2; utilization, 82, 84; vision *vs.* reform, 393–6; *see also* biomedical model; medicare system

health consciousness: access to information, 9–10; awareness of, 7–8, 12–13; concept, 7–8; and consumerism, 11–12; m-health, 10–11; products and services, 10–12; self-assessment, 8
health determinants. *see* determinants of health; social determinants of health
health diaries, 93–5, 178, 381
health disparities. *see* disparities in health
health expectancy, 87–9, 175
health indicators. *see* indicators
health inequities, 166; *see also* disparities in health; inequalities in health
healthism, 385–6
health lifestyle: and consumption, 236, 237, 255; definition, 250; discrimination towards patients, 238; disparities in health, 248; fundamental points, 254–6, 263; and health promotion, 234–5, 239–41, 243–7; intersectionality, 258–62; and life course perspective, 256–7, 258–62; marketing of, 255; as new public health, 236, 237, 241; and personal health, 243–6, 248; relational theory of, 250–7, 263; responsibility in, 236–43; self-test, 244; and social gradient, 237–8, 239; and social location, 237–8, 241, 253, 257; structure-agency issue, 247–50, 256, 263; *see also* health behaviour; lifestyle behaviour
"health lifestyle theory," 254–6
health literacy, 114–15, 140–1
health maintenance, and lay beliefs, 270–81
health professionals. *see* medical profession
health promotion: in Canada, 106; *vs.* consumerism, 12; and ethnicity, 214; example, 235; and government, 234, 236, 242–3, 245–6, 387; health lifestyles and behaviours, 234–5, 239–41, 243–7; individualized and individualization of, 234–43; and m-health, 10–11; personal health, 243–4, 245–6; policy, 389–92, 399–400, 401; and salutogenic model, 67, 102–3; social determinants of health approach, 102; traditional approach, 101–2

health reserve (of health capital), 256, 257, 274–5
health sociology: in Canada, 23–6; concept and goal, 6–7, 21, 23; development, 22, 23–4, 26; healthy societies and people, 377–81; mixed-method approach, 380–1; shift from medical sociology to, 18, 21–3
health status: as concept, 74; and determinants of health, 120–1; indicators, 75–81, 84; personal, 65, 93–6; population, 65–6; and self-rated health, 79; and social determinants of health, 24–5, 134; and socioeconomic status, 114
health status designation, 74–5
health surveys, 24
health trajectory, 258
health trutherism, 359–60
Health Utilities Index (HUI), 80–1
healthy futures, 374
healthy immigrant effect, 206–10
healthy societies and people: policy in Canada, 388–93; and pursuit of health, 393–409; responsibility in, 384–8; sociological view, 377–81
heart attacks, and gender, 169–70
hegemonic masculinity, 186, 188
helping networks, 270, 295–7, 299–301
heredity and genes, 107, 217
heroic medicine, 317
hidden health-care system: health belief systems, 281–5; lay beliefs, 270–81; overview, 268–70; and pain, 301–8; self-care beliefs and behaviour, 270, 285–95; social support and helping networks, 270, 295–301
Hippocratic Corpus, 13
holism, 372
Holmes-Rahe Life Event Inventory, 297–9
home care, in Canada, 296
hospitalization, and gender, 178, 179
Hospital Medicine, 318–19
House, M.D. (TV program), 325
human-rights based approach to health care, 387
humoral theory, 317

iatrogenesis, 336–8, 340–1
iceberg, as metaphor, 267–70
Illich, Ivan: on medicalization, 332, 334–5, 336–7, 340–1, 346; on self-care, 385

illness: absence of, 272–3; biomedical view, 6; causality, 273, 276–8; continuum, 72–3; determinants of health, 125–8; and employment stress, 137–8; and ethnicity, 216–22; and gender, 177–8; *vs.* good health, 72–5; indicators, 69, 81–4; and lay beliefs, 272, 275–81; meaning, 68, 69; social construction, 6; and society, 4–5, 30; thematic conceptions, 275–80; *see also* disease; sickness
illness behaviour, 25, 293
illness management, and lay beliefs, 270–81
illness narrative accounts, 93–4, 95–6, 302, 304–5, 381
immigrants: in Canada, 193–4; formal health care, 209–10; and gender, 209; healthy immigrant effect, 206–10; social determinants of health and health status, 207–8, 209, 210; use of health care, 212–13; *see also* ethnicity
incidence rate, 81
income: guarantee of, 161–2; inequality, 152–5, 157–8, 161–2; and life expectancy, 155–6; Mincome experiment, 162; and personal health, 135–6, 155, 156–7; and population health, 153–8, 161; rich-poor divide, 153, 155; social determinants of health, 134–6, 141–2; social gradient in health, 155; within-country effects, 157
income adequacy, 155
income inequality hypothesis, 155–6
indicators: in diagnosis, 68; diaries and narrative accounts, 93–6; good health and wellness, 84–9; health status, 76–81, 84; illness, 69, 81–4; importance, 78; integrative approach, 96–7; and life expectancy, 82, 87–9; mixed-methods approach, 89–90; morbidity and mortality, 81–2, 83; population health, 75–81; prevalence and incidence rates, 81; self-rated health as, 77–80; validity and reliability, 77, 78, 80
individualization, 236–43, 367–8
inequalities in health: Aboriginal peoples, 204; in Canada, 159; and disparities in health, 204; gender, 45–8, 171, 191; income, 152–5; intersectionality, 227; medicare

system, 397–9; multi-dimensional aspect, 227; policy, 160–2, 396–9; public perception, 152; redress of, 396–9; reduction of, 159–62, 396–7; and social determinants of health, 160–1, 163, 382–3; and social factors, 133; social gradient, 159; structures of, 131–2; *see also* disparities in health; social inequality
infant mortality, 135, 136, 148
infectious disease, reduction, 329
informal care: home care and social support, 295–7; iceberg metaphor, 269; responsibility in, 384–6, 387; self-care as, 287; as system, 289, 290; *see also* hidden health-care system
information about health, 8–10, 350–1
informational support, 295
institutions, 16, 30–1, 39–40
instrumental support, 295
The Integrated Pan-Canadian Healthy Living Strategy, 392
integrative medicine, 364, 372–5
intercultural care, 203
interest groups, and policy, 401
intersectional analysis, 228–9, 380–1
intersectionality. *see* specific topic
intersectoral approach, 400–1
intimate partner abuse, 187–8
Inuit, 198; *see also* Aboriginal peoples

knowledge development in medicine, 315, 316, 320

Laboratory Medicine, 319–20
labour. *see* employment
Lalonde, M., and 1974 report, 106, 389
lay beliefs: chronic illness, 276; description and study, 270–1, 280–1; good health and wellness, 272–5; and health behaviour, 271; in hidden health-care system, 270–81; illness and sickness, 272, 275–81; origins of, 281; *vs.* professional belief system, 281–5; role, 310
Lay Concepts of Health Inventory, 271
lesbian, gay, bisexual, and transgender (LGBT), 172
life chances, 250, 255–6, 383–4
life choices, 249, 255–6, 384
life course perspective: Aboriginal peoples, 199, 206; concept, 57, 58–61, 378; and determinants of health, 123–4; and disease, 74; disparities in health, 163–5; education and

health, 140; and ethnicity, 222–3; and gender, 189–91; and health lifestyle, 256–7, 258–62; for individuals and society, 166; intersectional model, 379–80; social determinants of health, 379–80; and socioeconomic status, 59, 162–6, 379–80
Life Event Inventory, 297–9
life expectancy: in Canada, 88, 174; and gender, 174–7; *vs.* health expectancy, 88–9; and income, 155–6; indicators, 82, 87–9; rich-poor divide, 134; and wellness, 88
lifestyle, description, 234
lifestyle behaviour: as determinant of health, 107–9, 124; factors in biosocial reality, 259–60, 261; and health promotion, 234–5; impact on health, 108–9; physical activity, 230–1; unhealthy behaviours, 229–34; *see also* health lifestyle
life trajectories, impact on health, 58–9, 164–6
logic of practice, 251–2
longer life and health, 83–4, 87–8
Longitudinal Survey of Immigrants to Canada (LSIC), 207, 209

machine metaphor, 324–6
Manitoba, obesity, 232
marketing, 255, 368–72
Marmot, Michael: on inequalities, 132, 134, 161, 398; social gradient in health, 142–3, 147, 159
masculinity, 185, 186–7, 188
materialism, 148
measurement of health. *see* indicators
medical consumerism, 11–12
medical dominance. *see* dominance
medical gaze, 51–2, 319, 342, 351
medical harm and errors, 336–9
medical ideology, 37
medical-industrial complex, 38–40, 345–6, 348–9
medicalization: Aboriginal peoples, 200–1; biomedical technologies, 350; clinical iatrogenesis, 336–9, 340; conflict approaches, 335–41; cultural iatrogenesis, 341; definition, 314; and demedicalization, 333; description, 331–2; of deviance, 331–2; dominance of, 331–6; emergence, 334–5; Foucauldian approaches, 341–2, 346; and gender, 180; and health-care system, 314–15; and information,

350–1; levels of, 332–3; and medical screening, 345; and patient safety, 338–40; pharmaceutical industry, 336, 342, 344, 345–50; positive aspects, 342–3; and risks, 333, 343–4; *vs.* salutogenic view, 406–9; as social control, 331–2, 335; social iatrogenesis, 340–1; and sociocultural processes, 333–4; and surveillance, 343–5; women, 46–7
"medically unexplained physical symptoms" (MUPS), 303
medical pluralism. *see* pluralism
medical profession: and Aboriginal peoples and minorities, 201–4; and conflict paradigm, 36–7, 39, 41; and disease diagnosis, 69; dominance of physicians, 329–30; responsibility, 386; and safety culture, 338–40; in self-care, 289; women in, 330–1; *see also* physicians
medical screening, 345
medical sociology: contribution of, 17; criticism, 19–20, 29; development, 13–15, 17; dominant issues, 15–17; as field of study, 13–14; "in" and "of" perspectives, 18–19, 20–1, 22–3; limitations, 17; medical pluralism, 356–64; and morbidity patterns, 14–15; scope of, 15–18; shift to health sociology, 18, 21–3; and structural functionalism, 33–4; traditional view, 3, 22
medical suppliers, 39–40
medicare system: importance, 391–2; inequalities and disparities, 397–9; introduction and impact, 387–8, 397–8; objective and results, 398–9; principles, 387; repair of, 395
medication, errors with, 338
medicine wheel, 204, 205
medico-centric bias, 19–20, 29
men, 45, 185, 186–7, 188; *see also* gender
mental health, 42–3, 177, 215
m-health, 10–11
Mincome experiment, 162
mind–body connection, 372
mind–body dualism, 49–50, 53–4, 322
mobile devices and technologies, 10–11
morality and moral values, 404–5
morbidity: definition, 14, 81; as iceberg, 267, 268–9; as indicator of illness, 81–2; and medical sociology, 14–15

mortality: in Canada, 145; as indicator of illness, 82, 83; infants, 135, 136, 148; from medical harm, 337; rates, 82, 83; reduction, 329; and self-rated health, 78; and social class, 134; social gradient, 144–5; *see also* death
multiculturalism, 371
Multiple Risk Factor Intervention Trial (MRFIT), 239
mutual aid, 287–8, 299
mystery of health: and good health, 2–3, 377–8; mixed-method approach, 380–1; psychological resources, 260–1; structure–agency issue, 249–50, 263

narratives of illness, 93–4, 95–6, 302, 304–5, 381
National Forum on Health, 394
National Population Health Survey (NPHS): description and goal, 91; and disability, 83; and gender, 171, 178; immigrants and ethnicity, 207, 211, 215; morbidity in Canada, 81–2; physical activity, 231; and self-rated health, 79
nature, and society, 49–50
neo-liberalism, 39, 236, 245–6
neo-materialism, 148
A New Perspective on the Health of Canadians (Lalonde report), 389
new public health, 236, 237, 241, 245, 343
normal health, 64
nurses, 330–1

Oakley, Ann, 46–7, 335
obesity, 112, 231–3
onanism, 334
Ottawa Charter for Health Promotion, 5, 389, 390–1, 393

pain: in Canadians, 306; chronic illness work, 308–9; and ethnicity, 211–12; as experience, 301–2, 305–10; and fibromyalgia, 302–5, 306–7; in hidden health-care system, 301–8; meaning and measurement, 69–70, 302–4, 306–8; narrative accounts, 302, 304–5; public aspect, 307
Parsons, Talcott, 31–5, 294, 342
pathogenesis, 102–3, 128
pathological lesion, 318

patriarchy, 45, 46, 178, 185–6
perceived health, 77
perceived susceptibility of illness, 279–80
performance orientation of good health, 272
personal determinants of health, 104–6, 382
personal health: health lifestyle and behaviour, 243–6, 248; and income, 135–6, 155, 156–7; promotion, 243–4, 245–6
personal health status, 65, 93–6
personal ideas. *see* lay beliefs
personalized medicine, 351
pharmaceutical industry: influence on health care, 345–50; and medicalization, 336, 342, 344, 345–50; and physicians, 347; and policy, 401; and research, 347–9
pharmaceuticalization, 346
physical activity, as lifestyle behaviour, 230–1
physical capital, 253
physical environment, as determinant of health, 109–13
physical reductionism, 322–3
physicians: and conflict paradigm, 37; development of biomedicine, 315–19; dominance of, 329–30; and gender, 178–80; influence of pharmaceutical industry, 347; and integrative medicine, 373; rating of, 10; *vs.* self-rated health, 78; services offered, 22; women as, 330
pluralism: and culture, 356–8; definition, 356; ethnicity and consumerism, 367–72; health as social construction, 356–7; in health belief system, 282, 356, 361–2; integrative medicine, 364, 372–5; persistence of, 358–61; revival explanations, 359, 365–8; sociological perspective, 356–64; stereotypes of marginality, 361–2; *see also* alternative medicine
policy: barriers to, 401; description and goal, 388; health promotion, 389–92, 399–400, 401; implementation issues, 399–402; and inequalities, 160–2, 396–9; initiatives in Canada, 388–93; intersectionality in, 400–1; population health, 389–92; salutogenic model of health, 393; shortcomings, 392–3;

and social determinants of health, 400, 401–2, 408–9
political economy, 36, 148
politics, and inequalities, 160–1
popular health, 281–5
population aging, 115–16, 118, 365–6
population health: biomedical model, 328–9; determinants of health, 106–19; and health expenditure, 313–14; health promotion, 102–3; and income, 153–8, 161; indicators, 75–81; inputs and outcomes, 75–6; mixed-method approach, 380–1; models, 84–5; policy initiatives in Canada, 389–92; social determinants of health, 65, 104–5, 107; surveys in Canada, 90–3; violence against women, 187–8; and welfare regimes, 161; and wellness, 84
population health status, 65–6
postmodern condition, 366–7
power, 45–6, 52
"pragmatic acculturation," 368
precarious employment, 137
prevalence rate, 81
preventative self-care, 291–2
professional health, belief systems, 281–5
psychosocial factors and explanations, 151–3, 259–60, 261
public health: expenditure, 327, 328; and health lifestyle, 236, 237, 241; new public health, 236, 237, 241, 245, 343
pursuit of health, 368, 377, 393, 404

quality of life, 87–8

race, and biology, 217–18; *see also* ethnicity
racialization, 201–2, 215, 218
racism, 196, 201–3, 219
randomized control trial (RCT), 364
reactive self-care, 293
reciprocal assistance, 287–8, 299
reductionism, 322–3
reform in health-care in Canada, 26, 393–6
regimen and control, 326–8
regulatory self-care, 291
relational theory, 250–4, 256–7, 263
religion, and ethnicity, 220–2
religiosity, 221
research, 347–9
resource for living, health as, 274–5

responsibility: Canadian initiatives, 388–93; for health lifestyle, 236–43; health promotion, 399–400; personal (informal care), 384–6, 387; professional (formal care), 386; public, 386–8; and self-care, 384–5
restorative self-care, 293–4
risk: and CAM, 367; and determinants of health, 126; and gender, 186–7, 188; and medicalization, 333, 343–4
risk-taking hypothesis, 186–8
role accumulation hypothesis, 183
roles, 31, 32, 183–4, 294–5
role strain hypothesis, 183–4
Romanow Royal Commission, 391–2
Roseto, Pennsylvania, and the "Roseto effect," 220–1

safety culture, in medicalization, 338–40
salutogenesis, 102–3
salutogenic model of health: and determinants of health, 102–4, 126–8; and dimensions of health, 380; and good health, 3, 66–7, 103, 377–8; and health promotion, 67, 102–3; as indicator, 85–7; *vs.* medicalization, 406–9; for policy making, 393; as vision, 393–4; and wellness, 85–6
screening, 345
self-care: criticism, 385–6; definition and range of practices, 287, 289–91; and digital technologies, 294–5; government in, 289; and health behaviour, 291–2; main characteristics, 294; as model of health, 289; as responsibility, 384–5; typology, 291–3
self-care beliefs and behaviour: and alternative model of health care, 288–91; and chronic illness, 311; dimensions of, 291–5; in hidden health-care system, 270, 285–95; mutual aid and self-help groups, 287–8; overview, 285–6; self-health management, 286–7, 310–11, 385
self-help groups, 288
self-medicalization, 343
self-rated health, 77–80, 207
self-treatment, 287
sense of coherence, 85–7
sense of healthiness, 71
seriousness of illness, 280

SES (socioeconomic status). *see* socioeconomic status
sex (biological), 171–3; *see also* gender
sex- and gender-based analysis (SGBA), 172–3
sexual intercourse, as unsafe activity, 233–4
sex workers, 44
sickness, 68–70, 72, 96, 275–81; *see also* disease; illness
sick role, 32, 294–5
sick role behaviour, 293–4
signs (of disease), in diagnosis, 68
Sinclair, Brian, 201–3, 338
skeptics, 357
smoking, 229–30, 240–1, 253, 271, 340
social acceptability hypothesis, 184–5
social capital, 253
social class, 133–4, 159–60, 254; *see also* social location
social cohesion, 220–1
social construction: of age, 115, 118; concept, 5; and healing, 356, 357; and health, 4–7, 51–2, 356–7, 378; of illness, 6; and knowledge, 320; medical pluralism, 356–7; symbolic interactionist paradigm, 41, 43; wellness as, 12
social determinants of health: and biosocial reality, 260, 262; definition, 102; direct and indirect effects, 246–7; and disparities in health, 133–42; and education, 114, 139–42; and employment, 25, 136–9, 141–2; and ethnicity, 213–16, 222; factors and categories, 260–1; and gender, 48, 180–2; global action on, 394; and health promotion, 102; and health sociology, 24–5; and health status, 24–5, 134; immigrants, 207, 209; importance, 128–9; and income, 134–6, 141–2; and inequalities, 160–1, 163, 382–3; intersectionality in, 141–2, 163, 246–7; and life course perspective, 379–80; origins, 13; personal and structural determinants, 104–6; policy, 400, 401–2, 408–9; and population health, 65, 104–5, 107; reflections on, 381–6; *see also* determinants of health
social environment, 113–19
social epidemiology, 15–16
social exclusion, 132–3, 196–7, 238, 239
social factors: and biological factors in health, 258, 259; in biosocial reality, 259–60, 261; and health status, 24; and inequalities, 133; and wellness, 71
social gradient in health: of Academy Award nominees, 146; in Canada, 145; concept and research in, 142–7; and employment, 143, 147; explanations of, 147–53, 162–3; and health lifestyle, 237–8, 239; and income, 155; and inequalities, 159; in life course, 165–6; and mortality, 144–5; and social status, 142–4, 152–3; and socioeconomic status, 145–9, 151–3, 165–6
social iatrogenesis, 340–1
social inequality, 131–2; *see also* inequalities in health
social institutions, 16
socialization process, 149–50
social location: and disparities in health, 383; and health lifestyle, 237–8, 241, 253, 257; intersectional analysis, 228; women, 228–9; *see also* social class
social medicine, 38
social organization, 16
social patterning, 16
social production, health as, 240
social roles, 31, 32, 183–4, 294–5
social status, 134, 142–4, 152–3
social structure: description, 249; factors in biosocial reality, 259–60, 261; health lifestyle and behaviour, 253; logic of practice, 251; and structural functionalism, 30–1; structure–agency issue, 249–50, 251, 256
social support: as determinant of health, 118–19; effect, 296–7; and gender, 185; in hidden health-care system, 270, 295–7, 299–301; major findings, 300; negative aspects, 300
society, 4–5, 30, 49–50
socioeconomic status (SES): and common cold, 59; definition, 133; and disparities in health, 133, 134, 159–61, 382–3; and ethnicity, 219–20; and exclusion, 132–3; and health status, 114, 134; and infant mortality, 148; intersectionality in, 141–2, 162–6; and life course perspective, 59, 162–6, 379–80; and life trajectories, 164–5; rich-poor divide, 152–3, 155; and social gradient in health, 145–9, 151–3, 165–6
sociological imagination, 29–30, 61, 247, 378
sociology: alternative paradigms, 378–9; origins, 14; structure-agency issue, 248–50, 251; theoretical paradigms, 29–30, 56–7, 378–9; view of health, 6, 378; *see also* health sociology; medical sociology
sociology of the body paradigm, 50–5, 57, 378, 380; and determinants of health, 106–7; relational theory, 250–1
specific etiology, 323–4
stability and changeability of illness, 280
Strategies for Population Health: Investing in the Health of Canadians, 391
stress, and social support, 296–9
structural amplification, 140
structural determinants of health, 104–6, 181–2, 382
structural functionalist paradigm, 30–5, 56, 378, 380
structure–agency issue, 247–50, 251, 256, 263, 383–4
suburbs and sprawl, health problems in, 111–13
suicides, Aboriginal peoples, 199
support. *see* social support
Surveillance Medicine, 343–5
susceptibility of illness, 279–80
symbolic interactionist paradigm, 41–4, 56, 69–70, 378, 380
Syme, Leonard, 239, 240
symptom orientation of good health, 272
symptoms, 69–70, 210–12, 317, 318

tanning beds, 242
theoretical paradigms, as framework, 30
"thrifty gene," 217
Traditional Chinese Medicine (TCM), 43, 357

unemployment, 114, 136–7, 142, 147
United States, 134, 329, 337, 338, 398
universal health insurance. *see* medicare system
unsafe sex, as unhealthy behaviour, 233–4
urban areas, health problems, 110–13
urban health penalty, 111

visible minorities, 193–4, 215; *see also* ethnicity

Weber, Max, 41, 249, 321, 373
welfare regimes, 161
well-being, health as, 274; *see also* wellness
wellness: components, 71; concept, 4; and consumption, 12, 403; crossing of cultures, 368–9; as dangerous ideology, 405–6; *vs.* health and good health, 3–4; indicators, 84–9; and lay beliefs, 272–5; and life expectancy, 88; meaning, 68, 70–2, 85, 96, 404; and population health, 84; as pursuit, 368; salutogenic model, 85–6; social components, 71; as social construction, 12; values and morality in, 403–5; *see also* good health
Whitehall Studies, 142–3, 238
Winnipeg Regional Health Authority, 39–40
women: biomedical view, 46–7; and caregiving, 189; causality of illness, 276–7; medicalization, 46–7; in medical profession, 330–1; roles, 183–4; and self-care, 287; social locations, 228–9; in sociology, 44–5; violence against, 187–8; *see also* gender
work. *see* employment
World Heath Organization (WHO): Aboriginal peoples, 200–1; alcohol use, 230; alternative medicine and CAM, 362, 368; meaning of good health, 70; obesity, 231, 232; population aging, 116–18; reduction of inequalities, 160; social determinants of health, 102, 394; tanning beds, 242